Principles and Practice of Research
Strategies for Surgical Investigators

"Principles and Practice of Research"

Strategies for Surgical Investigators

Edited by
Hans Troidl   Walter O. Spitzer   Bucknam McPeek
David S. Mulder   Martin F. McKneally

With 37 Illustrations

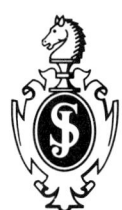

Springer-Verlag
Berlin Heidelberg New York London Paris Tokyo

Hans Troidl
Department of Surgery
University of Cologne
Surgical Clinic Merheim
D-5000 Cologne 91
Federal Republic of Germany

Walter O. Spitzer
Department of Epidemiology and
 Biostatistics
McGill University
Montreal, Quebec
Canada H3A 1A2

Bucknam McPeek
Department of Anaesthesia
Harvard University
Massachusetts General Hospital
Boston, Massachusetts 02114
U.S.A.

David S. Mulder
Department of Surgery
McGill University
Montreal General Hospital
Montreal, Quebec
Canada H3G 1A4

Martin F. McKneally
Division of Cardio-Thoracic
 Surgery
Albany Medical College of
 Union University
Albany, New York 12208
U.S.A.

Library of Congress Cataloging in Publication Data
Principles and practices of research.
  Includes bibliographies and index.
  1. Surgery—Research—Methodology. I. Troidl,
Hans, 1938–   . [DNLM: 1. Research. 2. Surgery.
WO 20 P957]
RD29.P75 1986   617'.0072   86-13896

© 1986 by Springer-Verlag New York Inc.
All rights reserved. No part of this book may be translated or reproduced in any form without written permission from Springer-Verlag, 175 Fifth Avenue, New York, New York 10010, U.S.A.
The use of general descriptive names, trade names, trademarks, etc. in this publication, even if the former are not especially identified, is not to be taken as a sign that such names, as understood by the Trade Marks and Merchandise Marks Act, may accordingly be used freely by anyone.
While the advice and information in this book are believed to be true and accurate at the date of going to press, neither the authors nor the editors nor the publisher can accept any legal responsibility for any errors or omissions that may be made. The publisher makes no warranty, express or implied, with respect to the material contained herein.

Media conversion by David Seham Associates, Metuchen, New Jersey.
Printed and bound by Arcata Graphics/Halliday, West Hanover, Massachusetts.
Printed in the United States of America.

9 8 7 6 5 4 3 2 1

ISBN 3-540-16340-9 Springer-Verlag Berlin Heidelberg New York
ISBN 0-387-16340-9 Springer-Verlag New York Berlin Heidelberg

This book is dedicated to our children and our students. Each in their own way have added enormously to our lives. By their questions they have encouraged us to ask *why* rather than only *what*. They have not been satisfied with simplistic answers, but have forced us to examine what we know and how well we know it. Their inquiring minds have encouraged us to improve our own knowledge that we might better meet their hunger for honest, forthright help as they build their lives and careers.

Foreword

For some readers, the title of this book will immediately raise the question, what exactly is meant by surgical research? In the very broadest sense the term can be taken to include all endeavors, however elementary or limited in scope, to advance surgical knowledge. Ideally, it refers to well-organized attempts to establish on a proper scientific basis, i.e., to place beyond reasonable doubt, the truth or otherwise of any concepts, old or new, within the ambit of surgery, and, of course, anaesthesia.

The methods used to achieve that end vary enormously, depending on the issue being investigated. They comprise a wide range of activities in the wards, outpatient clinics, operating rooms or laboratories, such as simple clinical or operative observations and clinical or laboratory investigations involving biophysics, biochemistry, pathology, bacteriology, and other disciplines. Well-planned animal experimentation is exceedingly important and it is well to remember the old truism that every surgical operation is a biological experiment whose results, unfortunately, are not always as carefully documented and analyzed as they should be. When the findings of any clinical, operative or laboratory study are being considered, stringent statistical methods must be applied to ensure that any conclusions rest on a statistically sound basis.

Surgery provides an almost unlimited range of topics for research. Much of what is practiced and taught in surgery consists of traditional concepts passed from surgical teacher to surgical trainee by example, by word of mouth, or by standard texts, without ever having been submitted to really objective assessment. Every year we see scores of promising new ideas emerging on the surgical scene to challenge orthodoxy. Although these innovations are often greeted with great optimism, a factual basis for that enthusiasm is sometimes far from secure and much further work is frequently required to discover whether we are dealing with genuine advances or not.

The most exciting and attractive scenario for surgical research is unquestionably one that depicts a successful attempt by a researcher to establish the accuracy of some bold innovation for which he himself is responsible. Joseph Lister, demonstrating by clinical trial that wound suppuration could be combated by antiseptic measures, comes to mind along with Lester Dragstedt showing by experimental and clinical studies that vagotomy could play a valuable role in the treatment of peptic ulcer disease.

In all well-developed countries, and most notably in the United States, there is now strong pressure on surgeons in training to engage in a period of research in order to foster a critical attitude towards the appraisal of the results of surgical treatment, and stimulate a continuing interest in combining investigative work with clinical practice.

Hitherto, acquainting the tyro researcher with the methods appropriate to his or her particular project has usually depended on the guidance of more experienced colleagues working in the same field, and on the acquisition of a gradually increasing understanding of how to conduct research as the result of being in a research environment. It is very surprising that there has been no textbook to which the young researcher could turn to secure a more systematic presentation of the various matters of importance in undertaking surgical research. Hans Troidl, David Mulder, Martin McKneally, Walter Spitzer, and Bucknam McPeek are to be congratulated most warmly on their great perspicacity in recognizing the claimant need for a work providing this sort of information and, even more, on the supremely effective way in which they have met that need by the production of their new book.

Principles and Practice of Research covers its subject in an unusually comprehensive way that includes not only the conduct of research in general, but also the special faciltities and problems encountered in several personal attributes that are conducive to success in research, such as a certain amount of open-mindedness combined with the enthusiasm and determination needed to carry a project through to its ultimate conclusion despite the various obstacles that may be encountered en route. Not to be forgotten in this connection is the decisive role played by sheer good luck in achieving a successful outcome in research — as is true of many other activities in life. An important subsidiary matter in the prosecution of investigative work is how subsequently to present an account of that work and its results, most effectively, at meetings or discussion groups and in publications; this book offers very helpful advice on all these points. Very appropriately, a concluding section affords an inspiring appraisal of future prospects in surgical research by that great surgeon-researcher, Francis Moore of Boston, whose contributions to surgical knowledge are legion.

I have no doubts that *Principles and Practice of Research* will be very widely read and greatly appreciated, not only by surgical trainees starting on research work, but also by experienced researchers and established surgeons who will welcome the wealth of information it provides on every facet of surgical research. Since research in anaesthesia medicine, obstetrics, gynaecology, and other fields of clinical activity follow essentially the same principles, this book should prove equally helpful to beginning or established investigators in other branches of health care. It cannot, in my judgement, fail to secure an assured place in the libraries of all medical schools, departments of surgery, and clinical departments the world over, as well as in the studies of many individual purchasers.

University of Leeds   J.C. Goligher
Leeds, England

Acknowledgment

Our wives have supported us in so many ways.

As editors we owe a special debt to the authors of this textbook. They have cheerfully given of their time to share their experience in diverse fields with us and with you the reader. Like almost all truly able people they are busy, most are overcommitted with active lives of scientific inquiry.

We are especially grateful for the foresight and generosity of Wolfgang Schmidt-Von Rohrscheid, of the Pfrimmer Corporation, who made possible the Eppan Conference on Surgical Research in November of 1984. At this conference the editors were fortunate to obtain the advice of leaders in various fields of surgery from many countries in Europe, North America and Asia.

We are particularly grateful to our colleagues at the University of Cologne, Harvard University, Albany Medical College, and McGill University who have generously assumed some of our own duties and thus made it possible for us to work on this project during the last 18 months.

We have benefited from thoughtful discussions and the sound advice of many of our colleagues, in particular, Dr. Norbert Boenninghoff, Dr. Jurgen Klein, Dr. Michael Schweins, Dr. Andreas Paul, Dr. Lothar Koehler, Dr. Burkhard Viel, Dr. Bertil Bouillon, Dr. Klaus Roeddecker, Dr. Rudolf Menningen, and Dr. Andreas Dauber. Dr. Norbert Boenninghoff in particular has helped us with many sections of the manuscript.

Our special thanks and deepest gratitude must go to the distinguished Canadian scientist and editor, Dr. N.J.B. Wiggin. We cannot adequately express how much we have enjoyed his wit, wisdom, and good fellowship. Most of the uniformity and clarity of expression are due to his artistic sense of the English language and his inciseful clarity of thought.

The fact that this book will appear within less than 24 months after conception is due largely to the grace and skill of Mrs. Elna Stacey. In addition to managing the preparation of the manuscript and dealing with so many authors and editors from across the globe, Mrs. Stacey has taught us each more than we can imagine about organizational skills, the differential importance of tasks and how to maintain a completely even keel in the presence of computer failures, scholars who do not return phone calls, authors who are late with promised manuscripts, and editors who want to redo work long since completed.

As Elna said, "There is a time when editors and authors must sit back and enjoy what they have written"; we hope that you will join us in this process.

Misses D'Ailleboust, Ward, Deer, Skye, and Cohan have cheerfully worked on this manuscript through numerous drafts.

Contents

Foreword
J.C. Goligher vii

Acknowledgment ix

Contributors xv

Introduction
H. Troidl 1

I. The Rationale of Surgical Research
Edited by D.S. Mulder 5

1. Historical Evolution: Methods, Attitudes, Goals
   A.V. Pollock 7
2. Philosophy of Surgical Research
   R.L. Cruess 18
3. Roles for the Surgical Investigator
   R.C.-J. Chiu and D.S. Mulder 20
4. The Development of the Surgical Investigator
   D.C. Sabiston, Jr. 26
5. Facilitating Scholarship: Creating the Atmosphere,
   Setting, and Teamwork for Research
   M.F. McKneally, D.S. Mulder, A. Nachemson, F. Mosteller, and B. McPeek 36

II. Starting the Research Process
Edited by H. Troidl and M.F. McKneally 43

1. Systematically Reviewing Previous Work
   S. Wood-Dauphinee and B. McPeek 45
2. Endpoints for Clinical Studies: Conventional and Innovative Variables
   S. Wood-Dauphinee and H. Troidl 53
3. Statistics Demystified
   M.S. Kramer and H. Troidl 69
4. Organizing a Clinical Study
   L. Del Greco, J.I. Williams, and D.S. Mulder 88
5. Some Things You Should Know About Computers
   G.G. Bernstein and R.G. Margolese 96

6. Ten Tips on Preparing Research Proposals
   W.O. Spitzer 106

7. Critical Appraisal of Published Research
   M.T. Schechter and F.E. LeBlanc 112

8. Ethical Principles in Surgical Research
   D.J. Roy, P. Black, and B. McPeek 118

III. Selected Strategies of Research
   Edited by B. McPeek and W.O. Spitzer 133

1. The Marburg Experiment
   W. Lorenz and H. Troidl 137

2. Animal Experimentation
   W.H. Isselhard and J. Kusche 149

3. A Case Study of the Evolution of a Surgical Research Project
   R.C.-J. Chiu and D.S. Mulder 162

4. Clinical Research
   B. Walters and D.L. Sackett 166

5. Multicentre Collaborative Clinical Trials in Surgical Research
   R.G. Margolese 180

6. Evaluation of the Diagnostic Process
   M.T. Schechter 195

7. Health Services Research: Focus on Surgery
   J.I. Williams and W.R. Drucker 207

8. Selected Non-Experimental Methods: An Orientation
   W.O. Spitzer 222

IV. Reporting Your Work
   Edited by B. McPeek and W.O. Spitzer 231

1. Writing an Effective Abstract
   B.A. Pruitt, Jr. and A.D. Mason, Jr. 233

2. The Ten-Minute Presentation
   M. Evans and A.V. Pollock 236

3. The Longer Talk
   B. McPeek and C. Herfarth 240

4. Presenting Your Work at International Meetings
   T. Aoki and J-H. Alexandre 246

5. Chairing Panels, Seminars and Consensus Conferences
   M.F. McKneally, B. McPeek, D.S. Mulder, W.O. Spitzer, and H. Troidl 249

6. The Poster Session, Audio Visual Aids
   Y. Reid and K-H. Vestweber 254

7. Writing for Publication
   N.J.B. Wiggin, J.C. Bailar III, C.B. Mueller, W.O. Spitzer, and B. McPeek 268

8. What to Do When You Are Asked to Write a Chapter for a Book
   B. Lewerich and D. Götze 276

V. International Perspectives on Surgical Research
   Edited by H. Troidl and M.F. McKneally 279

1. Surgical Research in Canada
   D.S. Mulder 281

2. Contributions from France
   J-H. Alexandre 289

3. Traditions and Transitions in Germany
   H. Troidl and N. Boenninghoff 293

4. Japan's Integration of Eastern Values and Modern Science
   T. Aoki, K. Hioki, and T. Muto 299

5. New Initiatives and Ideas in Spain
   P.A. Sánchez 306

6. Orderly Evolution to a Better Future in Sweden
   S. Fasth and L. Hultén 318

7. The Confluence of Private and Public Resources in Switzerland
   F. Largiadèr 324

8. Historical and Organizational Influences Upon Surgical Research in the
   United Kingdom
   R. Shields 327

9. Research Challenges and Solutions in the United States
   M.F. McKneally 336

10. Common Characteristics and Distinctive Diversity in Surgical Research: An
    International Analysis
    M.F. McKneally, H. Troidl, D.S. Mulder, W.O. Spitzer, and B. McPeek 344

VI. Opportunities in Surgical Research
    Edited by H. Troidl, D.S. Mulder, B. McPeek, and W.O. Spitzer 357

1. Future Horizons in Surgical Research
   F.D. Moore 359

Appendix A. The Declaration of Helsinki 369

Appendix B. Books on the Handling and Care of Animals 371

Index 373

Contributors

Jean-Henri Alexandre
Professor of Surgery, Chairman of Surgery, Université de Paris, Clinique Chirurgicale de l'Hôpital Broussais, Paris, 75014 France

Teruaki Aoki
Associate Professor, (Lecturer), Chief of Gastrointestinal Division, Department of Surgery II, Jikei University School of Medicine, 3-25-8, Nishishinbashi, Minato-Ku, Tokyo, Japan

John Christian Bailar III
Lecturer in Biostatistics, Department of Biostatistics, Harvard School of Public Health, Boston, Massachusetts 02115 U.S.A.

Gary G. Bernstein
Telecommunications Manager, McGill University, Montreal, Quebec, Canada H3A 1A4

Peter McL. Black
Associate Professor of Surgery, Harvard Medical School, Associate Visiting Neurosurgeon, Massachusetts General Hospital, Boston, Massachusetts 02114 U.S.A.

Norbert Boenninghoff
Department of Experimental Surgery, II Department of Surgery, University of Köln, D–5000 Köln, Federal Republic of Germany

Ray Chu-Jeng Chiu
Professor of Surgery, McGill University, Senior Surgeon in Cardiovascular and Thoracic Surgery, Montreal General Hospital, Montreal, Quebec, Canada H3G 1A4

Richard L. Cruess
Dean, Faculty of Medicine, McGill University, Professor of Surgery, McGill University, McIntyre Medical Sciences Building, Montreal, Quebec, Canada H3G 1Y6

Linda Del Greco
Faculty Lecturer, Department of Epidemiology and Biostatistics, Faculty of Medicine, McGill University, and Faculty Member of the Kellogg Centre, Montreal General Hospital, Montreal, Quebec, Canada H3G 1A4

William R. Drucker
Professor and Chairman, Department of Surgery, University of Rochester, School of Medicine and Dentistry, Rochester, New York 14642 U.S.A.

Mary Evans
Research Coordinator, Scarborough Hospital, Scarborough, North Yorkshire Y012 6QL United Kingdom

Stig Fasth
Associate Professor, Department of Surgery II, Sahlgrenska Sjukhuset, University of Göteborg, S-413 45 Göteborg, Sweden

John C. Goligher
Emeritus Professor of Surgery, University of Leeds, Leeds, United Kingdom

Dietrich Götze
University Medical School Heidelberg, Springer-Verlag, D-6900 Heidelberg 1, Federal Republic of Germany

Christian Herfarth
Professor and Head, Department of Surgery, University of Heidelberg, Chirurgische Universitätsklinik, D-6900 Heidelberg, Federal Republic of Germany

Koshiro Hioki
Associate Professor (Lecturer), Department of Surgery, Kansai Medical University, Fumizonocho Moriguchi, Osaka 570 Japan

Leif Hultén
Professor and Chairman, Department of Surgery II, Sahlgrenska sjukhuset, University of Göteborg, S-413 45 Göteborg, Sweden

Wolf H. Isselhard
Professor of Experimental Surgery, Director, Institute for Experimental Medicine, University of Köln, D-5000 Köln 41, Federal Republic of Germany

Michael S. Kramer
Associate Professor of Pediatrics, and of Epidemiology and Biostatistics, McGill University Faculty of Medicine, Montreal, Quebec, Canada H3A 1A2

Jurgen Kusche
Head, Biochemical and Experimental Laboratory of the II Department of Surgery, University of Cologne, D-5000 Köeln, Federal Republic of Germany

Felix Largiadèr
Professor of Surgery and Chairman, Department of Surgery, Director of Visceral Surgery, University Hospital, CH-8091 Zürich, Switzerland

Francis E. LeBlanc
Professor and Chief, Division of Neurosurgery, Department of Clinical Neurosciences, Foothills Hospital, University of Calgary, Calgary, Alberta, Canada T2N 2T9

Bernhard Lewerich
Springer-Verlag, D-6900 Heidelberg, Federal Republic of Germany

Wilfried Lorenz
Head, Institute of Theoretical Surgery, Centre of Operative Medicine I, Klinikum Lahnberge, D-3550 Marburg, Federal Republic of Germany

Richard G. Margolese
Associate Professor of Surgery, Associate Director, McGill Cancer Centre, McGill University Faculty of Medicine, Montreal, Quebec, Canada H3T 1E2

Arthur D. Mason, Jr.
Chief, Laboratory Division U.S. Army Institute of Surgical Research, Fort Sam Houston, San Antonio, Texas 78234-6200 U.S.A.

Martin F. McKneally
Professor and Chief, Division of Cardio-Thoracic Surgery, Albany Medical College of Union University, Albany, New York 12208 U.S.A.

Bucknam McPeek
Associate Professor of Anaesthesia, Harvard University Anesthetist, Massachusetts General Hospital, Boston, Massachusetts 02114 U.S.A.

Francis D. Moore
Moseley Professor of Surgery, Emeritus, Harvard Medical School, Surgeon-in-Chief, Emeritus, Peter Bent Brigham Hospital, Countway Library, Boston, Massachusetts 02115 U.S.A.

Frederick Mosteller
The Roger I. Lee Professor of Mathematical Statistics, Chairman, Department of Health Policy and Management, Harvard School of Public Health, Boston, Massachusetts, 02115 U.S.A.

C. Barber Mueller
Professor Emeritus of Surgery, McMaster University Medical Centre, Department of Surgery, Hamilton, Ontario, Canada L8N 3Z5

David S. Mulder
Professor and Chairman, Department of Surgery, McGill University, Surgeon-in-Chief, Montreal General Hospital, Montreal, Quebec, Canada H3G 1A4

Terukazu Muto
Professor and Chairman, First Department of Surgery, Niigata University School of Medicine, Niigata 951 Japan

Alf Nachemson
Professor and Chairman, Department of Orthopedic Surgery I, Sahlgrenska, sjukhuset, Göteborg, Sweden S-41345

Alan V. Pollock
Consultant Surgeon, Scarborough Health Authority, Scarborough Hospital, Scarborough, North Yorkshire Y012 6QL United Kingdom

Basil A. Pruitt, Jr.
Commander and Director, U.S. Army Institute of Surgical Research, Fort Sam Houston, Texas, San Antonio, Texas 78234-6200 U.S.A.

Yolanda Stassinopoulos Reid
Director, Preventive Services Initiative, Office of Disease Prevention and Health Promotion, U.S. Department of Health and Human Services, Washington, DC, 20201 U.S.A.

David J. Roy
Director, Centre for Bioethics, Clinical Research Institute of Montreal, Montreal, Quebec, Canada H2W 1R7

David C. Sabiston, Jr.
James B. Duke Professor of Surgery and Chairman, Department of Surgery, Duke University Medical Center, Durham, North Carolina 27710 U.S.A.

David L. Sackett
Professor of Medicine, Professor of Clinical Epidemiology and Biostatistics, McMaster University, Hamilton, Ontario, Canada, L8N 3Z5

Pedro A. Sánchez
Clinical Chief of Pediatric Cardiac Surgery, Centro Especial Ramon y Cajal Madrid, 28034 Spain

Martin T. Schechter
Assistant Professor, Department of Health Care and Epidemiology, Director, Clinical Research Support Group, Faculty of Medicine, University of British Columbia, Vancouver, British Columbia, V6T 1W5

Robert Shields
Professor of Surgery, University of Liverpool and Honorary Consultant Surgeon, Royal Liverpool Hospital and Broadgreen Hospital, Liverpool L69 3BX United Kingdom

Walter O. Spitzer
Professor and Chairman, Department of Epidemiology and Biostatistics, Strathcona Professor of Preventive Medicine, Professor of Medicine, McGill University, Montreal, Quebec, Canada H3A 1A2

Hans Troidl
Professor and Chairman, II, Department of Surgery, University of Köln, Surgical Clinic Merheim, D-5000 Cologne 91, Federal Republic of Germany

Karl-Heinz Vestweber
Oberarzt, II, Department of Surgery, University of Köln, Surgical Clinic Merheim, D-5000 Köln 91, Federal Republic of Germany

Beverly Walters
157A Beverly Street, Toronto, Ontario, Canada M5T 1Y7

Norman J.B. Wiggin
Scientific Editor, 82 Rothwell Drive, Ottawa, Ontario, Canada K1J 7G6

J. Ivan Williams
Professor, Department of Epidemiology and Biostatistics, McGill University, Scientific Director, Kellogg Centre, Montreal General Hospital, Montreal, Quebec, Canada H3G 1A4

Sharon Wood-Dauphinee
Associate Director and Assistant Professor, School of Physical and Occupational Therapy, McGill University, Montreal, Quebec, Canada H3G 1Y5

Introduction

H. Troidl

Early in my career as an academic surgeon, Professor Hamelmann encouraged me to venture from my home department at the University of Marburg to visit other academic surgical departments in Germany. I was immediately struck by the variety of approaches to similar clinical challenges and surgical research problems. When my good fortune took me to other university centers in Europe, I was particularly impressed by Professor John Goligher's philosophy and approach to surgical scholarship in Leeds. During the several months I subsequently spent working with him in 1973, I learned as much as I could about his way of doing clinical research and found his and other British perspectives especially valuable because my previous experience in Germany had been largely confined to basic laboratory research. The following year, Professor Wilfried Lorenz of Marburg accompanied me to North America to visit basic research laboratories, clinical departments of surgery, anesthesia, and clinical research centers. We consulted researchers at the National Institutes of Health, Cornell University, and the University of California at Los Angeles, and clinicians at Albany, Chicago, and the Mayo Clinic.

When I left Marburg to become first assistant to Professor H. Hamelmann in the Department of Surgery at Kiel, I continued my laboratory research activities while I acquired further experience as a clinical surgeon. During this period, the necessity for an academic surgeon to be a exemplary clinician, a skilled and uncompromising technician in the operating theater, an inspiring teacher, and a competent researcher, *simultaneously*, was brought home to me.

Once again, I was struck by the similarity of the unanswered questions in surgery and anesthesia, no matter where they arose in the world. The problems had common themes, but the solutions proposed were very different in different cities and countries, whether they were related to the organization of medical care, levels and sources of funding, or the design of research studies. Even the organization of research facilities varies not only between countries, but within countries; differences among the individual units of a single university or hospital are the rule, not the exception.

As I travelled and corresponded with friends in other centers, I realized that some of the ideas and solutions developed in Sweden had relevance to the problems we faced in Marburg and Kiel. Some of the ideas I discovered in North America, the United Kingdom, or Japan could be profitably brought home to Germany. My colleagues at home showed me that only a little modification was sometimes required to make them applicable and useful in Marburg. I was delighted to find that colleagues around the world were curious to know how we cope with problems in Germany, and that new friends in Boston and Montreal were not only open to sharing their problems but very receptive to ideas and potential solutions that my colleagues and I had worked out in Germany.

When I became Professor of Surgery at Cologne, I instituted an open door policy. I invited senior scholars to visit us in Cologne and arranged for my younger colleagues to be exposed to leaders and new ideas elsewhere. A number were able to present the results of their own work and to learn, first-hand, the techniques that I had discovered for myself, earlier.

My most trusted colleagues and I gradually recognized that while research problems had much in common around the world and many scientists had developed fruitful strategies and tactics for dealing with the problems associated with surgical research, there was no readily accessible source of information about much of the methodology that was evolving so rapidly. The idea of a book on feasible technology for research in surgery and other clinical disciplines became compelling. It would cover the principles of experimental design, biostatistics, epidemiology, starting and finishing research, and the diffusion of results.

Many a scholarly undertaking, whether it is a book or a research project, starts with an idea. Taking the idea from conception to fruition is often aided by interactions with friends—with whom I am still blessed!

The first step toward converting my idea of a book into a reality took place on October 14, 1984 in a chalet nestled in the hills near St. Adolphe, north of Montreal. My friend and host, Professor Walter Spitzer, spent half the night arguing with me about a possible Table of Contents. Early in the morning, we reached a consensus and quickly wrote down the headings and subheadings. When we called our mutual friend, Professor Jack McPeek in Boston, he immediately pronounced a benediction on our plan and agreed to work on it with us without hesitation. Professor Martin McKneally was the next to hear from us at four in the morning—it's hard to contact busy surgeons at any other time of the day. He was already up preparing slides for a paper and enthusiastically joined our growing team as soon as he had heard the details. Within a few hours, Walter and I succeeded in reaching Professor David Mulder in Montreal to find that he needed no persuasion before volunteering to contribute his considerable effort and resources.

Over a period of years, most clinical scholars develop an appreciation of the elements of experimental design and the recruitment and management of research resources. The acquisition of this knowledge is unpredictable in different academic settings and all too often is a matter of trial and error learning under the supervision of senior colleagues who have also learned by the trial and error method. It need not be so, because a much better understanding and consensus about scientifically acceptable methodology has been developing around the world.

The editors of this book share my concern about this state of affairs and my commitment to doing something about it. Each are scholars with a special responsibility for advancing research. Three of us are clinical surgeons charged with the care of patients, the supervision of research laboratories, and the development of younger surgical research colleagues in Albany, Cologne, and Montreal. One is a professor with a long track record of clinical epidemiologic research and teaching who now directs the affairs of the major Department of Epidemiology and Biostatistics at McGill University. One is an anesthetist, clinician–teacher, and research administrator at the Massachusetts General Hospital and Harvard University. Each is single-minded about helping colleagues with research problems and establishing an atmosphere and facilities to advance applied science. The underlying motive of all is to improve the care of patients through better understanding of relevant biological phenomena. We all give priority to the task of nurturing the academic growth of younger associates. A significant number of individuals who are world experts in their fields have joined our undertaking. Investigators in clinical disciplines, epidemiology, biostatistics, and the basic medical sciences have created a complementary ensemble of chapters giving advice on how to make research the creative, exciting, stimulating, intellectual endeavor it should be.

We offer practical suggestions and describe approaches and methods that have a proven record of success. The treatments prescribed for some of the most common ailments that afflict many well-intended clinical research endeavors are straightforward, but not simplistic or superficial. Most chapters are the product of collaborative efforts among clinicians and methodologists. Although the exposition of each topic is by no means exhaustive, sources of additional information are provided.

I sincerely hope that this book will help many of my colleagues, especially those who are newer in the field of clinical investigation, to avoid the errors and frustrations I have encountered in my search for a deeper understanding of clinical surgical research. The rewards and excitement of seeking and finding new knowledge can only be accelerated and enhanced by having a roadmap in hand when you start on your journey of discovery.

Cologne, Germany
August 1986

SECTION I

The Rationale of Surgical Research

1

Historical Evolution: Methods, Attitudes, Goals

A.V. Pollock

"Research" said Benjamin Jowett, the great Oxford classical scholar of the 19th century, "Research! A mere excuse for idleness, it has never achieved and will never achieve any results of the slightest value" (1).

The Philosophy of Research

I want to start with a proposition that is unscientific because it cannot be refuted. Let us call it an axiom. It is this: our forefathers, at least as far back as the fifth century BC, were no less intelligent than we are. Why is it then that biological and medical research is, with a few exceptions, a product of the last century? I suggest that the answer lies in certain attitudes of mind (Kuhn would call them paradigms) that have enslaved intellects in every century.

Observation alone can lead to fallacies. We still say that the sun rises in the east and sets in the west. What could be more natural to observers in medieval times than the supposition that the sun travels around a stationary earth? It took the genius of Nicolaus Copernicus to refute this theory. The observation was correct, but the ancient proposition ignored the movements of the planets—a new hypothesis was needed and Copernicus supplied it. The essence of a scientific statement is that it can be falsified by further observation and a new statement can then take its place. Newton gave the world several propositions that explained nearly all astronomical events, but Einstein sought the exceptions, and relativity explains not only those observations supported by Newton's hypotheses, but also others. Among living philosophers of science, I want to mention two whose views conflict to some extent, Karl Popper and Thomas Kuhn (2).

Popper proposes that the distinction between science and nonscience is that it is possible to falsify a scientific proposition. We can accept as a matter of faith that God created the universe because it is a proposition that cannot be refuted. When, however, the birth of the world is dated to 6000 or 7000 years ago, that is a falsifiable hypothesis and therefore a scientific statement. Popper sees criticism as one of the chief functions of a scientist. He traces disagreement back to the pre-Socratic philosophers of Greece—Thales, Anaximander and Anaximenes. They marked the beginning of the tradition of subjecting speculation to critical discussion which is the basis of the scientific method. In Popper's view, it comprises the following steps:

1. Seek a problem
2. Propose a solution
3. Formulate a testable hypothesis from that proposal
4. Attempt to refute the hypothesis by observations and experiments
5. Establish a preference between competing theories.

In Popper's words:

"All this means that a young scientist who hopes to make discoveries is badly advised if his teacher tells him: 'Go round and observe' and that he is well advised if his teacher tells him: 'Try to learn what people are discussing nowadays in science. Find out where difficulties arise, and take an interest in disagreements. These are the questions which you should take up'. In other words, you should study the problems of the day. This means that you pick up, and try to continue, a line of inquiry which has the whole background of the earlier development of science behind it" (3).

Kuhn, in contrast, does not believe that scientific knowledge progresses steadily by criticism of established hypotheses and claims that *ordinary* research seeks only to solve *puzzles* within the framework ("paradigm") of the existing accumulation of scientific knowledge. This steady state of puzzle-solving is interrupted from time to time by *revolutions* that arrive suddenly, irrationally and intuitively and establish a new paradigm within which the new scientists do their ordinary research and attempt to solve new puzzles.

In biological and medical research, in which neither Popper nor Kuhn took much interest, it seems to me that we can accept both these philosophies. We can set about solving puzzles and advance knowledge by setting up a hypothesis and devising observations and experiments to refute it. McIntyre and Popper (4) suggested the following 10 rules for medical practice:

1. Our present conjectural knowledge far transcends what any person can know, even in his own specialty. It changes quickly and radically and, in the main, not by accumulation but by the correction of erroneous doctrines and ideas. Therefore, there can be no authorities. There can, of course, be better and worse scientists. More often than not, the better the scientist the more aware he will be of his limitations.
2. We are all fallible, and it is impossible for anybody to avoid all mistakes, even avoidable ones. The old idea that we must avoid them has to be revised. It is mistaken and has led to hypocrisy.
3. Nevertheless, it remains our task to avoid errors. But to do so we must recognize the difficulty. It is a task in which nobody succeeds fully—not even the great creative scientist who is led, but quite often misled, by intuition.
4. Errors may lurk even in our best-tested theories. It is the responsibility of the professional to search for these errors. In this, he can be helped greatly by the proposal of new alternative theories. Thus we should be tolerant of ideas that differ from the dominant theories of the day and not wait until those theories are in trouble. The discovery that a well-tested and corroborated theory, or a commonly used procedure, is erroneous may be a most important discovery.
5. For all these reasons, our attitude towards mistakes must change. It is here that ethical reform must begin. For the old attitude leads to the hiding of our mistakes and to forgetting them as fast as we can.
6. Our new principle must be to learn from our mistakes so that we avoid them in future; this should take precedence even over the acquisition of new information. Hiding mistakes must be regarded as a deadly sin. Some errors are inevitably exposed—for example, operating on the wrong patient, or removing a healthy limb. Although the injury may be irreversible, the exposure of such errors can lead to the adoption of practices designed to prevent them. Other errors, some of which may be equally regrettable, are not so easily exposed. Obviously, those who commit them may not wish to have them brought to light, but equally obviously they should not be concealed since, after discussion and analysis, change in practice may prevent their repetition.
7. It is therefore our task to search for our mistakes and to investigate them fully. We must train ourselves to be self-critical.
8. We must recognize that self-criticism is best but that criticism by others is necessary and especially valuable if they approach problems from a different background. We must therefore learn to accept gracefully, and even gratefully, criticism from those who draw our attention to our errors.
9. If it is we who draw the attention of others to their mistakes, we should remind ourselves of similar errors we have made. We should remember that it is human to err and that even the greatest scientists make mistakes.
10. Rational criticism should be directed to definite, clearly identified mistakes. It should contain reasons and should be expressed in a form that allows its refutation. It should make clear which assumptions are being challenged and why. It should never contain insinuations, mere assertions, or just nega-

tive evaluations. It should be inspired by the aim of getting nearer to the truth; and for this reason it should be impersonal.

Whether the surgeon is solving puzzles or refuting hypotheses, he has three disciplines to help him: the laboratory, animal experiments and clinical practice. They are interdependent. There are many problems in clinical practice that can only be solved with the help of the disciplines of the biochemical and microbiological laboratories. There are questions that can only be answered ethically by animal experiments, but laboratory and animal research is sterile unless it has a potential for affecting clinical practice.

The History of Surgical Research

Clinical research was to all intents and purposes non-existent until 50 years ago due to a combination of the following:

Respect for the doctor–patient relationship. There was a time when the doctor was almost universally regarded as being all-seeing and all-knowing and this attitude persists in some parts of the world. As a consequence, a physician could never admit that his diagnosis was conjectural, his treatment ineffective. He could never confess ignorance.

Inaccurate diagnoses. Diagnostic precision has been one of the hallmarks of medical research in the last hundred years. It began with the revolution introduced by microbiology and was extended by radiology and the more recent advances in diagnostic imaging techniques, biochemistry and immunology.

Ineffective remedies. When physicians were powerless to influence the course of most diseases, it did not occur to them to do clinical research. One placebo was as good as the next, and it was merely discourteous to question the practice of others.

Reverence for authority. Until the late nineteenth century, the task of ordinary scholars was to study and interpret other people's writings; the outstanding virtue was reverence for authority. The approach to learning was conceptual rather than empirical. Sir Dominic John Corrigan (5), writing in *The Lancet* in 1829, had this to say about Harvey's discovery of the circulation of the blood: "Such, however, is the power of prejudice that no physician past the age of forty believed in Harvey's doctrine, and that his practice declined from the moment he published this ever-memorable discovery". Although a few original thinkers have challenged authority in every age in spite of opposing social pressures, it is only recently that respect for logical thinking has been accompanied by skepticism and the pursuit of pragmatism.

Lack of statistical tests. In therapeutics, one of the strongest forces for change has been the testing of remedies in clinical trials in which the fundamental requirements are comparison of treatment regimens and evaluation of differences in outcome by the application of methods based on the mathematics of probability.

Games of chance were the original stimulus to sixteenth century Italian philosophers, including Galileo, to attempt to give mathematical expression to probabilities (6,7). In the following century, Blaise Pascal corresponded regularly with a fellow mathematician, Pierre de Fermat, on the same subject in relation to card games, not scientific research. Jacob Bernoulli's *"Ars Conjectandi"* was published in 1713. He proved that the more often a test is repeated the greater is the probability that the result will be within certain limits.

In eighteenth century France, Abraham de Moivre published "Doctrines of Chance" and what was known as "The Petersburg Problem" was widely discussed, i.e., if a coin comes down tails several times, is it more likely to come down heads next time? In 1785, the Marquis de Condorcet declared in his "Essay on the application of mathematics to the theory of decision making" that probability calculus "weights the grounds for belief and calculates the probable truth of testimony or decisions".

One of the most important late eighteenth century French mathematical philosophers was Pierre Simon, Marquis de Laplace. He gave a series of lectures in 1795, and published "Analytical Theory of Probabilities" in 1812. In the latter, he wrote "The theory of probabilities is fundamentally only good sense reduced to calculation."

During the eight centuries between the compilation of the Doomsday Book, in which William the Conqueror evaluated his new kingdom and the nineteenth century, there was no systematic collection of vital statistics on a national scale anywhere in Europe. The Societe Royale de Medecine made one of the first attempts to record births and deaths in 1776, but it was not until the early nineteenth century that a reliable system was introduced in France, followed by other European countries. By 1880, individual cards had taken the place of highly fallible lists in the compiling of statistics. The Hollerith punch card sorting machine was first used in a national census in the United States of America in 1890.

It soon became evident that epidemiological studies were stultified by the inaccuracy of death certificates. Even as late as the beginning of the twentieth century, Sir Josiah Stamp (8) was able to write: "The government are very keen on amassing statistics. They collect them, add them, raise them to the nth power, take the cube root, and prepare wonderful diagrams. But you must never forget that every one of these figures comes in the first instance from the village watchman, who puts down what he damn well pleases."

In 1853 William Farr, who had been a student in Paris of Pierre-Charles-Alexander Louis (the exponent of the "numerical method"), cooperated with d'Espine in developing the anatomically-based system that formed the foundation of today's International Classification of Diseases.

Louis' numerical method, however, achieved no acclaim until relatively recently. In 1835 he published a paper, translated as "Research on the effect of blood-letting in several inflammatory maladies" (9) whose main conclusion was that blood-letting had little therapeutic value. The paper attracted adverse comment in the French Academy of Sciences and Francois Double issued a report condemning the use of statistical methods in clinical medicine, and extolling Morgagni's aphorism "*Non numerandae sed perpendendae*"—facts must be weighed, not counted.

Nevertheless, Simon-Denis Poisson wrote in 1837 that if a medication had been successfully employed in a large number of similar cases, and if the number of cases where it had not succeeded was small compared with the total number of cases, it was probable that the medication would succeed in a new trial.

By 1870, statistical analysis of whole populations was well-advanced, but the problems of sampling had not been tackled. Then, the new science of microbiology eclipsed interest in the application of statistics in medicine for a long time, and the development of statistical methods for analyzing samples shifted to brewing and agriculture. The word "random" was applied in a statistical sense at the end of the nineteenth century, and "randomize" in 1936.

The Evolution of Random Control Clinical Trials

It is in the nature of man to compare things—you find yourself doing it all the time. The weather is wetter, dryer, warmer, colder than you remember for the time of year. So it is in therapeutics. If patients do well, the regimen you are using is better than the one you used last year, and better than the one used by your colleagues. You have unconsciously selected a control against which to judge your results. Confusion and false claims can arise, however, if you choose the wrong method of controlling your observations.

Historical Controls

Most of the really great advances in therapeutics have been made by contrasting the results of a new regimen against those of previously documented treatment. The enormous benefits of general anaesthesia, the reduction of surgical wound infection by asepsis, the cure of many infections by penicillin and numerous other advances, have needed only careful documentation and comparison with previous experience to become accepted. If one were to make a rule, it would be this: if the new treatment is immeasurably better than the old, historical controls are not only sufficient, they are the only ones that satisfy the demands of ethics. Once it had been shown that penicillin could cure subacute bacterial endocarditis, a previously uniformly fatal disease, it was unacceptable to do other than treat all cases with penicillin. Random control trials are only justified if there is a therapeutic dilemma. Ignorance is essential.

False conclusions can, however, be reached by the inappropriate use of historical controls. This is particularly true if the results of surgical treatment for a disease are compared with previous experience with medical treatment. The bias in such a study is that of selection. The surgeon will only operate on patients who are fit enough to have the operation; the results cannot be compared with those for *all* patients in a previous medically treated series. An example of this bias was published in the *New England Journal of Medicine* in 1948 (10). Linton reported more favorable survival figures in patients with cirrhosis of the liver treated by portacaval anastomosis than in those in a control group treated medically in previous years. The patients who had the operation were those who survived long enough to be operated on; those who died before operation, or never became fit for operation, were not included in the report. The conclusions reached by this trial were subsequently repudiated by the Boston Liver Group (11). This group randomized patients fit enough for operation to standard medical treatment or to surgery (portacaval anastomosis). The results were not significantly different in the two groups, but vastly superior to those in an unselected group of patients not fit enough to be recruited into the trial.

Contemporary Non-Random Controls

Many questions about aetiology and epidemiology can only be answered by comparing a group of people subject to certain risks with another group that is not. Sometimes the evidence from such comparisons is sufficiently compelling to demand acceptance. This is true, for example, of the association of cigarette smoking and bronchial carcinoma, or of exposure to asbestos dust and mesothelioma. Often, however, epidemiological reseach using such controls raises more questions than it answers. The classical example of the confusion that may arise is the continuing controversy about the relationship between diet and atherosclerosis.

In therapeutics, all contemporary non-random comparative studies are suspect because the outcome of any disease or operation depends on so many factors. The sample of the population in the study group may differ from that in the control group in the incidence of risk factors, in an uneven distribution of the variables associated with treatment, and in variations in the method of assessment of events. Although the conclusions reached in such studies can only be tentative, they may form the basis for hypotheses to be tested in random control trials.

An example of such a study was published by Normann and his colleagues (12). The two surgical departments of Ulleval Hospital in Oslo followed different regimens for the treatment of perforated appendicitis. In one department, appendectomy was completed by the insertion of a drain into the appendix fossa; in the other, it was followed by 2 days of peritoneal dialysis. In the drainage group the complications included 1 death, 6 pelvic abscesses, 1 intraperitoneal abscess, 4 cases of paralytic ileus, re-laparotomies and 1 faecal fistula, i.e., a total complication rate 17 out of 77. In the lavage group, complications comprised 1 death, 3 pelvic abscesses, 1 paralytic ileus and 1 re-laparotomy for a total rate of 5 out of 78. Firm conclusions about the superiority of peritoneal dialysis are not justified, however, because of the strong likelihood of important undisclosed variables.

Random Controlled Clinical Trials

It was Ronald Aylmer Fisher who first recognized that many of the pitfalls of non-random trials could be avoided if the allocation of subjects to each arm of a trial was decided strictly at random and the investigator had no control over the randomization process (13). Fisher, a mathematician and a biologist, studied physics under James Jeans at Cambridge but decided on a career in biology. In 1919, he was appointed statistician to Rothamsted Agricultural Experimental Station where field trials had been carried out since 1843 but had never been subjected to statistical analysis. Fisher undertook the task not only of analyzing past trials but of designing new trials free from bias. He wrote widely on various aspects of the statistical analysis of trials and worked out the exact probability test that bears his name. In 1925, he published "Statistical Methods for Research Workers" (14) which dealt with the design and analysis of controlled trials. His second book, "The Design of Experiments" (15), appeared 10 years later when he was Galton Professor at University College, London.

When Fisher published "The Design of Experiments", Bradford Hill was working on a series of papers published in *The Lancet* in 1937 and in a book entitled "Principles of Medical Statistics". Now as Sir Austin Bradford Hill, he is a member of the central staff of the Medical Research Council and his name is synonymous with the proper ethical and statistical design of clinical trials. He, if anyone, deserves the name of father of the controlled clinical trial. His book renamed "A Short Textbook of Medical Statistics" (16) is now in its tenth edition, has been translated into several languages, and is a source of inspiration to clinical investigators throughout the world. One of Bradford Hill's greatest achievements was the organization of the Medical Research Council cooperative trial on the treatment of tuberculosis by streptomycin in 1947 (17). Because streptomycin was in short supply and could not be offered to all sufferers from tuberculosis, it was ethically justifiable to test it in a random control trial, in which the control group was treated by the best standard methods. The principle of central randomization, was introduced for the first time in this trial and it was a brilliant success.

The Development of Ethical Standards

(The Declaration of Helsinki (1964), as revised in Tokyo in 1975, is included as Appendix A of this textbook).

It was Bradford Hill who enunciated the famous aphorism: "The ethical obligation always and entirely outweighs the experimental" (18).

There are two inalienable rules of medical practice which apply whether or not you are conducting a controlled clinical trial. The first is that an investigation or treatment that is not in the best interests of the patient, or whose potential risks outweigh the potential benefits should never be advised. In the context of controlled trials this means that you may only participate if you are truly ignorant of the respective merits of the two (or more) arms of the trial. If you think that one arm is better than the other, you must not take part.

The second rule is that no investigation or treatment should ever be made or given without the patient's consent. The simple noun, consent, is rarely mentioned these days without the adjective "informed" attached to it, but the nature and extent of the informing is seldom apparent.

Informed Consent

Some years ago, Epstein and Lasagna (19) examined the process of obtaining informed consent. They enlisted 44 volunteers, to each of whom they proposed administering a tablet for headache. The subjects were not told the tablet was aspirin but an explanation of the actions and side effects of the drug was given to half of them in 178 words, and to the other half in 852 words. The comprehension score in those given the shorter explanation was 67%; 14% refused the "treatment". In the group given the longer explanation, 35% understood the information; 45% refused the "treatment".

What do we mean by informed consent? If it means anything at all, it must mean that we explain to the patient what we propose doing and why, that we inform him or her of the risks and benefits of the proposed investigation or treatment, and that we review the risks and benefits of not accepting what is proposed. These requirements apply equally to laying on a stethoscope or taking out a stomach; the difference lies in the amount of information the patient needs. When we have taken a history, we are usually content to say "Now, perhaps you will go and get undressed; I would like to examine your chest". When, on the other hand, we have made a diagnosis of carcinoma of the stomach, with the patient's consent to every step along the diagnostic pathway, we sit down and explain that, having weighed the risks against the benefits, our advice is to accept laparotomy with a view to gastrectomy. Gastrectomy, we will say, is a major operation, not devoid of complications including the possibility of death; the alternative is increasing illness and discomfort culminating in death.

Most patients will accept the advice and we will act in accordance with it—*always* in the best interest of the patient. We usually ask the patient to sign a document in which he or she acknowledges having been informed of the nature of the treatment advised, and we will countersign it. It must be emphasized that this document alone does not protect you, the doctor, from legal action and your only defense against an accusation of battery or negligence is that you honestly behaved at all times in such a way as to leave no doubt that your treatment was intended to benefit the patient.

In the United Kingdom the legal duty of a doctor has been explained by Mr. Justice Bristow (20) in the following words: "The duty of a doctor is to explain what he intends to do and its implications, in the way a careful and responsible doctor in similar circumstances would have done. . . But he ought to warn of what may happen by misfortune however well the operation was done if there is a real risk of a misfortune inherent in the procedure. . . In what he says any good doctor has to take into account the personality of the patient, the likelihood of the misfortune and what in the way of warning is for the particular patient's benefit.

In other countries the legal duty is similar and is, in many cases, defined by statute. In *Canterbury v Spence* (21), the landmark decision of the US Courts of Appeals, four propositions were enunciated:

1. The root premise was the concept that every human being of adult years and sound mind had the right to determine what should be done with his or her own body.
2. Consent was the informed exercise of a choice and that entailed an opportunity to evaluate, knowledgeably, the options available and the risks attendant upon each.
3. The doctor, therefore, had to disclose all material risks, "material" being determined by the prudent patient test: "when a reasonable patient in what the physician knows or should know to be the patient's position would be likely to attach significance to the risk or cluster of risks in determining whether or not to forgo the proposed therapy".
4. The doctor, however, had a "therapeutic privilege" enabling him to withhold from his patient information as to risk if it could be shown that a reasonable assessment of the patient would have indicated to the doctor that disclosure would have posed a serious threat of psychological detriment to the patient.

Chalmers (22) has commented that in the United States of America it is lawyers, not physicians, who determine medical policy. Lawyers have not yet entered the research field because they have been too busy making a living out of the ordinary practice of medicine but, when they do, there could be chaos because in law the best thing for the patient is what is done by the ordinary doctor in the community. The validation or rejection of a treatment in a controlled clinical trial will become more and more difficult.

Consent to Randomization

What information do you give a woman who consults you with a carcinoma in her breast when you are participating in a random control clinical trial comparing adjuvant chemotherapy with no adjuvant chemotherapy after total mastectomy with axiliary dissection?

There are two possible ways to inform her. The first is to tell her that there are at least a dozen acceptable ways of treating her, ranging from wide excision of the lump to extended radical mastectomy, with or without internal prosthetic replacement, with or without pre- or postoperative radiotherapy, with or without short term (e.g., one week of cyclophosphamide) or longer term (e.g., cyclophosphamide, methotrexate and 5-fluorouracil for 6 months) postoperative chemotherapy, and with or without hormonal manipulation (e.g., tamoxifen). You will then explain the advantages and disadvantages inherent in each treatment. By this time she, if not you, will be thoroughly confused. You might then say that you favor total mastectomy with axiliary dissection, that you are taking part in a multicenter trial of adjuvant chemotherapy, and that you would like her to give permission to have her postoperative management decided by chance. In so doing, you establish contracts between you and the patient not only for treatment but also for research. This approach is demanded by the Declaration of Helsinki, although the amendment agreed to in Tokyo in 1975 allows for circumstances in which the psychological welfare of the patient requires the investigator to opt for less than a full explanation that the treatment is being decided by chance.

The second attitude toward informed consent in a randomized clinical trial is this: each of the alternative treatments is thought to offer patients equal benefit; some doctors advise one, some the other. Accordingly the doctor's duty is to inform the patient only about the treatment to which the patient has been randomized. This is the view held by the organizers and clinicians in the British–French trial of carotid endarterectomy versus medical treatment for transient ischaemic attacks (23). Justification of this attitude is difficult and only possible when the treatment options are a matter of indifference to the patient. In a trial on methods of abdominal wound closure from my department (24), for example, we did not find it necessary to inform our patients that the material used to close the aponeurosis would be decided at random, and might be monofilament steel, monofilament nylon or polyglycolic acid.

The treatment options may not, however, be a matter of indifference to the patient. A working party of the Cancer Research Campaign (CRC) in the United Kingdom deliberated for 2 years without reaching unanimous agreement about the method of seeking informed consent for a trial of conservative (lumpectomy) versus radical (mastectomy) treatment of patients with breast carcinoma in which both options were accompanied by axiliary node sampling and followed by radical radiotherapy (25). The working party finally recommended that patients should be fully informed about the randomization process and both treatment options *before* being randomized, and that women who chose one option over the other should be excluded from the trial.

There are both ethical and scientific drawbacks to the CRC recommendations. From the ethical standpoint, the patients cannot be said to be fully informed unless they are also told that other operations and other postoperative regimens are available and that their value has been neither proved nor disproved. From the scientific point of view, the women who agree to be randomized are a self-selected group and the results cannot necessarily be generalized to the treatment of all patients with breast cancer.

Zelen (26) recognized that obtaining informed consent to randomization is the sticking point for many doctors and most patients, and that it retards recruitment of patients into perfectly ethical trials. He suggested, therefore, that randomization should precede consent. The patients in the control group should be offered, and consent to, the best standard treatment; those in the "experimental" group should be fully informed of the nature of the investigation and give consent to the new treatment. If the patient refuses the new treatment he or she should be given the best standard treatment, but the outcome should be attributed to the experimental, not the control, arm of the trial.

Zelen's design also raises difficulties. From the ethical point of view, when the patients in the control group are not told that they have been *randomly* allocated to the group, they are not fully informed and cannot decide for themselves to choose the alternative treatment. On the practical side, it is theoretically possible that the outcome of the disease in a patient who has been fully informed may differ from the outcome in one who has merely consented to what he or she is made to think is the best treatment in the opinion of his or her doctor. There is evidence that psychological factors influence the progress of cancer (27).

Patients must be retained in the arm of a trial to which they have been randomized even if they do not get the treatment prescribed in that arm. This may dilute the results, and the outcome of these patients may have to be analyzed separately, but in their allocated group and not as part of the control group. It is just as unethical to publish the results of a biased trial as it is to fail to obtain consent to a trial.

The Ethical Aspects of Stopping a Trial

In trials on the treatment of most cancers, the last outcome event (recurrence or death) will be years after the recruitment of the patients, and no ethical problems arise. It is different, when the outcome is more immediate and you, as the investigator undertake interim or sequential analyses of the results. You cannot agree to participate in a controlled clinical trial unless you are ignorant of the respective benefits of the treatment options. Any suggestion of a preference for one or another must debar you from participation, because you would be offering half your patients what you regard as suboptimal treatment. You must be willing to enter members of your own family into the trial.

Accordingly, you start with the conviction that the chances of your next patient receiving treatment A or treatment B are 50:50, and the chances that A is better than B, or B better than A, are also 50:50. Then a patient receiving treatment A dies, or suffers some other disaster. The chances that treatment A is equivalent to B are now less than 50:50. Another adverse event occurs in group A, and another, and another. Your belief that the two treatments are equivalent is now thoroughly shaken, although statistical testing shows that the result could easily have arisen by chance. Finally, your repeated interim analyses show that just one more death or other negative event in group A will tip the balance into statistical significance—the magic $P < 0.05$.

It is clear that such behavior is quite unacceptable and could bring controlled clinical trials into disrepute. Martin Fincke, professor of criminal law at the University of Bielefeld, wrote a book—quoted by Burkhardt and Kienle (28)—in which he claimed that a doctor treating patients in a controlled trial would be guilty of manslaughter if he continued to apply one treatment after he had begun to think the other was better. However, a trial stopped before statistical significance is reached is a trial wasted. If it was ethical to start the trial, it must be ethical to bring it to a convincing conclusion.

The dilemma can be resolved in three ways:

1. In many trials, the clinician can be kept ignorant of which of the treatments under investigation each of his patients is having. This is the principle of the "double-blind" trial, and it is applicable when no external distinguishing signs are apparent. In a trial of one drug against another the control and experimental substances can be made to look alike, and be numbered consecutively, i.e., not labeled A and B. In a trial of two operations for peptic ulcer, the doctor following the patient's subsequent progress can be denied access to details of the operation. In some trials, however, it is impossible to "blind" the assessing doctor; e.g., when medical and surgical treatments are being compared.
2. Repeated interim analyses are bad statistically, because analyzing results 10 times will increase the chance of finding $P < 0.05$ on one occasion to 1 in 5, and ethically, because a difference in the efficacy of treatments that has arisen by chance will tend to bias you toward the apparently better treatment. The rule must be that the clinicians involved in any trial must not do interim analyses, and the trial coordinator who does them must not communicate the findings to the clinicians. Nevertheless, the discovery that actual harm has been caused by one treatment should be communicated immediately. This applies particularly to evidence of toxicity of a drug.
3. "Play-the-winner" randomization. Failure of treatment A in one patient means that a future patient is allocated to treatment B, whereas failure of treatment B determines allocation to treatment A. This method, although ethically and statistically acceptable, is seldom practiced, mainly because it demands continuous monitoring of outcome events that may not occur soon enough for the method to have its proper impact.

Monitoring the Ethics of Controlled Clinical Trials

The doctor's duty to each patient must always come first. It is only within the framework of this duty that controlled trials are proper and numerous measures exist to safeguard each patient's welfare. National and international rules are laid down for the conduct of clinical trials; financial support will not be provided for unethical trials; and, in most countries, peer review bodies judge, and, if necessary, amend the protocols of clinical trials to ensure their ethical acceptability. In the United Kingdom, the recommended composition of Hospital Ethical Commitees is 2 senior and 1 junior hospital doctor, 2 general practitioners, 1 community physician, 1 nurse and 1 lay person. In the United States, Institutional Review Boards perform a similar function.

The U.S. Food and Drug Administration (FDA) was created by Congress in response to a public demand, articulated by President John F. Kennedy that: "The physician and the consumer... have the assurance from an impartial scientific source, that any drug or therapeutic device on the market today is safe and effective for its intended use." In 1970, the FDA published a set of rules defining "adequate and well-controlled" investigations which were subsequently tested and upheld in the United States Supreme Court (29). The rules stipulate that:

1. There should be a clear statement of the objectives of the study.

2. The study should embody a method of selection of subjects that:
   a. provides adequate assurance that they are suitable for the purpose of the study,
   b. assigns the subjects to test groups in such a way as to minimize bias, and
   c. assures the comparability in test and control groups of pertinent variables.
3. The protocol should contain an explanation of the methods of observation and recording of results and the steps taken to minimize bias on the part of the subject and the observer.
4. The investigators should make a comparison of the results in such a fashion as to permit quantitative evaluation. Four types of comparison are recognized:
   a. no treatment control,
   b. placebo control,
   c. active treatment control, and
   d. historical control.
5. The investigators should give a summary of the methods of analysis and appropriate statistical methods.

Conclusions

Controlled clinical trials must always be ethically acceptable to an independent observer. The essential requirements are ignorance by the investigator of the relative superiority of one or other arm of the trial; assurance that the ill effects of a new treatment are understood, that they are not serious in relation to the seriousness of the disease being studied and that patients are warned about them; consent of patients to accept the treatment recommended; avoidance of bias; and, finally, honest and accurate recording, analysis and reporting of results.

References

1. Sutherland J, editor. The Oxford Book of Literary Anecdotes. Oxford: Clarendon Press, 1975:253.
2. Lakatos I. Falsification and the methodology of scientific research programmes. In: Lakatos I, Musgrave A editors. Criticism and the growth of knowledge. Cambridge: Cambridge University Press, 1970.
3. Popper K. Conjectures and refutations: the growth of scientific knowledge. London: Routledge & Kegan Paul, 4th ed. 1972:129.
4. McIntyre N, Popper K. The critical attitude in medicine: the need for a new ethics. Brit Med J 1983;287:1919-23.
5. Corrigan DJ. Aneurysm of the aorta. Singular pulsation of the arteries—necessity of the employment of the stethescope. Lancet 1829;i:586-90.
6. Murphy TD. Medical knowledge and statistical methods in early nineteenth century France. Med Hist 1981;25:301-09.
7. Westergaard H. Contributions to the history of statistics. London: P.S. King & Son Ltd., 1932.
8. Stamp J. Quoted by: Dunea G. Swallowing the golden ball. Brit Med J 1983;286:1962-63.
9. Gaines WJ, Langford HG. Research on the effect of blood-letting in several inflammatory maladies. Arch Intern Med 1960;106:571-79.
10. Linton RR. Porta-caval shunts in the treatment of portal hypertension, with special reference to patients previously operated upon. New Eng J Med 1948;238:723-27.
11. Garceau AJ, Donaldson RM, O'Hara ET, Callow AD, Muench H, Chalmers TC and the Boston Inter-Hospital Liver Group. A controlled trial of prophylactic portacaval-shunt surgery. New Eng J Med 1964;270:496-500.
12. Normann E, Korvald E, Lotveit T. Perforated appendicitis—lavage or drainage? Ann Chir et Gynae Fenn 1975;64:195-97.
13. Yates F, Mather K. Ronald Aylmer Fisher 1890-1962. Biographical Memoirs of Fellows of the Royal Society 1963; 9:91-129.
14. Fisher RA. Statistical Methods for Research Workers. Edinburgh: Oliver & Boyd, 1925.
15. Fisher RA. The Design of Experiments. Edinburgh: Oliver & Boyd, 1935.
16. Bradford Hill A. A Short Textbook of Medical Statistics. London: Hodder & Stoughton Educational, 1977.
17. Medical Research Council. Streptomycin treatment of pulmonary tuberculosis. A Medical Research Council investigation. Brit Med J 1948;2:769-82.
18. Bradford Hill A. Medical ethics and controlled trials. Brit Med J 1963;1:1043-49.
19. Epstein LC, Lasagna L. Obtaining informed consent. Arch Intern Med 1969;123:682-88.
20. Chatterton V Gerson, The Times, 7 February 1980, per Bristow J. Quoted in: Legal correspondent, the limits of consent. Brit Med J 1983;286:182-83.
21. Law Report, House of Lords. The Times (London) 1985 Feb 22:28.
22. Chalmers TC. In: Tygstrup N, Lachin JM, Juhl E, editors. The randomized clinical trial and therapeutic decisions. New York: Marcel Dekker Inc, 1982.

23. Warlow C. Is informed consent always needed? Lancet 1982; 2:1280.
24. Leaper DJ, Pollock AV, Evans M. Abdominal wound closure: a trial of nylon, polygloycolic acid and steel sutures. Brit J Surg 1977;64:603-06.
25. Cancer research campaign working party in breast conservation. Informed consent: the ethical, legal and medical implications for doctors and patients who participate in randomized clinical trials. Brit Med J 1983;286:1117-21.
26. Zelen M. A new design for randomized clinical trials. New Eng J Med 1979;300:1242-45.
27. Papaioannou A. Informed consent after randomization. Lancet 1982$_z$:828.
28. Burkhardt R, Kienle G. Controlled clinical trials and medical ethics. Lancet 1978;2:1356-59.
29. Young RSK. Role of the FDA in cancer therapy research. Clin Oncol 1981;8:447-52.

Further Reading

Shapiro SH, Louis TA. Clinical trials. New York: Marcel Dekker Inc, 1983.

2

Philosophy of Surgical Research

R.L. Cruess

Contemporary surgeons are able to offer individual patients and society therapeutic interventions that help to prolong life and make it more meaningful. These interventions are the result of a better understanding of human disease that has converted possibilities that were unthought of merely one generation ago into realities. Unless you are completely satisfied with all the forms of therapy currently available to surgeons and other clinicians you *must* favor surgical and other clinical research in its broadest terms. No further justification for research on surgical problems is required.

The philosophy of surgical research is somewhat more complex. While one can insist upon its necessity, it does not immediately follow that research should be actually carried out by surgeons. There are, however, valid reasons why it should be.

Without an ongoing and regularly updated scientific basis for the practice of surgery, surgeons become mere technicians. John Hunter became a surgeon in the late 19th century, when surgery was a craft rather than a science. By the time he died, he had incorporated science as an essential part of surgery and had founded a tradition of investigation that has remained unbroken. The pride of surgeons in their skills and knowledge, and the intellectual satisfaction they gain from surgery are derived from this tradition.

Surgeons are more inclined than others to pose questions about the surgical aspects of the diseases they treat. The nutritional problems and requirements of surgical patients were only defined when they were investigated by surgeons; the therapeutic intravenous solutions in current use were developed in surgical research laboratories. Modern joint replacements are the result of surgeons' investigations of the problems posed by the arthritic patient and surgeons have participated actively in identifying the causes of that arthritis. Much of our present understanding of epilepsy developed in response to questions posed by neurosurgeons interested in the disease. There are a host of other examples of how the welfare of patients has benefited from the questions surgeons ask as they practice surgery.

A major reason for maintaining and expanding surgical research is the essential contribution it makes to the training of academic surgeons. Whether or not traning in research should be mandatory for all surgeons is debatable, but there is no doubt about its absolute necessity in the training of the academic surgeon. It is the only way in which the inquiring mind needed for academic creativity can be developed. The shifts among the centers that have influenced surgeons and surgical care during the last 150 years have been uniformly based on whatever form of investigation was at the forefront at any particular time and the involvement of any given center in the contemporary research endeavor. The European centers that had such great influence in the late 19th and early 20th century, the renowned centers in the United Kingdom, and the great academic centers in North America were all built around research laboratories and inquiring minds.

Francis Moore, in his presidential address to the Society of University Surgeons, outlined one of the serious problems facing all surgeons carrying out research. "The surgical investigator must be a bridge tender, channelling knowledge from biologic science to the patient's bedside and back again. . . . Those at one end of the bridge say that he is not a very good scientist and those at the other end say that he does not spend enough time in the operating room" (1).

The increasing complexity of both research and surgery poses serious problems for anyone attempting to maintain an identity in both camps. Sub-specialization in surgery is recognized by all as a partial solution, but even if one's practice is restricted to a small number of procedures or diseases, it is hard to remain at the forefront. To be competitive in the world of science, a scholar must maintain a continuous presence in the laboratory, or risk falling dangerously behind. The easy problems have been solved; the animal laboratory and the microscope are no longer adequate tools to provide exciting solutions like those of bygone years. Engineering, molecular biology, immunology, and in-depth epidemiology are the disciplines required today and they are not for the amateur.

The answers to this dilemma are varied and depend upon individuals, circumstances, and even specialties. Some specialties are closer to their allied research disciplines than others. Engineering and orthopedics appear to co-exist happily and surgeons can maintain reasonable levels of expertise in both if they are conscientious. The same is true of neurophysiology and neurosurgery. The technical aspects of microsurgery are amenable to rather traditional forms of research training. These examples are, however, rare and most surgeons find that they must obtain in-depth training in some branch of modern biomedical science if they wish to follow the splendid traditions of surgical research.

One frequently utilized solution is to form a partnership with a basic scientist who relates well and easily with what one might call the "surgical personality". There are many successful surgical laboratories in which the surgeon and the career scientist have a truly symbiotic relationship that provides great benefits to the discipline of surgery. Such individuals can play key roles in the education of surgeons; they come to appreciate the problems faced by surgeons and to understand the knowledge base required.

Another solution, which is much less satisfactory, is for the surgeon to pose the question, sub-contract the investigation to a basic scientist, and take very little part in the research process. This approach usually does not have an impact on the practice of surgery or the education of surgeons as those in which surgeons are active participants, but where there is virtually no alternative the results are clearly beneficial for mankind.

Surgical research, like other clinical research, is essential. There is almost certainly not a single living surgeon or other clinician who is satisfied with all aspects of contemporary surgical and clinical management. It follows that surgeons and other clinicians must carry out research.

During his Lister Oration in 1968, Lord Florey stated; "We need people engaged in the practice of medicine to try to solve, on a well-organized basis the problems thrown up by practical medicine" (2).

As a simple statement of need about the philosophy and justification for surgical and other clinical research, this appears entirely appropriate.

References

1. Moore F. The university and american surgery: presidential address, annual meeting of the society of the university surgeons. Boston: 1958;44:6.
2. Florey H. Lister Oration. Edinb.: J Royal Coll Surg 1968;13:106-111.

3

Roles for the Surgical Investigator

R.C.-J. Chiu and D.S. Mulder

"A surgical investigator is a bridge tender, channeling knowledge from biological science to the patient's bedside and back again. He traces his origin from both ends of the bridge. He is thus a bastard and is called this by everybody. Those at one end of the bridge say he is not a very good scientist, and those at the other say that he does not spend enough time in the operating room. If only he is willing to live with this abuse, he can continue to do his job effectively" (1).

The above observation, attributed to Dr. Francis D. Moore, captures the essence of both the role and the dilemma of the surgical investigator. The increasing difficulty experienced by the surgical investigator in playing his or her role well is partially responsible for what Dr. C. Rollins Hanlon, Director of the American College of Surgeons, has called a "deteriorating situation in surgical research that has been troublesome for some years and is now verging on crisis" (2).

The Dilemma of the Surgical Investigator

A surgeon who wishes to pursue active research faces many difficult questions, the foremost being how to maintain excellence both in the practice of surgery and in investigation. It is now generally accepted that to maintain operative competence, especially in performing complex procedures such as open heart surgery, a surgeon has to have a certain minimal case load. This requirement, combined with increasing sophistication in technology and in competition for research funding, makes it difficult for the investigator to dedicate enough time and effort to research to remain competitive. These conflicting time-demands are aggravated by changing patterns of medical financing that may pressure investigators to generate funds by expanding their clinical practice. Government intervention in the practice of medicine compounds the associated administrative chores. Finding a solution to this chronic and deepening time-dilemma requires the joint efforts of surgical investigators and the institutions that nurture surgical research.

Another question surgical investigators often face is how "basic" should their research orientation be? Researchers studying transplantation immunology, a surgically relevant problem, may quickly find themselves studying the function of suppressor T-lymphocytes; to understand that, they must appreciate the nature of cell surface receptors; grasp the function of the receptor fully, and impress the granting agency that they possess adequate scientific depth. They must learn how to analyze the molecular structure of its protein components. At this point, they will wonder whether they are stretching the limits of competence too far. When will whatever results they obtain become decreasingly cost-effective in relation to their investment of time and effort? There is no doubt about the importance of basic and fundamental research for the progress of surgery, but how basic should such research be for the individual clinical investigator?

Dr. Walter F. Ballinger denies the existence

of real "basic" research in surgery. He defines surgical research as a type of applied physiology. A surgical investigator uses biochemistry, biophysics, mathematics or electronics for his research and "may flirt with problems of radiation physics, but he will not become an expert radiologist or physicist because of his flirtation, and for this he may be criticized" (3). Dr. Francis D. Moore has also cautioned against allowing surgical research to become too basic and has written about "the very urgent and elegant work of applied science." These outstanding leaders in surgical research have re-emphasized the role of surgical investigators as "bridge tenders" and warned them not to go so far from the bridge that they lose sight of it.

Despite such admonitions, a much more liberal definition of what can be classified as surgical research has been adopted in many institutions and has given rise to a number of perplexing questions. The term surgical investigation is now used to describe:

1. Research done by anyone on any subject, provided it is done within the jurisdiction of a Department of Surgery. This could include the work of someone with a Ph.D. in molecular biology, appointed as an assistant professor of surgery, on the molecular structure of a cortisol-binding protein, published in a journal of biochemistry. Is this really "surgical" research?
2. Research on any subject provided it is done by a surgeon. Would a surgeon's work on improving the safety of a sailboat qualify as surgical research?
3. Research done by anyone, provided the subject is relevant to surgical problems. An individual with a Ph.D. in nutrition might make an important contribution by studying the nutritional support of patients with major burns. If their appointment is in the Department of Medicine, would the work still count as "surgical research"?
4. Research done by surgeons on such surgical problems as devising a new instrument for operative procedures. Is this definition not excessively narrow?

Any discussion of the role of a surgical investigator has to reflect this wide range of views about the meaning of "surgical research" today.

The Spectrum of Surgical Investigators

Several categories of surgical investigators play specialized roles in large departments of surgery:

1. *Tightrope walkers* are the real bridge tenders, trying to balance a commitment to clinical surgery with a research effort. They miss the operating theater if they are in the research laboratory every day, but if they operate all the time they feel guilty about ignoring the laboratory. Administrators or colleagues may feel that they do not generate sufficient funding for the department or institution, while grant review committees wonder whether full-time researchers should be supported. In the face of growing competition on both fronts, these investigators belong to the most endangered species of scholars although they best fit the classical description of academic surgeons and play the most important and indispensable role of bridging the gap between patient care and basic science.
2. *Benchmen* are either basic scientists or clinicians who devote time exclusively to investigation. They have either established or can develop the expertise required to pursue an in-depth program that may lead to major advances in surgery. They are indispensable in the many major projects where a team approach is taken. They may be more competitive in obtaining research grants but more dependent on the institution for personal support. They function best in an environment where there is good interaction between clinicians and scientists. Lack of clinical input and isolation from their colleagues, however, may make benchmen nominal "surgical" investigators, even if they work within a Department of Surgery.
3. *Occasional surgeon-investigators* are found among the many busy "cutting" surgeons who try to find time and money to do some research. They have no difficulty in maintaining clinical excellence and their research efforts, although limited, brings mental stimulation and interaction with other investigators to everybodies mutual benefit. Their efforts make it easier for them to follow advances in surgical science and may make

them more critical and better teachers. They are, however, in a constant struggle to find time for research. The few hours reserved each week for the lab will be constantly interrupted by emergency calls, unscheduled meetings, and other demands. They are not very competitive in acquiring grants. They may find it possible to do meaningful research only by proxy, through research assistants, residents and fellows. Even the provision of adequate supervision for these trainees may require an extraordinary effort by a very busy, and often exhausted, clinical surgeon. It might be more practical to devote themselves to clinical research that could be coordinated or integrated with clinical practice. Alternatively, they could join forces with benchmen.

4. *The organizer and the team leader*. Some investigators are best suited to the role of organizer, either in a department or in a laboratory. As administrators, they would be wise to follow the dictum of Detley Bronk, former president of Rockefeller University, to "find the right man or woman to back him or her up and stay out of the way" (4). A team leader, in contrast, would have to be able to contribute actively to the formulation of research ideas, and to commit enough time to supervise the research team properly. The lack of such supervision has led to many frauds and scandals in recent years (5). Team leaders who wish to receive credit for the achievements of the members of the team must also be prepared to share the blame for their misconduct. The problems such team leaders face are also related to the considerable time-demands on them by a multitude of responsibilities. Senior investigators may have many administrative duties within and outside the institution, in addition to clinical work. They may be in demand as visiting professors, lecturers or consultants, and the number of scientific meetings they have to attend multiply every year. Lack of adequate time for supervision, combined with the ambition of some trainee investigators who are trying to get ahead in a "publish or perish" atmosphere, produces a fertile ground for fraud and scandal (6). The team leader who provides strong leadership not only catalyses the team, but also provides a role model for associates and trainees.

Some academic surgeons go through many metamorphoses during their careers as they pass from one to another of the categories listed above. They may devote much of their time to research as benchmen after their training, but as their clinical practices build they move to being tightrope walkers, then to occasional surgeon-investigators, and eventually to being organizers or team leaders. This evolution has both positive and negative aspects, but it illustrates the dynamic changes the role of a surgical investigator can undergo.

The Scope of Research by a Surgical Investigator

For surgeons who are not basic scientists, the orientation of research is likely to be determined by a number of considerations. Scientific curiosity has a tendency to lead its possessor towards more and more basic issues. The truism that "the results raise more questions than answers" is as applicable to surgical research as to any other research and the desire to have answers to the questions so raised tends to lead the investigator away from clinical surgery. This trend should not be totally discouraged because doing so would not only carry the danger of dampening healthy scientific curiosity, but might also forestall the disclosure of a fundamental phenomenon of nature that might, like many others, be the basis for a major breakthrough in surgery. The lure of probing ever deeper should be controlled by an awareness of the danger of reaching beyond one's own expertise into an area that is best left to scientists trained specifically for that field.

Another practical consideration is the desirability of recognition by one's peers. If an investigator's work is published mainly in basic science journals, the investigator may not receive peer recognition from surgical colleagues. This, in turn, may affect the investigator's career pattern and change his or her future direction of research. Surgical investigators must, therefore, consider their own expertise and career objectives to determine how "basic" they wish to become in carrying out their own research.

The Role of Surgical Investigators in Grant and Journal Review

The attitudes of reviewers for granting agencies and surgical journals are closely related to the issues just discussed under the scope of surgical research. There are a number of reasons why applications and manuscripts by surgeons are said to be of "low scientific merit" by some detractors. In some instances, "peer review" of the grant application is not carried out by a real "peer". Surgeons who wish to study post-trauma sepsis may find that their application for grant support was sent to a "Committee on Infectious Disease and Immunology" and subsequently for review by a bacteriologist whose area of expertise is the bacterial cell membrane. It is recognized that the peer review process cannot be perfect, even if it is the best method available for assuring the quality of the scientific research. Nevertheless, the least that should be done is to engage real "peers" who have experience with and understanding of surgical problems. Surgical investigators should be adequately represented in such review committees. A commitment by senior surgical investigators to devote time and effort to such endeavors is essential to present the surgical point of view and to ensure the support of good surgical investigations. That having been said, it must be conceded that many surgical grant applications and papers do not embody the principles of good experimental design and analysis outlined in this book.

Criticism of the quality of certain surgical journal articles may partly be the result of an excessive proliferation of journals, and partly a reflection of the difficulty of obtaining high quality reviews for the manuscripts. The latter may be due, in great measure, to the many demands on the time of senior surgical investigators. It is also due to lack of careful attention to elements of rigorous scientific methodology.

For many investigators, a thoughtful and detailed comment by grant and manuscript reviewers is a very useful and educational experience. Constructive suggestions and criticisms by recognized experts can clarify a hypothesis, improve an experimental design, sharpen the accuracy of data analysis, and in so doing, contribute to the continuing research training of investigators. Surgeons or surgical investigators, who are so pressed for time that they reject an application or manuscript with a cursory paragraph or an abusive note, deeply discourage and embitter rejected authors. It is the responsibility of granting agencies and journal editors to evaluate their reviewers and drop those who are not committed to or capable of performing the task properly.

Peer review duties are generally undertaken by senior scientists on a voluntary basis. Although the continuation of such devotion is desirable and praiseworthy, the remuneration of reviewers may have to be considered in the future if it will lead to better reviews and valuable additional education for investigators. This issue has been receiving increasing attention from scientists in all disciplines in recent years (7), but the problem may be more acute for many surgical investigators because of the especially heavy and urgent demands on their time.

The Role of the Surgical Investigator in Surgical Education

Surgical investigators play a vital role in the education and training of students, surgical residents and surgeons. They are uniquely qualified and situated to instill a critical scientific attitude that will equip trainees to analyze and selectively absorb the large quantities of new information they will encounter during their careers. Once again, the surgical investigator serves as a bridge tender in bringing professional surgical and scientific training together. As mentors, surgical investigators have a major hand in discovering and guiding their proteges, the future surgical investigators.

Dr. George T. Moore once commented on the lack of creativity among surgeons (8). He felt that the surgical training environment is unfavorable for creative endeavor, because of the pressure it imposes on residents to develop clinical skills and to become master technicians. Dr. John Gibbon advocated having surgical trainees spend some time, seldom less than a year, working under supervision in a laboratory. During this period, the trainee will discover whether research holds any particular appeal. Supervisors will also quickly learn whether such beginners are self-starters. "The man with potentialities as an investigator will see problems that need solution and will outline methods of approaching these problems. The methods he proposes may be inadequate because of his experience, but the fact he recognizes the incompleteness of his knowledge in a certain area, and that he formulates an attack upon the problem indicates that he is a potential investigator. On the other hand, the individual who spends the year intelligently and faithfully carrying out the suggestions of his supervisor, adding little or nothing of his own to the solution of the problem under consideration is not the man to continue to do research . . . both he and his mentor will have a good idea at the end of that period as to whether he has the capacity for research. If he has not, the time will have not been misspent, because the year's experience will enable him to be a more critical reader of surgical literature during the rest of his professional life" (9). These insights are as valid today as when they were uttered more than two decades ago.

The Role of the Surgical Investigator in a Department of Surgery

The primary role of surgical investigators is to push forward the frontier of knowledge to improve the surgical care of patients; their three functions of care, teaching, and research in an academic surgical department are the expression of this fact. In return for important contributions, they require support from their departmental chairmen and colleagues.

The research productivity of surgical departments is largely determined by the degree of commitment to research by their chairmen, and there are many cases to illustrate this relationship. A young surgical department attempting to establish excellence in research will quickly find that it is an expensive undertaking. While the clinical service and staff generate funds as a by-product of their activities, research and research investigators are a financial burden. They are likely to be the first to go when demands on the financial resources of the departments become acute. A mutually supportive, collaborative attitude on the part of both clinical staff and investigators prevents jealousy, competition, and isolation. The department can nurture the productivity and excellence of surgical investigators by recognizing the dilemma they face in apportioning adequate time to both surgery and research. On their part, surgical investigators must avoid arrogance and recognize that their best results will be achieved in a milieu built in partnership with their clinical colleagues. Without that, they may be investigators, but not "surgical investigators".

The Ideals of a Complete Surgical Investigator

The ideal of surgical investigators is to be superb tenders of the bridge joining the science and the art of surgery. To be investigators, they must be good scientists who recognize that research starts with an idea—a working hypothesis. Claude Bernard (10) pointed out many years ago, that an idea comes as a particular feeling, a *quid proprium* that constitutes the originality, the inventiveness, or the genius of each individual. A new idea appears as a new or unexpected relation that the mind perceives among different things. Surgeons with such gifts should be encouraged, and they do lean towards research. Research ideas, however, are not innate; they do not arise spontaneously. They only arise, *a priori*, from an event or problem observed by chance in the course of caring for patients, or following some experimental venture, or as corollaries of an accepted theory.

To be able to develop and pursue ideas that will bring benefit to patients, the investigator has to be exposed to, and be able to discover, problems. Once an idea or hypothesis is crystallized, a background of proper scientific training will enable the investigator to reason logically, develop appropriate experimental designs, carry out an investigation, and analyze and interpret the results. These matters are covered in other chapters of this book, but it is important to bear in mind that "an experimenter puts questions to nature, but as soon as she speaks, he must hold his peace; he must note her answer, hear her out and in every case accept her decision . . . he must never answer for her nor listen partially to her answers by taking, from the results of an experiment, only those which support or confirm his hypothesis . . . this is one of the great stumbling blocks . . ." (10). The results obtained by research are brought back to the operating room or the patient's bedside, or become the basis for further research.

In summary, the life of a surgical investigator is very demanding and is replete with competing priorities and dilemmas. And yet, the consummate surgical investigator is blessed with a career that encompasses the humanity associated with care of the sick, the artistic satisfaction of delicate surgical operations, and the joy of creation and discovery.

References

1. Moore FD. The university in American surgery. Surgery 1958;44:1.
2. Hanlon CR. Decline of surgical research. Bullet Amer Coll Surg, 1985;70:1.
3. Ballinger WF, II. Surgical research as a discipline. In "Research Methods in Surgery". Ballinger WF II, editor. Boston: Little, Brown & Co., 1964:3.
4. Bronk D. Science 1965;150:1794.
5. Culliton BJ. Fraud inquiry spreads blame. Science 1983;210:937.
6. Genest J. Clouds threatening medical research. Ann Roy Coll Phys Surg Canada 1985;18:323.
7. Bailar JC, III, Patterson K. Journal peer review: the needfor a research agenda. N Engl J Med 1985;312:654.
8. Moore GT. Surgeons, age and creativity. Surg Gynec & Obst 1960;110:105.
9. Gibbon JH Jr. The road ahead for thoracic surgery. J Thorac Cardiovasc Surg 1961;42:141.
10. Bernard C. An introduction to the study of experimental medicine. Translated by Green HC. N.Y.: Dover Publ. Inc. 1957:33.

4

The Development of the Surgical Investigator

D.C. Sabiston, Jr.

For centuries, the discipline of surgery has been fortunate in having a number of investigators whose contributions have been of basic scientific significance as well as practical clinical application. The great medical historian, Garrison, selected three surgeons whom he considered the greatest of all time—Ambroise Paré, John Hunter, and Joseph Lister (Fig. 1). It was Paré who re-introduced the ancient use of the ligature in the control of hemorrhage and placed it upon a firm, systematic, and practical basis. He also introduced the concept of the controlled experiment into surgery when he treated two wounded soldiers with similar wounds lying side by side in a tent near the field of battle. The first soldier's wound was managed by the standard method of routine cauterization with boiling oil. The second was managed by debridement, cleansing, and the application of a clean dressing. He commented that he spent a restless night, feeling that the second patient would do very poorly. However, his wisdom was demonstrated the following morning when he found the second patient to be essentially without systemic symptoms whereas the former had high fever, tachycardia, and disorientation. When he was congratulated on the outcome of his first successful case, he very humbly replied: "Je le pansait, Dieu le guerit" ("I treated him, God cured him"), a quotation that is inscribed on his statue.

To John Hunter is due the primary credit for the introduction of the experimental method by using animals to develop surgical techniques prior to their application to humans. His philosophy and practice are appropriately summarized in his often-quoted response to a question from Edward Jenner, the noted developer of smallpox vaccination. When Jenner was speculating with ideas concerning hibernation in the hedgehog, Hunter responded tersely, "I think your solution is just; but why think? Why not *try* the experiment?" (1). Joseph Lister will forever be remembered for his great concern with wound infections and the hazards they posed to the expansion of surgery. He was confident that wound infections could be prevented and was the first to apply the bacteriological studies of Louis Pasteur to clinical practice when he initiated aseptic surgery.

It is clear today that the original patterns of surgical training were established in Europe during the last half of the nineteenth century, particularly in the university clinics of Germany, Switzerland, and Austria. It was in this setting that the surgical giants, who were all-powerful in their respective schools, established the principle of stepwise assumption of responsibility in residency training programs, culminating in the concept of the chief resident. Most medical historians regard Bernhard von Langenbeck, Professor of Surgery at the University of Berlin (Fig. 2), as the father of our modern training programs. An extraordinary teacher, clinical investigator, and master surgeon, he is credited with devising 33 original operative procedures (2). At the famed Charite Hospital in Berlin, he attracted a remarkable group of trainees, including Billroth, Kocher, and Trendelenburg, among others (Fig. 3). Each was later to become the leader of his own school and a great contributor in his own right. Langenbeck was also the first to initiate a journal solely devoted to surgery, *Archiv fur Klinische Chirurgie*, which

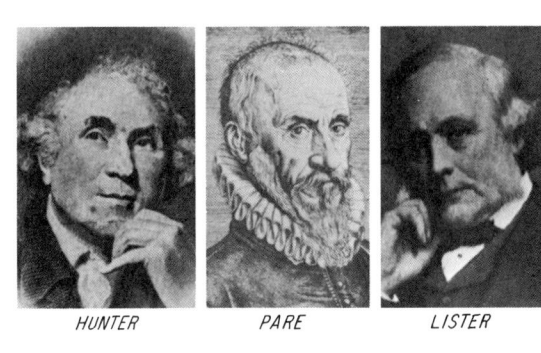

FIGURE 1. John Hunter, Ambroise Paré and Joseph Lister.

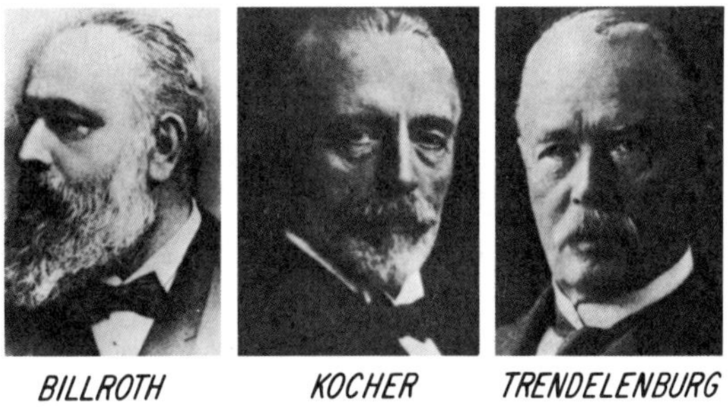

FIGURE 3. Students of Professor Bernhard von Langenbeck.

is also known as "Langenbeck's Archiv" (Fig. 4). After completing Langenbeck's program, Billroth became Professor of Surgery at Zurich and later at the University of Vienna where he was Chief Surgeon to Allegemeines Krankenhaus. Theodor Kocher was chosen to be Professor at the University of Berne at the amazingly early age of 31, and Trendelenburg was appointed to the Chair in Leipzig.

In the United States, the development of surgical residency training programs owes a clear debt to the Langenbeck-Billroth school, as introduced by William Stewart Halsted (Fig. 5). Generally regarded as the most outstanding surgeon in North America, Halsted regularly visited the major surgical clinics of Europe beginning

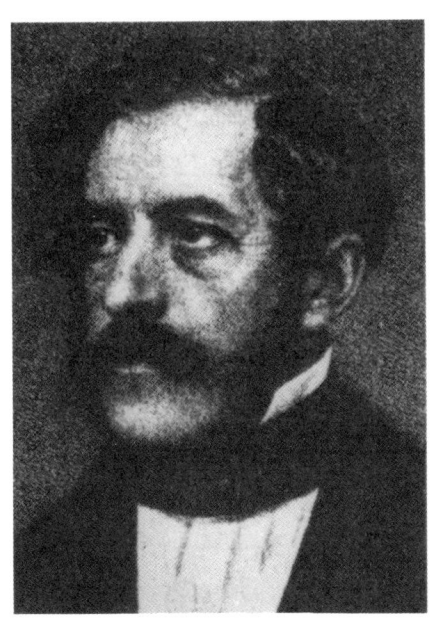

FIGURE 2. Bernhard von Langenbeck, Professor of Surgery at the University of Berlin.

ARCHIV

FÜR

KLINISCHE CHIRURGIE.

HERAUSGEGEBEN

VON

DR. B. LANGENBECK,

Geh. Medicinal-Rath und Professor der Chirurgie, Director des chirurgisch-ophthalmologischen Klinikums der Universität etc. etc.

REDIGIRT

VON

DR. BILLROTH, Prof. der Chirurgie in Zürich. und DR. GURLT, Docent der Chirurgie in Berlin.

ERSTER BAND.

Mit 6 Tafeln Abbildungen und 22 Holzschnitten.

7448

BERLIN, 1861.

VERLAG VON AUGUST HIRSCHWALD,

Unter den Linden, Ecke der Schadowstrasse.

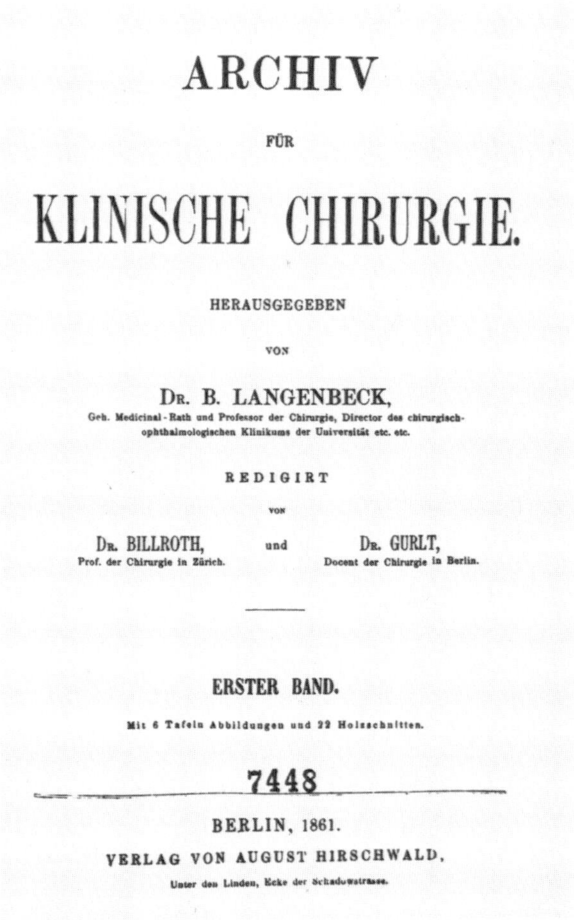

FIGURE 4. Title page of first issue of Langenbeck's *Archiv fur Klinische Chirurgie*.

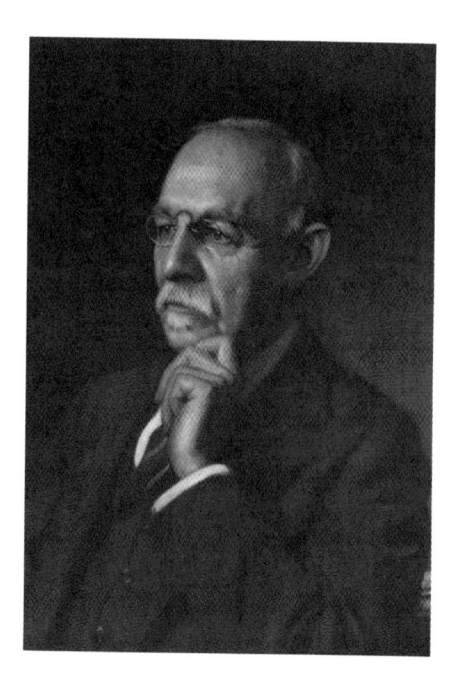

FIGURE 5. William Stewart Halsted

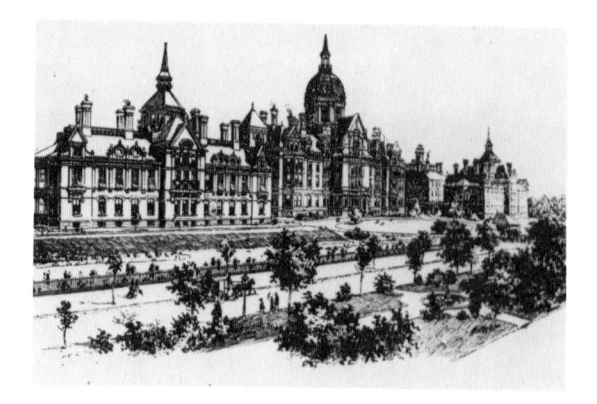

FIGURE 6. Original etching of Johns Hopkins Hospital as it appeared when built in 1889.

in 1878 and continuing throughout his life. He was immediately impressed by the progressive system of surgical training and became completely devoted to the concept that highly-selected, bright young trainees should begin as interns and gradually progress through the residency with increasing responsibility. It was his belief that, upon completion of the chief residency, the trainee should have essentially the same abilities as the teacher in the medical center. For this reason, many of his trainees were appointed directly to prestigious academic chairs immediately on completion of Halsted's training program at The Johns Hopkins Hospital (3) (Fig. 6). His astonishing success in the training of surgeons was later duplicated by several others, among whom the particularly notable were Blalock (4) (Fig. 7) and Wangensteen (5) (Fig. 8).

In describing his surgical residency training program, Halsted said: "It was our intention originally to adopt as closely as feasible the German plan, which, in the main, is the same for all the principal clinics . . ." He emphasized further: "Every facility and the greatest encouragement is given each member of the staff to do work in *research*." It is interesting that Halsted was deeply impressed with the contributions of those who involved themselves in original research, and specifically cited the discoveries of Hunter, Pasteur, and Lister as being the foundations of modern surgical practice.

In his classic address delivered at Yale in 1904 on "The Training of a Surgeon," Halsted said, "The assistants are expected in addition to their ward and operating duties to prosecute original

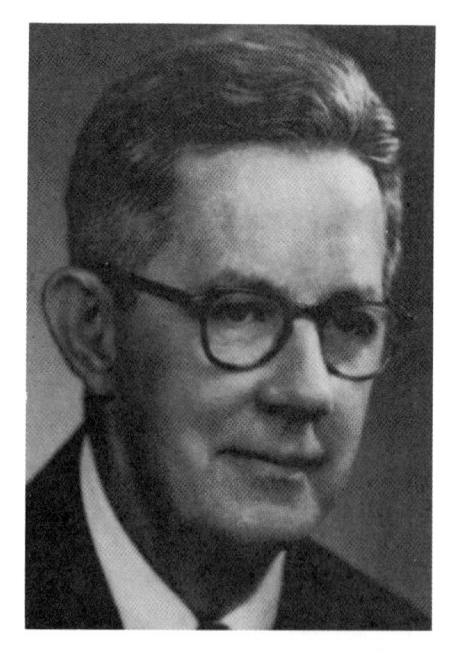

FIGURE 7. Alfred Blalock, renowned surgical investigator and teacher, trainer of many academic surgeons.

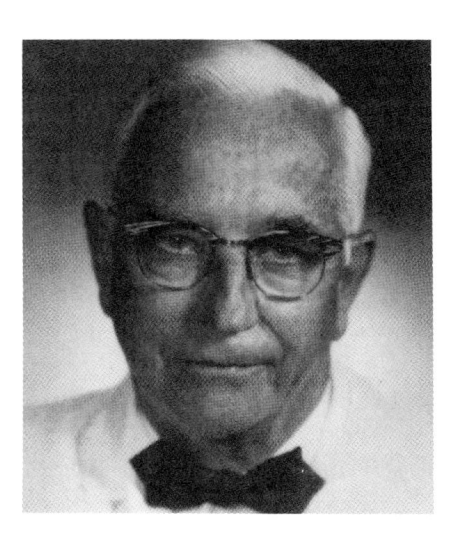

FIGURE 8. Owen H. Wangensteen, famed academic surgeon who trained many of the current leaders in Surgery.

investigations and to keep in close touch with the work in surgical pathology, bacteriology, and so far as possible physiology . . . Young men contemplating the study of surgery should early in life seek to acquire knowledge of the subjects fundamental to the study of their profession (3).'' It is now a historic fact that Halsted's men were subsequently appointed to the most prestigious academic posts and his concepts of surgical training, with emphasis on clinical excellence combined with research, rapidly spread and became widely adopted (6).

In a more recent generation, Alfred Blalock revealed his thoughts concerning surgical research in his Presidential Address to the American Surgical Association in 1956. In that frequently cited presentation, he said, "The only way an interested person can determine whether or not he has aptitude in research is to give it a trial . . . My point is that he should not shy away from it because of a misconception and fear that he does not have originality. As a medical student, I felt pity for the investigator, but later this changed to admiration and envy '' (7). Just as Halsted, his teacher in medical school, had done decades earlier, Blalock rapidly rose to a towering peak in the history of surgery as the result of his own achievements in clinical surgery, research, and the training of academic surgeons (4).

The responsibility for training surgical investigators is an obligation of all members of surgical faculties everywhere. More than two centuries ago, the noted literary scholar, Samuel Johnson, said, "Every science has been advanced to a perfection by the diligence of contemporary students and the gradual discovery of one age improving on another, either truths, hitherto unknown, must be enforced by stronger evidence, facilitated by a clearer method, or more ably elucidated by brighter illustrations." The distinguished Nobel laureate, Arthur Kornberg, in an essay entitled "Research—The Lifeline of Medicine" stated, "Advances in medicine spring from discoveries in physics, chemistry, and biology. Among key contributions to the diagnosis, treatment and prevention of disease, an analysis has shown that two-thirds of these discoveries have originated with basic observation, rather than applied research. Without a firm foundation in basic scientific knowledge, innovations perceived as advances frequently prove hollow and collapse." Surgical teachers will also be well advised to bear persistently in mind a comment of one of our greatest physiologists, Julius Comroe, who said, "I have always believed that a main responsibility of a faculty member is to be a talent scout—to determine the special abilities of medical students in clinical care, in teaching, or in research and then to encourage them to do the very best they can in their field of unusual competence. One field, of course, is research. I see no way for faculty to determine this special talent of their students unless students have contact with research while they are still in medical school." Quite clearly, it is highly desirable that students begin investigative work as soon as practicable. It is fascinating to review the major discoveries in medicine made by medical students. They include Andreas Vesalius (Fig. 9) who prepared his great anatomical text "De Humani Corporis" (Fig. 10) while a medical student. It was published four months after his graduation as a doctor of medicine from the University of Padua.

Other major discoveries in the field of medicine made by medical students include the first microscopic observation of the function of the capillary circulation by Jan Swammerdam, in 1665, when he noted erythrocytes flowing through the capillary network. In 1799, Humphry Davy, then a 19-year-old medical student,

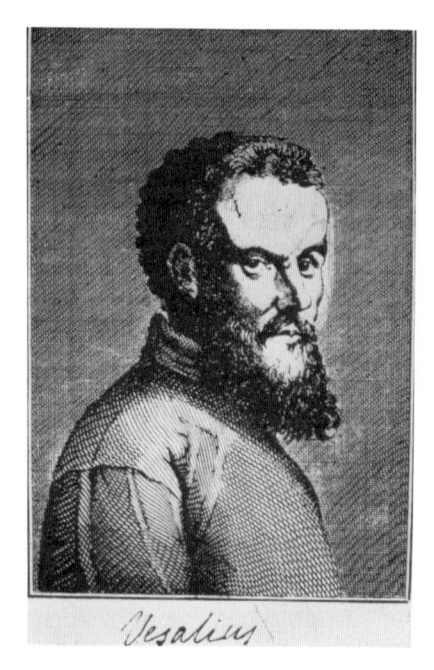

FIGURE 9. Andreas Vesalius, famed scientific anatomist.

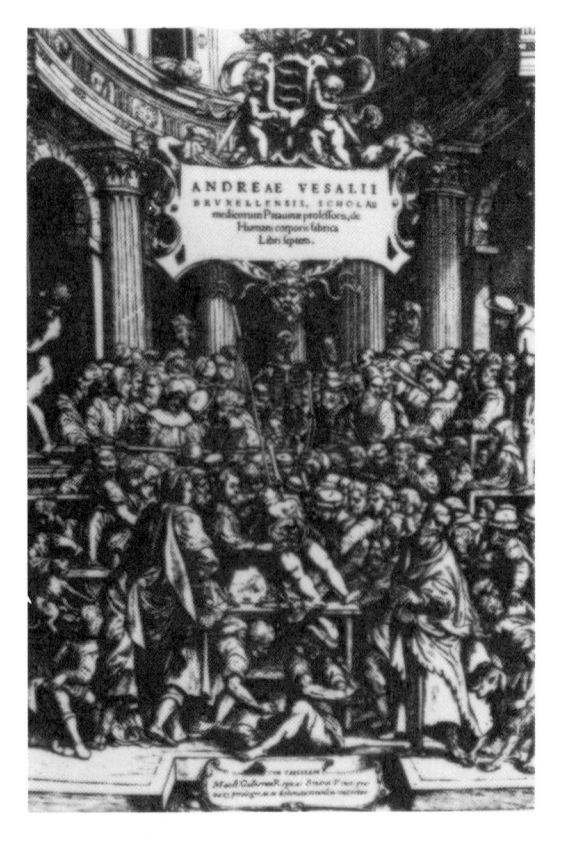

FIGURE 10. Frontispiece from Vesalius' *Fabrica* published in 1543.

prepared and inhaled quantities of nitrous oxide and discovered its marked analgesic effect. In 1846, while a Harvard medical student, William T.G. Morton administered ether as an anaesthetic at the Massachusetts General Hospital. While a student of Virchow, Paul Langerhans was the first to describe the islets in the pancreas that now bear his name. Similarly, Ivar Sandstrom, a medical student at the University of Uppsala, was the first to discover the parathyroid glands which he described in a monograph documenting his observations. The discovery of insulin, pioneered by Banting and Best, is another example. Best was a medical student at the time of this extraordinary discovery for which he and Banting received the Noble Prize. Jay MacLean was a second year student working in the physiology laboratory of William H. Howell when he discovered heparin in 1916.

A superb example of a major discovery by a surgical resident occurred in 1929 when Werner Forssmann passed a ureteral catheter through a vein in his left arm after having failed to convince another to volunteer for the experiment, and, with great courage, passed it into his heart. Once the catheter was in his heart, Forssmann pondered whether or not he would later be believed unless he had objective proof of this daring human experiment. Consequently, he arose from the operating table, walked up several flights of stairs, had a chest radiograph taken (Fig. 11) and then returned to remove the cath-

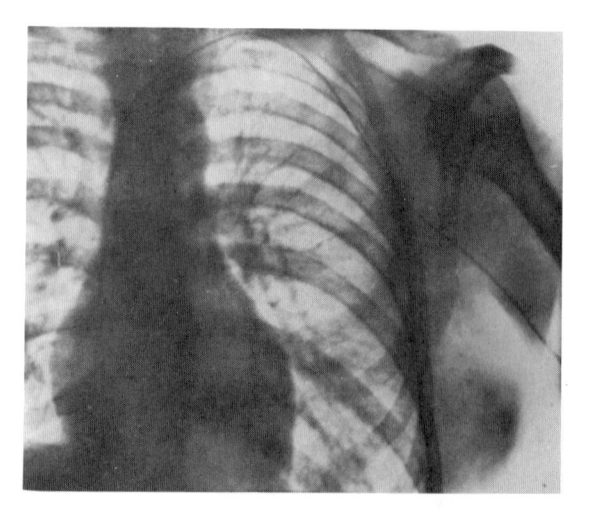

FIGURE 11. Chest film showing catheter inserted in the left antecubital vein where Werner Forssmann passed it into his own heart.

eter. His forthright honesty is reflected in the last sentence of his report in which he apologized to his readers since, he stated, a week later when he removed the bandage from his forearm he had a superficial wound infection. He felt he must have inadvertently broken sterile technique during that historic procedure (8).

Louis Pasteur is well known for his famous quotation: "Chance favors the prepared mind." Modern educational systems now approach complex subjects at a much earlier period in the student's life and child prodigies are becoming much more frequent. Although such individuals account for only a small percentage of those who become scientific investigators, a stepwise progression of education remains the usual and most reliable means of becoming a productive investigator. Many medical students now begin original investigation while in college and continue while medical students. The MD–PhD programs have exerted an influential role in the training of medical investigators. Research fellowships taken after receiving the medical degree have been of paramount significance. Many surgical residency training programs have fostered the concept of spending one or more years in research, and in some the numbers have approached 100 percent. This is true of our own program where nearly all trainees spend two full-time years working in basic research with a member of the faculty, or a group of researchers, or in a position in a laboratory elsewhere. Such programs have been the source of most of the recent academic surgical appointees in medical schools and medical centers.

The provision of *stipends* for these young investigators is a matter of considerable importance. In the United States, the National Institutes of Health have traditionally been the primary sponsor of such awards in addition to awards for the support of the actual research (Fig. 12). Other countries usually have a similar source of funds for distribution upon appropriate application. Universities, private foundations and industries have also been supportive in providing resources for such traineeships in countries around the world.

The desirability and results of experience in research during surgical residency programs are emphasized in a recent study. President Sanford of Duke University requested all the Departments in our School of Medicine to provide a statement summarizing the current positions of all post-graduate trainees who had finished residency training programs at the Duke University Medical Center during the past 15 years.

During this time, there were 64 consecutive trainees in the General and Cardiothoracic Surgical Residency Program at Duke who completed the chief residency. Of these, 53 currently hold full-time academic positions in departments of surgery throughout the country and 11 are in the private practice of surgery. Therefore, 82% entered full-time academic surgery and 18% became practitioners of surgery. Each was sent a letter requesting his personal views on the role of research in the training of surgeons for careers in an academic setting as well as for those in the practice of surgery outside a teaching center.

The format of the training program at Duke is that the first two years are devoted to basic surgical training in general surgery with rotations in the surgical specialties. At the end of the second clinical year, the residents enter general or cardiothoracic surgery, or one of the other surgical specialties, and continue until the chief year is completed (Fig. 13). While it is clearly *not* required, in most instances the residents, particularly in general and cardiothoracic surgery, spend two full-time years in basic research on surgically related problems. Most of these Research Fellows work with members of our surgical faculty who, in addition to holding appointments in the Department of Surgery, have qualifications permitting them to hold a joint

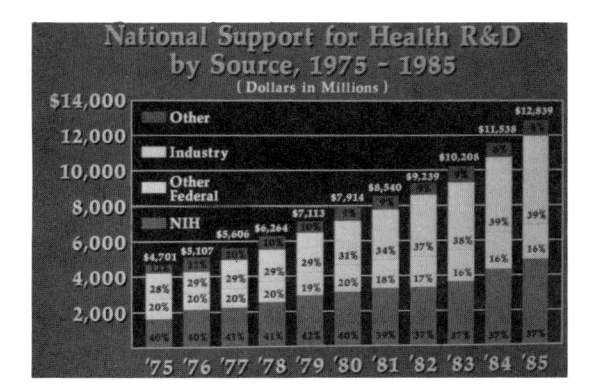

FIGURE 12. National support for health research and development by source, 1975-1985. (Source: NIH Data Book, U.S. Department of Health and Human Services, 1985)

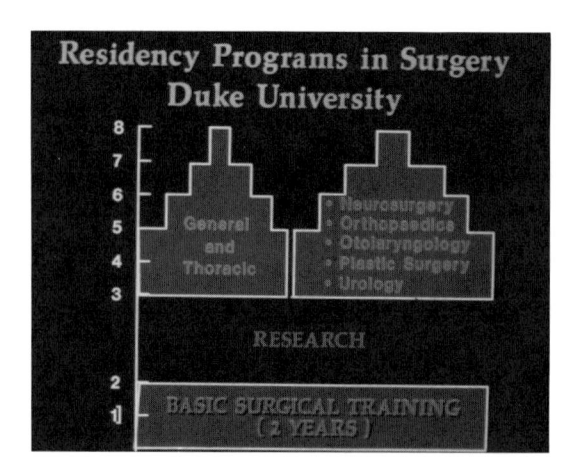

FIGURE 13. Residency Training Program at Duke University Medical Center. In the block entitled RESEARCH, the Residents spend two or more years in basic scientific investigation on a full-time basis as a Research Fellow.

appointment in one of the basic science departments of the medical school. Of the 64 residents completing the program, several elected not to take the full-time research experience and were under no obligation to do so. It is important to emphasize that research time is not required since it is generally agreed that this experience should be *elective;* a *requirement* to spend time in the laboratory is generally unwise.

Each of the chief residents in the study was requested to provide his view on the role of research in the training of surgeons for careers in an academic setting, as well as for those in the practice of surgery outside a teaching center. It seems preferable to quote representative responses of the residents directly. A selection has been made to reflect the views of the entire group. A distinct majority viewed a research experience as being almost essential in the development of the complete surgeon, whether the future career choice was academic surgery or clinical practice.

Dr. Dana K. Andersen, Associate Professor of Medicine and Surgery and the first American Surgical Association Fellow at State University of New York, Downstate Medical Center, said:

"I am convinced that a substantial period of time devoted to research is of considerable help to residents who intend to pursue clinical careers away from the academic setting. It is a rare surgical resident who, lacking investigative training, achieves the level of maturity that is shown by residents who pursue a research experience in depth. Furthermore, residents in surgical practice readily admit research experience has been not only valuable, but is specifically helpful in their efforts to evaluate clinical experience and in their ongoing need to critically evaluate the literature."

Dr. Robert W. Anderson, Professor of Surgery at Northwestern and Chief of Cardiothoracic Surgery at the Evanston Hospital responded:

"I believe that a period of research experience is valuable for anyone training to be a surgeon. Most of the significant advances that have been made in the field are the results of the experimental process and an orderly evaluation of results gathered from this process. It may not be economically possible for every surgeon in training to spend time in the laboratory and conduct independent research, but I believe it is possible for every surgeon to become exposed to the methods and techniques of contemporary surgical research upon which their professional careers largely depend. It became clear to me as an examiner recently for the American Board of Thoracic Surgery that very few of the candidates have any concept of the experimental background that has provided the foundation for the current practice of cardiovascular and thoracic surgery. Although many were able to quote lists of data and facts when presented with a problem, few were able to demonstrate any sound physiologic reasoning in the analysis of these problems. They appear to lack any historical perspective and were, for the most part, both unfamiliar and disinterested with ongoing investigative efforts that may completely alter the current practice of surgery in certain areas within the foreseeable future. I think that by preparing the minds of *all* surgical trainees by exposing them to a research experience we would not only make their own lives more interesting and productive, but improve the overall state of medicine."

Dr. Kenneth P. Ramming, Professor of Surgery at the University of California-Los Angeles, who has special interest in the field of surgical oncology, wrote:

"In any endeavor such as medicine, and particularly surgery, one cannot compete either in the marketplace or in the academic area without knowing at least the techniques and implications of disciplined scientific thought and the scientific method. Research experience is a requisite for the complete physician, and particularly for the complete surgeon. It forces him, sometimes reluctantly, into areas in which he may not feel initially comfortable. Accomplishment in such areas develops a whole new level of confidence, which is so important to successful surgical endeavor."

Dr. Kent W. Jones, in surgical practice in Salt Lake City with a part-time appointment at the University of Utah Medical School, writes:

"Research training taught me the importance of precise techniques, and the accurate results that this precision provides, not only in obtaining evidence on an experimental basis, but also in assessing clinical results."

Several other respondents currently in full-time academic surgery replied with highly positive views regarding the value of research. For example, Dr. Andrew S. Wechsler, Professor of Surgery at Duke, wrote:

"The laboratory is an intellectually enriching experience. It teaches one to develop disciplines that are readily applicable to clinical surgery in the manner of requiring scientific data prior to making conclusions, to learning before making such decisions and in becoming aware of one's own cognitive processes. I do not think that a surgeon who has spent a couple of years in the laboratory approaches clinical decision-making in the same manner as one who acts on a purely pragmatic basis. For those who invest time in investigational areas in the laboratory, it is likely that they will approach clinical problems with a new and fresh outlook."

Dr. William C. Meyers, Assistant Professor of Surgery at Duke, responded:

"When I entered the program I had very little interest in spending time in the laboratory. This was primarily due to the fact that I had never spent such time before, due to the emphasis on pure clinical training at my medical school. However, I did have an important desire to be 'the best' and this meant training in an academic environment, at least initially. I think that only with research experience can a clinician properly place into perspective his own experience and not spring to conclusions on the basis of a small experience or little data."

From Stanford University, Dr. Walter D. Holder, Jr., Assistant Professor of Surgery, who holds an intermediate view, responded:

"For those who follow the full-time practice of clinical surgery, I feel that residency research experience is very helpful in some circumstances and is generally positive. But for the majority, it does not contribute substantially to them in their eventual practice. In view of my current professional activities, I have found my research training experience to be invaluable. Without that experience I am certain that I could not have attained the position I now have nor could I be doing the many activities that I now enjoy."

Dr. William A. Gay, Jr., Professor and Chairman, Department of Surgery, University of Utah, writes:

"The practicing surgeon, as well as the surgeon who finds himself in a purely academic atmosphere, will find a research experience beneficial. In addition to the traditional concept of being able to better appreciate the research-oriented surgical paper more critically, it is my strong belief that the experience in basic research allows the individual to develop what I call scientific maturity."

Dr. Samuel A. Wells, Jr., Professor and Chairman of the Department of Surgery at Washington University-Barnes Hospital in St. Louis, said:

"An experience in the laboratory is helpful for anyone interested in a career in clinical medicine. I do not think, however, that it is a necessity. I do feel that the best surgeons are those who have spent time in the laboratory, and from personal experience, I feel that the care of my patients is better because of the research experience that I have had. Had I not spent time in the laboratory, I doubt that I would have pursued a career in academic surgery. My concerns in earlier years were whether or not to spend a career in investigative laboratory work or to pursue a clinical career. Fortunately, I was able to balance these to some degree but consider myself more of a clinician than a laboratory investigator."

As the young surgeon plans a career in academic surgery, it is wise for him or her to reflect upon the present fabric of the field and to recognize that the *biological* basis of modern surgical practice has become increasingly significant. Depth in the fields of physiology, pathology, biochemistry, immunology, pharmacology, biostatistics, genetics and other emerging areas of research are each of special importance. It is difficult to make significant advances in the surgical sciences without in-depth knowledge of one or more of these disciplines, including the ability to perform and utilize the appropriate laboratory techniques associated with the field. Close association over a significant period of time with a recognized investigator or team bears considerable emphasis and should be thoughtfully planned in advance in consultation with acknowledged contributors in the field, as well as the Director of the Surgical Residency Training Program.

Although a career in academic surgery is demanding, it is also the source of much excitement and many pleasures. Alfred Blalock stated this point very well when he said: "No satisfaction is quite like that which accompanies productive investigation, particularly if it leads to better treatment of the sick. The important discoveries in medicine are generally simple, and one is apt to wonder why they were not made earlier. I believe that they are made usually by a dedicated person who is willing to work and to cultivate his power of observation rather than by the so-called intellectual genius. Discoveries may be made by the individual worker as opposed to the current practice of a large research team. Simple apparatus may suffice; all the analyses need not be performed by technicians; large sums of money are not always necessary. Important basic ideas will probably continue to come from the individual. Whether by accident, design or hunch, the diligent investigator has a fair chance of making an important discovery. If he is unwilling to take his chance, he should avoid this type of work" (4).

Finally, for all those planning to enter investigative surgery, it is very helpful to bear continuously in mind a quotation from the physician who is generally regarded as being the greatest worldwide, in the first half of this century, William Osler (Fig. 14). His astonishing career was characterized by tremendous happiness and achievement. While in his thirties, he became Professor and Chief of the Department of Medicine at McGill University and the Montreal General Hospital in Montreal. Shortly thereafter, he was offered and accepted the leading post in internal medicine in the United States at the time, at the University of Pennsylvania. He was there for several years and was offered the position of Physician-in-Chief and Professor of Medicine at the newly formed Johns Hopkins Hospital and Medical School, in 1889, where he was given a large number of beds totally under his control. These beds were endowed and could be occupied by patients of any economic group upon the choice of the Physician-in-Chief. As a result, Osler was able to introduce medical students to the ward and, for the first time in the history of medicine, he made it possible for students *to perform* clinical examinations on patients. He was a also distinguished medical scholar, the editor of an extraordinary textbook of medicine that endured for more than half a century, a skilled diagnostician, a superb speaker, and a clinical scientist of great renown. In 1905, Osler was offered the highest post in world medicine, the Regius Chair at the University of Oxford in England.

When requested to respond to the question of why he had been so successful in his career and why he was well known by his friends and colleagues to be an exceedingly happy individual who thoroughly enjoyed all aspects of the medical profession, Osler simply said (9):

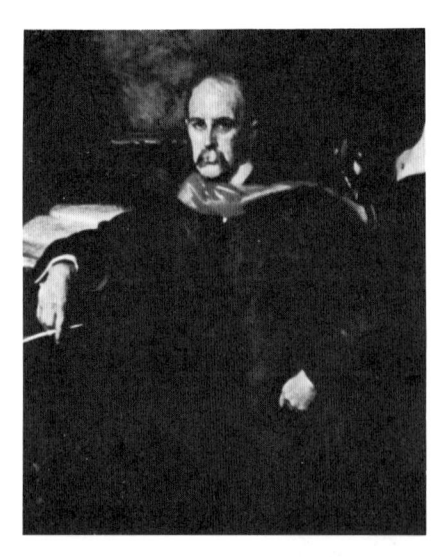

FIGURE 14. Sir William Osler, Regius Professor of Medicine at the University of Oxford, England.

"It seems a bounden duty on such an occasion to be honest and frank, so I propose to tell you the secret of life as I have seen the game played, and as I have tried to play it myself . . . This I propose to give you in the hope, yes, in the full assurance that some of you at least will lay hold upon it to your profit. Though a little one, the master-word looms large in meaning. —WORK—It is the open sesame to every portal, the great equalizer in the world, the true philosopher's stone, which transmutes all the base metal of humanity into gold. The stupid man among you it will make bright, the bright man brilliant, and the brilliant student steady. With the magic word in your heart all things are possible, and without it all study is vanity and vexation. The miracles of life are with it . . . To the youth it brings hope, to the middle-aged confidence, and to the aged repose . . . It is directly responsible for all advances in medicine during the past twenty-five centuries."

References

1. Gloyne SR. John Hunter. Edinburgh: E. & S. Livingstone Ltd., 1950:60.
2. Garrison, FH. History of medicine. Philadelphia: W.B. Saunders Company, 1929.
3. Halsted WS. The training of the surgeon. In Surgical papers by Halsted WS. Baltimore: The Johns Hopkins Press, 1924; II:512-431.
4. Sabiston DC Jr. Presidential address: Alfred Blalock. Ann Surg 1978; 188:255.
5. Wangensteen OH. Teacher's Oath. J Med Educ 1978;53(6):524.
6. Carter BN. The fruition of Halsted's concept of surgical training. Surgery 1952;32:518.
7. Blalock A. The nature of discovery. Ann Surg 1956;144:289.
8. Forssmann W. Experiments on myself. Klin Wochenschr 1929;8:2085.
9. Osler Sir William. Acquanimitas with other addresses. Philadelphia: P. Blakiston's Son and Co. Inc., 1932.

5

Facilitating Scholarship: Creating the Atmosphere, Setting, and Teamwork for Research

M.F. McKneally, D.S. Mulder, A. Nachemson, F. Mosteller, and B. McPeek

Sir William Osler, the legendary clinician–scholar–teacher, has identified patient care, teaching, and research as the three traditional functions of an academic clinical unit. He noted that scientific investigation, the most recent of the three, was often the first to suffer when resources were strained (1).

Academic surgeons everywhere find that their demanding roles as leaders in clinical care, teaching, and administration constantly encroach on whatever time is available for investigation. If they are heads of academic departments, they have to create an environment that fosters clinical and laboratory investigation as the basis for successful research. To do this, they need the support of all surgeons in their units, of physicians in other departments, and of hospital and university administrators. Unless all pull together, the effort will fail.

In addition to leadership that places high priority on academic productivity and sets a personal example of encouragement for scholarly research, investigators require protected time, appropriate clinical and research facilities, and suitable support in terms of money and interested colleagues. Some research projects may require great expenditures of time and money, but most can be carried out by one or two inquisitive clinicians with the encouragement and assistance of a handful of colleagues.

Much valuable research can be accomplished with an observant, educated eye, careful thought, a pen, and a notebook rather than electron microscopes, scintillation counters, mainframe computers, and a large staff dedicated to the project. The complexity of surgical problems does, however, require the collaboration of such scientific colleagues as biostatisticians, pathologists, and clinicians from other specialties. Each member of the team brings specific skills to the search for solutions to research problems. Because clinicians are best equipped to appreciate the needs of patients, they must provide skillful leadership in any research that is focussed on a clinical problem.

Surgery offers dramatic interventions to correct physiologic derangements, to repair or replace damaged organs, and to prevent loss of function or life. Patients accept present risk, pain, and disability if doing so offers them the hope of an improved quality of life in the future. The practice of surgery has characteristics that parallel those of the scientific method: the surgeon formulates a diagnostic hypothesis, undertakes an intervention to alter the course of a disease, and submits specimens for pathologic confirmation of the validity of the diagnosis. Although the main objective of this process is to produce an improved outcome for the patient, such a rigorous confirmation of diagnosis is not regularly possible in any other field of clinical medicine. As a consequence, surgeons have an opportunity to practice their art in a scientific and scholarly fashion frequently denied other specialists, who must mount special studies to achieve the endpoint observations regularly available to surgeons. Thus, surgeons are uniquely placed to contribute to the understanding and conquest of disease.

Surgical leaders organize their units to provide the atmosphere, personnel, facilities, and support required to bring the scientific approach to problems faced in the operating room, the intensive care unit, the surgical floors, and the outpatient area. Many investigators conduct their research almost exclusively in the surgical unit and only return to the experimental laboratory to explore hypotheses that cannot be evaluated in human patients.

A surgical operation, like a scientific experiment, needs a carefully organized team comprising surgeons, anesthesiologists, nurses, perfusionists, and other specialized assistants. The team recognizes that its responsibility extends beyond the provision of outstanding care for today's patient to the advancement of knowledge and improved care for tomorrow's patients. Surgeons appreciate the importance of team work based on shared objectives and respect for the role played by each member. Close understanding, cooperation and personal interest are as important for patient care as they are for research. They are fostered by full discussion of research hypotheses and timely updates on both clinical and research progress.

Anesthesiologists can insure timely and complete collection or recording of specimens, data and observations because they are not confined to the limits of a sterile operating field. The Anesthesia Department of the Massachusetts General Hospital has set a notable example of the value of interdepartmental collaboration in the scientific analysis of pharmacologic interventions in hemodynamic problems encountered during cardiac surgery (2).

Junior personnel, like senior members of the team, derive added satisfaction from their day-to-day work when they see it as part of a quest for a solution to a larger problem. Juniors watch their seniors, observe their habits of observation and scholarly inquiry, and learn how to provide both clinical and research leadership. In the process, they contribute greatly to the research effort as they build clinical and academic careers for themselves. Surgical or anesthesia residents assigned to full-time research sometimes act as the data managers in the operating room as part of their scientific experience.

In the cardiac operating room, perfusionists can serve as data collectors for research projects because they are familiar with the details of the surgical procedure and have well-established roles in recording the details of cardiopulmonary bypass. They made a very significant contribution in the recording of data for the randomized coronary artery surgical study conducted by the U.S. National Heart, Lung, and Blood Institute (3).

Patient care must always be uppermost in the minds of a surgical team; research activities must never interfere with good care. Specially designed procedures can make it easy and convenient for research to proceed. The team develops a protocol, data collection procedures, and forms needed to insure that research will not intrude on patient care. Besides adequate numbers of people, simple steps like posting an outline of the protocol or the data collection steps on the wall of the operating room may enable research to proceed unobtrusively. For example, Naruke's maps of the mediastinal lymph nodes and the node station sampling required for inclusion of patients in the Lung Cancer Study Group protocols are posted in thoracic surgical operating rooms in all of the participating hospitals. This facilitates the collection of uniform data about each patient and the use of standard international nomenclature (4).

Much good research originates in intensive care units and recovery rooms where opportunities exist for data collection on patients whose physiologic status is being actively monitored with invasive recording equipment. Some projects focus on the intensive care unit, per se, while others use the data collected there as short-term outcome measures for operating room interventions. Extraordinary examples of the effectiveness of clinical research in intensive care settings are provided by the work of Cerra (5) at the University of Minnesota, and of Civetta (6) in Miami on complex metabolic, pulmonary, economic, and ethical problems.

Surgical floors, outpatient clinics, and private offices play important roles in the scientific study of patients. In the course of their daily rounds, clinicians encounter an abundance of unsolved problems in patient care. Academicians perceive such problems as challenges to formulate researchable hypotheses as the first steps toward finding solutions. Comparisons of postoperative analgesic regimens, postoperative anticoagulants in the prevention of pulmonary embolization, the efficacy and cost of preventive perioperative antibiotic treatment, early discharge and home care programs, and enteral versus parenteral nutrition are a few examples of productive research performed in surgical units. The results not only provide better care for tomorrow's patients, but the process of gathering and analyzing the data has already been an enriching experience for all those who worked in the units involved.

A research team may be large or small. The members and their roles depend on the research protocol. In clinical research settings, residents, nurses, ward clerks, technical personnel from the laboratory, or members of the pump team participate in the collection of research data. A modest salary supplement for assisting in research can convert a nurse or technician into a colleague who collects clinical information with faithful attention to the research protocol. This inexpensive and productive technique may make it unnecessary to hire full-time data-collection personnel. It also has a galvanizing effect on the participants because it transforms their daily work into a project with a broader scientific purpose. Adding even $1,000 a year from research funds to the salary of a nurse in an intensive care unit can turn him or her into an on-site scientific colleague equipped to collect patient-related data. Participation in the scientific analysis of a patient care problem (e.g., decubiti, infected central line sites, the timing of a tracheostomy, etc.) helps to prevent "burn-out" in nurses, and others who care for patients, by expanding their horizon. Their understanding and enthusiasm can be further enhanced by promoting their active, personal involvement in scientific meetings.

Basic Science Research

The research laboratory, unlike clinical units, has research as its primary focus. Nevertheless, if the basic science laboratory is to have a real role in a surgical department, it must be as closely integrated as possible with the clinical side. This, in turn, is mainly a question of departmental atmosphere, the importance attached to basic research, and its input into clinical surgical decisions by the chairmen and their principal associates. Clinicians who are encouraged to become participants in basic research and who feel welcome in the laboratory will gradually find their way there.

Much also depends on geography and architecture. If the basic science laboratory is far from the clinic or is difficult to get to, it will not retain the interest of clinicians and will gradually become divorced from patient care. In many departments, the basic research laboratory comprises one or two rooms located within the surgical unit adjacent to patient areas. This makes it easy for research-oriented surgeons and anesthesiologists to take a problem from the operating room to the basic laboratory to test hypotheses and develop potential treatments. The latter can then be tested in clinical trials in the operating room, the intensive care unit, or on the surgical floors. Many useful basic projects do not require enormous expenditures. Great research units are simply larger versions of this basic model.

The McGill University Surgical Clinic is an integral part of the Montreal General Hospital Research Institute and was built with the primary goal of providing basic laboratory space in immediate proximity to clinical teaching units. This research unit contains animal care facilities, an animal operating suite, and appropriate preparation space. Each of its three operating rooms is fully equipped with anesthesia machines, monitoring equipment, and heart-lung machine, and can cater to virtually any operative procedure. Supervision of postoperative recovery and long-term care by a veterinary surgeon are provided. Office, laboratory, and conference space are also available to meet the needs of investigators, residents, and students in the department of surgery. The research facility is on the same floor and immediately adjacent to two major general surgical teaching units within the Montreal General Hospital. Weekly rounds in the research unit are coordinated by the director of the surgical clinic. The proximity of the research and clinical teaching units promotes regular interaction between the residents and surgeons who are working on the clinical services with all the individuals who are currently involved in research projects. The physical presence of the research laboratories immediately adjacent to the clinical area overtly acknowledges the importance of research in the activities of this surgical department.

Responsibility for the success of both clinical and basic research ultimately rests with the departmental chairman. Chairmen must use their positions in the hospital and university to obtain the resources of salary, protected time, space, facilities, and support personnel required by investigators. Chairmen must convince each individual clinician of the importance of supporting an active research program. They function as role models, facilitators, and expeditors of research. Although the demands on the time and energy of departmental chairmen frequently preclude continuation of their own active research programs, everyone within the department, hospital, and university must recognize the chairman's abiding commitment to research.

Collaborative relationships are of crucial importance to surgical scholars. Department chairmen must actively foster an atmosphere that makes it easy for surgeons and their colleagues in other fields to work together on projects of joint interest. The entire department must welcome and encourage such collaboration, and join with other departments, the hospital, and the university to make it a mutual and pervasive endeavour. For example, when a choice has to be made between two equally qualified endocrine physiologists of equal interest to the Department of Physiology, the dean and the physiology chairman might favor the appointment of the one whose field is gastrointestinal hormones because that would complement the research activities of a surgical scholar already on the faculty. An institutional and departmental strategy of fostering collaboration and giving strong support to joint research programs increases the scientific vigor of the whole intitution.

Department chairmen will work hard to avoid the physical or intellectual isolation of individual scholars that leads to stagnation. Most investigations profit from the intellectual stimulation, and enjoyment that occures to scholars when they work as a team on a joint project. Scholars frequently look to skilled clinicians for this collaboration because of their outstanding skills of observation and insight into the relative importance of clinical problems. Surgeons, internists, anesthesiologists, pathologists, radiologists and other medical specialists bring different perspectives to a problem, give valuable help in the interpretation of clinical and laboratory findings, and suggest fruitful directions for further research. Such on-going critical review and comments focus the relevance and precision of scholarly work.

The results of some research are so clear that virtually no effort is required to design and analyze confirmatory studies. Warren, Bigelow, and Morton needed no clinical trial in 1846 to convince the world of the importance of the discovery of anesthesia (7). Most effects are not so striking. Limitations on size and feasibility require most surgical scholars to have the regular collaboration of a biostatistical colleague in the design and analysis of their research project.

Since mastery rather than acquaintance with a field of expertise is a requirement for excellence in research, it is essential that the biostatistical collaborator be a full-scale partner in the research endeavor. The relationship should begin with the formulation of the hypothesis to be tested and move on to careful, cooperative planning of the experimental design. A joint grant application is frequently the result. Continuing collaboration by the biostatistical partner will help to solve problems in data collection and insure that the chosen analytic methods extract all the information embedded in the data, accurately and efficiently.

Clinicians who have received some training in statistics must realize that, valuable as this experience may be in developing a certain level of insight, it may be analagous to spending a single year as a resident in surgery or internal medicine. It does not qualify one to provide professional advice in biostatistics on which clinicians and their colleagues can depend. Statistics is a professional field, and a half-trained statistician may be only slightly less dangerous than a half-trained surgeon. Nevertheless, a growing number of statisticians who are experienced in medical science, and a smaller number of clinicians who are well-trained in biostatistics and epidemiology, have made significant contributions to bridging the gap between the two.

Statisticians who are well adapted to collaborative surgical research intuitively start with questions about patient referral patterns and the probability that patients and their physicians will accept proposed treatment alternatives. The first thought of surgeons who have become full partners with biostatisticians in design and analysis is to meet with their statistical colleagues to "brainstorm" about a project. They realize that the scientific methodologist is uniquely adept at formulating answerable questions from the presentation of clinical problems. Problems in experimental design and analysis are more easily prevented at the time of protocol writing than resolved after the control errors have been committed. When the clinician hears the biostatistician referring to "our patients" and "our treatments," he can be certain that the partnership has been established. The role of collaborators as true partners is clearly recognized by their status as co-investigators on grants and as co-authors of published papers.

Like biostatisticians, physiologists, pharmacologists, biochemists or other basic scientists may join with clinicians in joint endeavors. Alternatively, they may participate as independent investigators who focus their efforts on testing hypotheses that deal with aspects of a common problem in which the clinician plays a less prominent role. This latter is usually the least productive form of collaboration. An example would be a pharmacologist who undertakes a study of catecholamine levels in an amputated atrial appendage provided by a surgical colleague who is unaware of the scientific questions asked or the design used by his nominal associate.

Productive interactions require an investment of time and effort by all parties to the collaboration. Surgical investigators need to be aware of the costs of collaboration in terms of creative time and energy. Clinicians sometimes feel that the small amount of time they ask a basic science collaborator to devote to a surgical research project is a relatively trivial claim on the co-investigator. Surgeons, and other clinicians, may forget that all able people are very busy and most are over-committed. Teaching, administration, and other projects already underway may leave many basic scientists with only 10% of their time for their own creative work. Asking that half or all of this creative time be devoted to a new surgical project takes on fresh meaning when viewed in this context.

During the past decade, as many Ph.D. basic scientists have been appointed to clinical departments in the U.S.A. as have entered basic science departments in American medical schools (8). These basic science colleagues must develop their own programs of research to allow them to aquire substantial academic credentials in their own fields, as well as the intellectual and scientific independence they need to collaborate with clinical investigators as true partners (9). Clinical investigators must recognize this truth and assist their basic science colleagues in maintaining their growth and earning intellectual reputations in their own fields. This is particularly important for surgical chairmen and surgical scholars to remember when a basic scientist is employed in the research division within a department of surgery. Isolation within a clinical department is inimical to the maintenance of skills and the career development of a basic scientist and will eventually have detrimental effects on the surgical projects. Chairmen must make every effort, therefore, to provide appropriate joint appointments in the relevant science departments so that basic science collaborators can stay at the leading edge of their fields. To achieve this, appropriate opportunities and time must also be assured to permit the active participation of these individuals in the life of their basic science departments.

The "Marburg Experiment," discussed in Section III, Chapter 1, provides an interesting approach to real collaboration between basic and clinical scientists. In Marburg, Germany, two scholars are linked together on a long-term basis to undertake joint exploration of the scientific and clinical problems faced. Through constant review and direct personal exposure to the techniques and problems of the other, each partner develops insight, asks new qustions, and contributes a sympathetic but critical review of research procedures and results. The Marburg approach recognizes how difficult or even impossible it is for surgeons to maintain expertise in a basic science even if they have dedicated several years to full-time training and research in that field. This model has now been adopted in a number of centers and has produced excellent results.

Residents in surgery and in anesthesia contribute stimulation, technical help, and focus to a variety of research projects. Many academic programs require a one- or two-year exposure of all or selected residents to training in the scientific discipline of research and scholarship in their fields. This experience enriches the education of clinicians, whether they continue in research or support research through clinical leadership. At McGill University, every surgical resident devotes a minimum of one year to clinical or basic surgical research in the University Surgical Clinic or in another department, such as pathology, anatomy, physiology, or immunology. This year of surgical scholarship comes after the completion of a two-year core clinical training program, and before the senior clinical years of a general surgical residency. During this year away from clinical responsibilities, surgical residents work with a surgeon or a basic scientist on a project that is suited to their ability and interest. They review the literature and formulate a study program or experiment that relates to their mentor's ongoing research. The resident who attends formal lectures in biostatistics, anatomy, physiology, and pharmacology, and successfully completes a good research project and thesis during this year of surgical scholarship is awarded the degree of Master of Science in Experimental Surgery. During this year, residents with a special talent for research frequently decide to enter academic surgery as a career. Appropriate candidates continue their research training for as long as three years to obtain the degree of Doctor of Philosophy in Experimental Surgery. The residents who are selected for this advanced research training subsequently return to the clinical surgery program for two more years. They then ordinarily assume academic positions with a major commitment to surgical research.

Every surgical resident in the training program of the Montreal General Hospital is encouraged to carry out a clinical research review with a member of the faculty during each academic year. Each resident, therefore, approaches clinical problems under the supervision of an experienced surgical teacher. The results of these clinical reviews, or of laboratory research by other residents, are presented each year at a special convocation. All residents are also encouraged to present their work at national and international meetings and are given financial support to attend such meetings if their papers are accepted for presentation.

Graduate students and medical students often impart a special stimulus to a research program by emphasizing and expanding the basic science aspects of a project. Their presence in the clinic and laboratories heightens the atmosphere of academic inquiry, enhances their own education and has a marvelously stimulating effect on the curiosity of their teachers. Research seminars expose students to clinical scholars, basic scientists, exciting investigations, and residents who are striving to advance their level of surgical knowledge. Student research fellowships during the summer months allow selected students to expand their exposure to research that awakens an interest in some that eventually leads to lifetime commitments to surgical science.

Many academic departments provide clerical and support assistance that is specifically dedicated to the academic side of surgeons' lives. Academic secretaries and other assistants help with the gathering of reference material and the preparation of manuscripts, illustrations, audiovisual aids, presentations, reports, and grant applications. Separation of this function for research and teaching allows it to enjoy a priority comparable with that given patient care and protects the secretarial staff from the uncomfortable conflicts that might otherwise arise.

A quiet, well-equipped, well-staffed writing and reference center within the surgical department can be a powerful incentive for the production of manuscripts and reports. Such centers contain key reference material; maintain files on grant deadlines, meeting dates, and summaries of telephone and personal conferences with collaborators; and serve as operational foci for the planning and documentation of research.

Collaborative Research

Research collaboration between surgical units or research teams from different institutions is especially effective in the solution of certain clinical problems. The inter-institutional collaborative projects of the Randomized Coronary Artery Surgical Study, the Lung Cancer Study Group, and the National Surgical Adjuvant Breast Project described in Section III, Chapter 5 are notable examples of such collaboration.

These programs have drawn together surgeons, anesthesiologists, statisticians, internists, radiologists, pathologists, and other scientific personnel to produce well-focused questions and provide well-documented answers to problems that could not be resolved in any one institution. By developing, refining, and following joint protocols, the investigators have made significant advances in the definition of disease, the standardization of optimal care, the establishment of minimal criteria for reporting, and the elimination of inappropriate application of surgical or adjuvant remedies.

Although we have discussed some of the special arrangements that have proven effective in some great academic centers, one must not forget that some of the most important and significant clinical research is performed by individual scholars working quietly in small departments or small clinics—sometimes virtually alone, but more often in partnership with interested colleagues from other fields.

Much more important then great financial or technical resources is an inquiring mind that looks at problems in terms of potential solutions and a spirit that is determined tomorrow's patients will receive better care than today's.

Complex problems and the fun of working together with friends provides the motivation for collaboration in research: synergistic interactions among partners provide powerful stimuli to investigators who might otherwise be frustrated in attempts to find solutions. Surgeons, other clinicians, and basic scientists share the thrill of finding solutions to human problems in the clinic and laboratory. Clinicians can have the excitement of using the sharp leading edge of science as a sword against diseases they cannot conquer by traditional clinical approaches.

What more powerful incentive could there be for a full commitment to collaborative research?

References

1. Osler, Sir William: The collective essays of Sir William Osler. The classics of medicine. Birmingham, Alabama: The Medical Library, 1985.
2. McIlduff JB, Daggett WM, Buckley MJ, Lappas DG: Systemic and pulmonary hemodynamic changes immediately following mitral valve replacement in man. Cardiovas Surg 21;1980:261–266.
3. The principal investigators of CASS and their associates: The National heart, lung, and blood institute coronary artery surgery study (CASS). Circulation 63 (Suppl I): 1981.
4. Naruke T, Suemasu K, Ishikawa S: Lymph node mapping and curability at various levels of metastasis in resected lung cancer. The Journal of Thoracic and Cardiovascular Surgery, 1978;76:832–839.
5. Cerra FB, Mazuski J, Tusly K, et al. Nitrogen retention in critically ill patients is proportional to the branched chain amino acid load. Critical Care Med 1983; Oct 11 (10):775–778.
6. Civeta JM, Hudson-Civetta JA. Maintaining quality of care while reducing charges in the I.C.U.: ten ways. Annals of Surgery 1985;202:524–532.
7. Bigelow HJ. Insensitivity during surgical operations produced by inhalation. Boston Medical and Surgical Journal 1846;35:309–317.
8. Fishman AP, Jolly P. Ph.D.'s in clinical departments.Career opportunities in physiology. Ramsay DJ, editor. Bathesda, MD.: American Physiological Society, 9–12.
9. Saba TM. An academic career in a basic medical science department of physiology. Physiologist 1981;24:16–20.

SECTION II

Starting the Research Process

From Idea to Results

Good research ideas are rare and priceless treasures; but even when one lies glowing in your mind, translating it into the reality of a feasible research project may seem just as insurmountable a challenge to you as it does to most of us. Clinical observations frequently cause thoughtful surgeons to formulate fruitful hypotheses that beg to be tested. They often beg in vain because, many things other than the relentless demands of patient care conspire to block the next few steps.

Reviewing the literature requires an investment of time to search, collate, copy, and classify material; we cannot evade it. No one wants to repeat work already done, or repeat mistakes others have already made. Orienting and reformulating an idea into a researchable question requires an understanding of feasible design strategies that will satisfy the appropriate criteria of scientific rigor. The clinical investigator must think through issues, such as the nature of the interventions to be studied, the target variables, and the length of follow-up within the context of biological and clinical realities. Ethical principles must guide every aspect of the work. Those who overlook such statistical considerations as measurement, sample size, analytic approach, clinical significance, and probabilities do so at their peril.

Formulating and writing a detailed protocol and preparing a formal research grant application are tasks you must perform before you can contemplate embarking on any but the smallest project. Most large research projects require resources that will only be granted after written documentation of a viable and promising research plan. Even if you are a newcomer to research, do not be discouraged by the list of steps you have to take to achieve reliable results. In this section, we offer a plan to help you take each successive step. Your ideas will become research questions to which you will have the satisfaction of obtaining credible answers through your own research.

1
Systematically Reviewing Previous Work

S. Wood-Dauphinee and B. McPeek

Many of us tend to regard reviewing previous literature as an unexciting chore, perhaps because well-read laboratory chiefs appear to consider the research review as a low-priority activity to be delegated to a research assistant or the most junior member of the team. For many, the excitement lies in carrying out a new experiment to add more information to what already exists. They regard poring over old research reports as a boring or less creative step. This is a major error in thinking. The accumulation of evidence is an important goal underlying all scientific inquiry. This is as true of surgery as of theoretical physics. An individual study is seldom an isolated event, but rather part of a continuum in which each new endeavor builds upon preceding work. New findings lose much of their value if they are not linked with the accumulated wisdom, both theoretical and empirical, of earlier reports.

Quite apart from any associated research findings, the methods used by previous scholars may suggest fresh ideas. Some may present approaches to problem-solving that have not occurred to you. Attention to previous design and analytic methods may help you to avoid difficulties that plagued earlier efforts.

On a practical level, a thorough critical appraisal of existing literature provides background information for developing a research proposal, a grant application, or a report for publication.

A research review in surgery is likely to lead to one of four products:

1. It may bring together what is known of a specific research area and lead directly to new work designed to test a specific hypothesis or add to the knowledge base.
2. It may analyze data from previous studies in a new way to answer new research questions.
3. It may summarize what is known in an area of surgery and appear in a journal in its own right as a "state of the art" paper. Such a review will not only be of interest to those working in the specific field, but will also be particularly helpful to other specialists who wish to bring themselves up to date, quickly.
4. It may inform clinical decisions made by individual surgeons about the care of patients, or by chiefs of units about policy matters.

Approaches to Reviewing the Literature

Most literature reviews are unsystematic and largely narrative presentations of studies and their findings; the methods employed in the studies are discussed selectively and informally.

Equally able reviewers disagree about basic issues and occasionally arrive at diametrically opposite conclusions. With little concern for scientific rigor, reviewers frequently turn to a mindless vote-count. When some studies show a positive treatment effect, others no effect, and still others a negative effect, the reviewer counts the number supporting each result and selects the majority view. This procedure ignores the size of the effect found and the strength of the research design. If the number of previous studies is large, the traditional reviewer easily gets lost.

Despite the subjectivity, scientifically questionable validity, and inefficiency of the traditional narrative approach to reviewing the literature, most scholars in medicine and surgery still use this antiquated procedure.

Over the last 15 years, new methods have been developed. Although they are not widely known to clinical scientists, they are significant advances in the methodology of reviewing scientific literature that bring it into the mainstream of modern science.

G.V. Glass (1,2) has written about three levels of data analysis. The first, or *primary analysis,* is the original analysis of data from a research study. This is what most of us think of as research, and articles describing such work form the bulk of medical communications.

Secondary analysis, as described by Glass, is the re-analysis of original data to bring current statistical methods to bear on them or to answer new questions. We can learn much from secondary analysis. Better ways of looking at the data gathered in a project may be suggested after they have been published. For example, a variety of useful secondary analyses of the data collected by the University Group Diabetes Project (UGDP Study) in medicine (3) advanced our understanding of how diabetes should be treated. Similarly, new hypotheses can be tested by the imaginative re-analysis of data already collected for a similar or even an entirely different purpose. Secondary analysis can be particularly useful in dealing with volunteer case reports where volunteer reporting bias may have produced an effect if the data were collected prospectively. McPeek and Gilbert (4) used secondary analysis of published data to disprove a new hypothesis concerning postoperative jaundice following repeated exposure to halothane.

Meta-analysis, like secondary analysis, uses existing data but it focuses on the quantitative integration of findings across a group of independent studies and provides a more scientific alternative to the traditional narrative method of literature review. It is only during the last 15 years that scholars, particularly in the social sciences, have developed the notion of quantitative meta-analysis in a robust way.

There is no question that meta-analysis is a major advance, but we must remember that it is a comparative observational study with all the strengths and weaknesses of observational studies. We celebrate the fact that we now have a way to review work systematically, but guard against trying to extend it too far.

In thinking about meta-analysis, we lean heavily on three principles. First, *develop a strategy*. Bear in mind that the most effective review strategies and analytic techniques arise from the answers to the specific questions that are leading you to make the review. What do you want from the review? Do you seek a broad exploration of available information on a subject, or do you want to test specific hypotheses? Is an overall answer desirable, or are you interested in identifying interactions between specific treatments, patient populations, or settings, like hospitals or clinics? Are you interested in the feasibility of implementing a new program locally? If the plan is for an exploratory review, you ask what is known about a particular area of research, a specific disease, a clinical problem, or a treatment, such as an operation or an element of pre- or postoperative care. Your strategy will be to include diverse studies to increase the chance of uncovering interesting findings that may lead to new directions for future research. Unless you know what you are doing at the start, you may finish with a simple recitation of previous findings that does little to advance research, contribute fresh insight, or inform decisions.

The second principle is that *conflicting results must be carefully investigated*. When we find dozens of previous studies, we hope that most of them will agree. If they do, a review is easy, but this rarely happens. Conflicting findings have several potential explanations. There may be substantial differences between operations with the same name. Follow-up care may be quite dissimilar. Perhaps the treatment works poorly for some kinds of patients and well for others, or is effective in certain hands or settings and not in others. These explanations can only be uncovered through the careful study of the narrative reports of patients, treatment descriptions and details of hospital, clinical or laboratory procedures. A letter or telephone call to the authors may uncover new postpublication information or insights that clarify the analysis.

The third principle is that *we often need formal, quantitative, analytic methods to identify small effects across studies* that are not apparent through simple inspection of the results of the studies individually.

Beware! Drawing inferences about findings uncovered from exploratory analyses can be risky. Searching among many research studies for factors significantly related to outcome will lead to some false positives—statistically significant relationships due only to chance. If you examine many separate relationships, each at the .05 level of significance, you should not be surprised to discover that 1 in 20 is significant due entirely to chance—a finding consistent with probability theory.

To appreciate the impact of such chance selection, consider the political example of bellwether counties. Every four years, there is a national presidential election in the United States. Sometime during the campaign preceding the election, journalists always seem to discover a bellwether county, a county that has an incredibly good record of voting for the winner in past elections. Somehow, somewhere, a small county has voted for the winning presidential candidate every four years since the election of 1824. With great enthusiasm, reporters descend on the residents of this county to ask them about their preferences in the current election on the presumption that this information offers a sound prediction of who will win this year.

Think about this for a moment. In any election, roughly half the counties will have given a majority vote to the winner. We could expect that half of these counties preferred the winner in the previous election as well, and so forth. Since there are some 3,000 counties in the United States, we should find several that have seemingly impressive records just by chance. Moreover, about half of the latter counties can be expected to be on the winning side in the next election although we cannot predict which. If we had started by looking at a single county, a record of picking the winner correctly 19 out of 20 times would be impressive, but if we screen 3,000 we ought not to be surprised to find several such counties and should be rather amazed not to find at least one.

If several treatments are compared, sample variation alone may make some look better than others even when they are truly equivalent. Similarly, when institutions are compared for success with an operation, sampling variation will make some look much better than others even if they are equal in excellence. For example, in the United States National Halothane Study (5) 34 institutions were compared for standardized surgical morality rates and they appeared to differ, initially, by a factor of 24; after allowance was made for sampling variation, the ratio between the highest and lowest was only 3:1.

One way to prevent a review from *over-capitalizing on chance* is to break the data into parts. Half of the studies can be used to generate hypotheses about effective treatments or to predict treatment success; the other half can be used to test the hypotheses so generated. If the entire set of studies has some systematic bias, this procedure cannot eliminate it. Regardless of how you perform the review, your inferences will only be as valid as the underlying studies.

If your review is aimed at testing a previously established hypothesis, you must specify the hypothesis precisely, before you start. This may lead you to an early decision as to whether your review should look across studies to aggregate treatments (like operations), to aggregate patients, or to aggregate settings (like clinics or hospitals).

In surgery, we ordinarily view the outcome of a clinical research study as being the result of interactions between the treatment, the patient, and the setting, compounded by random error. Reviews can answer many diverse questions, but we commonly seek answers to three:

1. What is the *average effect* of the treatment?
2. Are there *particular* patient *groups* or settings where the treatment works especially well?
3. *Can we implement* it in our department?

To answer the first question, we compare patients who receive the treatment with similar people who do not.

The second question asks for interactions. Do particular combinations of treatments and patients work especially well or poorly? For example, suppose a surgeon believes that a particular operation is especially valuable for elderly men while any one of several operations is as effective in younger men. A single research design that crosses different operations with patients of various age groups can test this hypothesis. But what do you do if no study systematically considers all of the combinations of operations and patients that you wish to examine? Examining the studies as a group may provide such information. For example, one study may have looked at large numbers of elderly men and other studies at large groups of younger men. Taken together, these studies may give the reviewer some information about whether or not interactions exist, i.e., a collection of studies can sometimes shed light on complex interactions when studies considered individually do not.

The third question concerns implementation. Strictly speaking, studies tell us only what happened to the patients or the participants in the investigation. We are ordinarily interested in generalizing these findings to similar patients under our care. If we know from the start that a review is to inform a local policy decision, the reviewer will look for studies that bear particularly on the local circumstances. Information can be sought that would help us to decide how an operation is likely to work in our hands, at our hospital, on our kinds of patients.

Conducting the Search

This book is not the place to teach adults how to use libraries, and yet, an amazing revolution has taken place in the way libraries work all over the world. Scholars and research workers, even those connected with major universities and research institutes, are likely to be surprised at the extent of this transformation. Although catalogs and bound indexes of periodical literature still exist, one uses a computer in most research libraries today. Rather than searching printed indexes by year for separate subject headings, a user asks a computer to search entire data bases for many different terms and years, simultaneously. The computer provides rapid retrieval of citations and, prints out the bibliographies and frequently, brief abstracts of the papers it finds. You or I, working by hand, might require several days to perform a search the computer accomplishes with fewer errors in a few minutes. Although this quiet revolution started in large research libraries located in major centers, it is rapidly progressing to small libraries around the world.

In most research libraries, you first consult a reference librarian who helps you formulate search instructions and interact with a computer. Newer systems that allow scientists to communicate with bibliographic services by telephone and microcomputer from their own offices or laboratories are also becoming widely available. The cost varies according to the data bases used, the computer time consumed, and the number of citations retrieved (6,7). The computer ordinarily prints out a brief selection of the results of a search, e.g., the first 5 or 10 citations found, and a tally of the number that satisfied the search request. You have the opportunity to review the print-out and modify the instructions, if necessary. If your search request would yield 1,500 references and drown you in a flood of paper, you may prefer to modify the search instructions to seek only those in your own language, published in the last 10 years or involving human subjects.

You may find on reviewing the sample print-out that the references being identified are not what you wanted and that your search instructions have to be revised to seek other citations. You can also review a sample of any citations supplied to see whether you are on the right track. This repetitive, exploratory process with instant feedback lets you refine your search instructions until you get what you really need.

Selecting Studies for Inclusion

When you are faced with a wealth of possibilities, how do you select studies for inclusion? The answer depends on the availability of previous research reports, the number and frequency of different designs, and the specific questions driving your review. The simplest course is to include everything you can find. It has the advantage of avoiding criticism for neglecting some work or including one study while excluding another, but it does present some problems. What do you do if you have located 1,100 studies? Such an embarrassment of riches would almost certainly sink the project and some way of cutting down the number would be appropriate, e.g., a random sample of all the studies available could be drawn and used for your review.

While it is important to include a wide variety of research designs and treatment variations, if a particular study clearly has obvious, substantial, fundamental flaws, it ought to be excluded. Wrong information is much worse than no information. When studies have been excluded, the reviewer should state why.

You may have trouble finding some studies, e.g., in North America, it may be difficult to have a paper translated from the original Hungarian, and monographs have a habit of being out of print. A decision about how much digging is warranted may have to be made on the basis of the title or an abstract.

Another possible approach is to stratify your sample. You divide the available studies into categories and then select some studies from each category for review. This procedure guarantees inclusion of each important type of study in your review while requiring you to analyze only the shorter list of selected studies in detail.

For example, experimental design has often been found to be a strong predictor of research outcomes. In a review of almost 100 studies of portocaval shunt surgery, Chalmers (8) found a clear negative relationship between the degree of control in a research design and the level of success attributed to the surgical interventions; the higher the degree of control, the less enthusiastic the investigators were about an operation's effectiveness. Similar findings were obtained by Gilbert, McPeek, and Mosteller (9,10) in a study of innovations in surgery and anaesthesia. Such results support the "Law" enunciated by the famous statistician, Hugo Muench, that nothing improves the performance of an innovation more than the lack of controls (11). Some papers suggest that this rule is not universal (12–14) but there is a great deal of evidence that it often applies in medicine and surgery.

Research design is not the only basis for stratification. You may wish to stratify by geography, treatment, type of operation, type of clinic or hospital, or the socio-demographic or clinical characteristics of patients.

Publication bias is another matter for consideration. Most reviews in medicine and surgery include only published studies located in libraries accessible to everyone. They are easy to find in indexes and you save time and money by omitting unpublished reports. Moreover, the leading refereed journals have reasonably strict requirements for publication. Studies published in prestigious journals are likely to have been more carefully executed and to have undergone more rigorous review, and scholars generally have more faith in the results they report.

However, the strategy of using only published studies has a serious drawback. Authors are more likely to submit work with statistically significant findings and editors are more likely to publish it than research yielding nonsignficant results. As a consequence, a reviewer who focuses only on published studies will likely overstate treatment effects. A careful reviewer will want to make a special effort to uncover unpublished work by contacting other scholars known to be working in the field, by tracking down unpublished theses, and by searching for government reports and printed reports of conferences. The reviewer who is able to include information from these sources *can estimate the effect of publication bias* and adjust his conclusions accordingly. If unpublished information is not considered, a careful reviewer will want to warn readers against this potential source of systematic error.

Let us suppose we have arrived at a population of studies to review. We can expect that the studies differ. They differ somewhat in design. They differ in size. Some will be large, but many in medicine and surgery are likely to be small, unfortunately. Some will come from large hospitals, others from small clinics, some from cities, others from rural areas. As we read them, we will uncover variations, sometimes subtle, in treatment, in patient populations, and in the measures used to assess outcomes. If the studies agree, there will be no problem reviewing the work. This rarely happens. Ordinarily, we find conflicting findings. Sometimes the treatment works well, sometimes poorly. What do we make of all this?

An important first step is to examine any variation you find. Look at the range of outcomes to see if calculating an average effect will be a useful approach. Do the differences in outcomes seem to be due to random sampling around a single population average, or could the variation indicate several groups? Are several different treatments masquerading as a single operation? Is the vagotomy-pyloroplasty reported from Boston the same as that studied in Cologne? Why are the results reported from Scotland better than those from Canada? Are the patients really similar? What are their socio-demographic and clinical characteristics? While populations that are relatively homogeneous are best for study purposes, we can sometimes address differences with statistical methods.

By using meta-analysis, we can encompass studies with various research designs and with different approaches to the statistical analysis of results, provided they report findings in sufficient numerical detail to furnish the data necessary for a quantitative analysis.

Now, *consider the various end-points or outcome variables used to assess treatment effects.* If you are reviewing the literature on surgical approaches to vagotomy and are specifically interested in the effects of selective vagotomy with antrectomy in patients with duodenal ulcers, that operation must be one of the independent variables in each report. An important advantage of meta-analysis is that it can take several different dependent variables into account (15). In our example, the effects of selective vagotomy with antrectomy could include such outcome measures as mortality, recurrence, pain, or quality of life.

Analysis and Interpretation

A major feature of *meta-analysis* is that, in the analysis of the results of many studies, the unit of analysis is not an individual patient or clinic, but a study. To compare studies, we must measure a treatment impact for each study. The two most common measures are statistical significance and effect size.

Most research about the effectiveness of treatments asks the question, Do the differences between the treatment and the control groups exceed those we expect due to chance alone? If each of several studies compares treatment and control groups, we can take the *p-values* as measures of statistical significance to interpret the effectiveness of treatment.

This strategy has two problems. Many studies in medicine and surgery have rather few participants in each of the comparison groups, i.e., they are small. Small investigations are said to have weak power because *their ability to detect real differences between groups* is small. If a weak study reports a difference, we can assume that the difference is substantial. However, if a weak study reports no significant differences, the reader must wonder whether the findings indicate that there are truly no important differences or only that the study is too small to detect differences that do exist. Relying on a *p-value* may, therefore, be misleading.

The sample size issue can cut the other way too. Occasionally, one sees a study in medicine with very large sample sizes. Tests of significance, like the *p-value*, are heavily influenced by sample size and in a truly large study very small or even trivial differences can appear statistically significant. Significant does not mean important!

Effect sizes provide a simple estimate of how valuable a treatment is. Let us say that we wish to compare the main results between the treatment group and the control group. If the information is reported in each of the individual studies, an average effect size for the entire group of studies can easily be calculated. For each study, we need to know the mean of the treatment, the mean of the control group, and the standard deviation of the control group. With an average effect size across a number of studies, we have a single summary value for the effectiveness of the treatment studies. In 1976, Glass and Smith (16) computed the average effect size for psychotherapy treatment across 400 separate studies to be .68. They concluded that, on average, psychotherapy is beneficial since the average patient receiving psychotherapy was approximately two-thirds of a standard deviation more improved than the average control group member (2).

A comparison of proportions will give another measure of effect size. For example, one could compare the proportion of people who live longer than 5 years following different treatments for cancer. The effect size for proportions is calculated by simply subtracting the proportion surviving in the treatment group from that surviving in the control group.

Frequently, your chosen measure of effect size will depend on what numerical information is reported in the various studies. For example, if the standard deviation of the control group is not reported or cannot be calculated, a mean-score effect size cannot be computed.

Another method of looking at the overall impact of treatment is to try to combine the significance tests from many separate studies into one comprehensive test of a null hypothesis for the studies as a whole. Rosenthal (17) has described nine ways to accomplish this. To illustrate one technique, consider the method of adding *Z-scores* (standard normal deviates). If each study has two comparison groups, there is a *Z-score* associated with each reported *p-value*. The *Z-scores* from each individual study are simply added across studies. The sum of the *Z-scores* is divided by the square root of the number of studies. The probability associated with this total score gives an overall level of significance for the studies under review.

Combined significance tests are simple to compute and generally require only that we know the sample size and the probability level or the level of a test statistic, such as the value of T, Z, or F, for each individual study. The larger the overall sample size, the more likely it is that a given underlying effect size will be detected as statistically significant. For example, assume that patients with duodenal ulcer treated by vagotomy and antrectomy have slightly better results than those receiving vagotomy and pyloroplasty. If the two operations are repeatedly compared in very weak trials (small sample sizes for each group), many of the studies will not show statistically significant differences between the two operations even if they exist. A traditional informal reviewer who did only a vote count would almost certainly fail to see the true effectiveness of vagotomy and antrectomy. A careful reviewer who combines the studies by adding Z-scores is much more likely to find that the overall statistical test is significant because the small numbers of patients in each weak study combine to become a much larger number of patients and produce a meta-analysis of greater power than any of the smaller studies taken individually.

Presentation of Results

There are no hard and fast rules about the format for presenting the findings of a review employing meta-analysis. The format depends, to some extent, on the purpose of the final product and the organizational framework of the individual reviewer. Coope (18) has suggested that such reviews should follow an outline similar to the one used for primary research, i.e., (1) an **Introduction** defining the problem to be addressed and identifying the controversy in the literature; (2) a **Methods** section describing how the articles were selected, the sources tapped, and the kind of information collected about each study; (3) a **Results** section presenting the statistical procedures and findings; and (4) a **Discussion** section containing a summary of the findings, a comparison with other related work, and a statement of the direction future research might take.

References

1. Glass GV. Primary, secondary, and meta-analysis of research. Educ Res 1975;5:3–8.
2. Glass GV. Meta-analysis: an approach to the synthesis of research results. Res Sc Teach 1982;19:93–112.
3. University Group Diabetes Program (UGDP) Study. Journal of Diabetes 1970;19:Suppl 2:740–850.
4. McPeek B, Gilbert JP. Onset of postoperative jaundice related to anesthetic history. Brit Med J 1974;3:615–617.
5. Moses LE, Mosteller F. Afterword for the study of death rates. Chapter IV-8 in The National Halothane Study; a study of the possible association between halothane anesthesia and postoperative hepatic necrosis. Bunker JP, Forrest WH Jr., Mosteller F, Vandam LD, editors. Washington, D.C.: U.S. Government Printing Office, 1969:395–408.
6. Hewett P, Chalmers TC. Using MEDLINE to peruse the literature. Controlled Clinical Trials 1985;6:75–84.
7. Hewett P, Chalmers TC. Perusing the literature: methods of assessing MEDLINE and related databases. Controlled Clinical Trials 1985;6:168–178.
8. Chalmers TC. The randomized controlled trial as a basis for therapeutic decisions. Chapter 2 in J. Lachin, Tygstrup N, Juhl E, editors. The Randomized Clinical Trial and Therapeutic Decisions. New York: Marcel Dekker, 1982.
9. Gilbert JP, McPeek B, Mosteller F. Statistics and ethics in surgery and anesthesia. Science 1977(a);198:684–689.
10. Gilbert JP, McPeek B, Mosteller F. Progress in surgery and anesthesia: benefits and risks of innovative therapy. Chapter 9 in Costs, risks and benefits of surgery. Bunker JP, Barnes BA, and Mosteller F, editors. Oxford University Press, NY: 1977(b);124–169.
11. Bearman JB, Loewenson DB, Gullen WH. Muenchs postulates, laws and corollaries. Biometrics Note 4, Bethesda, MD: Office of Biometry and Epidemiology, National Eye Institute, NIH, 1974.
12. Stock WA, Okun M, Haring M, Witter R. Age difference in subjective well-being: a meta-analysis. In Evaluation Studies Review Annual. Light RJ, editor. Beverly Hills, CA: Sage 1983;8:279–302.
13. Straw RB. Deinstitutionalization in mental health: a meta-analysis. In Evaluation Studies Review Annual. Light RJ editor. Beverly Hills, CA: Sage 1983;8:253–278.
14. Yin RK, Yates D. Street level governments: as-

sessing decentralization and urban services. Los Angeles, CA: Rand Corp, 1974.
15. Ottenbacher KJ, Peterson P. The efficacy of vestibular stimulating as a form of specific sensory enrichment. Clinical Pediatrics 1983;23:418–433.
16. Smith ML, Glass GV. Meta-analysis of psychotherapy outcome studies. American Psychology 1976;32:752–760.
17. Rosenthal R. Combining results of independent studies. Psychological Bulletin 1978;85:185–193.
18. Cooper, HM. Scientific guidelines for conducting integrative research reviews. Review of Education Research 1982;52:291–302.

Further Reading

Light RJ, Pillemer DB. Summing up—the science of reviewing research. Cambridge, Mass., Harvard University Press, 1984.

2

Endpoints for Clinical Studies: Conventional and Innovative Variables

S. Wood-Dauphinee and H. Troidl

Two well-dressed gentlemen who on their way home from a party where they had obviously dined and wined too well. One was on his knees systematically examining the sidewalk beneath a streetlight. His friend volunteered helpfully: "I'm sure I heard your keys drop back here where it's dark!" The searcher replied: "I know, but what's the use of looking back there where I can't see when it's so much easier here in the light?"

This chapter discusses flashlights for finding keys in the dark. Surgical treatment is not always dramatically lifesaving. Its aim is to improve quality of life and halt the ravages of disease that quietly and relentlessly erode comfort and dispel happiness. Patients come to surgeons for relief from discomfort and pain of gallbladder disease or heartburn that accompanies reflux esophagitis, not to have their abnormal laboratory findings corrected.

As surgeons, we inquire about decrease in discomfort following surgery, note improvement in appetite or ability to sleep throughout the night and record any such changes on our patients' charts. When data are collected for research purposes, however, such information is conspicuous by its absence. We collect mortality figures, length of hospital stay, pH of gastric secretions, and other similar data.

Because pain, functional limitation, and overall well-being are difficult to measure, we turn to variables we can measure even if they have little bearing on the disease process or the symptoms that brought the patient to see us in the first place. The fact that an outcome variable is easy to measure reliably, does not enhance its usefulness if it measures the wrong thing.

Resorting to such measures is also unnecessary because it really is possible to measure the effects of treatment in terms of variables like discomfort, disability, and dissatisfaction; to document the true value of surgery; and to assess the effectiveness of innovative treatment.

Variables in General

Variables are measurable attributes of patients or of the process of care that vary from one individual to another. Identifying the differences or changes in particular variables in groups of patients subjected to different treatments to discover what causes them is the essence of clinical research.

Patient variables include sociodemographic characteristics like age, sex and marital status; clinical information like the type and stage of disease, signs, and symptoms; and laboratory measurements like hematocrit, body weight, or x-ray findings. Patient variables also include physical, emotional and social functioning; personal aspects of daily living; and attitudes towards life, illness and the health care process (1).

Table I lists patient variables of potential use in surgical studies. They may be described by direct observation, by noting a related behavior that appears to reflect an underlying trait, or by self-reporting by the patient. They are usually recorded as "present", "absent", or as a number denoting the degree of deviation from specified criteria.

Treatment variables are interventions by health professionals intended to effect a cure,

TABLE I. Examples of patient variables in surgical studies.

Sociodemographic	Clinical	Sociopersonal
Age	Diagnosis	Physical performance
Sex	Stage of disease	Emotional performance
Marital Status	Localization of disease	Cognitive performance
Socioeconomic Status	Disease specific signs	Social performance
Educational level	Disease specific symptoms	Beliefs
Occupation	Co-morbidity	Attitudes
Religion	Complications	Health status
Place of residence	Laboratory data	Quality of life
Nationality		
Ethnic origin	Radiographic data	
Employment status	Angiogram information	
	Endoscopic information	

prolong life, alleviate suffering, improve function, or otherwise ameliorate the quality of life. They include pharmaceutical, surgical, rehabilitative and other approaches to care, and the way such approaches are organized and delivered to patients. They are usually documented in terms of operative procedure, therapeutic regimen, length of hospital stay, or the skill and experience of those providing treatment. Examples of some treatment variables related to surgical studies are listed in Table II.

The selection of appropriate patient and treatment variables depends on the question under investigation, the nature of the clinical disorder and the cultural setting of the study. Care must be taken at the outset to identify and record clinical variables related to prognosis, e.g., if tumor stage and location are known to affect outcome, they must be included.

The interaction between patient and treatment variables is the focus of primary interest. Treatment variables are said to be independent because they can be manipulated by the investigator and are presumed to alter certain patient variables. Patient variables that change and reflect the effect of a therapeutic intervention are called **dependent** or **outcome** variables.

Outcome Variables in Clinical Studies in Surgery

In 1967, White (2) listed five outcome variables that describe much of the spectrum of health states: death, disease, discomfort, disability, and dissatisfaction. Death has been used as an endpoint in many intervention studies because preventing premature death is an eminent therapeutic, goal, and death is easily recognized and reported. When death occurs in relation to a surgical intervention, the major issues are the specific cause of death and whether it could have been prevented. The duration of survival following an operative procedure for a condition known to lead eventually to death, and operative or late mortality are obviously useful outcome variables, but if they are the only endpoints measured, other important consequences for those who survive may be missed.

Disease manifests itself as a combination of physical signs, subjective symptoms, and abnormal test-results. Such deviations from normal may be the result of the disease process, its complications, or of therapy. When the impact of health care is being assessed, the aspects of morbidity that are of interest will vary with the nature of the disease. In cancer, local recurrence and distant metastasis are significant; in peripheral vascular disease, information on distal pulses, flow rates and pain during ambulation is required; in urological conditions, data on urinary output, glomerular filtration rates, or frequency are required. Whether a doctor is attempting to cure or palliate, one or more manifestation(s) of the particular disease may be selected as endpoints for a surgical study.

Discomfort is such a salient feature of disease that it merits its own category. Discomfort includes symptoms like pain, nausea, dyspnea,

TABLE II. Examples of treatment variables in surgical studies.

Related to surgery	Related to adjunct Treatments
Type of surgery	Anesthetic technique
Extent of surgery	Post surgical nursing care
Timing of surgery	Drug therapy
Skill of the surgical team	Chemotherapy
Use of mechanical devices	Radiotherapy
	Physical therapy
	Nutritional therapy

depression, anorexia, anxiety, and fatigue, and is clinically important to both patient and physician. The presence, absence or severity of discomfort is a meaningful outcome for investigators trying to determine the effects of a surgical procedure. Although measures of discomfort were seldom used as outcome variables in older studies, relief of discomfort is now appearing in the literature and is being advocated as a criterion of successful treatment (3,4).

Disability (5) refers to a decrease in the normal competence of individuals to perform activities like caring for themselves, moving about their environment, and going about their daily lives at home, at work or during recreational or social pursuits. Outcome variables reflecting the physical dimensions of disability have been reported in the surgical literature (6–8) for many years but endpoints relating to social and emotional components have been much less common. This discrepancy reflects not only the difficulty of assessing the social and emotional components of disability, but also the absence of their consideration in traditional medical education programs where disease was viewed in terms of a biomedical model; treatment was directed at modifying biologic mechanisms and outcome measures were chosen accordingly (9). Because the multidimensional characteristics of disease and response patterns are now better understood, the newer health models include physical, emotional and social components. Studies using all of them as endpoints are now appearing in the surgical literature (10–14).

Dissatisfaction with the process of care, or its results, has been widely discussed in the literature and its measurement is currently regarded as a necessary component in any evaluation of quality of care (15). Several scales have been designed for the purpose (16–18), but patients' perceptions of surgical care and its results are just starting to be addressed in reports of surgical studies (19,20).

Selecting Outcome Variables

Assessing the outcome of a disease process or its treatment has long been a major preoccupation of investigators. A study of the literature reveals that our understanding of the causes and mechanisms of disease is growing constantly and that the positive accomplishments of therapeutic interventions are numerous. Feinstein (21) has pointed out, however, that much of the information used to substantiate these achievements has been gathered from clinical information that only provides anatomical, physiological or biochemical data about disease. Fletcher and Fletcher (22) determined that 90% of published articles documenting outcomes of disease used biologic data obtained by diagnostic tests. Although clinical phenomena form much of the basis of medical practice, relatively little attention has been paid to them.

Measurement of clinical parameters is appropriate because surgery involves an agreement by patients to accept the risk and pain associated with surgery in the hope that it will alleviate their symptoms and improve their quality of life. Patients threatened by cancer submit to radical operations to evade or delay premature death, even though the radical surgery may be followed by a significant decrease in the quality of their lives. Because it is difficult to convey to patients what their lives will be like following an operation, variables designed to record the course of recovery after operation must be included as endpoints in studies of treatment. For instance, almost every operation is followed by a recovery phase during which the patient feels worse and quality of life variables recorded during this period would make the operation seem less effective. This problem can be overcome by making measures of patients' status at specific points during the course of recovery. Armed with such concrete information, surgeons can give patients a more accurate picture of what to expect following an operation.

Physiologic or anatomic variables, such as arterial blood gas determinations, hemoglobin or electrolyte levels, and tumor size, are important parameters in tracking the course of a disease or searching for more efficacious treatment. They hold little meaning for patients unless they are related to significant clinical events in their lives (9,23). Accordingly, the evaluator of a treatment should choose outcome variables that reflect patient-important values as well as the usual laboratory findings.

Advocating clinical data as outcome measures raises the issue of "hard" versus "soft" data. Traditionally, hard data were chosen because they were "objectively" acquired and "quantifiable" in terms of an established scale, and could be "accurately" reproduced or stored for analysis (24). Standard hard data include: death or survival and information obtained through radiography, CT scanning, endoscopy, cardiac catheterization, biochemical analysis, etc. Patients' reports of symptoms or their attitudes toward illness and the health care system, and measures of functional capabilities are considered imprecise, variable and non-reproducible, i.e. suspect or "soft". In truth, extensive evidence suggests that much of the "hard" information in the literature is softer than we like to think (25). Many of the outcomes regarded as being soft are really as solid as, or more reliable than, those long accepted as hard.

Several methods exist to acquire harder data in the traditionally "soft" areas (21,26,29). One way uses procedures developed through social science research for the design of standardized questionnaires and indices. This approach, like other research endeavors, requires special skills and knowledge. Data on such clinical signs as heart murmurs, joint swelling, organ enlargements, and blood pressure are made more consistent or reliable by repeated assessment by the same person or by two or more individuals in accordance with specified criteria or standards. A similar routine can be used for diagnostic tests. The new system for staging dysplastic changes in biopsy specimens from patients with ulcerative colitis illustrates the use of this approach to develop standards or criteria (30).

Reproducibility of results is enhanced by recording the precise findings of the physical examination and the clinical impression or the diagnosis inferred from the findings. Reporting hematuria, flank pain, and abdominal mass is more conducive to agreement than simply stating a diagnosis of renal carcinoma, and it provides data for comparisons of initial findings in groups of patients subjected to different interventions.

Assessments made with simple aids like tape measures, pupil gauges, eye charts, or goniometers are more reproducible than casual estimations. These more precise findings can be verified by checking them against existing records of other clinical examinations or the results of diagnostic tests. Patient evaluations or test interpreters should be "blind" to the treatment regimen of the patient and to the specific purpose of the study, if possible. Ways of making clinical data more reliable are summarized in Table III.

TABLE III. Suggestions for making clinical data more reliable.

Repeat evaluation and assess agreement
Evaluate according to specified criteria
Record precise physical findings
Use appropriate assessment aids
Use "blind" evaluations
Verify findings against other data sources

Adapted from Sackett et al. 1985, page 39

Some types of "hard" data are based on endpoints that occur infrequently and, as a consequence, large sample sizes are required to obtain statistical significance. If, for example, death is chosen as the principal outcome variable in the study of a surgical procedure and it occurs only rarely, a large number of patients will be required (25). You can choose other more frequent outcomes, provided they are related to the primary objective of the study (25). A study comparing survival following different surgical approaches to ruptured appendix might use in-hospital mortality as a principal endpoint. If relief of symptoms rather than improving survival is the aim of a surgical intervention in patients with pancreatic carcinoma, endpoints reflecting a change in pain and short-term well-being are appropriate.

You may be strongly tempted to generate a list of all the relevant outcome variables for your study and measure each of them. You will find this not only time-consuming and expensive, but potentially fatiguing for your patients. It also has methodological and statistical implications. If you use multiple endpoints, the probability of your finding one that demonstrates a difference increases. If you assess 20 endpoints and set .05 (1 in 20) as the level of statistical significance, at least one should demonstrate such a difference by chance alone. Statistical procedures are available to correct the problem just described, but they dramatically increase the sample size requirements and complexity of your study (31).

Few guidelines are available, but the advice of one author is to "choose as many as necessary and as few as possible" (32). The most widely accepted procedure is to select one variable from the group of possible dependent variables and make it the primary focal point for assessing the treatment effect (26,33). A few of the other outcome variables may be added to reflect different impact areas of the intervention.

TABLE IV. Guidelines for selecting endpoints

Make sure your endpoints are related to the primary objective of your study.
Choose endpoints that have a high probability of being influenced by the intervention.
Be certain your endpoints will occur frequently among the patients under study.
Incorporate socio-personal and clinical as well as laboratory outcomes.
Choose as few endpoints as possible to achieve the study objective.
Be sure your endpoints are important for future clinical management.
Be certain your endpoints can be accurately measured.
Make sure the endpoints chosen can be reproduced by the other investigators.

For example, if you are comparing dialysis and kidney transplantation for endstage renal disease, you could choose quality of life as the principal endpoint and document specific symptom relief and length of survival as subsidiary outcomes. Establish a hierarchy of outcomes, choose the most relevant and add a few others according to their importance.

The outcome variables chosen by other investigators are in the literature, but your own clinical expertise and knowledge of the intervention and your study's objectives are your best guide to what is pertinent and important. Remember to consider how common the outcome is in terms of future clinical management, how likely it is that the outcome will be influenced by the intervention being assessed (34), and how measurable the outcome currently is. Table IV lists the guidelines for selecting study endpoints.

Methodologic Criteria of Measuring Instruments

Although the term measuring instrument is commonly associated with mechanical devices, it is also used to describe laboratory tests, physical tests, questionnaires, and scales and indices of various types. Carefully developed evaluation protocols, i.e., standardized measuring instruments, should include information about the methodologic criteria that must be met to ensure satisfactory measurement. Reliability, validity, precision, applicability and practicality are some of the criteria (35–37).

Reliability

Reliability is the extent to which a measure obtains similar results when the presence or magnitude of a stable characteristic is repeatedly determined. Some degree of variation, or error, attributable to the measuring instrument or the individual making the observation is unavoidable; there is always some disagreement among clinicians about physical findings or the interpretation of laboratory data (38,39). Measuring errors can lead to serious consequences like missed diagnoses, mislabeling of patients (40), and incorrect study conclusions. A measure is said to be reliable when the variation or random fluctuation due to errors in measurement is small.

Test-retest reliability refers to the stability of a result when the measure is repeatedly determined under similar conditions.

When human judgement is required to assess the presence of a physical finding, interpret laboratory data, score a scale, or complete a questionnaire, both **inter-rater reliability** (the ability of more than one rater to obtain similar results) and **intra-rater reliability** (the ability of one rater to obtain similar results when a test is repeated under identical conditions) become important.

One study of rater reliability (41) compared surgeons' agreement in assessing the physical signs and clinical status of 8 patients with acute ulcerative colitis. Three surgeons agreed 51% of the time on whether the patient was improving but >90% of the time on whether surgical intervention was indicated. A study (42) assessing the results of surgery for peptic ulcer revealed that the surgeons involved agreed on the presence, absence, or severity of symptoms >90% of the time, but on the success of the surgery in <66% of the assessments. Communication and feedback substantially improved the latter level of agreement. These were not incompetent doctors, but the data show that agreement in medicine is less frequent than we like to think.

When a measuring instrument includes several items summed to a total score, we must ask how the items are related to each other and to the whole instrument. An example of such an instrument would be one that contained a number of items reflecting the severity of pain. **Internal consistency** is the degree to which the various items within the instrument, designed to measure the same characteristic, are scored similarly by respondents.

TABLE V. Assessment of instrument reliability.

Method	For estimation of	Measure
Test-retest	Stability of results	Laboratory data
		Presence, absence or severity gradings of physical signs
		Questionnaires, scales or indices assessing symptoms, function, well-being or satisfaction if the characteristic is stable
Inter-rater reliability	Reproducability of results by different raters	Diagnostic test interpretations
		Presence, absence, or severity of physical signs
Intra-rater reliability	Reproducability of results by a single rater over repeated observations	Questionnaires, scales or indices assessing symptoms, function or well-being
Internal consistency	Relation of individual components of an instrument to each other and to the overall content of the instrument	Multiple item questionnaires, scales or indices assessing symptoms, functional capacity, well being or satisfaction

Although each type of reliability-testing is not appropriate for every type of instrument or intended use (Table V), a standardized instrument or procedure should provide information on the aspects of reliability that are applicable. Reliability is usually expressed as a decimal value <1. It indicates the proportion of information a score contains rather than the amount of random error within it. Although no universally acceptable values are set, reliability is considered high if the coefficient is .80 or above, moderate if it is between .60 and .79, and questionable if it is below .60 (43). When two or more large groups are compared, an instrument with a reliability coefficient of .50 may be sufficient if it is likely that the intervention will cause considerable differences in the outcomes of the groups receiving it compared to those who do not (37).

Validity

Validity is the extent to which an instrument actually measures what it claims to measure, i.e., the relation between what is observed and reported, and the real situation.

For laboratory measures, ensuring validity is less difficult than it is for measures assessing abilities, attitudes or behaviors. In the laboratory, quality control techniques are used to establish and maintain accuracy. For example, each instrument is calibrated by comparing its accuracy with a known standard. In some laboratories, 50% of all the tests performed are for calibration purposes (23); in some countries, analytical variance is monitored through inter-laboratory surveys, and certification is dependent upon satisfactory performance (44).

The validity of clinical observations can be similarly established by comparing the observed measure to some accepted standard. For example, the pulse rate obtained by palpation and a watch can be compared to the heart rate recorded simultaneously by an ECG monitor; the existence of a peptic ulcer, suspected on the basis of a clinical history, can be confirmed by direct viewing through a fiberoptic endoscope.

For many clinical measures, such as pain, functional ability, and quality of life, there are no physical criteria by which to judge validity. They are, however, appropriate outcome variables in clinical studies and instruments like questionnaires, scales and indices must be employed. Establishing the validity of such instruments is achievable by using methods already available (Table VI).

Content validity expresses how well the instrument measures or represents the various components of the characteristic being assessed. For example, if you are responsible for teaching a course in surgery and for evaluating how much your students have learned, the examination you set for them should contain a good cross-section of the components of the course if this measure of their performance is to have content validity. **Face validity** is what the instrument appears to measure upon inspection, i.e., its credibility. A close examination of the individual components

TABLE VI. Approaches to assessing the validity of paper instruments.

Type of validation	Purpose	Procedure
Content	To estimate whether the instrument represents the spectrum of content of the characteristic being measured	Inspection of instrument Professional judgement
Criterion related	To compare the results of a new instrument with a criterion or "gold standard"	Comparison or correlation scores from the two measures
Construct	To assess the meaning of an instrument in terms of its hypothesized or theoretical basis	Comparison with external variables related to the construct

and over-all content of an instrument will disclose what is being measured and what the responses will mean (37). By considering the content of an instrument, you can judge whether an intervention can cause changes that will be reflected in the scores you will obtain. Trying to measure something that the proposed intervention cannot possibly alter is a waste of time, money and effort.

Criterion-related validity is based on a comparison of the results obtained by an instrument with an independent outcome that reflects the same characteristic and is already formally validated and/or highly accepted.

Melzack (45) has developed a pain questionnaire that is now the standard reference measure although it is cumbersome and time-comsuming. If another investigator developed a much shorter form that obtained results that correlated well with those obtained with the original version, when the two were administered concurrently, it would be said to have **concurrent validity.** If the measures obtained with an instrument when it is being validated agree closely with criterion measures obtained at a later date, rather than concurrently, the measures obtained with the instrument are said to have **predictive validity.** For instance, if students' scores on a written examination in surgery predict how well they will perform in the operating theater, the examination scores are said to have predictive validity.

For many clinical outcomes no criterion or "gold standard" is available. Nevertheless, instruments to measure such outcomes can be developed and tested for their **construct validity.** A construct is an attribute, such as health status, that cannot be measured independently but can be evaluated by looking at a combination of variables. This combination can then be tested as an instrument to determine how closely the scores obtained with it correlate with behaviors believed to be related to the attribute. An example would be assessing an instrument designed to measure "independence" by looking at self-care styles, indoor and community mobility, and employment or financial status. If the correlation is positive and its magnitude is reasonable, construct validity is deemed to be present.

A common approach to ascertain construct validity is to determine whether the measurement scale under assessment discriminates between subjects with values that should be high and subjects with values that should be low. For instance, a quality of life index should easily classify ostensibly healthy adults holding down a job from adults with advanced irrevocable chronic disease who are bedridden in an institution. If the scale also converges, this suggests construct validity. It means that the new data-gathering instrument yields similar scores when you expect then to be similar. For instance, a "trauma impact index" should yield similar scores for accident victims sustaining comparable injuries and short term clinical sequelae. All minor incidents should get a low score. Or, all major multi-organ incidents associated with shock and loss of consciousness should yield high scores. Construct validity is butressed if the scale is sensitive, that is, its score changes with known changes in the attribute it is measuring, especially over time. Measures obtained with instruments that have been construct validated and widely accepted can be considered valid.

Precision

The precision of a measuring instrument is its ability to distinguish differences or to determine gradations of change in the characteristic being studied. It is based on qualitative judgments, such as assessing the presence or absence of a physical sign, and the quantification and ordering of degrees of change, such as classifying the health status of a patient as much improved, slightly improved, unchanged, slightly worse or much worse (35).

Precision is sometimes referred to as sensitivity (46), but sensitivity, as commonly used in relation to diagnostic tests, only denotes the proportion of subjects with a given disease who give a positive test result for that disease (23). As such, sensitivity only covers the qualitative component of precision (35).

The level of precision required in an instrument depends on how it will be used in a specific study (35). If you only need data about the presence or absence of pain after back surgery, the instrument you use only needs to be precise enough to determine this directly. If you need to know the intensity of the back pain, choose an instrument with this degree of precision.

In controlled studies, precision requirements are related to the clinical changes that may occur following an experimental intervention. If the group receiving the intervention is expected to do "much better" than the control group, a high degree of precision is not necessary. If the anticipated difference is small, greater precision is required. The aim is to choose an instrument that is able to detect differences regarded as being both real and clinically important.

Few older published reports on measuring instruments discussed their precision unless various instruments designed to measure the same outcomes were being compared (47). Now that the importance of grading patient response is recognized, precision is receiving more attention (46). Nevertheless, the precision of most instruments still has to be appraised by the intended user on the basis of their content and how they are scored (35).

Applicability

The **applicability** of a measuring instrument is the appropriateness of its use with the proposed study population. For example, the Quality of Life Index (48) was initially developed for cancer patients, but was subsequently validated on patients with other chronic diseases of varying severity in several geographic areas and in three languages. This kind of information allows you to assess whether the instrument is appropriate for your intended use.

Another concern about applicability is whether the outcome measure you choose should be specific to the disease or intervention you are studying, or whether a more general measure would be adequate. For instance, assessments of the quality of life are currently being reported following cardiac, orthopedic, or other surgery and the question arises, do we need disease- or system-specific instruments to assess this construct? Although no answer is currently available, disease-specific measures would probably be more valid and more precise.

The prevalence of the outcome variable has a bearing on the applicability of an instrument to your proposed study sample. One group of investigators found, in the course of constructing a battery of functional status measures for use in a general population, that <1% of participants reported any limitations in such basic physical activities as personal care or indoor mobility (49). This outcome variable should obviously not be chosen for a study in such a population, nor operative mortality as the primary endpoint in a study comparing different types of hip arthroplasty.

Practicality

The final criterion, **practicality** of the measure, only becomes important when you have decided the instrument is acceptable in terms of its other properties. You should assess it from your patients' and your own point of view.

Can good compliance be anticipated or is the burden unreasonable for patients? Does the measure involve a painful procedure? Will obtaining the information take so long that patients will become fatigued? Are there so many questions that patients will never answer them all if the instrument is self-administered? Is the instrument anxiety-provoking because it invades privacy or raises sensitive issues? The answers to these and other similar questions are particularly important if it is necessary to evaluate patients on several occasions in order to obtain complete data profiles. Serious consideration of these aspects of the instrument should reduce losses due to patient withdrawal or refusal to be evaluated.

The burden for you and your colleagues should be similarly assessed. What type of data collection procedure does the instrument de-

TABLE VII. Considerations for determining the usefulness of an instrument for your research project.

Has the instrument been shown to be reliable enough over time or between observations for the intended use?

If the instrument has multiple items, has the relationship among the items been evaluated?

Does the content of the instrument reflect what you hypothesize the intervention will alter and therefore what you wish to measure?

If a gold standard or criterion is available how does the instrument relate to it?

Has validity been demonstrated either through wide acceptance and use, or by formal construct validation testing procedures?

Does the instrument and its scoring system seem precise enough to detect anticipated clinical changes?

Has the instrument been developed or used in a patient population similar to yours?

Is the instrument practical in terms of patient compliance and professional burden?

mand? Does it need patient evaluation or direct observation? Are interviews required or can patients do a self-assessment? If it is to be administered by someone other than the patient, what kinds of skill or knowledge must this person possess? Is this individual already available or would it require intensive training beyond that necessary to achieve rater reliability? Is a chart audit or other information retrieval necessary? For laboratory measures, is the instrument available or would it have to be purchased specifically for the investigation? How expensive is it? For paper instruments, are they available and standardized in the language of the patients? Is the instrument easily understood and scorable or does it require complicated mathematical manipulations or coding reversals for computation? Can the data be stored and interpreted easily? Each additional procedure increases the difficulty, the time requirement, and the possibilities for human error. In sum, mode of data collation, its cost, and burden it imposes must be taken into account.

Do not consider creating a new instrument unless you have the necessary time, resources and expertise because it is a difficult procedure and a scientific investigation in its own right. Table VII is a list of guidelines for determining the usefulness of an instrument for your research.

Instruments for Appraising Endpoints

Measures of Symptoms

In practice, clinicians evaluate signs and symptoms separately and then aggregate the results to arrive at a diagnosis. In research, individual signs and symptoms are evaluated to determine whether and how they are influenced by the care process.

Because, pain is one of the most distressing symptoms and the one for which relief is most often sought, medical practitioners frequently wish to assess it as an outcome of a therapeutic intervention. Many attempts to measure pain failed until Melzack and colleagues (50–52) developed a theoretical model on which to base an instrument. In 1975, Melzack (45) reported the properties and scoring methods of the McGill Pain Questionnaire (MPQ) for measuring the relative intensities of the sensory, affective and evaluative qualities of pain. Patients are asked to choose from among specific groups of descriptive adjectives, those that most closely describe their pain. Since intensity is the most prominent feature of pain, a separate scale is used to record its intensity at the time the question is posed. This Present Pain Intensity (PPI) Index is recorded on an equal interval scale of 1 to 5 with each number representing a descriptive word in the range of mild to excruciating (52). Completion of the MPQ provides three scores: the Pain Rating Index (PRI) based on the rank values of the words and their assigned points; the total number of words chosen; and the PPI.

The MPQ has been widely used in clinical studies of several pain syndromes (3,4,53–57). It takes an interviewer 15 to 20 minutes to administer it on the first occasion but up to 50% less time for repeat evaluations. Patients find it acceptable and comply readily. A recent review (58) of the psychometric properties of the MPQ has found that (1) acceptable reliability has been demonstrated even when the instrument is administered to patients retrospectively; (2) the number and variety of studies in which the scores obtained with the MPQ have been used as an outcome variable support its face validity; (3) construct validation studies have confirmed its theoretical framework in terms of its ability to distinguish the sensory, affective and evaluative dimensions of pain; (4) the practice of forming representative scores of the qualities of pain just cited has been rationalized; and (5) criterion validity has been confirmed in terms of its concurrent, predictive and discriminant aspects. The Present Pain Intensity Index, alone, can be administered in <1 minute and may be an acceptable alternative to completion of the entire Questionnaire (59).

Increasing attention is being given to nausea as a side-effect of chemotherapy for cancer. Although many assessment procedures have been reported and none of the new scales and indices being developed can currently be regarded as well-standardized (60), Melzack and co-workers (61) have proposed a Nausea Questionnaire that looks potentially useful. Words chosen from categories of ranked descriptors are used to measure the subjective qualities and intensity of the nausea experienced. An Overall Nausea Intensity Scale similar to the present Pain Intensity Index and a visual "no nausea" to "extreme nausea" analogue scale are included to provide three measures of the subjective features and intensity of nausea. The three assessments correlate closely with each other and with the responses to specific chemotherapy drugs as judged by physicians and nurses. The Nausea Rating Scale demonstrates satisfactory internal consistency and discriminates between the effects of drugs known to provoke severe nausea and those that stimulate a much milder response.

Visick (8) proposed another approach to the assessment of symptoms as outcomes following gastrectomy for peptic ulcer. In 1968, Goligher and colleagues (62) published the results of a study in which they used a modification of the Visick instrument that attempted to clarify the criteria for each symptom category without altering the overall concept of Visick's classification scheme. Since then, other minor modifications have been made (63) and the instrument has been applied to patients with gastric cancer (64). Hall and colleagues (42) have assessed its intra-observer reliability and have found high agreement on the absence or presence and severity of symptoms, but quite low agreement on the overall Visick gradings before extensive discussion with the raters. After discussion, inter-rater agreement was acceptably high, but the raters' gradings were quite different from those made by the patients on themselves. Hall and colleagues concluded that the most reliable method of assessing the status of the ulcer patient after surgery is simply to record the presence or absence of specific symptoms.

Measures of Physical Function

Although the appraisal of functional performance is common in patients who are elderly or undergoing rehabilitation, many other patients have a disease, disorder or injury that leads to temporary or permanent structural or functional impairment. The addition of a functional descriptor to other clinical outcome measures provides greater insight into the overall results of any surgical intervention.

Many measures of functional performance focus on the activities and skills of daily living (ADL). The Katz Index of ADL (65,66) was developed through studies of large numbers of patients with various diagnoses. Six ADL dimensions—bathing, dressing, toileting, transferring, continence and feeding—are used, and scoring is on an ordinal scale that bifurcates according to whether or not the patient can perform a task independently. The Index takes account of the number of activities the patient can perform and the order in which self-care capabilities are lost or regained. The theoretical basis of the instrument is the authors' contention that the pattern of recovery from a disabled state parallels the normal sequence of development in a child. Functional abilities are categorized by an overall score that ranges from A (independent) to G (dependent). A high coefficient of reproducibility has been reported (67) and concurrent validity has been demonstrated (47) by comparing the instrument to two widely accepted ADL Scales, the Barthel Index (68) and the Kenny Self-Care Evaluation (69). Although the Katz Index is the least sensitive of the three to change (47), it has been widely used to describe and classify the functional performance of patients in clinical studies.

Various scales have been devised to assess specific joints and their function pre- and postoperatively (70–72).

Kettlekamp and Thompson (73) have developed a Knee Scale that combines clinical expertise, biomechanical principles and statistical analysis. Two scales were developed and tested on post-osteotomy and post-arthroplasty knees, and compared with each other and with a previously determined clinical classification. The one chosen sums to 103 points. It contains items on pain, function, range of motion, instability and deformity; is short and easy to complete; and contains only clinical variables obtained routinely during a knee examination. Although relatively little information is available about the validity or reliability of this instrument, it has been used in clinical studies and has demonstrated change between the pre- and postoperative states (74–76).

In 1961, Karnofsky (77) developed what has become one of the most widely used clinical scales for measuring the overall ability of patients to perform physical activities. The scale comprises 11 categories that cover the functional spectrum from dead to normal with scores that range from 0 to 100. The categories are major groupings that classify the patients' current performance in relation to self-care, general activities, and work. The scoring can be completed by the patient or a health care professional in a few minutes. Professional inter-rater reliability has been shown to range from moderate (78) to low (79), especially when the scores are corrected for chance agreement, and there is considerable disagreement between the patients' self-ratings and the physicians' ratings (79). Hutchinson and colleagues (79) feel that the defects in the scale could be easily corrected by providing specific criteria and having only one performance activity in each category.

Measures of Well-Being

Instruments designed to assess well-being are based on the World Health Organization concept of health (80) that includes physical, social and psychological dimensions. Their objective is to produce a single summary score for an attribute that is multidimensional (81). To capture the full spectrum of daily functioning, several investigators have developed measures of health status (36,82,86).

One such measure, the Sickness Impact Profile (SIP) (83), is based on the concept that sickness-related dysfunction is manifested by behavioral changes that are quantifiable. The physical and psychosocial dimensions of the SIP encompass 136 items grouped into 12 categories (87). Each item is a first-person statement of a specific dysfunction currently being experienced as a consequence of illness and each has been weighted on the basis of an estimate of the relative severity of the stated dysfunction (88). The SIP can be administered by an interviewer or the patient, and is reported to be acceptable to patients even though it takes 20–30 minutes to complete. It has also been validated in Spanish (89) and used with a Spanish-speaking population (90). It has been used in studies of low back pain, cancer, arthritis and hip replacement (11,87,90–92), and has demonstrated consistently acceptable levels of inter-rater and test-retest reliability and internal consistency in test trials and field applications (93,94). The SIP distinguishes groups of patients with small degrees of clinical distinctiveness and is a useful measure of the behavioral impact of illness.

Assessing quality of life as an outcome of a disease process or a therapeutic intervention is currently popular in the literature, but its use as an endpoint in comparative studies is mainly recommended in chronic conditions when insignificant differences in survival are anticipated or when a treatment is known to increase survival while incurring substantial morbidity (95).

Quality of life is difficult to define, but it includes physical, social and psychological components (96). The physical component includes self-care, mobility, common daily activities, sexuality and freedom from discomfort. Social functioning involves relationships with family and friends, leisure, recreational and work activities, and the fulfillment of social and cultural roles. Psychological functioning has cognitive, perceptual and emotional constituents that include how a patient copes with a perceived problem in order to diminish the associated stress.

Even when defined, quality of life is still difficult to measure. Most attempts to assess it rely on narrative documentation (97–99); a variety of instruments (11,14,100,101), and proxy measures such as the total time spent in hospital during the final months of life (102), or the ability to work (13,103). More precise measurement of this construct has received considerable attention and it is currently viewed as an "emerging science" (103). Well-standardized instruments are already available (10,48,105,107,108).

A Quality of Life (QL) Index devised by

TABLE VIII. Psychometric properties of measuring instruments for clinical endpoints

Instrument	Reliability	Validity	Precision	Practicality
McGill Pain Questionnarie (MPQ)	xx	xx	x	x
Nausea Questionnaire	x	x		xx
Visick	x			xx
Katz Index (ADL)	xx	xx	x	xx
Knee Scoring Scale		x	x	x
Karnofsky	x	xx		xx
Sickness Impact Profile (SIP)	xx	xx	xx	x
Quality of Life (QL) Index	xx	xx	x	xx

xx = Criterion fulfilled
x = Criterion partially fulfilled

Spitzer and co-workers (48) has a questionnaire format that addresses five equally-weighted factors related to the patient's mood, perception of his or her own health, self-care ability, work capability, and social interaction with family and friends. The main part of the QL Index sums to 10 points but there is also a one-dimensional visual analogue scale that portrays the overall estimate. The QL Index can be administered by the patient, an interviewer, or a health professional who knows the patient well in <5 minutes. It was initially developed for cancer patients, but has been subsequently validated for patients with other diseases in several geographic settings and has been found to be acceptable to patients and health care providers. Its content validity was assured by incorporating the perceptions of both sick and well people during its development (81). The QL Index's construct validity; ability to discriminate between very sick and relatively well individuals; sensitivity to change over time (109); and inter-observer reliability in English, French and German have been demonstrated. It is currently in use in several studies and its value has been reported (10).

Table VIII is a summary of the known psychometric properties of the measuring instruments described in this chapter.

Final Comment

The instruments described in this chapter were compared to flashlights for illuminating the dark areas where the "keys" will be found. We are convinced there is much to be learned in this area which will be helpful to patients and to investigators.

Our conviction about the importance of broadening the choice of endpoints in surgical studies does not imply that mortality and technologically acquired data should be ignored or abandoned, since they make significant contributions to advancing our understanding of disease. We suggest, however, that the validity and reliability of these so-called "hard" measures be questioned because the difference between them and those labeled as "soft" are not nearly as great as we are inclined to believe. Information on functional capacity, overall well-being, and quality of life will increase our comprehension of the impact of disease and the results of treatment.

References

1. Spitzer WO, Feinstein AR, Sackett DL. What is a health care trial? J Am Med Assoc 1975;233:161–163.
2. White KE. Improved medical care statistics and health services system. Pub Health Reports 1967;82:847–854.
3. Graham C, Bond S, Gerkovich M, Cook M. Use of McGill Pain Questionnaire in assessment of cancer pain replicability and consistency. Pain 1980;8:377–387.
4. Melzack R, O'Fiesh JG, Mount BM. The Bromptom Mixture: effects on pain in cancer patients. Can Med Ass J 1976;115:125–129.
5. World Health Organization. International classification of impairments, disabilities, and handicaps. Geneva: World Health Organization, 1980.
6. Criteria Committee of the New York Heart Association. Diseases of the heart and blood vessels.

Nomenclature and criteria for diagnosis. Boston: Little Brown and Company, 1964:112–113.
7. Karnofsky DA, Burchenal JH. Clinical evaluation of chemotherapeutic agents in cancer. In Macleod CM, editor. Evaluation of chemotherapeutic agents. New York: Columbia University Press, 1949;191–205.
8. Visick AH. A study of the failures after gastrectomy. Edinburgh: Ann Royal Coll Surg, 1948;3:266–284.
9. Fries JF. Toward an understanding of patient outcome measurement. Arthrit Rheum 1983;26:697–704.
10. Gough R, Furnival CM, Shilder L, Grove W. Assessment of the quality of life of patients with advanced cancer. Eur J Cancer Clin Oncol 1983;19:1161–1165.
11. Sugarbaker PH, Barofsky I, Rosenberg SA, Gianola FJ. Quality of life assessment of patients in extremity sarcoma clinical trials. Surgery 1982;91:17–23.
12. Troidl H, Kusche J. Lebensqualitat nach gastrektomie: ergebnisse einer randomisierten studie zum vergleich oesophago-jujunostomie nach Schlatter mit dem Hunt-Laurence-Rodino Pouch. In Rohde H, Troidl H. Das magenkarzinom. Methodik klinischer studien and therapeutischer ansatze. New York: Georg Thieme Verlag Stuttgart 1984.
13. LaMendola WF, Pellegrini RV. Quality of life and coronary artery bypass surgery patients. Soc Sci Med 1979;13A:457–461.
14. Williams NS, Johnston D. The quality of life after rectal excision for low rectal cancer. Br J Surg 1983;70:460–462.
15. Lebow JL. Consumer assessment of the quality of medical care. Med Care 1974;12:328–337.
16. Hulka BS, Zyzanski SJ, Cassel JC, Thompson SJ. Scale for the measurement of attitudes toward physicians and primary medical care. Med. Care 1970;5:429–435.
17. Mangelsdorff AD. Patient satisfaction questionnaire. Med care 1979;17:86–90.
18. Taylor PW, Nelson-Wernick E, Currey HS, Woodbury ME, Conley LE. Development and use of a method of assessing patient perception of care. Hosp Health Serv Admin 1981;26:89–103.
19. Light HK, Solheim JS, Hunter GW. Satisfaction with medical care during pregnancy and delivery. Am J Obstet Gynecol 1976;122:827–831.
20. Pineault R, Contandriopoulos A-P, Valois M, Bastian M-L, Lance J-M. Randomized clinical trial of one-day surgery: patient satisfaction, clinical outcomes, and costs. Med Care 1985;23:171–182.
21. Feinstein AR. An additional basic science for clinical medicine: IV. The development of clinimetrics. Ann Intern Med 1983;99:843–848.
22. Fletcher RH, Fletcher SW. Clinical research in general medical journals. A 30-year perspective. N Engl J Med 1979;301:180–183.
23. Fletcher RH, Fletcher SW, Wagner EH. Clinical epidemiology - the essentials. Baltimore: Williams & Wilkins, 1982.
24. Feinstein AR. An additional basic science for clinical medicine: II. The limitations of randomized trials. Ann Intern Med 1983a;99:544–550.
25. Feinstein AR. Clinical biostatistics XLI. Hard science, soft data, and the challenges of choosing clinical variables in research. Clin Pharmacol Ther 1977;22:485–498.
26. Feinstein AR. Clinical biostatistics XLV. The purposes and functions of criteria. Clin Pharmacol Ther 1978;24:479–492.
27. Feinstein AR. Clinical biostatistics XLVI. What are the criteria for criteria? Clin Pharmacol Ther 1979;25:108–116.
28. Department of Clinical Epidemiology and Biostatistics, McMaster University. Clinical disagreement: II. How to avoid it and how to learn from ones mistakes. Can Med Assoc J 1980;123:613–617.
29. Sackett DL, Haynes RE, Tugwell P. Clinical epidemiology. A basic science for clinical medicine. Toronto: Little Brown and Company, 1985.
30. Riddell RH, Goldman H, Ransohoff DF, Appelman HD, Fenoglio CM, Haggett R, Ahren C, Correa P, Hamilton SR, Morson BC, Sammers SC, Yardky JH. Dysplasia in inflamatory bowel disease: standardized classification with provisional clinical applications. Human Path 1983;14:931–968.
31. Smythe HA, Helewa A, Goldsmith CH. Selection and combination of outcome measures. J Rheumatol 1982;9:770–774.
32. Abramson JH. Survey methods in community medicine. Edinburgh: Churchill Livingston, 1979.
33. Pocock SJ. Current issues in the design and interpretation of clinical trials. Br Med J 1985;290:39–42.
34. Bombardier C, Tugwell P. A methodological framework to develope and select indices for clinical trials: statistical and judgmental approaches. J. Rheumatol 1982;9:753–757.
35. Jette AM. Concepts of health and methodological issues in functional assessment. In Granger CV, Gresham GA, editors. Functional assessment in rehabilitation medicine. Baltimore: Williams and Williams, 1984:46–64.
36. Sackett DL, Chambers LW, MacPherson AS, Goldsmith CH, Maculey RG. The development and application of indices of health: general methods and a summary of results. Am J Public Health 1977;67:423–428.

37. Ware JE, Brook RH, Davies AR, Lohr KN. Choosing measures of health status for individuals in general populations. Am J Public Health 1981;71:620–625.
38. Department of Clinical Epidemiology and Biostatistics, McMaster University. Clinical disagreement: I. How often it occurs and why. Can Med Assoc J 1980;123:499–504.
39. Koran LM. The reliability of clinical methods, data and judgment. N Engl J Med 1975;293:642–646,695–701.
40. Haynes RB, Sackett DL, Tugwell P. Problems in the handling of clinical and research evidence by medical practitioners. Arch Intern Med 1983;143:1971–1975.
41. Graham NG, de Dombal FT, Goligher JC. Reliability of physical signs in patients with severe attacks of ulcerative colitis. Br Med J 1971;2:746–748.
42. Hall R, Horrocks JC, Clamp SE, de Dombal FT. Observer variation in results of surgery for peptic ulceration. Br Med J 1976;1:814–816.
43. Makrides L, Richman J, Prince B. Research methodology and applied statistics. Part 3: measurement procedures in research. Physiotherapy Canada 1980;32:253–257.
44. Whitehead TP. Quality control techniques in laboratory services. Br Med Bull 1974;30:237–242.
45. Melzack R, The McGill Pain Questionnaire: major properties and scoring methods. Pain 1975;1:277–299.
46. Deyo RA, Inui TS. Toward clinical applications of health status measures: sensitivity of scales to clinically important changes. Health Serv Res 1984;19:275–289.
47. Donaldson SW, Wagner CC, Gresham CE. A unified ADL form. Arch Phys Med Rehabil 1973; 54:175–180.
48. Spitzer WO, Dobson AJ, Hall J, Chesterman E, Levi J, Shepherd R, Battista RN, Catchlove BR. Measuring the quality of life of cancer patients. A concise QL-Index for use by physicians. J Chron Dis 1981;34:585–597.
49. Stewart AL, Ware JE, Brook RH. Construction and Scoring of Aggregate Functional Status Measures: Vol. I. Rand Health Insurance Experiment Series. R-225 1-1-HHS. Santa Monica: Rand, 1982.
50. Melzack R, Wall PD. Pain mechanisms: a new theory. Science 1965;150:971–979.
51. Melzack R, Casey KL. Sensory, motivational, and central control determinants of pain: a new conceptual model. In Kenshalo D, editor. The skin senses. Springfield: Springfield, 1968:423–439.
52. Melzack R, Torgerson WS. On the language of pain. Anesthesiology 1971;34:50–59.
53. Melzack R, Jeans ME, Stratford JG, Monks RC. Ice massage and transcutaneous stimulation: a comparison of treatment of low back pain. Pain 1980;209–217.
54. Melzack R, Taenzer P, Feldman P, Kinch RA. Labour is still painful after prepared childbirth training. Can Med Assoc J 1981;125:357–363.
55. Melzack R, Vetere P, Finch L. Transcutaneous electrical nerve stimulation for low back pain. Phys Ther 1983;63:489–493.
56. Prieto EJ, Hopson L, Bradley LA, Bryne M, Geisinger KF, Midax D, Marchisello PJ. The language of low back pain: factor structure of the McGill Pain Questionnaire. Pain 1980;8:11–19.
57. Taenzer P. Postoperative pain: relationships among measures of pain, mood and narcotic requirements. In Melzack R, editor. Pain measurement and assessment. New York: Raven Press, 1983:111–118.
58. Reading AE. The McGill Pain Questionnaire: an appraisal. In Melzack R, ed. Pain measurement and assessment. New York: Raven Press, 1983;55–61.
59. Finch L, Melzack R. Objective pain measurement: a case for in creased clinical usage. Physiotherapy Canada 1982;34:343–346.
60. Morrow GR. The assessment of nausea and vomiting. Past problems, current issues and suggestions for future research. Cancer 1984;84(suppl):2267–2280.
61. Melzack R, Rosberger Z, Hillingsworth ML, Thirlwell M. Measurement of nausea: three valid indices. Can Med Assoc J 1985;133:755–759.
62. Goligher JC, Pulvertaft CN, de Dombal FT, Conyers JH, Duthie HL, Feather DB, Latchmore AJC, Shoesmith JH, Smiddy FG, Willson-Pepper J. Five-to-eight-year results of Leeds/York controlled trial of elective surgery for duodenal ulcer. Br Med J 1968;2:781–787.
63. Emas S, Fernstrom M. Prospective, randomized trial of selective vagotomy with pyloroplasty and selective proximal vagotomy with and without pyloroplasty in the treatment of duodenal, pyloric and prepyloric ulcers. Am J Surg 1985;149:236–243.
64. Troidl H, Menge K-H, Lorenz W, Vestweber K-H, Barth H, Hamelmann H. Quality of life and stomach replacement. In Herfarth CH, Schlag P, editors. Gastric cancer. Berlin: Springer Verlag, 1979:312–317.
65. Katz S, Ford AB, Moskowitz RW, Jackson BA, Jaffe MW, Cleveland MA. Studies of illness in the aged. The Index of ADL: a standardized measure of biological and psychosocial function. J Am Med Assoc 1963;185:914–919.
66. Katz S, Downs TD, Cash HR, Grotz RC. Progress in the development of the Index of ADL. The Gerontologist 1970;10:20–30.
67. Sherwood SJ, Morris J, Mor V, Gutkin C. Compendium of measures for describing and assess-

ing long term care populations. Boston; Hebrew Rehabilitation Center for the Aged. In Kane RA, Kane RL. Assessing the elderly. A practical guide to measurement. Lexington, MA: Lexington Books, D.C. Heath & Co. 1981;45.
68. Mahoney FI, Barthel DW. Functional evaluation: the Barthel Index. Md St Med J 1965;14:61–65.
69. Schoening HA, Iversen IA. Numerical scoring of self care status: a study of the Kenny self care evaluation. Arch Phys Med Rehabil 1968;49:221–229.
70. Harris WH. Traumatic arthritis of the hip after dislocation and acetubular fractures: treatment by mold arthroplasty. J Bone Joint Surg 1969;51-A:737–755.
71. Larson CB. Rating scale for hip disabilities. Clin Orthop Rel Research 1963;31:85–92.
72. Neer CS, Watson KC, Stanton FJ. Recent experience in total shoulder replacement. J Bone and Joint Surg 1982;64-A:319–337.
73. Kettlekamp DB, Thompson C. Development of a knee scoring scale. Clin Orthop Related Research 1975;107:93–99.
74. Hejgaard N, Sandberg H, Hide A, Jacobsen K. Prospective stress radiography in 38 old injuries of the ligaments of the knee joint. Acta Ortho Scand 1983;54:119–125.
75. Murray DG, Webster DA. The variable axis knee prosthesis. J Bone Joint Surg 1981;63-A:687–694.
76. Short WH, Hootnick DR, Murray DG. Ipsilateral supracondylar femur fractures following knee arthroplasty. Clin Ortho Related Research 1981;158:111–116.
77. Karnofsky DA, Burchenal JH. The clinical evaluation of chemotherapeutic agenst in cancer. In Evaluation of chemotherapeutic agents. Macleod CM, editor. N.Y.: Columbia University Press, 1949;191–205.
78. Yates JW, Chalmer B, McKegney FP. Evaluation of patients with advanced cancer using the Karnofsky Performance Status. Cancer 1980;45:2220–2224.
79. Hutchinson TA, Boyd NF, Feinstein AR. Scientific problems in clinical scales as demonstrated in the Karnofsky Index of Performance Status. J Chron Dis 1979;32:661–666.
80. World Health Organization: Constitution of the World Health Organization. In Basic Documents. Geneva: World Health Organization, 1948:2.
81. Boyle MH, Torrance GW. Developing multiattribute health indexes. Med Care 1984;22:1045–1057.
82. Brook RH, Ware JE, Davies-Avery A, Stewart AL, Donald CA, Rogers WH, Williams KN, Johnston SA. Overview of adult health status measures fielded in Rand's Health Insurance Study. Med Care 1979;17(suppl 7):1–131.
83. Gilson BS, Gilson JS, Bergner M, Bobbitt RA, Kressel S, Pollard WE, Vesselago M. The sickness impact profile. Development of an outcome measure of health care. Am J Public Health 1975;65:1304–1310.
84. Grogono AW, Woodgate DJ. Index for measuring health. Lancet 1971;2:1024–1026.
85. Kaplan RM, Atkins CJ, Timms R. Validity of a quality of well-being scale as an outcome measure in chronic obstructive pulmonary disease. J Chron Dis 1984;37:85–95.
86. Patrick DL, Bush JW, Chen MM. Toward an operational definition of health. J Health Soc Behav 1973;14:6–23.
87. Bergner M, Bobbitt RA, Carter WB, Gilson, BS. The Sickness Impact Profile: development and final revision of a health status measure. Med Care 1981;19:787–805.
88. Carter WB, Bobbitt RH, Bergner M, Gilson BS. Validation of an interval scaling: the Sickness Impact Profile. Health Serv Res 1976;11:516–528.
89. Gilson BS, Erickson D, Chavez CT, Bobbitt RA, Bergner M, Carter WB. A Chicano version of the Sickness Impact Profile (SIP). Cult Med Psychiatry 1980;4:137–150.
90. Deyo RA, Diehl AK. Measuring physical and psychosocial function in patients with low-back pain. Spine 1983a;8:635–642.
91. Deyo RA, Inui TS, Leininger J, Overman S. Physical and psychosocial function in rheumatoid arthritis. Arch Intern Med 1982;142:879–882.
92. Deyo RA, Inui TS, Leininger JD, Overman SS. Measuring functional outcomes in chronic disease: a comparison of traditional scales and a self-administered health status questionnaire in patients with rheumatoid arthritis. Med Care 1983;21:180–192.
93. Bergner M, Bobbitt RA, Pollard WE, Martin DP, Gilson BS. The Sickness Impact Profile: validation of a health status measrue. Med Care 1976;14:57–67.
94. Pollard WE, Bobbitt RA, Bergner M, Martin DP, Gilson BS. The Sickness Impact Profile: reliability of a health status measure. Med Care 1976;14:146–155.
95. Schipper H. Why measure quality of life? Can Med Assoc J 1983;128:1367–1370.
96. Newton M. Quality of life for the gynecologic oncology patient. Am J Obstet Gynecol 1979;124:866–869.
97. McLeod RS, Fazio UW. Quality of life with continent ileostomy. World J Surg 1984;8:90–95.
98. Bennett RC. Long term follow up of surgical adrenalectomy for breast cancer. Aust NZ J Surg, 1983;53:415–519.
99. Meyers S. Assessing quality of life. Mt. Sinai J Med 1983;50:190–192.

100. Drettner B, Ahlbom A. Quality of life and state of health for patients with cancer of the head and neck. Acta Otolaryngol 1983;96:307–314.
101. Trudel L, Fabia J, Bouchard J-P. Quality of life of 50 carotid endarterectomy survivors: a long term follow-up study. Arch Phys Med Rehabil 1984;65:310–312.
102. Scharschmidt BF. Human liver transplantation: analyses of data on 540 patients from four centres. Hepathology 1984;4(suppl I):958–1019.
103. Westaby S, Sapsford RN, Bentall HH. Return to work and quality of life after surgery for coronary artery disease. Br Med J 1979;2:1028–1031.
104. Schipper H, Levitt M. Measuring quality of life: risks and benefits. Cancer Treatment Reports 1985;69:1115–1125.
105. Priestman TJ, Baum M. Evaluation of quality of life in patients receiving treatment for advanced breast cancer. Lancet 1976;2:899–901.
106. Coates A, Dillenbeck CF, McNeil DR, Kaye SB, Sims K, Fox RM, Woods RL, Milton GW, Solomon J, Tattersall MHN. On the receiving end—II. Linear Analogue Self Assessment (LASA) in evaluation of aspects of the quality of life of cancer patients receiving therapy. Eur J Cancer Clin Oncol 1983;19:1633–1637.
107. Selby PJ, Chapman J-A-W, Etazadi-Amoli J, Dalley D, Boyd NF. The development of a method for assessing the quality of life of cancer patients. Br J Cancer 1984;50:13–22.
108. Morris JN, Suissa S, Sherwood SW, Wright SM, Greer D. Last Days: a study of the quality of life of terminally ill cancer patients. J Chron Dis 1986;39:47–62.
109. Schipper H, Clinch J, McMurray A, Levitt M. Measuring the quality of life of cancer patients: the functional living index—cancer: development and validation. J Clin Oncol 1984;2:472–483.

3

Statistics Demystified

M.S. Kramer and H. Troidl

Most clinical investigators approach statistics in one of three ways: (1) total avoidance; (2) mindless "number crunching" often facilitated by ready access to microcomputers with statistical software packages; or (3) blind faith in the advice of statistical consultants. Unfortunately, none of these approaches is particularly conducive to research of high quality and utility.

The main objective for this chapter is to provide the surgical researcher with sufficient background to become an informed consumer of biostatistics. The discussion is not intended to replace either professional statistical advice or standard texts. Our emphasis is on conceptual understanding, rather than technical facility; the use of algebraic notation and mathematical formulas will be kept to the strict minimum required for clarity. We have included a number of clinical examples to illustrate the concepts discussed, including several from general surgery and the surgical subspecialties. Careful reading of the chapter should help demystify a subject for which unfamiliarity all too often leads to one of the unfortunate consequences cited above.

Introduction

Variables

The attributes or events that are measured in a research study are called *variables*, since they vary (take on different values at different times in different subjects). Variables are measured according to two broad types of measurement scales: continuous and categorical.

Continuous variables (also called dimensional, quantitative, or interval variables) are those consisting of continuous integers, fractions, or decimals, in which equal distances exist between successive intervals. Age, systolic blood pressure, and serum sodium concentration are all examples of continuous variables.

Categorical variables (also called discrete variables) are those in which the measured attribute or event is placed into one of two or more discrete categories. Categorical variables may be either *dichotomous* (2 categories) or *polychotomous* (3 or more categories). Examples of dichotomous variables include vital status (dead vs alive), treatment (surgical vs medical) in a two-arm clinical trial, yes vs no responses to a question, and sex. Polychotomous variables can be either nominal or ordinal. *Nominal variables* consist of named categories that bear no ordered relationship to one another, e.g., hair color, identity of operating surgeon, or country of origin. With *ordinal variables,* the categories are ordered or ranked. Unlike continuous variables, the intervals between categories need not be equal. For example, post-operative pain might be measured using the following four ranked categories of severity: none, mild, moderate, and severe.

The different types of variables are summarized in Table I.

TABLE I. Types of variables (with examples).

I. Continuous (systolic blood pressure)
II. Categorical
    A. Dichotomous (vital status: dead vs alive)
    B. Polychotomous
        1. Nominal (country of origin)
        2. Ordinal (severity of post-operative pain: none, mild, moderate, severe)

Most clinical research studies involve measurement of variables in *groups* of study subjects. The groups are defined by certain characteristics of interest for the study, such as the presence or absence of a certain disease or the use of one kind of treatment versus another. The primary statistical analysis often consists of a comparison of a given variable of interest (e.g., survival, blood pressure, or post-operative infection) between the study groups. When the study variable is continuous, the overall value for the group is usually taken as the average (or *mean*) value for the individuals in the group. When the variable is categorical, the comparison between groups is based on the *rate* (proportion) of group members having the attribute.

Populations and Samples

Neither an investigator nor the public he or she intends to benefit is exclusively interested in results that apply *only* to the subjects participating in a given study. Unless the study subjects are representative of some *target population* of interest, the results will have little meaning. Since, for reasons of feasibility, the entire target population can rarely be studied, some sampling procedure, whether explicit or implicit, must usually be employed. Inferences about the target population will be valid only to the extent that the sample is *representative* of that population.

The best way of ensuring representativeness is by *random sampling,* in which a random number table or some other procedure based on pure chance (e.g., rolling a die or flipping a coin) is used to create the study sample. When random numbers are used, a 50% sample can be obtained by selecting all subjects corresponding to even (or odd) numbers. (For a 10% sample, those whose numbers are divisible by 10 are chosen, etc.) *Systematic* (e.g., alternate, every tenth) *sampling* may result in a representative sample, but if there is any inherent ordering in the population, the sample may be distorted (non-representative). The most common method of sampling is called *convenience sampling,* in which a group of study subjects who either happen to show up or are readily accessible to the investigator are chosen for study. For feasibility reasons, convenience sampling is often unavoidable, but it then becomes difficult to identify the target population such a sample represents.

Another important aspect of sampling is *sampling variation,* which refers to the chance variation in a sample statistic such as the mean (for continuous variables) or rate (for categorical variables). A small sample thus might, just by chance, have a mean or rate that differs considerably from that of the entire population, even if the sample is truly random. Repeated small samples from the same population are likely to exhibit considerable sampling variation. In contrast, repeated samples that are large enough to include almost all members of the population would yield sample means or rates that are very close to the population value and to each other. In other words, sampling variation is inversely related to the sample size.

Descriptive vs Inferential Statistics

Descriptive statistics are intended to summarize a set of individual measurements for a study sample. No contrasts or statistical inferences are made; the data are presented for their own sake. Continuous variables are described by summary measures of central location and spread. Mean urine output and median survival time are examples of central location statistics. Standard deviation and percentile ranges are the kinds of statistics used to describe spread. Rates (e.g., survival rate or treatment success rate) are the descriptive statistics most commonly used for categorical variables.

Inferential statistics is a process by which data from samples are used to make inferences about populations. It comprises two principal activities: (1) parametric estimation and (2) significance testing. In *parametric estimation,* inferences are drawn about *parameters*[*] (mathematical descriptors such as the rate, mean, or standard deviation) in a population based on *parametric estimators* obtained in a sample. This activity includes the calculation of *confidence intervals* around sample means and rates. *Significance testing* is the major focus of inferential statistics and consists of the calculation of the P values (probabilities) that

---

[*]Many people use the term "parameter" as a synonym for "variable". Although this is common in everyday parlance, we will avoid it in this chapter and restrict the use of "parameter" to its accepted statistical meaning.

have become so important in modern scientific investigation.

It must be emphasized that statistical inference is not the same thing as *analytic inference*. In analytic inference, we are concerned with how representative the study sample is of the target population and the absence of bias in the design and execution of the study. Statistical inference, on the other hand, *assumes* the sample is obtained randomly (and is therefore representative). It is based purely on sampling variation and concerns the role of chance in extrapolating the sample results to the population.

TABLE II. Age distribution of 250 post-cholecystectomy patients.

Age (years)	Number (%) of Patients
16–20	2 (0.5)
21–25	2 (0.5)
26–30	5 (2.0)
31–35	9 (3.6)
36–40	17 (6.8)
41–45	31 (12.4)
46–50	83 (33.2)
51–55	46 (18.4)
56–60	35 (14.0)
61–65	20 (8.0)
Total	250 (100)

Descriptive Statistics and Data Display

Continuous Variables

Perhaps the most informative method for summarizing and displaying a set of measurements for a continuous variable is by constructing a *frequency distribution*. This is accomplished by categorizing the continuous data (i.e., breaking down the range of observed values into a series of successive categories) and counting the number of study subjects whose measurements fall within each category. The frequency distribution can be displayed in either tabular or graphic form. The usual graphic form is the *histogram*, a bar graph in which the rate for each category is proportional to the *area* of the corresponding bar. If the investigator wants the *heights* of the bars to reflect the rates for each category, he or she needs to ensure that the *width* of each bar (i.e., the upper minus the lower limit for each category) is the same.

Suppose, for example, that you want to describe the age distribution of 250 patients undergoing cholecystectomy in your surgical department within a given time period. If you choose ten 5-year age categories, the results might look like those shown in Table II. The corresponding histogram appears in Figure 1. Because there is a total of only 9 patients in the three youngest age categories, it might be advisable to "collapse" them into a single category, 16–30 years. In that case, the height of the corresponding histogram bar should be 3, rather than 9, so that the total area of the bar remains proportional to the overall rate for the enlarged category:

$$[(3)(15) = 45 = (2)(5) + (2)(5) + (5)(5)]$$

In addition to these tabular and graphic methods, continuous variables can often be sum-

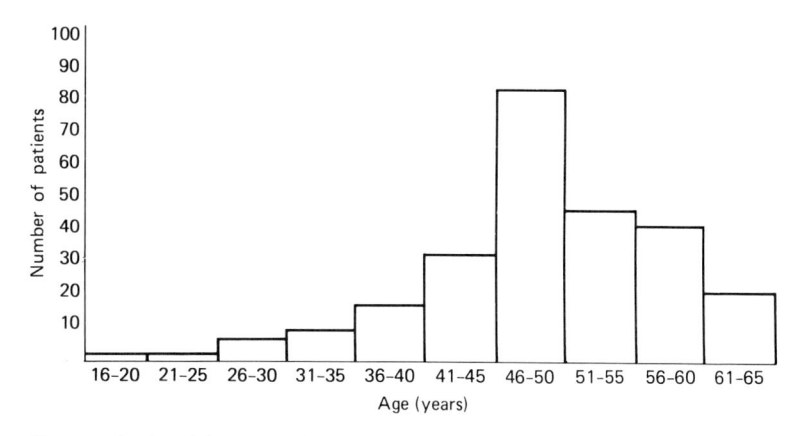

FIGURE 1. Age histogram for 250 post-cholecystectomy patients.

marized using simple statistics that describe the distribution of individual values in the sample. Two major characteristics of the distribution are usually described: central tendency and spread.

Three measures are in common use for describing central tendency: the *mean,* the median, and the mode. The mean (or average) is the sum of all values divided by the number of values. The *median* is the value of the middle member of the group. The *mode,* the measure of central tendency, used more often, is the value that appears most often. The calculation of each of these three measures is illustrated below for the serum creatinine measurements (in mg/dl, arranged in ascending order) in a sample of 15 patients:

0.3, 0.6, 0.6, 0.7, 0.8, 0.8, 0.8, 0.9, 1.0, 1.0
1.1, 1.3, 1.4, 1.6, 2.1

mean = 15.0/15 = 1.0 mg/dl
median = 8th value = 0.9 mg/dl
mode = 0.8 mg/dl

Four types of statistics are commonly used to describe the spread of a distribution: range, percentile ranges, variance, and standard deviation. The *range* is the interval between the lowest and highest value in the distribution. A *percentile range* is an interval between two percentile points. Thus the inner 90 percentile range includes all values between the 5th and 95th percentile; the inner quartile range includes those between the 25th and 75th percentiles. The *variance* is defined as follows:

$$\text{variance} = \frac{\Sigma(x_i - \bar{x})^2}{n - 1}$$

where x_i = the individual values,
$\bar{x}$ = the mean (average) value of the study group,
n = the sample size (the number of subjects in the study group),
and Σ = the Greek symbol used to denote summing all the $(x_i - \bar{x})^2$ for each x_i in the group

The *standard deviation* (SD) is the square root of the variance:

$$SD = \sqrt{\frac{\Sigma(x_i - \bar{x})^2}{n - 1}}.$$

The quantity $n-1$ is called the *degrees of freedom.* The rationale for its use is based on the fact that, for a given mean $\bar{x}$, $n-1$ x_i's are considered free or independent, since the nth value of x is determined by $\bar{x}$ and all the other x_i's. The standard deviation can also be expressed as a proportion, or percentage, of the mean value. This entity $SD/\bar{x}$ is called the *coefficient of variation.*

The range and percentile ranges can be used for any distribution, regardless of its shape. The standard deviation is best reserved for sample data that are distributed fairly symmetrically around the sample mean, because it is affected by extreme (very high or very low) values. It is most appropriate when the distribution is what statisticians call *normal.*

The *normal,* or *Gaussian, distribution* is the most important distribution in statistics. This is the well-known bell-shaped curve that not only describes the distribution of many traits (e.g., height, blood pressure, and intelligence) in the general population, but also serves as the basis for the inferential statistics of means to be discussed on pages 77–78.

The standard deviation is a particularly useful descriptor of spread for data that are normally distributed, because the proportions of values that lie within intervals defined by multiples of the SD are known:

68.3% lie within ± 1 SD from the mean
95.4% lie within ± 2 SD from the mean
99.7% lie within ± 3 SD from the mean

Despite these attractive properties, it must be emphasized that the term "normal", when used to describe this distribution, has absolutely nothing to do with the usual clinical connotation of the word indicating absence of disease.

There is one other statistic that is often encountered in the medical literature as a descriptor of spread: the *standard error of the mean* (SEM), which is defined as

$$SEM = \left(\frac{SD}{\sqrt{n}}\right)$$

where n is the sample size (number of subjects in the study group).

Because the SEM decreases with increasing sample size, it is *not* a good descriptor of the spread of a distribution, despite its popularity. A large sample with a high standard deviation may have a small standard error. Since the standard error is always smaller than the standard deviation, it tends to give the impression that the spread of the data is less than it really is. Consequently, it may be favored by authors who wish to minimize, rather than illustrate, the variability of their data.

The SEM is actually the SD of a distribution of *means* obtained in repeated sampling from a population. As we shall see later, it is important in making inferences based on sample means. As a descriptor, however, its use should be avoided.

Categorical Variables

A categorical variable is best described by the rate, or proportion, of study subjects falling within each category of the variable. Suppose you are interested in describing the outcome in the sample of 250 cholecystectomy patients mentioned earlier. If the outcome of interest is the (dichotomous) presence or absence of right upper quadrant pain 6 months postoperatively, the result can be expressed as a proportion or percentage. Thus if 140 patients are pain-free at 6 months, the overall rate for the sample is 140/250, or 56%. Although such a result could be represented visually in a table or graph, a single rate or percentage is usually sufficient to convey the information. The proportion of patients still experiencing pain is, of course, $1 - 140/250 = 110/250$, or $100 - 56\% = 44\%$.

When rates for a polychotomous variable are described, tables and graphs are often helpful. Suppose, for example, that your 6-month follow-up variable comprises the following four ordinal categories: more pain, no change (from pre-operative pain status), less pain, and no pain. (Assume that this scale has specific criteria that produce reproducible, valid measurements.) The hypothetical results in the 250 study patients can then be described as follows: 15/250 (6%) with more pain, 25/250 (10%) with no change, 70/250 (28%) with less pain, and 140/250 (56%) (as above) with no pain. The sum of the proportions must equal 1, and that of the percentages, 100%. When many categories are involved, the use of a table, histogram, or pie chart can often aid the reader to appreciate the relative proportions in each category. A pie chart achieves the same effect as a histogram by dividing a circle into slices that correspond in size to the respective proportions.

Hypothesis Testing and P Values

Formulating and Testing a Research Hypothesis

There are four steps in the execution of a research project (see Table III). The first is the statement of a *research hypothesis*. The research hypothesis is what the researcher thinks might happen. It can usually be posed in the form of a statement or question. Consider the example of a clinical trial of medical vs surgical (coronary artery bypass grafting) therapy in patients with left main-stem coronary obstruction. The research hypothesis might be expressed as a statement, "Surgery leads to longer survival than medical therapy" or as a question: "Does surgery lead to longer survival than medical therapy?"

The second step in carrying out a research project is the *design* of a study that will test the research hypothesis adequately and without bias. This aspect has already been dealt with in Chapter 2 of this Section. After the design has been carefully laid out, the study is begun and the *data* are *collected*—the third step. The fourth step is the *statistical analysis* of the data.

In the conventional approach to testing for statistical significance, the researcher usually examines the data obtained in the study with respect to a *null hypothesis*. The null hypothesis is a theoretical construct, postulating that there is no difference between the study groups. When two groups are being compared, the null hypothesis states that the two groups are random samples from the same target population.

Note that the null hypothesis is usually quite different from the research hypothesis. The investigator plans the research because he or she thinks a difference exists between the two groups or is suspicious enough that it might exist to make such a study worthwhile. The null hypothesis is an artificial "straw man" that provides a reference for examining the significance

TABLE III. Four steps in research.

1. Statement of research hypothesis
2. Study design
3. Data collection
4. Statistical analysis

of the data actually obtained. For our coronary bypass example, the null hypothesis is that there is no difference in survival among patients with left main stem coronary obstruction who receive surgery and those who receive medical therapy.

The null hypothesis can be the same as the research hypothesis if the researcher believes, or wants to demonstrate, that there really is no difference between the two groups. In general, however, the research and null hypotheses are entirely different. Once this distinction is clear, the testing of the null hypothesis becomes the basis for assessing the statistical significance of an observed difference.

Testing the Null Hypothesis

Our discussions shall be restricted to the consideration of data obtained from two study groups (samples). We wish to determine whether the difference obtained between the two groups is statistically significant, that is whether their underlying target populations are different. We begin testing the null hypothesis by assuming it is true, i.e., that the two groups are both random samples from the same target population. We then calculate the probability of obtaining a different at least as large as the observed difference between the two study groups under that assumption. In other words, we calculate the probability of obtaining the observed difference *by chance* if the two groups are random samples from the same population. This probability is called the *P value*.

If P is less than a certain amount (by convention, .05), we consider the null hypothesis to be sufficiently unlikely to reject it. Conversely, we are unwilling to reject the null hypothesis if P is $> .05$ because we do not consider it sufficiently unlikely. Rejecting the null hypothesis means that we conclude that the two study groups are not random samples from the same population, i.e., that they arise from two different populations. The P value "cut-off point," or threshold, for rejection of the null hypothesis, should be established *a priori*. This threshold is called the α-*level* and is conventionally set at .05.

Although .05 has come to be the accepted α-level for most studies in the medical and scientific literature, there is nothing "magic" about it. The difference between a P value of .04 and .06 is very small. The sensible scientist will keep such distinctions in their proper place and will not discard results if the P value is above .05, nor automatically accept them as proven merely because the P value is below .05. It is a fact of life, however, that the difference between P values of .04 and .06 can result in a paper being accepted or rejected for publication.

We may be wrong in rejecting the null hypothesis even if $P < .05$, but we consider the probability of being wrong acceptably low. A P value of .05 simply indicates that the results obtained could have occurred by chance 5% of the time when the null hypothesis is true. Once out of every 20 times, on average, rejecting the null hypothesis when the P value is .05 will result in an error, i.e., we will be rejecting the null hypothesis when it is true. This type of error is called a *Type I error* and we run the risk of making it whenever we reject the null hypothesis. The lower the P value, the lower the risk. With a P value of .001, there is only one chance in a thousand of making a Type I error.

Because clinical investigation is usually expensive and time-consuming, studies are often used to answer several questions at once, i.e., to test several hypotheses. Interventions may be compared for multiple outcomes, or a variety of clinical, sociodemographic, or treatment factors may be examined for their effects on one or more outcomes. When many tests of significance are performed, some significant differences are likely to arise by chance. In fact, for every 20 independent tests of the null hypothesis, one, on average, will result in statistical significance just by chance. If 100 tests are carried out and 10 are associated with P values $< .05$, it is impossible to know which of the 10 are mere chance findings and which represent "truly" significant differences.

To protect against a plethora of Type I errors, some statisticians advocate dividing the α-level required to reject the null hypothesis by the number of tests performed. Because many of the outcomes are associated with one another the probability of their joint occurrence is usually greater than the product of their individual probabilities, i.e., they are not statistically independent. Consequently, such a procedure may be overly conservative and may tend to attribute true differences to chance. At the very least, the investigator should indicate the number of tests performed in addition to the number achieving statistical significance and should moderate his inferences accordingly.

Multiple hypothesis testing becomes an even greater problem when the research hypotheses arise *post hoc*, i.e., after the data are collected, rather than *a priori*. When descriptive statistics are used to *generate* hypotheses for statistical testing, the calculated P values do not accurately reflect the true probability of a difference occurring by chance. After all, it is virtually certain that *some* differences will occur by chance. Betting on a horse after a race is not usually rewarded at the ticket window. Similarly, performing a statistical test of significance on data because they "look" different will result in significant *P* values that bear no relationship to the chance occurrence of a difference hypothesized *a priori*.

Whether we are correct or not in rejecting the null hypothesis, an observed difference that is *statistically significant* may or may not be *clinically important*. Suppose that a study comparing serum sodium concentration in two groups of patients yields means in the two groups of 140.2 and 139.9 meq/l. The difference of 0.3 meq/l is clinically trivial, despite the fact that with large sample sizes such a difference might be statistically significant. The clinical importance of the observed difference is a *clinical*, not a *statistical*, decision. Never let a colleague, statistician, or editor convince you that a low (i.e., significant) *P* value can compensate for a difference that is too small to be useful to you or your patients. As we shall see shortly, clinically important differences can fall short of achieving statistical significance, just as clinically trivial differences can occasionally be statistically significant.

We have already discussed the important distinction between the research hypothesis and the null hypothesis. We have also indicated that the research hypothesis can be put in the form of a statement or a question. Let us now consider the *directionality* or *non-directionality* of the research hypothesis and what it implies in terms of testing for statistical significance (testing the null hypothesis).

In *directional* hypothesis testing, the research hypothesis implies not only that the two groups under investigation will be different but also indicates the direction of the difference. For example, in our study of surgical vs medical therapy for patients with left main-stem coronary disease, the research hypothesis is that surgery is *better* (leads to longer survival) than medicine. In *non-directional* hypothesis testing, the investigator still examines two groups of subjects for a difference but may have no *a priori* knowledge of which group will fare better. Asked in non-directional terms, our example would read as follows: *Which* treatment leads to longer survival, surgical or medical? It cannot be overemphasized that if the research hypothesis implies a certain direction, i.e., if the investigator has a strong suspicion that one treatment is better than the other or that the outcome will be better in one group, this must be stated *before* the research is actually carried out, in other words, *before* any data are collected.

The *P* values listed in most statistical tables are associated with *non-directional* testing of the null hypothesis, i.e., the probability of obtaining the observed difference whether Group 1 is better than Group 2 or vice versa. This is called a *two-sided* test of the null hypothesis. (It is also called a *two-tailed* test, because the distributions of test statistics that are used to test the null hypothesis often contain two tails, and the *P* value is equal to the area under the curve of these two tails.)

When the research hypothesis is *directional*, a *one-sided* (*one-tailed*) test of the null hypothesis can be used. It is essential that the observed difference be in the expected direction, i.e., the direction hypothesized in the directional research hypothesis. If the investigator suspects that Group 1 is better than Group 2, but the data show the reverse, the derived *P* value will be highly misleading. The investigator would then do better to refrain from reporting any *P* value and explain that the direction of the difference was opposite to the one hypothesized. To obtain a one-sided *P* value, we simply divide the *P* value listed in a two-sided statistical table by two.

When in doubt, it is better to use a two-sided test, since this is the more conservative approach. If the research hypothesis is non-directional, a two-sided test *must* be used. When the research hypothesis is directional and the results are concordant with the direction predicted, a one-sided test can be justified. This distinction can be important, because dividing a *P* value by two (for example, $P = .08$ to $P = .04$) can create a "statistically significant" (P < .05) result, which can often determine the fate of a scientific paper.

Type II Error and Statistical Power

So far we have talked about what happens when P is less than .05 and about rejecting the null hypothesis. When P is greater than .05 (or some other chosen α-level), we do not reject the null hypothesis. The fact that the chance probability of obtaining the observed difference is greater than .05 does not prove that the null hypothesis is correct, however. It merely says that the probability is not low enough to reject it. Failing to reject the null hypothesis does not validate it.

If P equals .10, for example, the probability of obtaining the observed difference, under the assumption that the null hypothesis is true, remains unlikely (this is equivalent to a horse with 9-to-1 odds winning a race), but by convention, we do not consider it unlikely *enough* to reject the null hypothesis. Whenever we accept the null hypothesis, i.e., whenever the P value is not low enough to reject it, we risk making another sort of error. This is called a *Type II error* and it can occur only when the null hypothesis is not rejected. This is important to remember. When we reject the null hypothesis, we run the risk of making a Type I error and the probability of our doing so is equal to the P value. When we do not reject the null hypothesis, we run the risk of a Type II error, i.e., the null hypothesis might still be untrue and the study groups are not samples from the same target population. These relationships are illustrated in Table IV.

As mentioned before, the magnitude of the observed difference may be clinically important even if it does not achieve statistical significance. This is especially likely to occur when the sample size is small. Suppose that our coronary artery bypass trial included only 3 patients in each group. Because sampling variation is very large with such small sample sizes (see earlier discussion), even if all 3 patients die in one group and all 3 survive in the other, the difference would not be statistically significant. Thus any investigator who wants to argue that two groups are *not* different merely needs to restrict the number of study subjects to guarantee that no statistically significant difference will be found. The argument remains unconvincing, however, because the risk of a Type II error is high.

The probability, β, of a Type II error can be calculated by constructing an *alternative hypothesis* in which the observed difference is compared to some difference determined *a priori* to be of potential clinical importance. 1-β is called *statistical power* and is the probability of detecting some specified, potentially important difference. If a researcher wants to "prove" the null hypothesis, i.e., if the research hypothesis is that no difference exists between the study groups, he or she needs to show that the probability of the alternative hypothesis being correct is very low. The higher the statistical power, the lower the risk of missing (failing to detect) a difference that is potentially clinically important. In other words, to *validate* rather than just fail to reject the null hypothesis, Type II error must be minimized. The probability of committing a Type II error is determined by the magnitude of the hypothesized difference under the alternative hypothesis, the magnitude of the observed difference, the sample size, and (for continuous variables) the variability of the data.

TABLE IV. The two errors of hypothesis testing (H_0 = null hypothesis).

	Truth	
Inference	H_0 False	H_0 True
Reject H_0	Correct	Type I Error
Do not reject H_0	Type II Error	Correct

Since sample size is the only one of these determinants that is directly controllable by the investigator, sample size is the most important consideration in the planning of a research project for an investigator who wishes to minimize the possibility of a Type II error and maximize statistical power.

Inferential Statistics of Means

Repetitive Sampling and the Central Limit Theorem

Suppose we chose a random sample from some infinitely large source population with known mean μ and standard deviation σ, determined the sample mean $\bar{x}$, replaced the sample, then chose another random sample of the same size, and so on.* What distribution would the *means* of those repeated samples have? It turns out that if n, the size of each sample, is large enough, then the $\bar{x}$'s form a normal distribution, regardless of the distribution of the source population. The mean of this *sampling distribution* of $\bar{x}$'s is the same as the population mean μ; its standard deviation (called the standard error of the mean, or SEM) is $\sigma/\sqrt{n}$.

These interesting and useful facts derive from the *Central Limit Theorem*, one of the main pillars of statistical theory. What requirements must be met for the Central Limit Theorem to apply? The main requirement is that n be large enough. How large is "large enough" depends on the distribution of the source population. If it is very close to normal, n can be as small as 2 or 3; if it is quite non-normal (particularly if highly skewed in one direction), n may have to be 50 or even 100.

These properties of the Central Limit Theorem would only be of theoretical interest if their application depended on actual repetitive sampling. In the real world of clinical investigation, the investigator has no chance to observe or make use of the distribution of means of repeated samples from a target population. The Central Limit Theorem, however, tells us the mean and standard deviation of the normal distribution that *would* result from repetitive sampling.

By comparing the actual mean obtained in a study sample with the mean and standard deviation of the theoretical sampling distribution of means, the investigator can determine the likelihood (i.e., the probability) of obtaining such a sample assuming that it originated from the source population of the theoretical sampling distribution. Thus, he (or she) can calculate a P value representing the probability that the sample mean observed would occur in random sampling from a source population with a given mean and standard deviation.

Unfortunately, the use of the normal distribution to test the statistical significance of a difference between a single sample mean and a known population mean depends on knowing the population standard deviation, σ. To test the significance of a sample mean when σ is unknown, a different sampling distribution, the so-called *t-distribution*, is required. The *t*-distribution was discovered by William S. Gosset, a statistician working at the Guinness Brewery in the early years of this century. To avoid a possible adverse reaction by his employer, Gosset published his observations under the name of Student. Most of Gosset's experiments involved small samples from unknown source populations, and he found that the normal distribution was unsatisfactory for making inferences about the means of his samples.

The *t* sampling distribution differs from the normal sampling distribution in that, although its mean is the same (namely, the population mean μ), its standard error, $s/\sqrt{n}$, uses the *sample* standard deviation s, rather than the population standard deviation σ. Like the normal distribution, the *t*-distribution is bell-shaped. Its two "tails," however, are higher than the tails of the normal distribution. Thus, the calculated *P* values, which correspond to the area under the curve of the tails, are higher (i.e., less significant) for a given difference between the sample and population means.

Unlike the normal distribution, there is a different *t*-distribution according to the number of

---

* Although avoiding excessive use of algebraic symbols is desirable, a certain minimum is required for clarity and economy of expression. The usual convention is to use small Roman letters to indicate sample statistics and small Greek letters for the correponding population parameters. The sample and population means are usually represented by $\bar{x}$ and μ, and the standard deviations by s and σ, respectively.

degress of freedom (n-1). For small samples, the difference from the normal distribution is quite marked. For large samples ($n \geq 30$), the t distribution is quite close to the normal distribution and the latter can be used for making inferences.

Statistical Inferences Using the t-Distribution

As mentioned in the last section, the t-distribution (or, for large samples, the normal distribution) can be used to test for a statistically significant difference between a sample mean and a known population mean. It can also be used to construct a *confidence interval* around a sample mean. Such a confidence interval consists of the sample mean plus or minus a multiple of the sample standard error and represents the range in which the investigator can be "confident" that the true population mean lies. A 95% confidence interval represents the range in which the population mean can be expected to lie 95% of the time, based on the sample mean and standard error. An investigator who wants to be more confident, e.g., 99%, needs to extend the interval. Formulas for calculating such intervals are provided in several standard biostatistics texts (1–4).

The most common use of the t-distribution is in testing the significance of a difference in two sample means. If one were to randomly choose two samples at a time from a given (hypothetical) source pouplation, replace the two samples, choose two new samples of the same size, and so on, the *differences* between the two sample means would be normally distributed, provided the source population and sample size do not grossly violate the assumptions of the Central Limit Theorem. In the real world in which an investigator wishes to test for a statistically significant difference between the means of two study groups, he (or she) uses the observed difference in means and the standard error of the difference. Under the null hypothesis that the two study groups represent random samples from the same source population, he can then test the observed difference using the t-distribution.

This is the so-called *Student's t-test* (after Gossett) for unpaired (or independent) samples. In effect, the t-test compares the magnitude of the observed difference to the variability of the difference as represented by the standard error. If the size of the difference is large with respect to its standard error, the calculated P value will be small ($< .05$), the null hypothesis is rejected, and the difference is declared statistically significant. The formula for the t-test, as well as instructions for using the t-tables for determining P values, are provided in the previously cited texts (1–4).

When two study groups represent matched pairs, the *paired t-test* is a statistically more efficient technique. A matched pair analysis of means is appropriate whenever (1) each subject from one study group is matched to a subject from the other group or (2) the same subject receives each of two study maneuvers. An example of the first type might be a comparison of blood pressure reduction with arterioplasty vs medical therapy in patients with hypertension caused by renal artery obstruction, in which the patients were pair-matched for age, sex, pretreatment blood pressure, and the presence or absence of pretreatment cardiac decompensation. The second type is represented by the crossover trial. In a clinical trial comparing two oral antihypertensive agents, for example, each patient might be tried sequentially on the two agents. Differential treatment of paired organs represents another example of this type, as illustrated by the use of one topical anti-glaucoma agent in one eye and a second anti-glaucoma drug in the other eye of patients with bilateral disease.

In the paired t-test, statistical significance is based on the differences observed between the two values for each pair. The pairing results in greater statistical efficiency, i.e., a smaller sample size is required to demonstrate statistical significance, because the variability between members of a pair is typically less than that of two unrelated subjects. By eliminating or greatly reducing all sources of intra-pair variability *other* than that caused by the study maneuver, any given mean difference will have a greater chance of achieving statistical significance. The formula for the paired t-test can be found in previously cited texts (1–4). Crossover trials require several additional statistical considerations, and the interested reader is referred to an excellent recent review (5).

Calculating of Sample Sizes

In the planning (design) stage of clinical investigation, one of the most important questions that the researcher needs to ask is "How many patients (or rats, tissue culture samples, etc.) do I need to study?" To be protected against a Type II error and, in particular, against obtaining a difference that may be clinically important but not quite statistically significant, the investigator must specify, in advance, the difference in means considered clinically worth detecting and the statistical power (1-β, where β is the probability of a Type II error) desired to detect this difference. The investigator must also estimate (perhaps by consulting the results of previous studies) the standard deviation expected in the sample. Formulas are provided in standard texts (1,2,4).

A far greater (often 2- to 4-fold) sample size is usually required to protect against Type II error than to demonstrate statistical significance. Consequently, the temptation to ignore Type II error is strong, especially when patients are involved, because the calculated sample sizes are smaller and therefore easier to achieve at a single center over a reasonable period of time. Despite its attractions, such a practice is perilous because the investigator may well find it impossible to make *any* inference at all.

Let us take another look at our study of arterioplasty vs medical therapy for renovascular hypertension. Suppose the surgeon-investigator specifies a difference of 10 mm Hg in diastolic blood pressure as a clinically important difference that is worth detecting. He estimates his sample standard deviation and, ignoring Type II error, calculates his required sample size. But suppose the study is then carried out with the calculated sample size and the results show a 9 mm Hg difference favoring surgery. Because the sample size calculation was based on a 10 mm difference, the 9 mm difference is not statistically significant. The surgeon may not consider the 9 mm difference as clinically important, but how sure can he be that the true difference (under the alternative hypothesis) is not 10 mm or even larger? Not very sure, unfortunately, and he is left in a situation where he can neither say there is a clinically important difference nor that there is not. The dangers of this Scylla and Charibdis can be avoided only by considering Type II error (statistical power) in the sample size calculation.

Many investigators, faced with the above results, would be tempted to enroll additional patients in the study in an effort to achieve statistical significance for the 9 mm Hg difference. There are two problems with such an approach. First, repeated significance testing increases the risk of detecting a significant difference by chance alone, i.e., of commiting a Type I error. If results are repeatedly analyzed, the P values calculated from the t-tests will underestimate the true risk of a Type I error (see the discussion of multiple significant tests). Second, if the null hypothesis is in fact true, subsequent results may show a difference smaller than 9 mm Hg, and the difference may fail to achieve statistical significance despite the larger sample size.

Nonparametric Tests

The t-test (paired or unpaired) is the significance test of choice in comparing two means, provided the requirements of the Central Limit Theorem are met. Unless sample sizes are quite small, however, the underlying source populations may exhibit considerable departure from normality without disturbing, to an important degree, the sampling distribution of means or difference in means. In statistical parlance, we say that the t-test is *robust*. Many investigators who have had some exposure to statistics have the quite mistaken notion that the t-test can only be used when source populations are normally distributed. Such is not the case.

When the requirements of the Central Limit Theorem are grossly violated, alternative analytic strategies are required. This is particularly likely to occur with small samples from highly skewed source populations. Variables with zero as the obligatory lower boundary often exhibit skewed distributions, with many low values and fewer and fewer high values extending out into a long tail. Examples include length of hospitalization and the dose of drug required to produce a given clinical effect.

Faced with a highly skewed distribution, the investigator has two main choices. He (or she) can either *transform* the native data in a way that normalizes the distribution (e.g., by taking their logarithms), or use a *non-parametric* test. Non-parametric tests differ from the *t*-test and other *parametric tests* because they do not depend on using sampling distributions of parametric estimators (such as the mean) obtained in samples to make inferences about the corresponding population parameters. In other words, they require no assumptions about underlying distributions.

To use a non-parametric test of two continuous variables, the actual magnitudes are ignored and only the *ranks* (i.e., relative magnitudes) are used to calculate statistical significance. In the unpaired test [the *Mann–Whitney U test* (1,6,7)], each member of one study group is compared to every member of the other group, and a "winner" is declared for each comparison. The total number of wins in each group (called the *U* statistic) is calculated and then compared to the totals that would be expected if the wins were distributed by chance. In the paired test the *Wilcoxon signed rank test* (1–3,6), the magnitude of the differences (ignoring the sign) between each matched pair are ranked, assigning the rank 1 to the smallest difference, and the sums of the ranks are compared in those pairs with positive differences and those with negative differences. Under the null hypothesis, these sums should be equal and the actual result can be referred to the chance-expected distribution of sums around a median of 0.

Although non-parametric tests of means have the advantage of requiring no assumptions, the use of relative magnitudes or ranks rather than actual values may result in a loss of statistical efficiency and, therefore, in more conservative statistical inferences. To maximize statistical efficiency, it is sometimes preferable to use the *t*-test even if prior logarithmic or other transformation of highly skewed data is required.

Comparing Three or More Means

So far, we have restricted our discussion to testing the statistical significance of a difference in two means. To compare the means of three or more groups, the investigator uses a procedure called a *one-way analysis of variance* (ANOVA). The assumptions are similar to those required for the *t*-test, and the null hypothesis is that the groups are equivalent, i.e., that they represent random samples from the same hypothetical source population. In essence, the procedure divides the total variance (the square of the standard deviation) of all study subjects into two portions: (1) that part accounted for by differences among the groups (the inter-group variance); and (2) that part accounted for by differences between subjects within the same group (the intra-group variance). The larger the former relative to the latter, the less likely it is that the differences among group means are due to chance.

The primary result of a one-way ANOVA is a *P* value representing a test of the null hypothesis. If $P < .05$, we conclude that the group means are not equivalent. If the investigator is interested in finding out which group or groups are responsible for the overall difference, pairs of groups can be compared two at a time, but *P* values must be adjusted to account for multiple testing. Different procedures are available for carrying out such secondary analyses, and the interested reader may wish to consult an appropriate reference (1).

Sometimes, an investigator may wish to study the effects of two or more treatments or other study factors simultaneously. In the example of arterioplasty vs medical therapy in renovascular hypertension, the investigator may be interested in studying the effect of gender, as well as treatment, on the outcome (diastolic blood pressure). Although a separate *t*-test could be performed for males and females, a *two-way analysis of variance* (ANOVA) provides greater statistical efficiency and an opportunity to test for gender effects independent of treatment. Provided the sample size is sufficient to yield adequate numbers in each subgroup, ANOVA methods can be extended (three-way, four-way, etc.) for larger numbers of study effects.

Control for Confounding Factors

In many clinical investigations, a simple comparison of two or more group means may be biased by confounding differences between groups. Consider once again our example of arterioplasty vs medical therapy for renovascular hypertension, in which the major outcome is diastolic blood pressure 6 months after initiating treatment. If the surgical group has lower pretreatment blood pressure, on average, than the medical group, a lower posttreatment diastolic pressure in the surgical group might be due to the pretreatment difference rather than the surgery. Such a confounding effect could even occur in a randomized trial in which patients were randomly assigned to medical vs surgical therapy if the random treatment assignment yielded a maldistribution of pretreatment blood pressures, unlikely as that would be.

We have already mentioned one way of controlling for such a confounding factor, namely pair-wise matching. For example, each surgical patient could be matched by pretreatment diastolic pressure (e.g., ± 5 mm Hg) with a medical patient, and a paired t-test could be used to test for a significant difference. A second strategy would be to stratify all study patients according to the confounder (e.g., 90–99 mm Hg, 100–109 mm Hg, and ≥ 110 mm Hg) and then compare the stratum-specific group means.

The most convenient strategy, in this day of prepackaged computer software programs, may be to *adjust* the group means according to the outcome each subject would have if he had the mean value of the confounder. (This adjustment assumes that the relationship between the confounder and the outcome is known, e.g., pretreatment and posttreatment diastolic pressures, respectively, in our example. Most frequently, a linear correlation is assumed. Linear correlation will be considered in greater detail on pages 84–86.) This procedure is called *analysis of covariance* (ANCOVA) or covariate adjustment and can be used for any number of continuous and dichotomous categorical variables (1, 8). It can be combined with the study of multiple study effects by using multiple-way ANCOVA.

Inferential Statistics of Rates and Proportions

Comparing Two Proportions

When the outcome variable under analysis is categorical rather than continuous, the main statistical procedure is a comparison of rates (proportions) rather than means. When there are two study groups and the outcome variable is dichotomous, the comparison is between two proportions. As an example, consider a comparison of postoperative wound infection rates in patients treated pre-operatively with broad-spectrum antibiotics and those treated with placebo. Suppose we randomized treatment assignment in 500 consecutive laparotomy patients, with 240 receiving the antibiotic and 260 receiving the placebo, and that the subsequent infection rates were 7/240 (2.9%) and 15/260 (5.8%), respectively. The data can be displayed in a 2 × 2 (four-fold) table, as shown in Table V. The row totals are the total numbers of patients receiving antibiotic and placebo; the column totals are the total numbers of patients with and without wound infections. In 2 × 2 tables, the greater the difference between two proportions (e.g., the proportions of antibiotic and placebo recipients with post-operative wound infections), the greater the association of the columns with the rows. In our example, we are interested in testing whether there is a statistically significant association between post-operative wound infection (columns) and pre-operative treatment (rows).

To test for such an association, we establish a null hypothesis of no association and then assess the probability that the observed association arose solely by chance. (This is equivalent to saying that the two treatment groups arose by random sampling from the same source population with a single infection rate.) Because the null hypothesis of no association indicates that the columns should be independent of the rows, we thus calculate the frequency we would *expect* in each of the four cells of the 2 × 2 table under the null hypothesis of statistical independence. If the observed frequencies differ sufficiently from the frequencies expected under the null hypothesis, we reject the null hypothesis and conclude that the columns and rows are not independent, i.e., that they are associated.

How do we calculate the expected cell frequencies? The probability that two independent events will both occur is the product of their individual probabilities. (For example, the probability of simultaneously obtaining a heads on a coin flip and a 6 on a die roll is (1/2)(1/6) = 1/12.) The probability of being in a given row is the same as the proportion of the total sample N lying in that row, i.e., r_i/N, the row total divided by the total sample size. Similarly, the probability of being in a given column is c_j/N.

TABLE V. Post-laparotomy wound infection after preoperative antibiotic vs placebo.

	Infection	No Infection	
Antibiotic	7	233	240
Placebo	15	245	260
	22	478	500

Thus the probability of being in a given cell (i.e., the two independent events of being in a given row *and* a given column) is $(r_i/N)(c_j/N)$, or $r_i c_j / N^2$. The expected cell frequency (E_{ij}) is then simply the probability of being in a given cell times the total sample size: $E_{ij} = (r_i c_j / N^2)(N) = r_i c_j / N$. For the example shown in Table V, the expected frequency for the upper left cell (antibiotic recipients with post-operative wound infections) is calculated as

$$E = \frac{(240)(22)}{500} = 10.6$$

In each cell of the table, we now have both an observed (O) and an expected (E) frequency. The only thing we lack is a statistical method for comparing the O's with the E's to see whether we should reject the null hypothesis.

χ^2 is a statistic with a known frequency distribution that allows us to calculate P values from observed (O_{ij}) and expected (E_{ij}) cell frequencies. It is defined as:

$$\chi^2 = \Sigma \frac{(O_{ij} - E_{ij})^2}{E_{ij}}.$$

It can be calculated by computing the expected frequency (E_{ij}) for each cell, subtracting it from the observed frequency (O_{ij}) in the table, squaring the resulting difference, dividing by the expected frequency, and then summing this ratio over all four cells in the table. [Various algebraically equivalent, but computationally more convenient, formulas for calculating χ^2 are found in most statistics texts (1, 3–9).] The larger the value for χ^2, the more the observed frequencies differ from those expected under the null hypothesis and the smaller (i.e., the more significant) the P value.

As with the *t*-distribution, a different χ^2 distribution exists for each different number of degrees of freedom. For χ^2, however, the number of degrees of freedom is based, not on the total sample size, but on the number of rows and columns:

degrees of freedom = $(r-1)(c-1)$,
where r = the number of rows and
c = the number of columns.

For a 2 × 2 table, degrees of freedom = $(2-1)(2-1) = 1$. This makes initiutive sense, because the marginal (row and column) totals are considered fixed in calculating the expected cell frequencies. With fixed marginals in a 2 × 2 table, the value in any one cell automatically determines the other three.

The theoretical χ^2 frequency distribution is a smooth, continuous curve. Because observed frequencies are discrete, so are the calculated values of χ^2. When N is very large, many more values are possible for O_{ij} and thus for χ^2, and the distribution of calculated values begins to approach the theoretical distribution. A wound infection rate of 7 out of 240 might represent any number from 6 1/2 to 7 1/2, i.e., a similar group of 2400 patients would have observed frequencies anywhere from 65 to 75. Some statisticians feel that when N is small, a *continuity correction* is required to compensate for the fact that the discrete possible values do not closely approximate the continuous distribution. In 1934, Frank Yates decided to subtract 1/2, arbitrarily, from the absolute value of each $O_{ij} - E_{ij}$ to provide a better approximation. The resulting χ^2 with continuity correction, (χ_c^2), is defined as follows:

$$\chi_c^2 = \Sigma \frac{(|O_{ij} - E_{ij}| - \frac{1}{2})^2}{E_{ij}}$$

where | | indicates absolute value (i.e., a minus sign becomes positive). χ_c^2 is then interpreted in the same way as the uncorrected χ^2.

The continuity correction results in smaller values for χ^2 and, consequently, in statistical inferences that are more conservative. In other words, the null hypothesis is less likely to be rejected. The lower risk of Type I error must be balanced against a greater risk of Type II error. For large samples, the continuity correction is probably unnecessary, but for small samples the P values obtained using χ_c^2 will be closer to the exact probability calculated using a purely stochastic (chance-based) model.

When expected cell frequencies are very small (< 5), the χ^2 test, even with the continuity correction, should be avoided. The statistical test of choice in such a situation is the *Fisher exact probability test* (1–3,9). The *P* values calculated with the Fisher exact test are derived from a pure stochastic model based on permutation theory. The test requires laborious computations if performed by hand but is expeditiously executed by programs that are readily available in most computer statistical software packages. The test first examines all the 2 × 2 tables possible by chance, given the fixed marginal (row and column) totals, then determines the number of such tables with results at least as extreme (i.e., with the rows and columns associated to at least as great a degree) as those observed. Since each table is equally likely to occur by chance under the pure stochastic model, the *P* value is simply the number of tables with equal or greater association divided by the total possible number of tables.

Calculating Sample Sizes

To ensure adequate statistical power to detect a given difference in proportions and exclude such a difference if no significant difference is found, statisticians usually rely on a formula based on the normal distribution. The normal distribution can be used as a basis for this calculation because the pure stochastic model produces a frequency distribution, called the *binomial distribution*, that closely approximates the normal distribution, provided the expected cell frequencies are all 5 or more.

Assuming an α-level of .05, the investigator must specify two additional components to permit the sample size calculation: p_1 and p_2; the proportions he or she estimates in the two groups, such that p_1-p_2 represents the minimum threshold for a clinically important difference; and 1-β, the statistical power desired to ensure that a difference as large as p_1-p_2 in the hypothetical source population will be detected. Once these components have been specified, the investigator may use a standard formula (1,2,9) or consult the derived tables provided by Fleiss (9).

Comparing Three or More Proportions

The χ^2 test is easily extended to comparisons of three or more proportions, although this is not the case with χ^2_c or the Fisher exact text. χ^2 is still defined as $\Sigma(O_{ij} - E_{ij})^2/E_{ij}$ and is interpreted at $(r-1)(c-1)$ degrees of freedom. When the outcome variable is ordinal, however, the χ^2 test does not take account of the inherent order among the categories used to measure the variable. It merely tests the signifance of the observed-expected differences across all the $r \times c$ cells of the table.

Consider, for example, a 6-month follow-up comparison of ankle swelling (none, mild, or severe) in patients with ligamentous injuries treated with surgery versus those treated conservatively (cast only). With a χ^2 test, none, mild, and severe are treated as simple nominal, non-ordered categories of swelling. Such a test of mere association between columns and rows may be statistically inefficient, because it fails to account for the *direction* of the association. For example, the χ^2 test makes no distinction between results showing more instances of severe swelling with casts and more instances of mild and no swelling with surgery (surgery clearly better than casts) and those showing more instances of mild swelling with surgery and *both* more instances of severe *and* more instances of non-swelling with casts (surgery more likely to produce intermediate results).

One alternative to the χ^2 test that does take order into account is the *Mann–Whitney* test. This test is the same non-parametric test described on page 80 and is based on comparing the ranks, or relative magnitudes, of all subjects in both groups. With only three categories in our example, there will be many ties, but the procedure may nevertheless provide an improvement in efficiency over the χ^2 test.

Control for Confounding Factors

Comparisons of proportions, like comparisons of means, can be biased by confounding differences between the study groups. For example, in our study of surgical repair vs casts in patients with ligamentous ankle injuries, a result showing less swelling in the surgically treated group at 6-month follow-up would be biased if the patients in that group were younger, on average, than those in the group treated with casts. Surgeons might be understandably reluctant to operate on older patients with such injuries, but the younger patients might be expected to do better regardless of treatment. Thus a fair test of the treatment effect should control for the confounding effect of age.

Because our discussion can be greatly simplified by focusing on dichotomous outcomes, we shall "dichotomize" ankle swelling as absent or mild, (clinically unimportant) vs severe, i.e., clinically important. One way of controlling for the confounding effect of age would be to pair-match surgically and non-surgically treated patients by age, e.g., ± 5 years. A matched-pair χ^2 test, called the *McNemar test*, can then be performed and the result can be interpreted in the same way as the usual χ^2 test (1–3,9,10). A second strategy would be to stratify the study group by age category (e.g., ≤ 40 years vs > 40 years) and then calculate the stratum-specific χ^2's or an overall χ^2 weighted by the size of the individual strata, the *Mantel-Haenszel χ^2 test* (1,9,10).

In the case of multiple confounders, two multivariate adjustment techniques are most commonly used: *discriminant function analysis* and *multiple logistic regression*. The latter is generally preferable, because the validity of the former depends, to some extent, on the assumption of normally distributed source populations. Both techniques are beyond the scope of this chapter, but the interested reader will find excellent discussions in two recent texts (11, 12).

Linear Correlation and Regression

Linear Correlation

As we have seen, a comparison of proportions is really a test of association between two categorical variables: study group (e.g., antibiotic vs placebo) and outcome (presence or absence of postoperative wound infection). Even a comparison of means can be thought of as a test of association between a categorical variable (study group, e.g., surgery vs medical therapy for renovascular hypertension) and a continuous variable (the study outcome, e.g., post-treatment diastolic pressure). But how do we measure the association between two continuous variables? The usual strategy is to examine the extent to which the relationship between the two can be described by a straight line, that is, the extent of their *linear correlation*.

Linear correlation measures the degree to which an increase in one continuous variable is associated with an exactly proportional increase or decrease in a second continuous variable.

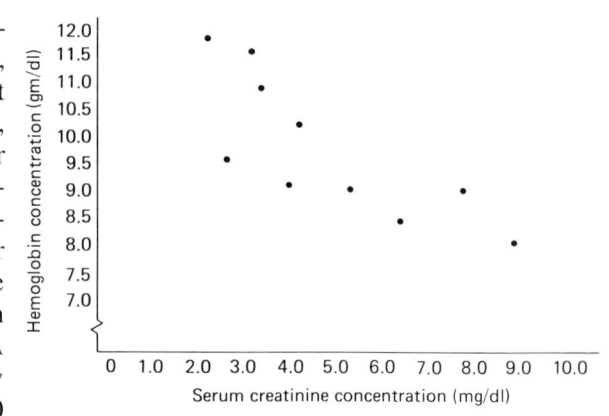

FIGURE 2. Hemoglobin and serum creatinine concentrations in 10 patients with chronic renal failure.

Consider the scatter diagram shown in Figure 2, which depicts the hemoglobin and serum creatinine concentrations in 10 patients with chronic renal failure. If every point fell exactly on a straight line, the two variables would be perfectly correlated.

The *Pearson correlation coefficient*, which is abbreviated by the letter r, is a descriptive statistic indicating the extent of linear correlation. It ranges in value from -1 to $+1$, with 0 representing no correlation, -1 a perfect inverse correlation (negatively sloping line), and $+1$ a perfect positive correlation (positively sloping line) between the two variables. For our hemoglobin-creatinine example, $r = -.78$, indicating a strong inverse correlation. It should be stressed that r indicates the extent of *linear* correlation only. Two continuous variables may have a very close relationship but poor linear correlation (e.g., a U-shaped or quadratic relationship).

Dependent and Non-Dependent Relationships

In examining the linear relationship between two continuous variables, we can often deduce, on biological grounds, whether one variable is *dependent* on the other or whether the two are *non-dependent*. In our chronic renal failure example, hemoglobin is being tested for its dependence on renal function (as represented by serum creatinine). We certainly do not believe that the creatinine depends on the hemoglobin; this type of dependency makes no biologic sense. Hemoglobin concentration is called the *dependent variable*, and serum creatinine the *independent variable*. (It is as if the creatinine were allowed to vary independently, and the hemoglobin then depended on the observed value of creatinine.) By convention, the independent variable is usually represented by the *x*-axis and the dependent variable by the *y*-axis.

In contrast to the dependent relationship between hemoglobin and creatinine, consider the relationship between blood urea nitrogen (BUN) and creatinine. The two are usually highly positively correlated because both are tests of renal function, even though other factors (e.g., state of hydration for BUN and muscle mass for creatinine) prevent the correlation from being perfect. Although both variables depend on renal function, neither depends on the other and the relationship between the two is non-dependent. In a graphical display of the relationship, either could be represented by the *y*-axis. The decision that a relationship is dependent or non-dependent arises from *clinical*, not *statistical*, reasoning.

Since the correlation between two variables is rarely perfect (i.e., r rarely equals +1 or -1), we are often interested in measuring the extent to which the relationship between the two is explained by a straight line. To do this, we make use of a concept known as *explained variance*.

We can interpret r in these terms by measuring the proportion of total variance in one variable that is due to its linear relationship with the other. (Variance was defined on page 72.) In our example of hemoglobin and creatinine, we can divide the variance in hemoglobin into: (1) a component due to the linear relatonship between hemoglobin and creatinine, and (2) a component due to undetermined causes, including random variation. It can be shown that r^2 equals the proportion of variance in either variable that is due to its linear correlation with the other. In our example, $r = -.78$, and $r^2 = .61$. Our interpretation of this value of r^2 is that the relationship between hemoglobin and serum creatinine "accounts for" 61% of the variance in hemoglobin.

Linear Regression

Linear regression is the process of fitting a straight line to bivariate continuous data. Given two continuous variables, *x* and *y*, we wish to determine the parameters *a* and *b* in the equation: $\hat{y} = a + bx$, where the $\hat{y}$ symbol indicates the estimated value of *y*, based on *x*. In this general equation for a straight line, a is the intercept (the value of *y* when *x* = 0) and *b* is the slope (the amount of change in *y* per unit change in *x*). Another name for *b* is the *regression coefficient*.

In our example of hemoglobin (*y*) and creatinine (*x*),

$$\hat{y} = 12.04 - .49x$$

This means that, on average, for every increase in serum creatinine concentration of 1 mg/dl, the decrease in hemoglobin concentration is .49 gm/dl, at least over the range of measurements shown in Figure 2. (It is hazardous to extrapolate the linear relationship between *x* and *y* beyond the observed ranges of *x* and *y*.)

Because the relationship between hemoglobin and creatinine is a biologically dependent one (we believe renal function, as represented by the serum creatinine, affects the hemoglobin concentration, rather than the converse), we have *regressed* hemoglobin on creatinine. This is the usual practice when we regress one variable on another, i.e., we regress *y* (the dependent variable) on *x* (the independent variable).

Interpretation of *r* and *b*

We now have two different descriptive statistics, or coefficients, to describe the extent of linear relationship between two continuous variables, *x* and *y*. The correlation coefficient *r* is useful for describing the degree of linear closeness (linear correlation) between *x* and *y*, irrespective of which is dependent or independent. A major advantage of *r* is that it remains the same regardless of units. In our example, $r = -.78$ whether creatinine is measured in mg/dl or mmole/l. The one disadvantage of *r* is that it is not useful for *predicting y from x*.

To predict *y* from *x*, regression is required. Unlike *r*, the value of the regression coefficient, *b*, will change with changes in the units in which *x* and *y* are measured. The value of *b* in our example would be entirely different from -.49 if creatinine were measured in mmole/l instead of mg/dl.

The extent to which a relationship between variables can be described by a straight line is denoted by *r*, whereas *b* is the rate of change in

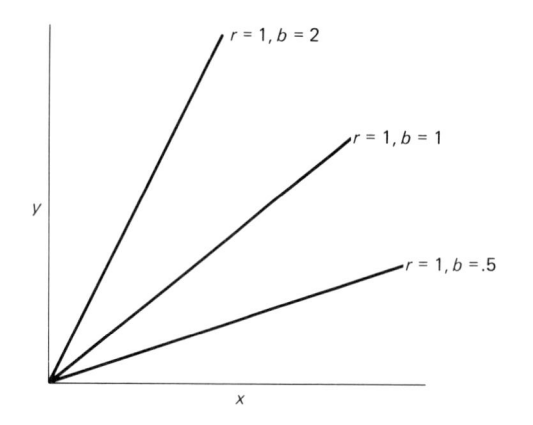

FIGURE 3. The distinction between r and b.

y for every unit rise in x. Interpretation of the two coefficients is contrasted by the three regression lines shown in Figure 3. Each of the three regressions is represented by a perfectly straight line, i.e., $r = 1$ for all three. The slope, b, differs considerably.

Thus r and b are descriptive statistics that denote different aspects of the linear relationship between two continuous variables, x and y. When $r = 0$ or $b = 0$, there is no linear relationship between and x and y. When values different than 0 are obtained in a study sample, we need to ask ourselves whether the difference might have arisen by chance.

Since r and b are calculated from samples, we must turn to inferential statistics to provide inferences about the linear relationship between x and y in the underlying target population. We can test for the statistical significance of r or b by postulating the null hypothesis that ρ (the population correlation coefficient) or β (the population regression coefficient) is equal to 0. Standard statistical tests (1,2,8) provide a formula for carrying out a t-test on either r or b (the result is the same with either coefficient). It should be emphasized, however, that the statistical significance of r or b is heavily dependent on the sample size. With very large samples, even small degrees of correlation may yield P values below .05.

Control for Confounding Variables

A third (or more) variable can confound the linear relationship between two continuous variables. Although matching or stratification can be used to control for such confounding factors, a powerful mulivariate statistical technique exists for simultaneous control of any number of confounders: *multiple linear regression*. Multiple regression also allows the investigator to assess the separate unconfounded effects of several independent variables on a single dependent variable.

The multiple linear regression technique models the dependent variable y as a linear function of all the independent variables (x_i's):

$$\hat{y} = a + b_1x_1 + b_2x_2 + b_3x_3 + \ldots + b_nx_n.$$

The x_i's may be any continuous or dichotomous variables, and the b_i's are the corresponding regression coefficients. Each b_i is adjusted simultaneously for the linear relationship between its corresponding x_i and every other x_i, as well as the linear relationship between the other x_i's and y. An overall r^2 can be calculated for the model; it represents the proportion of the total variance in y accounted for by its linear relationship with all the x_i's. Further details are available in standard texts (1,8,11).

Correlation Between Two Ordinal Variables

On page 83, we mentioned the two-group comparison for an ordinal variable using the Mann–Whitney U test. When two ordinal variables are measured in each study subject, the investigator may be interested in measuring the correlation between the two. In this situation, using the *Spearman rank correlation coefficient*, r_s, may be preferable to a χ^2 test. The Spearman technique compares the ranks for each of the two variables for each subject. The smaller the sum of the squared differences in ranks, the greater the correlation there is between the ranks, and the higher the value of r_s. The magnitude of r_s can vary between -1 and $+1$ and is interpreted in the same way as the usual Pearson correlation coefficient, r. The formula for computing r_s, as well as tables for testing its statistical significance, are available in standard references (2,8).

Concluding Remarks

Familiarity with statistical principles and techniques is invaluable for the researcher, from the earliest planning stages to the final proofreading of a manuscript already accepted for publication. Although many surgical investigators will choose to consult or collaborate with one or more statistical colleagues, some background is essential if such consultation or collaboration is to be both useful and efficient. Few statisticians are trained in the nuances of clinical medicine and the subtle processes that influence physicians' decisions. Statistically bereft clinicians who put themselves entirely at the mercy of a biostatistician do so at their own peril. The results may be mathematically sound but clinically irrelevant or, if relevant, incomprehensible and therefore of no practical value to a clinical audience.

The surgical researcher should know at least enough to be an informed consumer, if not a producer, of statistics. As a general principle, investigators should avoid using any statistical technique whose purpose *and* interpretation they do not understand. Although they usually need not be familiar with statistical theories and mathematical derivations, when these are required (e.g., in examining the validity of assumptions underlying certain tests), professional statistical help is essential.

References

1. Armitage P. Statistical Methods in Medical Research. Oxford: Blackwell Scientific Publications, 1971.
2. Colton T. Statistics in Medicine. Boston: Little, Brown and Company, 1974.
3. Swinscow TDV. Statistics at Square One. London: British Medical Association, 1976.
4. Ingelfinger JA, Mosteller F, Thibodeau LA, Ware JH. Biostatistics in Clinical Medicine. New York: Macmillan Publishing Co., 1983.
5. Louis TA, Lavori PW, Bailar JC, Polansky M: Crossover and self-controlled designs in clinical research. N Engl J Med 1984. *310:* 24-31.
6. Smart JV. Elements of Medical Statistics. Springfield: Charles C. Thomas, 1963.
7. Moses LE, Emerson JD, Hosseini H. Analyzing data from ordered categories. N Engl J Med 1984. *311:* 442-448.
8. Snedecor GW, Cochran WG. Statistical Methods, 7th Edition. Ames: Iowa State Unviersity Press, 1980.
9. Fleiss JL. Statistical Methods for Rates and Proportions, 2nd Edition. New York: John Wiley & Sons, 1981.
10. Kleinbaum DG, Kupper LL, Morgenstern H. Epidemiologic Research: Principles and Quantitative Methods. Belmont: Lifetime Publications, 1982.
11. Kleinbaum DG, Kupper LL. Applied Regression Analysis and Other Multivariable Methods. North Scituate: Duxbury Press, 1978.
12. Anderson S, Auquier A, Hauck WW, Oakes D, Vandaele W, Weisberg HI. Statistical Methods for Comparative Studies: Techniques for Bias Reduction. New York: John Wiley & Sons, 1980.

4

Organizing a Clinical Study

L. Del Greco, J.I. Williams, and D.S. Mulder

Introduction

Each year, a particular surgeon performs about 70 operations for aorto-femoral bypass grafting to restore blood supply to the extremities. Initially, he judged the success of the surgery in terms of survival and the saving of limbs. As methods for assessing blood flow in peripheral vessels, and diagnostic and surgical techniques improved, the proportion of patients under the age of 65 years increased. In the course of following his patients, particularly those under 65 years of age, questions arose in the surgeon's mind about the impact of this surgery on patients' return to work and sexual functioning.

Concern arises from the possibility that current surgical procedures damage the pelvic and autonomic nervous system. Alternative operations are more invasive, but the question that still arises "Do sexual dysfunction and nonresumption of principal activities, whether related to work or retirement, indicate that a comparative trial should be considered?" The surgeon has been gathering data on the patients and he or she wants to know, "How can a clinical research project be organized to address this question?"

The First Step: Establish the Scope of Study

The surgeon presented data on the clinical findings at several meetings (1), and colleagues raised a number of questions and issues. In response to the issues so raised, the surgeon changed the data collection procedures, and Table I summarizes the information gathered so far.

TABLE I. Clinical data gathered on aorto-femoral bypass patients preoperatively, postoperatively, and after one year.

Data gathered	Preoperatively	Postoperatively	One year
Survival	NIA	Hospital records	Hospital records
Blood supply in limbs	Physical exam; Ankle–Brachial Index	Same	Same
Levels of principal activities	Doctor–patient interview	Clinical observation	Doctor–patient interview
Significant prognostic indicators (age, smoking, comorbidity)	Doctor–patient interviews; information from referring physician	Clinical observation	Doctor–patient interview
Medications	Doctor–patient interview	Medical record	Doctor–patient interview
Sexual dysfunction	Doctor–patient interview; Urologic tests; Penile–Brachial Index		Doctor–patient interview; Urologic test; Penile–Brachial Index
Diagnosis and treatment plan	Arteriogram		
Complications–sepsis, wound infection	Doctor–patient interview	Clinical observation	Doctor–patient interview; Physical exam
Pain, Discomfort	Doctor–patient interview	Clinical observation	Doctor–patient interview
Quality of life	Assessed indirectly	Assessed indirectly	Patient reports

Initially, the surgeon relied on the patient interview, a physical examination, and clinical judgments formed about the responses of the patients to the bypass. Later, he introduced noninvasive laboratory studies and employed the Ankle-Brachial Index, routinely (2). As blood supply in the pelvic region became an issue, the surgeon began to ask the patients a series of questions suggested by a urologist. Still later, he experimented with the use of the Penile-Brachial Index (3). At this point, he is uncertain about the clinical usefulness of the data gathered for assessing outcomes.

When the surgeon reviewed the above information with a research consultant, they agreed that the scope of the study had to be established by defining the research questions as hypotheses, specifying the data-gathering instruments for putting key concepts into operation, and planning the collection and editing of data to ensure the reliability and validity of measurements. The task is to restrict the scope of the study to the patients and period of time required to answer the research questions and hypotheses.

The Definition of the Basic Terms of the Research Question

The basic terms of the research questions or hypotheses may include diagnosis, prognostic indicators, type of surgical intervention, complications, pain, physical functioning and quality of life. Each term requires two types of definition, conceptual and operational. A conceptual definition specifies the phenomena to be studied in theoretical or clinical terms that are consistent with the accepted usage of the terms in medical science. The operational definition is the set of rules for assigning numbers, henceforth called scores, to the phenomena to be observed and recorded. The scoring system should follow logically from the conceptual definition, so that the numbers assigned make sense and convey a meaning to the investigator.

It is common to have two or more measures for the same concept. Scores can be compared in terms of how well they fit the theoretical concept, their reliability and validity, and the time and cost of data collection.

It is clear that in this case, the primary outcome of interest is the restoration of the blood supply to the legs to assure physical functioning and minimize the likelihood of amputation or death. The clinical efficacy of aorto-femoral bypass grafting is beyond dispute.

During further discussions between the surgeon and the research consultant, it became clear that the surgeon could focus the research on changes in the patients' principal everyday activities, sexual functioning, and quality of life. He could focus on the physical capacity for activities or sexual functioning, or the actual levels of functioning and the patients' satisfaction with them.

Since age, co-morbidity, medications and smoking are prognostic indicators of outcome, the surgeon could establish a hypothesis on the likelihood of particular outcomes, given the presence or absence of the prognostic factors.

With respect to sexual functioning, impotence may be the result of inadequate blood supply to the pelvic region, operative injury to the parasympathetic nerves urologic problems, reactions to medication, other health problems, or psychological or other problems in sexual relationships. One approach is to classify patients, at the time of diagnosis, in terms of sexual activity. For those sexually active preoperatively, reduction in sexual function postoperatively could be related to possible nerve damage; if the preoperative sexual dysfunction appeared to be related to reduced blood supply, the capacity for erection and ejaculation should increase following surgery. In those with impotence related physiological problems, the surgery should have a minimal impact apart from any improvement in the blood supply. Accordingly, a research question can be asked about the level of sexual functioning in each of these groups following surgery, assuming that appropriate measures are available for each *key term*.

Separate research questions can also be formulated for principal activities, quality of life, and satisfaction with the surgery.

Limiting the Data to Be Gathered

As interest in the findings of the surgeon increased, colleagues posed more questions and suggested the gathering of interesting information on the clinical, personal, and social characteristics of the patients. Their specific suggestions included the use of new clinical measures, such as the Ankle-Brachial Index or a Penile-Brachial Index. As a consequence, considerable new information accumulated.

The term data-gathering instrument is used to signify any and all types of data collection aids, such as questionnaires, indexes, observation forms, mechanical devices as calipers, blood pressure cuffs, and thermometers.

When you are planning a study, you may be tempted to collect interesting information above and beyond what is required to answer your research question or hypothesis. But data are costly, not only in terms of the time and money required to produce them, but in terms of the problems of data management and analysis that increase with the volume of information you have to process. If you collect data without a specific purpose or question in mind, you will probably leave them unanalyzed.

The three general guidelines for limiting the urge to collect too many data are brevity, clarity and pre-coding.

1. **Brevity.** Restrict data collection to the information you need to answer your research questions or hypotheses and collect in the most efficient manner possible.
2. **Clarity.** Keep data collection as simple and straightforward as possible. Make your instructions for obtaining the information explicit so that there is no ambiguity about where the data are to be found or how they are to be recorded. The more judgments the data collector has to make, the greater the likelihood of error.
3. **Pre-Coding.** Establish rules for the classification, scoring and coding of data before collection so that the data-gathering forms can be pre-coded. If you leave such decisions to the end, you run the risk of ending up with information that is incomplete.

Reliability and Validity

The surgeon recognizes that much of the data he obtained from patient interviews and physical examinations reflected the questions he asked and the clinical judgments he made regarding the responses. He had a set of questions to ask, but he had not set them down in a standard form. He could have anticipated or assumed the answers to some of the questions. He also used the patients' responses to determine their levels of physical functioning, and did not employ exercise tests. He asked the questions the urologist had suggested but he wasn't always clear about their purpose.

The surgeon noted the strength of the peripheral pulse on a four-point scale devised for the purpose, but he hasn't checked the reliability of the scoring. After he introduced the vascular laboratory tests 3 or 4 years ago, readings for the Ankle-Brachial and Penile-Brachial Indices were taken for a large series of patients with vascular disease, but he hasn't tested their sensitivity and specificity as measuring instruments. He now gathers data for these indices for all patients, preoperatively and at the one-year follow-up. As a part of another research project, he will compare the preoperative data for the two indices with arteriograms to test their diagnostic accuracy.

The surgeon recognizes the limits of the approach he adopted for gathering data. Many of the data have been coded and entered into a computer file, but he has not yet explored the potential for using them to answer any of his research questions.

To be scientifically acceptable, an instrument must be reliable and valid. It is reliable when it performs consistently for the same person in different applications when the phenomena being recorded have not changed, and for different observers during simultaneous applications. The validity of an instrument is defined in terms of its accuracy. An instrument must be reliable in order to be valid, but a reliable measure may not be valid because the observers may simply be consistently reproducing errors. Chapter 2 of this Section discusses rsearch strategies for testing the reliability and validity of instruments. The key point is that you, as the researcher, are responsible for assuring the reliability and validity of the data collected in each of your projects.

The first task for the research advisor and the surgeon is to agree on which research questions and hypotheses are of central importance. The impact of surgery on sexual functioning, given the level of sexual functioning preoperatively, is a researchable question. It could be the focal point for a single study. A study may include two or more hypotheses, but it is generally advisable to have no more than three or four in a given study.

The operational measures could include physiological tests, scales or indices that are appropriate for the outcomes, and clinical judgments. Clinical investigators in the field of sexual therapy and counselling could be consulted about other possible measures. The reliability and validity of the measures should be established, and the investigators satisfiy themselves that the measures are sufficiently precise to detect clinically important changes in available sample sizes of patients. These steps define the boundaries of the study. The next stage is the specification of plans for collecting and managing the data.

Advantages and Disadvantages of Different Methods of Data Collection

Basically, four different data collection strategies are available for clinical research. They are the medical record, the self- administered questionnaire, the interviewer-administered questionnaire, and observation.

The Medical Record

The medical record of each patient contains the results of history taking, physical examination, laboratory tests, diagnostic consideration, interventions and follow-up. Health professionals are accustomed to making medical records, and a large number of records can be abstracted inexpensively over a relatively short period of time. However, if the medical record is entirely in narrative form, the reliability and validity of the clinical judgments it contains may not be known. Reports of particular laboratory or diagnostic tests may not be included in all the charts, i.e., they are incomplete for research purposes.

Researchers often introduce forms designed specifically for research purposes. The research medical record assumes that data will be recorded on a standardized form so that missing information can be quickly identified. Because clinicians often find it difficult to adapt to new forms and may be reluctant to complete research charts as well as existing medical records, some teams employ research nurses to gather the necessary information for all eligible patients. This requires the finding of research funds to pay their salaries.

Self-Administered Questionnaires

Patients and their partners could be asked to complete a questionnaire on background characteristics, past and present levels of physical functioning and activity, and structured questions on levels of sexual functioning and satisfaction.

The main advantages of this strategy are that many questionnaires can be filled out in a very short period and fewer field workers need to be employed. The main disadvantages are that the researcher can never be sure that each questionnaire was completed by the intended person and the response rate tends to be low, particularly if the questionnaire is administered by mail. A low response rate could bias the study's results and the completeness of responses has to be carefully monitored.

Interviewer-Administered Questionnaires

The surgeon, another health professional, or a trained interviewer can obtain additional information by interviewing the patient or a significant other person in the patients' life. The main advantages of the interviewer-administered strategy are that it yields a better response rate and allows the greatest flexibility in questionnaire construction and length. Its main disadvantage is its cost. Quality interviewers are usually paid well and travel expenses will be incurred if the interviews are conducted in the homes of interviewees spread over a large geographic area. Another problem is that interviewees may not be as honest in their answers as they would be on a self-administered questionnaire because of interactions with the interviewer that cause them to give socially acceptable responses.

Observation

If the researcher wishes to know whether the patient can perform certain basic physical activities, such as walking two blocks or climbing a flight of stairs without pain or discomfort, the patient can be asked to perform these activities in the presence of the observer, who then records the responses.

The advantage of the observational or measurement technique is that the problem of eliciting socially desirable answers is eliminated. There is, however, a problem in ensuring consistent results from the same rater, over time, and between raters. A further disadvantage is that the rater's presence may alter the subject's behavior and the results may indicate what the patient *can do* rather than what he or she usually does.

Multiple Method of Data Collection

Researchers may strive to include all the outcomes or variables considered important, and to rely on multiple sources for the required data. If you use multiple methods to gather data, you may have to rank-order the methods according to the relative importance of the information they are intended to produce. Should problems arise in employing all the methods equally well, you should focus your time and attention on those of primary importance in the testing of the research question or hypothesis.

Repeated Measures

You can gather the same data at two, or more, different times to monitor the patients' progress. The problem of maintaining high quality data increases each time you repeat a measure. Scheduled appointments may be missed, your commitment and that of your subjects may falter, and a pattern of fixed responses may systematically bias the results. Monitor the administration of repeated measures carefully to reduce the number of problems.

Data-gathering procedures must be acceptable to clinicians and health professionals, cause minimal disruption of patient care activities, and only collect information that is essential to the answering of your research question(s).

The problems of maintaining complete files of reliable and valid data increase exponentially with the complexity of your study. High quality data depend, to a great extent, on the vigor of the members of your research team and your clinical partners in intervention trials.

Multi-Center Trials

The surgeon performing the aorto-femoral bypass grafts wants to know whether the prophylactic use of antibiotics would reduce the subsequent requirement for their therapeutic use. Since the sepsis rate in such cases is <5%, 1000 patients would be needed in each treatment and control group to do a trial. Such a study would require the participation of a number of centers to obtain sufficiently large sample sizes to make the statistical test of differences in outcomes reliable.

Since the surgeons and clinical staff in each center have their own techniques, considerable time, effort, and fiscal resources would have to be expended to assure uniform data collection in all the centers. Usually, at least one center drops out of a multi-center trial, or is asked to withdraw by the coordinating committee responsible for monitoring the research procedures. The ratio of the resources required for data management to those needed for data collection tends to increase as more centers are included. The design, organization, and management of multi-center trials are discussed in greater depth and detail in Chapters 4 and 5 of Section III.

Recruiting and Deploying an Effective Research Team

All persons associated with a research project can be described as being either core or staff members. The core team comprises the investigator(s) and co-investigator(s) who are responsible for the designing, funding, quality and completion of the study; they do not necessarily engage in the day-to-day execution of the study. The research staff frequently consists of a research associate or coordinator who runs the study on a day-to-day basis, and research assistants who organize and deal with the field workers responsible for gathering and coding the data. Each research assistant's tasks also include the editing and supervision of the coding of data sheets. Finally, a data manager is responsible for preparing the data for analysis. The actual analysis is usually carried out or supervised closely by a statistician who may be a core or staff member or a consultant. Core members can also play an active role in data-gathering and management. Inputs from health professionals, such as surgeons, radiologists, pathologists, internists, physical therapists or nurses may be required on a core or staff level or both.

Training the Research Staff

Regardless of the level of professional expertise or experience of the persons involved in recording data, training personnel to behave in a standardized manner enhances reliability and validity. The goal is to have the phenomena under study recorded with minimal distortion arising from the expectations and subjective impressions of the research personnel. Ideally, the data gatherers should be unaware of the research questions and hypotheses and blind to the groups to which subjects have been assigned, when applicable. Subjective judgments on the part of the coders should also be minimized. The key to achieving this is to have explicit rules for data reduction that eliminate the need for subjective judgments as completely as possible.

Data must be not only reliable and valid, but complete. Missing information can be a major problem and alternate sources should be sought when required. All persons providing information for the project must appreciate the importance of its being complete and be trained accordingly.

Evaluation of the Research Staff

During training sessions, you can use simulated exercises and practice runs to evaluate the data collection process. This evaluation has two parts: (1) the assessment and correction of the performance of the members of the research staff, when necessary, and (2) the modification of procedures for collecting data to make them acceptable, straightforward, unambiguous, and easy for field workers to use. Comments and suggestions regarding forms and procedures from the team members can be used to improve data collection and management.

Pretesting the Study Procedures

To verify that the research study will proceed as planned and that the data-gathering instruments will perform as intended, always conduct a pretest, or dress rehearsal of the study in the field. The pretest is a critical step because it is impossible to anticipate all the potential detrimental factors that may come into play. The pretest trial offers you the opportunity not only to identify, but to correct for such factors. During the pretest, you can examine the three main components of the study: the data gathering instruments, the logistics, and the personnel. When you are examining the logistics, note whether the data can be gathered with few losses, i.e., can charts be retrieved, subjects accrued, and measures taken. When you examine the data-gathering instruments, determine whether they work in the field. For questionnaires, examine the vocabulary to make sure it is understandable to the subjects; find out whether the subjects are compliant and appear to be giving honest answers to all questions; and determine the length of the interview. You should also check the pre-coding schema for the questionnaire and determine the adequacy of its format and skip patterns. A 10.0% verification will indicate the quality of the work performance of personnel. Research personnel have to respect the dignity and rights of patients at all times; betrayal of the confidentiality of patients is sufficient reason for dismissal from the project.

There is no formula for determining the number of pretest subjects, but the accepted number seems to be between 30 and 50 regardless of the intended sample size. Since the pretest subjects are drawn from the same pool as the actual study subjects, a major consideration in determining the number of pretest subjects is their availability. You will want to avoid depleting a large proportion of the population on the pretest trial. Establishing the size of the pretest sample is, therefore, a subjective decision influenced by the availability of potential study subjects. To avoid contaminating the sample population, draw your pretest subjects from a hospital or region at some distance from your intended study area. There is no predetermined number of pretest trials; any number may be needed to convince you that the study can be conducted.

Cleaning the Data

The editing of questionnaires or clinical data sheets is the first step in cleaning the data. The field worker checks the questionnaire, or data sheet, line by line to ensure that all the appropriate items have been correctly completed. If there are any errors, the questionaries or data sheets must be sent back to the data gatherer for correction. This helps to eliminate the problem of missing data.

The next step is coding, the process of converting written answers into numbers suitable for analysis by computer. The codes for precoded items are transferred to the coding boxes first; open-ended items are coded, next. Each open-ended item is read and given a code number that corresponds to the answer. Make sure that special care is taken to code what is written and to avoid interpreting the answers. Each distinct response is given a new number; identical responses share the same code. This process is repeated for each item until all the open-ended items are coded. To ensure quality, a 10% sample of the questionnaires or data sheets are re-coded blindly—a process commonly referred to as double coding. By examining the accuracy with which the codes are assigned during the first and second codings, you can estimate the error rate for each item and for the entire data-gathering instrument.

Key Punching

The coded questionnaires or data sheets are now sent to keypunching to record the codes on 80-column cards or electronic files. Each code, to be meaningful, must appear in the correct column on the card or file. To ensure accuracy, have the keypunching done twice, examine the two outcomes for discrepancies and see that all identified discrepancies are checked and corrected.

When the data file returns from keypunching, examine it for further inaccuracies. For each question, there are possible values and out-of-range values. Examine each item for out-of-range values, and see that those that are found are subsequently corrected by reference to the questionnaires or data sheets. Errors can also occur when "possible values" that are logically impossible are keypunched. You can find such errors by comparing the coded answers to different questions. For example, a person cannot be female and have prostatic cancer. An extra character, an omitted character, or a blank space will change the position of all the characters that follow and change the codes and information they represent. When the procedures just outlined have been completed, the data are considered clean, or ready for pre-analysis.

Pre-analysis constitutes looking at the frequency distribution of the answers to each question. Because no interpretation is allowed during the orginal coding process, you may end up with as many different codes as there are people in the study. Analyzing such information would be meaningless. In such cases, review the codes and decide which can be collapsed to form broader, but logically sound, categories. Repeat this procedure for each question, if necessary. When the collapsed codes are corrected on the data file, it is ready for statistical analysis.

Budget Concerns

The collection and management of data are expensive undertakings, and there are numerous ways to cover the costs. Some physician-investigators collect and analyze data in their own small research projects and the principal cost is the time they spend on the project.

Diagnostic tests, laboratory work, and clinical examinations performed solely for research purposes are the most expensive data to collect. In some jurisdictions, the cost of such procedures can be charged against health insurance plans or be absorbed by the hospital or clinic; in others, research procedures must be covered by a research budget.

Data collected from individuals will include the responses to self-administered questionnaires, and face-to-face and telephone interviews. If you use rigorous follow-up procedures to assure a high response rate, self-administered questionnaires and telephone interviews usually cost about the same, whereas face-to-face interviews cost about twice as much.

Data gathering may include the collection of laboratory and other test results and the abstraction of data from clinical records. Research personnel can be salaried or paid for each piece of work completed. For example, a data collector could be paid a specified amount for each *complete* set of data for a given subject. This arrangement provides an incentive to make certain that all the required information is collected, and fits well with the strategy of paying nurses, residents and others to collect data in the course of their regular patient care duties. The data manager must be certain that the data forms are complete and that the data are of high quality. If you use this approach, the data collectors should be assured that if they work for a week at a reasonable pace, they can complete enough forms to earn a reasonable wage.

There will always be a certain number of subjects for whom data cannot be completed, because the information is missing, or the subjects have been lost to follow-up. Do not penalize data collectors for any loss of information that is beyond their control. Adjust the work schedule or rate of pay to allow for the expected percentage of their time they will have to spend on incomplete data.

Security and Confidentiality

The completed research record is the primary product of the research project. Its monetary value is related, in part, to the time and costs required to complete it, and the confidentiality of the information. Keep the "hard copies" of the research file in locked cabinets in locked rooms to which only one designated research worker has access. Once the data have been entered into a computer file, store the hard-copies safely, as a general rule, for one year, following data analysis. Destroy them then if it is appropriate.

Use identification numbers to collate the information on subjects and to protect confidentiality. A master list of personal identifiers and identification numbers for each subject is recommended. Record the identification numbers, but not the individual identifiers, on the data forms. If a person who is collecting information needs a name to find information, it can be included on a cover sheet which should be destroyed when the information is collected.

Enter data onto data processing cards, magnetic tapes, a computer disk or diskettes. Because such data processing files can be accidentally altered or destroyed, create master files and store them separately from the working file.

Once the data are edited and "cleaned," you can modify the data files as variables are recorded, transformed and created. Document every change made on the data file and keep one copy with the coding manual so that you can determine, at any time, how any score has been derived or modified. Keep back-up copies of the working files and update them as changes are made. Ensure the security of the data at each stage of data analysis.

You can store computer data files in archives, indefinitely, but if you have not used them within five years following the completion of your project, you probably never will. When your data are no longer used to answer questions, your project is complete. Ethical guidelines governing the confidentiality of personal information in research records justify destruction of all hard copies and computer files in the archives at this time.

References

1. Chiu RC-J, Lidstone D, Blundell PE. Predictive power of penile/brachial index (P.B.I.) in diagnosing male sexual impotence. Vasc Surg (in press).
2. Barnes RW. Hemodynamics for the vascular surgeon. Arch Surg 1980;115:216–223.
3. Barnes RW. Noninvasive diagnostic techniques in peripheral vascular disease. Am Heart J 1979;97(2):241–258.

5

Some Things You Should Know About Computers

G.G. Bernstein and R.G. Margolese

Introduction

In the interest of those who are just embarking on a "computerization" effort, we have simplified discussions by avoiding highly technical terms and omitting even important issues that have little relevance in the clinical research environment. Such technical terms as are used are defined in a glossary at the end of the chapter.

The computer is used as an aid in literature searches and data collection, analysis, and presentation. Typically, it fulfills these functions by means of such fairly general-purpose generic programs as "data management," "statistical analysis," "bibliographic reference management," "word processing," and "graphics presentation." All can now be purchased from a multitude of vendors.

The choice of appropriate equipment, programs, and staff is influenced by such specific factors as:

The complexity and variety of analyses to be performed;
The volume of data collected;
The number of researchers who will be using the computing facilities;
The potential requirement for simultaneous access to the data by a number of researchers;
The sharing of data with collaborators in other departments or hospitals;
Security and confidentiality of the data and programs.

In Part I we present tutorial-type discussions of the five main types of generic program used in research; in Part II we discuss the issues that should be taken into account when you are choosing the tools to match your particular environment. The theme throughout is "what to watch for".

Part I: General Purpose Programs

Most clinical research problems involve the collection of data, the entry of data into the computer and simple examination of the collected data to discover relationships. If we are considering the establishment of a trauma or other clinical registry, we would enter data describing selected elements of the patient's background (name, age, sex, previous medical problems, etc.), the nature of the injury (site, severity, etc.), treatments administered, and eventual outcome. The first stage of investigation might then be to ask simple questions like "How many gun-shot wound patients were admitted this month?" or "What was the average amount of time between the hospital's being notified of the injury and the administration of treatment?". This type of analysis can be accomplished using "database programs".

Subsequent treatment of the data usually involves the use of traditional statistical analysis test (analysis of variance, Student's t tests) to examine the validity of hypotheses formulated while relationships were being sought by means of the database program. If the hypotheses prove to be tenable, we can, and often do, prepare graphical representations of the data (histograms, bar charts, line graphs). The "general-purpose" computer packages (database, statistical, graphics etc.) that are available in abundance, enable the user to perform all these steps without any further programming.

The preparation of manuscripts is handled by "word-processing" programs that allow the entry of text, tables, graphic illustrations, and bibliographic lists—all prepared by appropriate programs—into the computer.

Once data are recorded by the database program, they can be manipulated by any number of "general-purpose" programs that require no specialized programming skills. Admittedly, it takes some effort to learn how to use the programs effectively, but most are so designed that you can become immediately productive after learning some basic concepts. As your confidence and requirements expand, it becomes an easy matter to execute increasingly complex operations. There are, however, a number of things that you should be aware of before you choose or use any of the foregoing types of program.

Databases

A database program allows you to collect information by stating the questions you want the computer to ask (e.g., "What is the patient's name?") and directs the computer to accept responses that you make from the keyboard and store them in an orderly fashion in its long-term memory device (the disk). The database program should also allow you to ask questions later about all the data you have entered (a "query" facility). It should be flexible enough to allow you to retrieve all or a subset of the data in a form that can be used by other general-purpose programs. For example, it should be able to deal with the instruction "Extract all patients from the database who have a diagnosis of lung cancer, along with data on their operative procedure, mortality, and postoperative complications. Ensure that these data are extracted in such a form that they can be given to the T-test program in my statpak software package. Conversely, the database program should be able to accept and operate on data generated by other programs. It should provide you with flexible commands that allow you not only to perform ad-hoc queries ("How many patients had breast cancer"?) but also to prepare standardized reports that summarize the data, e.g., a table listing the frequencies of occurrence and the stages, at diagnosis, of the various types of cancer found at your hospital.

The most flexible database programs are those that make no *a priori* assumption about the relationships between data. They do not assume, for example, that you will *always* want to print out the entire history file for a particular patient identified by his or her hospital number. They do, however, give you the freedom to explore the entire database to discover relationships for yourself. Such systems are called "relational database systems". Although they tend to operate more slowly then other database systems, (e.g. those used in hospital information systems) they provide much greater flexibility.

Relational systems usually require you to think about your data in the form of "tables". Each row of a table usually contains information about a single patient while columns contain information about discrete "variables", or data "elements", e.g.,

HOSPITAL #	NAME	DATE OF BIRTH	SEX
1234	Doe, John	31/03/1947	M
3754	Smith, Mary	23/12/1932	F

Relational database systems differ in the ways they allow you to define the data. It is important that you should be able to define

at least as many rows as there will be patients in your largest study;
a large number of columns — something between 250 and 500 is reasonable;
columns as numbers, letters or dates; and
at least one column (usually the one containing the patient's identification number) as a special (keyed) column that allows fast retrieval of all the data for a selected patient.

The best database programs allow you to define and gain access to a number of tables simultaneously, both at data-input-time and at query-time. A common technique is to define a demographic table in which each row has at least one column that uniquely indentifies each patient in that table; e.g., by hospital number. The database program should then allow you to formulate queries that span several data tables, e.g., "How many males (from a demographic table) with lung cancer (from a diagnosis table) had no surgical intervention (from a treatment table?"

The database query language allows you to make ad-hoc queries of the type "How many patients . . ." or "List all the patients who . . .". Modern query languages closely resemble ordinary English. A typical statement typed into the computer might be:

"Display NAME where AGE is greater than 40" (Displays the names of all patients whose age is > 40 years.)

or

"Display AVERAGE (AGE) where SEX = "M" and DIAGNOSIS = 2345" (Displays one value, the average age of all male patients who have been diagnosed with a disease coded by the numeric "2345".)

Most relational systems do a good job of allowing you to specify restrictions ("AND" and "OR" conditions) that apply to data in the same row, but few provide the capability of answering queries that compare one row against another. For example, only a few available systems (the more costly) could answer a query of the type "Display the first treatment (from the treatment table) that coincided with a decrease in the white blood cell count (from the "lab tests" table) for selected patients in the database". Such systems are often called "time-oriented" databases.

The database program should allow you to produce "standard reports" from the stored data. For example, a tumor registry will occasionally generate follow-up reports that list the names, addresses and disease classifications of all patients who have not been seen since a certain date. Database systems often have a "mini" programming language, (known as the "report generation language") which allows you to create simple programs which can be periodically reused without retyping.

Statistical Analysis Programs

Statistical analysis programs are usually sold in the form of "packages" ("statpak") containing many different programs, each of which performs one type of analysis. The usual procedure for using them is to extract data with the database program and then "submit" them to a particular test contained in the statpak. Most statpaks will also allow you to enter data directly from the terminal. You should ensure that the one you choose provides both capabilities.

Statistical data, like relational database data, are organized in rows and columns. Consequently, the same features (number of columns, rows, etc.) are important when selecting a statpak; some will deal with temporal data (e.g. survival tables).

The number of tests contained in a package and their accuracy and precision are important parameters to consider when you are selecting a statpak. Most well-known packages (SAS, BMDP, SPSS) provide sets of analysis programs that are both rich and reliable. Even so, it is sometimes necessary to purchase more than one statpak to obtain all the tests that you may wish to use in your environment.

Some statpaks allow you to perform "transformations" on the data contained in your tables. For example, it might be necessary to convert all data in a particular column to the logarithm of the data value before a particular test is done. It is usually a good idea to select a package that can carry out this type of operation, but also allows you to write small, specialized programs that augment the analysis being performed.

Word Processing Programs

Word processing programs enable you to:

enter text from the keyboard and store the text on the computer's disk;
retrieve and modify old text on the disk;
print text using different "formats"; e.g., smooth right margins, underlining; and
perform miscellaneous functions, such as the preparation of form letters and mailing lists.

Editing

The portion of the program that makes it possible to enter and modify text is called the "editor". A good editor allows you to move the "cursor" (a mark on the screen that indicates where the next character will appear) to any portion of the screen using the "arrow keys" and start entering text without any special commands. Other desirable capabilities are "scrolling" (moving text up, down and sideways on the screen), margin setting, and the choice of "inserting" (which causes existing text on the line to be moved further to the right) or to "overwriting" (which obliterates existing text). An "autowrap" capability (words at the right margin boundary are automatically placed on the next line as they are typed) eliminates the need for the typist to view the screen while inputting text.

Good editors allow you to search for all occurrences of certain words in the text (both forward and backward); search for and replace one word with another; and cut, remove, and relocate portions of text ("cut and paste"). You should be able to delete words, lines and entire paragraphs without executing multiple commands. It is also desirable to have a feature that allows you to undo or "undelete" an inadvertent deletion.

More advanced editors will allow you to edit more than one manuscript simultaneously and to move text from one document to another. This feature is often combined with another that displays portions of both files on the screen at the same time ("multi-windows"). Another very useful feature, not found in most editors, is the ability to perform cut and paste operations on columns rather than whole lines.

In some research environments an editor that supports the entry and display of Greek, French, German, or mathematical character sets is important. Mathematical equations or chemical formulae often require special capabilities, especially in printing.

Most research publications contain some graphical displays. Systems that allow graphs prepared by some other programs to be inserted directly into the text are now available. They eliminate subsequent manual "cut and paste" operations.

Some editors require that all text be fitted into the main memory of the computer. They should be assiduously avoided because they impose artificial constraints on the length of manuscripts that can be prepared. An editor that maintains its text in some "internal" or "private" format, must be able to transform it into a standard format that can be read by other programs.

Formatting

The formatting operations (centering, underlining, use of bold face, underlining, etc.) that prepare your text for final printing, employ two basic approaches.

(i) Special commands are embedded in the text and are recognized by another program that instructs the printer to produce the desired effect.
(ii) Keyboard commands that perform the formatting on the screen — "what you see on the screen is what you get on paper".

The first approach allows more numerous and flexible operations, but it requires mental visualization of the final output, takes longer to learn how to use, and usually presents difficulties in training clerical staff to use it effectively. The second approach allows you to perform more error-free formatting operations and requires considerably less training, but it causes long delays whenever reformatting is necessary. Another serious problem associated with some versions of this approach is that formats previously associated with text regions are not "remembered," and re-formatting becomes an arduous procedure whenever you change or the reprint the document: look for packages that provide the required memory. Some word processing packages combine the two approaches to allow the use of embedded commands to perform operations that are difficult to do on the screen or too time-consuming.

Most word processing packages include text centering, underlining, left and right margin justification, and/or filling, highlighting, control of output line spacing, and automatic pagination. In a research environment, formatting capabilities that provide for footnoting, automatic indexing, table-of-contents preparation, titling, subtitling, and flexible pagination parameters are a must. If the editor does not provide support for mathematical representations, you should ensure that the formatter you choose provides it.

Printing

The word processing package should allow you to choose the printer on which hard-copy will be produced. Avoid systems that tie you down to a particular printer or set of printers. The best systems cater to special effects (underlining, bold-face, italics, etc.), font selection (e.g. multinational, mathematical), proportional spacing, and graphics output.

The usual combination of one or more "draft-quality" (dot matrix) printers with a slower and more expensive "letter-quality" printer is changing now that several new and affordable printing technologies are on the market. The most flexible is the desk-top laser printer which provides letter-quality output, different type styles and sizes, cut-paper handling and collating, high-resolution graphics capabilities, and high-speed output (typically 8–12 pages per minute). Ink-jet printing provides many of these features at a lower cost, but it is slower and the quality of the product is not quite as good as it is with the laser printers.

Before selecting any printer you should ascertain whether your word processing program can take advantage of the special capabilities of the printer. It is disappointing to purchase a printer that can do proportional space printing and find out, later, that your word processing software cannot give it the commands required to make it work properly.

Additional Features

Most word processing packages offer several useful miscellaneous functions, such as spelling and grammar-checking programs, list processing programs (form-letters, labels) and mathematical programs. In the research environment, the spelling checker becomes the most valuable of these tools. You should try to find a system that not only provides a robust dictionary, initially, but also allows the addition of new words when they are found in the text. Systems that give you the option of modifying the text directly when errors are discovered, or of producing lists of "misspelled" words and their context, should be preferred.

Graphics Programs

Graphics programs accept data in tabular form and present them in a different format on special printing devices known as "plotters". Most modern programs will allow you to plot data in "X vs Y" format, as histograms (or bar charts), and as "pie charts", that depict the fractions of a whole population as slices of a pie. You should look for programs that do as much of the work as possible automatically; several existing programs will draw axes, label them, make "tickmarks", and draw graph headings, automatically. You can usually override any of the decisions made by the program if you are not satisfied with the result. Some of the more advanced programs will calculate and plot three-dimensional surfaces and automatically eliminate "hidden lines". They are useful for representing X vs Y vs time data, e.g. the effect of different doses of a drug (X) on different volumes of cells (Y) as a function of time (T).

The picture drawn by the program is usually viewed, initially, on the video display unit ("VDU") connected to your computer. Since all VDU's cannot portray graphics, you should make sure that the one you choose has this capability. All graphics VDU's do not operate in the same way—some programs will only work with certain VDU's—and you should choose your program and VDU accordingly. It is usually a good idea to try the program demonstrated on various VDU's, because the quality of the pictures varies.

Although you will invariably require a hard copy of the graphs displayed on the VDU, its quality is relatively unimportant if you are just trying to get a better "feel" for the relationships in your data. An inexpensive plotting device will meet such a need and also serve as a printer for non-graphic material; two types in common use are called "dot-matrix" and "ink-jet" printers. Ink-jet printers operate more quietly and produce better quality text and pictures than dot-matrix printers do. You may wish to consider a laser printer, which can also draw graphics, if you are committed to doing word processing on your computer. Although more expensive than an ink-jet printer, it produces higher quality output more quickly and reliably.

Graphics programs are becoming increasingly popular for the preparation of "presentation-level" graphics. Many researchers save a great deal of time by using the computer to prepare "poster papers". Programs to help you do this should have some form of "layout" capability, that allows you to move text around on the page and print it in different type styles, orientations and sizes. They should also provide certain standard graphics symbols (arrows, lines, boxes, circles) and the same layout freedom as with text. Some allow you to design your own graphics symbols and re-use them at any time.

The most popular device for producing a hardcopy of the presentation-level graphics is the "graphics plotter". It can draw high quality pictures on various sizes and kinds of paper and usually has replacable ink pens to permit variation in line-width and color; with appropriate pens, it can also be used to prepare transparencies for overhead projection.

Plotters with several pens to produce multi-color plots are not much more expensive than single-pen plotters but they produce more attractive results. Make sure your graphics program and your plotter will work well together. Choose a graphics program that provides all the features you require without tying you down to a single type of plotter.

Computers can also be used to prepare photographic slides of presentation level graphics. The most inexpensive method is to photograph the image on the VDU with a 35 mm Polaroid camera and film especially designed for this purpose. Better quality results are produced with more expensive units that process special electronic signals generated by the VDU.

Reference Management Programs

Reference management programs allow you to enter all your literature references and retrieve selected references for a manuscript, lecture or grant application. Such programs store the information in a format that makes it possible to identify such paramters as author, subject, keywords, journal, or date published. You can search for combinations that satisfy whatever criteria you enter, e.g. "all publications by J. A. Smith on the subject of immunotherapy published after 1982".

Some additional features to look for are the ability to

enter text (abstracts) in addition to the usual information;
modify previously-entered references;
print the stored data in different formats, e.g. index cards sorted by author or by subject;
read references transmitted from other computer bibliographic databases (e.g. MEDLINE) without requiring you to retype them; and
cite references in the body of a manuscript, automatically prepare the bibliographic reference list, and place it at the end of the manuscript in any of the common formats required by journals.

Reference management programs can be used to advantage for retrieving any information that requires indexing, such as a collection of surgical slides or x-rays. (Print the numbers of all slides in our collection that illustrate a particular surgical procedure and are at a level that can be presented to first year medical students.)

Different systems will operate at different speeds; the more flexible are usually slower.

Part II: Choosing the Computer

Computer Types

Computers can be categorized as:

(i) Very large—"Mainframes",
(ii) Medium-sized—"Minicomputers",
(iii) Small—"Personal Computers".

Which type you choose usually depends on your budget, how many people will need to use it simultaneously, the amount of data it must store permanently, and whether the data must be available to several users at the same time. Other factors, such as how fast the computer can process data ("power"), the ease with which special purpose programs can be written, the security requirements of your data, and the need for your computer to communicate with other computers or to read data directly from electronic equipment (e.g., blood gas machines), must also be considered.

Big Computers

Mainframe computers are the most expensive and should only be considered when the computing project is very large. They can support the simultaneous activity of hundreds of users, store vast amounts (trillions of characters) of data, process data more quickly than any other type of computer, and provide excellent facilities for preparing specialized programs. Several users can have simultaneous access to common data and communication with other computers is possible, though often difficult and expensive. Big computers cannot read data that originates from machines or patients.

Mainframes are most often found in the computing centres of universities and the administration departments of hospitals. In the university environment, their simultaneous use by many people performing different operations can slow performance or cause frustrating variations in "response times". Such centres are usually staffed with competent engineers, programmers and technicians, but access to their expertise is sometimes very limited and you seldom have the freedom to choose the general purpose programs most suited to your needs. Hospital administrative systems are geared to the business aspects of health care and almost never have the kind of programs researchers require or a staff that understands research problems.

You should only consider using a mainframe if you only use the computer occasionally, require some special purpose program only available on a mainframe, or need a type of processing that requires an exceptionally powerful machine.

Medium-Sized Computers

Minicomputers are scaled-down versions of mainframes that provide speeds and data storage capacities somewhere between those of mainframes and personal computers. They offer better communication facilities than mainframes and are capable of reading data directly from other equipment or patients. They cost considerably less than mainframes—$20,000 to $250,000 U.S.—and can frequently be shared by a small group of researchers (5–20) in a single department. Since the computer is under local control, the users generally have more say in the type of programs purchased and the type of support staff hired. General purpose programs for "minis" cost less than those for mainframes and are often more "user friendly".

Inconsistent response times militate against minis, but the problem is not as severe as it is with mainframes since more control can be exercised over the number of users who have access and the type of work they can do (some programs cause more slowing than others). A professional staff of 1 to 4, depending on the size of the mini and the amount of support desired, is usually required and adds to the cost. Annual machine maintenance contracts, usually purchased from the vendor, are an additional ongoing expense.

Minis are a cost-effective solution to computing problems arising in the research environment if there are enough users to share in the cost of purchase, ongoing support, and maintenance.

Small Computers

Personal computers (PC's)—(the least expensive of the three types—$1,500 to $7,500 U.S.) have the least power and storage capacity. Since they are usually used by one person, they provide very uniform response times and often outshine the performance of the other two types. Because of their low cost, it is possible to add computer resources as required, without making any large expenditure for a mini. All of the general purpose programs discussed in Part I can not only be purchased for PC's at a much lower cost than for multi-user computers, but also from a much wider assortment in the areas of database management, word processing and graphics presentation. In these areas, in particular, the better programs are very easy to use and often provide features not found in their mini or mainframe counterparts. Decisions about which programs and add-on devices to buy are easier to make because they do not affect other users. PC's can communicate with other computers, and acquire external data, but not as effectively or easily as minis.

Personal computers are not very suitable in situations calling for the sharing of data (such as central registries). If the need for some special programming arises, it is often much more difficult on a PC and the processing of patient databases containing more than 5000 records or the statistical analysis of similar quantities of data will be very slow.

Some important considerations are often overlooked when the decision is made to support an entire department's computing needs with PC's. As the needs increase, components (programs, special printer, screens, tapes) have to be added to each PC and what started out as a cost-effective plan may result in unnecessary duplication. The problem can be solved more effectively and cheaply by using a larger, shared machine or by connecting the smaller computers to form a network.

When PC's are appropriate, it is important to avoid a "Tower of Babel" syndrome where researchers in one department use many different types of machine; the more types there are, the more difficult the sharing of data, programs and expertise becomes. Decide on one system and coordinate your efforts.

The notion that only a large computer requires a professional staff is not entirely valid. What determines the number and type of professionals you require is the value you place on your own time. Good people will help you make the right choices and eliminate your spending great amounts of time solving technical problems having little to do with your research. Whenever the number of users of a shared computer or of multiple PC's is relatively large, you should consider investing in people.

Security

Sensitive data, (such as patient's files and letters) must be protected against unauthorized access. Where a single mainframe or mini computer is used simultaneously by a number of people, such protection is provided by special programs that must be run before you can gain access to the data—most require you to enter your name and a secret password. Other methods provide higher levels of security and prevent most users from reading your data, but the specialized computer staff will often have sufficient knowledge and privileges to allow them to view your data.

Security on PC's is usually accomplished by physical means, such as keeping the computer in a locked office. When this is not possible, sensitive data are copied onto a separate disk for storage in a secure place and then erased from the main disk. The most common threat to such security systems is the failure to perform the necessary operations.

Exchanging Data and Sharing Resources

Occasionally, you will want to move data from your computer to another in order to share them with someone else or because your computer is not powerful enough to process them. The simplest way to do this is to copy your data onto another disk and take it to the other computer *if* it is *identical* to yours, i.e., has the same kinds of disks and uses the same "operating system" (the computer's master program). Special programs sometimes exist to allow you to convert data so that they can be transferred between dissimilar systems, but they sometimes create as many problems as they solve. This, the most rudimentary form of "computer communications" or "networking" is rather inconvenient and solves only a few communication problems.

Most computers can transmit data over telephone lines by means of a special "communication program" and a device known as a "modem" that add to the cost of your system but provide greater convenience and flexibility. Both the sending and receiving computers must have these components and this approach is often the *only* one that will allow dissimilar systems to exchange data.

More sophisticated programs and communication devices allow you not only to exchange data but also to gain access to the capabilities of some other computer. Such systems, or true "networks" allow:

a number of computers to communicate with each other simultaneously—you don't have to await your turn if someone else is using another computer on the network;
the use of a program available on another computer without copying it into yours—a saving of both time and money;
the sharing of such devices as a large disk, or an expensive printer—avoids the duplication of expensive or infrequently used devices; and
the sending of a memo, note or other document, i.e., "electronic mail" by simply typing it on your keyboard and specifying the name of the user who is to receive it. This speeds up interpersonal communications, eliminates a lot of paper, and provides automatic filing and indexing of correspondence.

When all the computers to be connected are in one location, special cables that do not require modems or telephone lines can be used. Such a "local area network", or LAN, is very reliable and has the highest speed of communication.

Although the most sophisticated and reliable networks are currently provided by minicomputers, rapid progress in the PC field should make comparable PC networks available in the near future.

Buying the Computer

Although the discussion thus far provides a good starting point for evaluating your computing needs, it is usually wise to seek the advice of a computer professional regarding the selection and purchase of both hardware and software. If you decide not to hire one, then help may be available from the Computer Science, Electrical Engineering, or Biomedical Engineering Departments of your university. The types of programs you will need; the number of users you plan to support; the quantity of data to be stored;

the types of special devices (printers, plotters, VDU's, etc) and whether your needs would be better served by a mainframe, a shared minicomputer or one or more personal computers should be discussed. A shopping list and a budget should be drawn up before you start any discussion with any vendor.

If you decide that a mainframe would best suit your needs, you should speak to other researchers who are using mainframes that are already available. If you could rent mainframe time from several computing centers, you should try to determine which has the best information about availability, response time, and the programs at one's disposal. Try to determine whether a "Computer Users' Group" exists and how much it influences the computing center's policies. Find out what it would cost to use the kinds of programs you will be running most often. The purchase of a mainframe computer will rarely be necessary.

If your needs dictate the use of a minicomputer, you should get the names of two or three manufacturers whose products are already popular in your university or hospital. Minicomputers are usually purchased directly from the manufacturer's representative in your area and you should buy as much of the equipment and software you need as possible from the one vendor selected. Although this usually results in higher start-up costs, it inevitably saves money and time when problems arise with the hardware or software. A number of things should be borne in mind when you are choosing a minicomputer vendor, e.g.,

At a national level, how popular is this type of computer? How many different programs are available for it? What do these programs cost? Can you get good programs free?

Choose a well-established vendor. Do some checking on the financial status of the organization. Avoid newly formed "high-technology" companies selling "state-of-the-art" equipment unless you have good reason to believe they will still be in business 10 years hence.

Does the vendor provide maintenance services from a local office? Is support provided for all the programs you will buy? Will you be allowed to speak with the vendor's technical staff when problems arise? Are toll-free hotlines, easy-to-read catalogues, telephone ordering services, automatic documentation update services provided? Does the vendor sponsor and encourage the activities of a local user's group?

Personal computers are usually purchased from a walk-in store that specializes in such equipment or a special group that may exist in a university. Most of the criteria used in choosing a minicomputer are applicable when buying a PC but it is particularly important to be very careful when you are selecting the manufacturer; many large firms that at one time produced excellent products no longer exist.

In North America, two PC manufacturers, IBM and APPLE, currently hold most of the market. Although many other vendors sell similar products at lower prices and advertise them as being "compatible", this is not always the case. Ask for a demonstration of *all* the programs you intend to use before purchasing a "compatible" PC.

Technology is changing very rapidly. The major manufacturers have new products sitting in their warehouses awaiting a time when their unveiling will be optimally advantageous. Ask salespeople whether there are rumors about a newer machine being in the offing; a sudden lowering of the price of a given machine is usually an indication that a newer machine is about to be introduced.

Even though it costs less to repair a PC than any other type of computer, you should seriously consider purchasing an annual service contract. One can be obtained from third-party vendors in most major cities.

Glossary

cut and paste: An operation that involves deleting text from one region of a document and moving it to another.

database: A collection of information with a special organization that makes it easy to retrieve elements of the data.

database program: A computer program that is able to perform operations (add data, inquire about data) on a database.

disk: A magnetic device that is capable of storing computer data and programs indefinitely.

dot-matrix printer: A computer printing device that displays characters on paper by imprinting patterns of dots. The quality of the output is usually much lower than that of a conventional typewriter.

editor: A computer program that allows you to change text previously stored on a disk and add new text.

graphics resolution: The number of dots per inch displayed on the VDU when it is doing graphics. Low resolution devices produce images that are more "grainy" than those produced by high resolution devices.

hardware: All the electronic and mechanical components of a computer system, as distinguished from the computer programs, or "software".

ink-jet printer: A printer that produces characters on paper by spraying a fine jet of ink.

language interface: The language you use to instruct a program to execute a function. A "natural" language interface resembles the language used in ordinary speech.

laser printer: A printer that operates on the same principles as a photocopying machine to produce almost typewriter-quality results.

local area network: A group of computers located physically close to one another and communicating with one other by sending information at high rates over a special cable.

modem: An electronic device that allows computers to transmit data over long distances using telephone lines.

multi-windows: A capability provided by some programs that allows you to divide the VDU screen into several different regions in order to display data originating from different programs simultaneously.

network: A group of computers that can communicate with one another, simultaneously.

operating system: The master program that controls the operation of the computer. It usually has a name which is an acronym, e.g. UNIX, CP/M, VM, MS-DOS.

plotter: A device that draws images on paper.

proportional spacing: A printing technique that makes the space between characters proportional to their width to eliminate the "unnatural" look of print produced by conventional computer printers.

response time: The interval between the making of a request by the user and the delivery of a response by the computer.

software: Programs written for a computer.

statpak: A group of programs, each of which performs some particular statistical operation.

terminal: A self-contained device that combines a video display unit (VDU) and a keyboard. It is capable of being connected to a computer in contrast to a VDU and a separate keyboard built into the computer.

video display unit: A television-like device used to display characters and graphics.

6

Ten Tips on Preparing Research Proposals*

W.O. Spitzer

New or potential investigators with good research ideas often fail to take even the first step in exploring or implementing them. This usually happens when the required resources do not appear to be available. Young investigators and even mature clinicians with strong track records in teaching and service become unduly discouraged at the thought of writing a study protocol, submitting to peer appraisal, and overcoming all the real and imaginary "hurdles" associated with the preparation of grant applications.

Unfortunately, clinicians who practice outside universities and colleges and whose ongoing contact with the "real world" makes their work particularly relevant to the needs of patients are among those who are most easily discouraged. They assume they do not have the ability or the credentials required to generate the financial support their project needs and merits and they make no effort to seek it.

Although some skills are necessary, and there is a "right way" to do certain things, much of what is needed to prepare a research proposal is common sense. Seasoned investigators with long careers have learned most of what they need to know about writing grant applications from the comments, recommendations and objections of the peer reviewers of their earlier proposals.

The suggestions that follow are not intended as a "checklist" that will guarantee your success in "shaking the money tree" of research foundations and other research funding agencies. They are simply some tips learned over the years from colleagues and passed on to the reader. Anybody venturing into research is certain to make mistakes at first; the suggestions that follow may help you to avoid some predictable pitfalls.

Before you consider each of the ten points, it is important that you realize that undertaking research without a protocol is irresponsible, at best, and unethical at worst. Doing so is just as reprehensible as embarking on the construction of a building without approved blueprints from an architect. As a general recommendation, avoid initiating or participating in "off the cuff" or "informal" research when no effort has been made to develop a plan, rationalize it and commit it to writing in advance. Writing a grant proposal accomplishes all of these goals, whether it is funded on the first submission or not.

1. State Your Objective and Study Questions Clearly

When you come upon a good idea, an intriguing hypothesis, a burning question, or an important demonstration project, write your thoughts down, promptly. Then, preferably within days, carefully restate your project or study. Two important steps must now be taken; neglect of either will frequently jeopardize the quality of the rest of your work. First, write the broad objective of the study. Second, formulate the specific questions your research project seeks to answer.

Try to limit the questions to two or three; if

---

*Adapted from a paper by W.O. Spitzer published in Canadian Nurse, Volume 69, No. 3, 1973.

you find yourself writing more than five or six, your objectives may be vague and your concepts woolly. Questions should be phrased to permit objective and preferably quantitative answers. Here are some examples:

Example I

Objective. To determine whether the introduction of a system in which a senior general surgery resident functions as a consultant in the emergency ward of a teaching hospital would expedite the handling of patients with surgical problems.

Related Study Questions

1. Is the span of time from the arrival of a patient in the triage station in the emergency ward to a disposition (i.e., discharge home or admission to hospital) reduced?
2. Are calls to other senior surgical residents and to surgical attending staff in the hospital to come to the emergency room reduced after introduction of the on-site surgical resident compared to the previous situation?
3. Does an assessment of the quality of surgical care for non-elective conditions using a quantitative index developed specifically for surgical problems commonly seen in the emergency room, indicate any improvement following introduction of the new arrangement.

Example II

Objective. To determine whether a strategy of transporting trauma patients to hospitals that involves limiting intervention at the accident site or in transit to first aid and essential life-saving maneuvers is preferable to deploying surgeons with sophisticated equipment to accident sites to initiate more immediate and definitive treatment.

Related Research Questions

1. What are the rates of mortality and of serious residual morbidity for cases treated with the first versus the second approach after adjustments have been made for case mix and severity?
2. What are the direct and indirect costs of the first compared with the second approach?
3. What are the barriers to the feasibility of each approach in urban and rural areas? ("Urban" and "rural" will have been operationally defined very carefully).

Example III

Objective. To determine whether a specific preoperative bowel preparation in conjunction with intravenous administration of antibiotic X improves the results of aorto-femoral grafting in patients with selected types of aorto-iliac occlusive disease and abdominal aortic aneurysms.

Related Study Questions

1. What is the immediate post-operative morbidity (i.e., within 72 hours) of patients who receive the bowel preparation plus antibiotic X compared to those who receive antibiotic X alone?
2. What is the infection rate in the aortofemoral grafts within 30 days of the operation among patients in each of the arms of the study?
3. What are the 1-year and 5-year survival rates for patients in each arm of the study?
4. Do intervening dental procedures, minor operations, or viral or bacterial infections such as pneumonia or gastroenteritis, affect the survival and morbidity rates for patients in each arm of the study?

When you have rewritten your objectives and study questions several times, review them with colleagues whose opinions you respect. They are likely to give you candid comments on the clarity of your objective, the feasibility of the project, and whether your research questions are sensible and amenable to research.

2. Study the Background Literature and Summarize It in Your Proposal

It is important to determine whether the kind of study or project you propose has already been done. Those who are asked to review grant applications are usually very knowledgeable in the appropriate field and are aware of related work reported in the literature or in progress. It is unlikely that you will be granted support for a project that is equivalent to seeking to "reinvent the typewriter". Expert advice on how to review the literature is provided in Section II, Chapters 1 and 7.

When you have reviewed the literature, write it up briefly. If you are not breaking completely new ground, you should demonstrate how or why your project would shed new light on a problem already studied by others, how you will obtain new knowledge, or how you will test an innovative application of existing knowledge. If your emphasis is on application of existing techniques or knowledge, you should indicate the relevance of your work in such terms as "benefit to patients" or "greater efficiency attained".

3. Decide on General Strategy

Before you consider the detailed tactics you might adopt (e.g., selection of comparison groups, delineation of criteria, selection of samples, scoring techniques etc.), design your general strategy. Are you proposing a demonstration model? Will you be conducting a survey? Do you plan a true experiment? The nature of your objective and your research questions will usually suggest the proper strategy. When two or more approaches would be suitable your choice should be based on which is the most feasible and practical.

A common pitfall is to seek support from a research funding agency for a project that is clearly not research. If you are trying to establish a service or educational project, such as a counseling center for adolescents who have sustained serious skiing accidents, you should apply to granting agencies whose terms of reference include the provision of funds for service or educational programs on the basis of their merit rather than an agency whose primary focus is on research into the pathophysiology and treatment of trauma.

4. Identify the Most Appropriate Funding Agency

You should investigate whether accepted procedures or ethical considerations justify your applying to more than one funding agency for support for the same project. It is important to make a decision about possible sources of funds at this stage because the tactics you specify in your detailed research design may be influenced or even determined in part by the known policies of a funding agency. Most funding agencies publish their terms of reference and you should obtain and study them before proceeding.

5. Seek Expert Consultations

This is the time to consult some experts. Although you may have spoken with colleagues or other advisors when you formulated your objectives and study questions, you should now consult with resource persons, such as research methodologists, biostatisticians, or other experts in the field that concerns you. Too often, consultations are sought *after* a grant application has been rejected or the data have been gathered. By that time, it is usually too late for a consultation to be of much help to you. Consultation with the administration staff and with the director of the agency to which you are planning to apply is an invaluable but often neglected step. You can learn what is "fundable" under the agencies present guidelines, and obtain many valuable suggestions about your application. For a major grant or contract, it is worthwhile to do this in person.

At most institutions, there are experienced investigtors who have well developed skills in the field of "grantsmanship". Do not hesitate to enlist their support in planning your grant. A critical review of the finished grant by such an advisor can be extremely valuable, even if your consultant is outside your field.

When you seek expert advice about your research design, it is wise to consider some ethical questions. Are there any risks to patients or other individuals who may become study subjects? If there are, do they outweigh the potential benefits to such individuals or to the population in general? Will the study subjects be free from invasion of their privacy or any form of personal assault? Are reasonable safeguards incorporated in the design to protect the confidentiality of personal or clinical information? Is it ethical in your particular study to withhold some treatment from a control group?

The following commitment, in these or equivalent terms, should be included in your grant application: "The individuals and families involved in this investigation would enjoy freedom from assault; personal privacy, the ability to withdraw from the experiment at any time, and the confidentiality of all personal information obtained would be scrupulously protected. The applicants have carefully weighed the potential gains from the new knowledge that would be obtained from this investigation and have concluded that they vastly outweigh the risks to the individuals involved in this project. Consent to take part in this investigation will only be requested after full disclosure of the nature of the project and of any potential risks to the prospective participant associated with the delivery of health services in the proposed fashion."

Some agencies require a statement on ethics, i.e., approval of the project by a properly constituted ethics review commitee, in each proposal along with copies of the consent forms that will be used.

6. Specify the Criteria You Will Use to Evaluate the Answers to Your Study Questions and the Success of Your Project

Unless you indicate what kind of objective or quantitative answers to your research questions will constitute a particular verdict, your proposal may be regarded as a self-fulfilling prophecy. Specifying the criteria for judging the answers to research questions, *in advance,* usually distinguishes the disciplined and rigorous investigator from the wishful thinker who is "out to prove a point". If we refer back to question 3 under Example I, the criterion for success might be:

Criterion: Bowel preparation plus antibiotic X will be judged to be better than antibiotic X alone if two of the following three outcomes are demonstrated:

1. The immediate post-operative morbidity in the combined approach is not only less than that with antibiotic alone, but is <2%.
2. The rate of infection of patients treated with the combined approach is 20% less than it is in those treated with antibiotic alone within 30 days of the operation.
3. The 1-year and 5-year survival rates for patients treated with the combined approach are at least 20% better than they are in those treated with antibiotic alone.

Although negative findings in a study tend to be viewed as evidence that it failed, it may really have been successful if it provided strong, irrefutable evidence that settled a question. *The success of a study or project is not determined by the verdict it yielded, but by the quality of the evidence it produced.* Consequently, it is wise to spell out the criteria that will determine the success of your project separately from the criteria to be used in evaluating the answers to your study question.

7. Be as Brief and Clear as Possible

Reviewers of grants are not particularly interested in reading countless typewritten pages. Most successful grant applications for clinical or health care research projects are not longer than 10 to 15 pages. Unnecessary verbiage reflects unfavorably on the applicant's ability to think clearly and communicate effectively. Brevity, however, should not be carried to the point where you fail to communicate why your group is distinctive and able to make a significant contribution. If your proposal covers a large study involving several centers and a complex design, the detailed descriptions required may justify an application that is considerably longer.

Funding agencies take pride in identifying and supporting investigators who will be effective in solving problems. A helpful stratagem you can incorporate in the significance section of your grant application is to point out that your institution has already assembled most of the pieces of the puzzle. You can show, for example, with solid documentation, that you have access to all the patients needed for the study, most of the required laboratory equipment, and a well developed plan with a proven record of productivity; *all you need* is support to obtain the few missing pieces of the puzzle. In other words, the granting agency can underwrite a solution to the problem very economically by supporting your research plan to provide the last few pieces of the puzzle.

Although the suggested outline for grant applications provided in Appendix I will require modification for each study and may have to be changed to conform with different requirements in various countries, it may be useful in getting your thinking started and in assembling the information you will need.

8. Keep Appendices and Supporting Documents to a Minimum

Lengthy appendices, supporting documents, and bibliographies will produce a cumbersome application. The reviewer will usually feel compelled to read them and may well be irritated when he has finished if the appendices do not contribute much. An appendix or supporting document should only be included if the proposal cannot be understood without it and it is clearly inappropriate to include the information in the main body of the application, e.g., the precise format of an interview form. If you are in doubt, state what the document contains briefly in the text of your proposed and indicate that it is available on request. Do not attach it.

9. Be Realistic in Your Assessment of the Available and Required Resources

Do not propose to hire categories of professionals that are not available in your setting or community. If the execution of your project depends on non-existent human or other resources, or on equipment you cannot maintain, you should not be applying for support. On the other hand, identifying the person who will perform the task *by name* strengthens the proposal by its concreteness.

Ascertain what funds you will need for salaries, equipment, supplies, specialized services, consultants, and other items very carefully. Underestimating what you require will cause you unnecessary difficulties when you come to carry out your study. Deliberately overestimating the cost of the required resources will undermine your credibility during the first review or when you submit your annual progress report.

The peers who will judge the merits of your proposal and assess its progress when you submit renewal requests are usually aware that errors of judgment can be made in estimating the requirements for a study; most of them have experienced such embarrassments and are sympathetic. Reviewers can be expected to be reasonable about applications for amendments of budgets when such requests are sensible and caused by unforeseeable contingencies. It is much better to submit supplementary requests, if the need arises, than to "pad" a submission at the outset.

10. Prepare and Justify Your Budget Carefully

Most granting agencies provide preprinted application forms that include the required breakdown of requested funding into budgetary categories. Nevertheless many research proposals are submitted without adequate justification of the expenditures included in the various categories or without enough detail about the budget as a whole to enable the appraiser to link listed items of expenditure with the activities described in the project.

Your justification of your budget should explain the need for each individual for whom a salary (or wages) is requested, for every item of equipment, for each category of supplies, for travel, and for any other special requirements.

It is wise to identify any major expenditure for which the estimates are not firm. Should budgetary difficulties concerning an uncertain estimate arise later, prior identification of the potential problem will have paved the way for approval of any necessary amendment.

Conclusion

Preparing a research proposal and applying for its support need not be dreaded as an unavoidable tournament that must precede any rewarding research activity. Designing a project, exploring feasible approaches to its implementation, identifying the resources needed, and communicating all this information in a grant application are integral components of investigative activity. If you don't win the award the first time, you have still organized your project. Seek a detailed critique from the reviewers, revise your application and resubmit it. The whole process is intellectually challenging and can even be enjoyable.

Appendix I

Suggested Outline for a Research Protocol

A. Summary (300 words or less)
B. Main Protocol
   1. The objective and research question(s)
      (a) objective
      (b) question(s)—may be restated as a hypothesis or hypotheses if desired or appropriate
      (c) significance of the problem to health care or biomedical science
   2. Review of pertinent literature
   3. General strategy of the study, including a discussion of the rationale for the choice of method(s) (e.g., historical study, survey, experiment, etc.; use or not of comparison groups)
   4. Laboratory and/or clinical facilities (if applicable)
   5. Specific procedures or tactics
      (a) Kinds of information to be collected
      (b) procedures to be used in the collection of information
      (c) from whom will the information be collected
      (d) by whom
      (e) where
      (f) schedule for collection of information
      (g) copies of letters, recording forms, interview schedules, questionnaires, etc., should be included either in the text or appendixes as deemed appropriate
   6. Ethical considerations
   7. Methods of data preparation
   8. Method of analysis, including statistical techniques, if appropriate (for sections 6 and 7 justify any planned use of computers)
   9. Dummy tables, charts, and graphs
   10. Justification of budget
   11. Criteria for success of the project

Summary of Ten Recommendations

1. State objective and research questions clearly.
2. Use the literature review to justify the need for the proposed project.
3. Be clear about your general strategy.
4. Identify the appropriate funding agency.
5. Seek early consultation with experts.
6. Declare criteria for evaluating answers to the research questions *and* the success of project.
7. Be brief.
8. Keep appendices and supporting documents to a minimum.
9. Assess the resources needed to implement your project realistically.
10. Justify your budget carefully.

References

1. Apley AG. The Watson-Jones Lecture 1984: Surgeons and Writers. J Bone Joint Surg (Br) 1985:67;140–144.
2. Dixon J. Developing the evaluation component of a grant application. J Nurs Outlook 1982:30;122–127.
3. Jagger J. How to write a research proposal. Grants Magazine 1980;3(4);216–222.
4. Skodal HW. Research proposal: the practical imagination at work. J Nurs Adm 1985:15(2); 5–7.

7

Critical Appraisal of Published Research

M.T. Schechter and F.E. LeBlanc

Every year thousands of articles appear in the surgical literature. While many present the results of careful investigations based on good methodology, many others report studies whose results are either invalid because of defects in their conduct or analysis, or ungeneralizable to other settings because of biases in the way they were executed. This chapter describes a framework within which published research can be appraised and judged as to its validity and generalizability. We will examine a frequently encountered type of research, i.e., controlled trials of therapeutic interventions, According to six easily-remembered appraisal criteria: WHY, HOW, WHO, WHAT, HOW MANY, and SO WHAT.

Why

The critical appraiser should always begin by considering the reasons for the study and whether sufficient evidence is presented to justify it. In the absence of clear statements of the purpose of the study and of the study hypothesis at the outset, the reader may well consider moving on to another article, because such statements are essential for two reasons. First, the design of the study, which includes the population to be studied, the variables to be considered, and the method of analysis to be utilized, depends very heavily on the purpose of the study. Second, it must be possible for the reader to determine whether the hypothesis was specified in advance, i.e., *a priori,* or arose out of the data, i.e., *a posteriori.* The study hypothesis should also indicate whether the study is intended to be hypothesis-generating or hypothesis-testing.

In studies of therapeutic interventions, it should also be clearly stated whether the study is considering *efficacy* or *effectiveness*. Efficacy studies seek to determine whether an intervention provides a specific outcome under ideal circumstances, i.e., in properly diagnosed and properly treated patients who are compliant. Effectiveness studies seek to determine whether an intervention does more good than harm in patients under normal clinical circumstances, i.e., in patients who are diagnosed and treated, as in the community, and who may or may not comply, as in the community. In general, the outcome measures used in efficacy studies tend to be short-term and specific while those in effectiveness studies are longer term and more global. *While both types of study have their merits, it is the results of effectiveness studies that indicate whether a given intervention should be adopted.* Nevertheless, efficacy studies have their place in the early investigation of new therapies. Much of the methodology in the study, especially the population to be studied and the outcome to be assessed will be determined by which approach, i.e., efficacy or effectiveness, is chosen.

Consider for example, studies investigating coronary artery bypass surgery as a treatment for coronary artery disease. To study the *efficacy* of this intervention, one would ideally utilize a treatment group consisting of patients with clearly documented coronary stenoses, all of whom undergo coronary artery bypass surgery. To test efficacy, one would consider short term outcomes that this intervention is designed to produce, namely increase in myocardial blood flow, relief of anginal symptoms, etc. In such a study, anyone who was allocated to receive the surgery but did not actually receive it because of intervening illnesses say, would not be included in the treatment group because any subsequent benefit could not be attributed to the efficacy of the intervention itself. On the other hand, when one considers *effectiveness,* one is challenging not merely the intervention itself, but the *policy* of using this intervention in the study population. This is sometimes known as the "intent-to-treat" principle. In a study of the effectiveness of coronary artery bypass surgery, a wider spectrum of outcomes including long term survival, quality of life, level of function, etc., should be considered. In such studies, patients who are allocated to receive medical therapy but are given surgery at a later date, should be analyzed within the medical group since it is the policies of initial treatment with medical versus surgical therapy that are being compared.

How

The critical appraiser should endeavor to determine how the study was carried out. The types of study design that readers are most likely to encounter in relation to therapeutic interventions include (1) *case series* which simply report the results of a series of cases treated with a given intervention, (2) *before-after studies* in which the patients' condition before and after the intervention are compared, either in entire settings or within individuals, and (3) *controlled trials* which compare the results in a treated and an untreated control group. In controlled trials, the reader should carefully assess how the patients were allocated to the treatment or the control group. Was the allocation truly randomized? If randomization was not employed, could any biases have occurred in the allocation of the patients? Readers should be on the alert for *quasi-random allocation* in which patients are assigned to the treatment or control group on the basis of some seemingly random process such as birth date, chart number, day of week, etc. Subtle biases can be introduced in such situations and there is no reason why a true randomization could not have been utilized.

The reader should also attempt to determine what type of *blindness* was employed. *Single-blindness* refers to studies in which only the patient does not know whether the experimental treatment or the "control" therapy was received. When *double-blindness* is used, both the patient and the care providers are unaware of the allocation. *Triple-blindness* describes the situation where the patients, the care providers, and those who determine the outcome, are all unaware of what treatment was given. In studies of surgical interventions, blinding of the patients and care providers is not always possible but, at the very least, those who perform the outcome assessment can be blinded to the treatment the patient received. The reader should carefully assess whether any lack of blindness might have led to an expectation bias that distorted the results.

It is also important to determine whether significant prognostic variables were equally allocated to the treatment and control groups. Although most prognostic variables will be equally distributed in large studies employing randomized allocation, maldistribution can occur in small studies. Consequently, it is wise for investigators to use a method known as *prognostic stratification* in which patients are first stratified with regard to an important set of prognostic variables, and then randomized from each stratum. This method guarantees equal distribution of the prognostic variables to the treatment and control groups.

Consider for example, a clinical trial comparing two different treatments for astrocytomas. To make the comparison fair, the groups to which the respective treatments are applied should be comparable with regard to tumour grade as histological grade is a very important predictor of prognosis in this disease. Since the number of available patients is likely to be small, it is possible that a maldistribution could occur with simple randomization in which an excess of patients with grades III and IV astrocytomas might be allocated by chance to one of the treatments. To avoid this, prognostic stratification could be used in which patients entering the trial could be first stratified by the grade of their lesion and then randomized to treatment from within each grade. This would guarantee a more equitable distribution of the grades to the two treatment groups.

Who

One of the most important aspects of critical appraisal is understanding the type of patient studied. The reader must determine if the type of patient included in an investigation was sufficiently representative to allow the results to be applied to all patients in similar clinical situations. This representativeness can be assessed in several ways.

First, the source population from which the study sample was drawn should be clearly described and suitably representative. Are demographic details of the catchment area provided? Was the study sample drawn from a primary, secondary, or tertiary referral centre? Is there any evidence that the study sample includes only a small sub-sample of the entire spectrum of the disease?

Are clear and replicable inclusion and exclusion criteria specified, and do they match the goals of the study? If clear and replicable inclusion and exclusion criteria are not given, the readers can know neither exactly what type of patient has been studied nor to which of their patients the results can be applied. The inclusion and exclusion criteria should define a study population that matches the type of patient that the investigators intend should benefit from the results. The reader should compare the type of population that remains, after the exclusion and inclusion criteria have been applied, with the stated goals of the study to see if they match.

Do the authors account for every patient who was eligible for the study but did not enter it? Typically, patients who are eligible for a study, i.e., who meet the inclusion criteria and are not rejected by the exclusion criteria, are approached for informed consent and some decline. If the proportion of refusals is small, (i.e., < 10%,) it is of limited importance, but *volunteer bias* can occur if a significant proportion of eligible patients do not agree to participate. Participants tend to be more motivated, more compliant, and destined for better outcomes than those who decline to participate. Investigators should either recruit 90% of all eligible patients, as a minimum, or provide evidence that those who decline to participate had outcomes similar to those who did; either approach provides some evidence that volunteer bias was not a significant factor.

Finally, the reader should determine whether the baseline comparability of the treatment and control groups has been documented. Although randomization of large numbers of patients can be expected to provide relatively equal distributions, maldistributions of important prognostic variables can still occur, especially with smaller sample sizes. The investigators should provide an assessment of the baseline comparability of the two groups and if any prognostic variable has been maldistributed, it should be taken into account in the analysis.

What

This aspect of the critical appraisal centers on two questions: What intervention is under study? and What outcome measures are being assessed?

The investigators should provide a clear definition of the intervention because without it the reader cannot really know what is being assessed. Some measure of *compliance* should also be included. This may apply even in trials of surgical interventions where some components of care beyond the surgical procedure, such as follow-up care, self-care, adjunct medications, etc. may require the patient's compliance. How non-compliers were analyzed in the study deserves attention. In effectiveness trials, non-compliers should be analyzed within the treatment arm to which they were randomized; in efficacy studies, it may sometimes be more appropriate to omit non-compliers from the analysis. Investigators should attempt to monitor *contamination* (patients assigned to the control arm subsequently underwent the experimental intervention), *co-intervention* (additional therapies were made available to patients in either arm of the trial), as well as all side effects of the intervention.

It is critically important that all the patients who entered into the study be accounted for. All withdrawals (patients removed by the investigators) and drop-outs (patients removed of their own volition) should be documented and the reasons given for their departure. *Cross-overs* occur when a patient in one arm of the trial receives the intervention assigned to another arm of the trial, e.g., in studies of surgical versus medical treatment of coronary artery disease, patients originally assigned to medical therapy may deteriorate and subsequently undergo coronary artery bypass surgery. The reader should determine whether withdrawals, dropouts, cross-overs, and poor compilers were analyzed in accordance with the goals of the study. For example, in an effectiveness study of coronary artery bypass surgery, patients initially assigned to medical therapy who cross over and receive the surgical intervention should be analyzed within the arm of the study to which they were originally randomized.

With regards to the second aspect of this portion of the critical appraisal the reader should determine whether all clinically relevant outcome measures were used and whether they matched the goals of the study. For example, a study comparing two interventions may focus on the subsequent three-week mortality in the treatment and control groups. Even if such a trial showed an improvement in the three-week mortality with the intervention, it would still not provide any reassurance about the long-term survival of patients. Moreover, if the reader is deciding whether to use the intervention, he or she will to want to know if the quality of life is improved for those undergoing the intervention. Another important consideration is whether the measurement of the outcomes was precise. This may not be an issue if the outcome was length of survival because the endpoint (death) is clear, but if the outcome being measured was severity of pain, quality of life, improvement of clinical signs or symptoms, etc. the reader should determine whether a reliable and valid method was used to gather such information. Those who assess the outcome can usually be blinded to the patients allocation and provide an unbiased assessment of outcome. But the reader should ascertain whether the process of observation required to assess the outcome could, in itself, have influenced the outcome.

How Many

The reader should determine whether statistical significance was considered in the paper, whether statistical tests used were applied appropriately (see Section II, Chapter 3), and whether the authors considered the methods of analysis and the sample size requirements *prior* to initiating the study. It is well known that the more analyses one performs on a data set, the more likely one is to obtain a significant result by chance. Accordingly, a significant result obtained from a single prespecified analysis is much more meaningful than it would be if derived from a series of analyses suggested by the data. Similarly, the reader should check for the possibility of the *multiple comparisons problem*, which occurs when investigators consider several different outcome variables and, in so doing, increase the likelihood of a significant result arising by chance. In such instances, the investigators should adjust their alpha level according to well known methods (see Section II, Chapter 3).

In studies where no statistically significant differences are found between the treatment and control groups, it is critically important that the authors consider the possibility of a beta error (type II error) and estimate the probability of its occurrence. All too often, investigators conclude that there is no difference between the experimental and control treatment when all they can really conclude is that their study failed to detect a difference. If consideration of a type II error is not provided, the reader might well ask whether the study was large enough to detect important differences.

Small sample size frequently leads to trials whose power to detect important differences in outcome between treatment groups, is weak. Freiman and colleagues (1) found that in half of the articles that reported no significant differences between the therapies under study, a 50% improvement in performance could easily have been missed. The overall assessment of these authors was that the problem of type II error and small sample size was ubiquitous in the medical literature. When no statistically significant difference is found in a study, the reader who knows that the study was strong enough to have had a good chance of detecting a clinically important difference can conclude that the matter is fairly well settled. If the authors do not discuss the power of a trial, the reader has the right to suspect that the study was not large enough to detect important differences.

So What

The heading "So What" reminds the reader to form some overall conclusion about the importance of the information provided in the article and its relevance to his or her own clinical practice.

If differences were detected, was their CLINICAL SIGNIFICANCE discussed? Clinical significance refers to the magnitude of the difference observed between treatment and control groups measured in clinical (not statistical) terms. If a statistically significant difference is also clinically significant, it implies that a change in clinical behavior is warranted. For example, a study may observe survival rates of 55% in the treatment group and 50% in the control group. If large numbers of patients are involved, this difference may be statistically significant. However, if the intervention is exceedingly expensive or entails considerable morbidity, it may be hard to justify using it to obtain such a marginal gain in survival, i.e., the difference may be judged as being not clinically significant.

Were the patients included and analyzed in the study sufficiently representative to allow the results to be generalized to other patients? By considering the source population from which the study sample was obtained, the method by which patients were recruited, the inclusion and exclusion criteria, the possibility of volunteer bias, and the patients actually analyzed, the reader should be able to decide whether the type of patient studied was sufficiently similar to his or her own patients that the results can be applied to them. A simple rule of thumb is: THE TYPE OF PATIENT INCLUDED AND ANALYZED IN ANY STUDY IS THE ONLY TYPE OF PATIENT TO WHICH ITS RESULTS CAN BE APPLIED.

Was the intervention as performed in the study sufficiently representative that the results can be generalized to other settings? Is the intervention available in other settings? Were those who performed the intervention highly specialized? If the study involved highly motivated, highly trained, and compliant care providers, questions may arise as to how well the intervention will be performed on a community wide basis. This is particularly true in studies of surgical interventions performed in specialized settings by highly skilled surgeons, practiced in the technique under study, and supported by highly specialized adjunct care.

Do the outcomes assessed in the study provide an adequate basis on which to establish which of the therapies under study does the most good? If six-week mortality for example was the outcome variable of central interest, the reader may not consider the results sufficient justification for incorporating the intervention into his or her own clinical practice; he or she might very well prefer to await evidence that the benefit is not only a short-term reduction in mortality but also a long-term improvement in survival, morbidity, quality of life, level of function, etc.

In conclusion, the goals and hypotheses (the "WHY") upon which a study is based are inexorably linked to several crucial methodological components of the study design, namely the source population to be sampled, the inclusion and exclusion criteria, allocation methods, appropriate handling of various events (withdrawals, cross-overs, etc.), outcome assessment, methods of data analysis, and interpretation of clinical significance to name but a few. It cannot be overemphasized that a clear understanding of study goals and hypotheses is fundamental to good research methodology and astute critical appraisal.

Summary

Why

Is sufficient evidence presented to justify the study?

Is the purpose of the study clearly stated?

Is the study hypothesis clearly stated?

Is it clearly outlined whether the study is considering EFFICACY or EFFECTIVENESS?

How

What exactly is the study design?

If it is a controlled trial, is the allocation truly randomized?

If not, are there any biases in the allocation to treatment?

What type of blindness is employed? (Single, double, triple, etc.).

Was prognostic stratification used?

Who

Is the population from which the study sample was drawn, clearly described?

Are inclusion and exclusion criteria specified and replicable?

Do the criteria match the goals of the study?

Do the authors account for every eligible patient who does not enter the study?

Is the baseline comparability of the treatment and control groups documented?

What

What, exactly, was the intervention performed? Is it clearly defined and replicable?

Was compliance with the intervention(s) measured and were non-compliers analyzed appropriately?

Were contamination and co-intervention considered?

Were all patients who entered the study accounted for?

Were withdrawals, drop-outs, cross-overs, and poor compilers analyzed in accordance with the goals of the study?

What outcomes were assessed in the study?

Were all relevant outcomes utilized?

Could the process of observation have influenced the outcome?

How Many

What statistical significance considered in the study?

Were statistical tests applied appropriately?

Did the authors consider the methods of analysis and the sample size requirements prior to the study?

When no statistically significant differences were found, did the authors consider the possibility of a beta (Type II) error and estimate its probability?

Was the study large enough to detect important differences?

So What

If differences were detected, was their clinical significance discussed?

Were the patients entered and analyzed in the study sufficiently representative to allow the results to be generalized to other patients?

Was the intervention, as performed in the study, sufficiently representative that the results can be generalized to other settings.

Do the outcomes assessed in the study provide an adequate basis on which to establish which of the therapies under study does the greatest good?

References

1. Freiman JA, Chalmers TC, Smith H Jr., Kuebler RR. The importance of beta, the type II error and sample size in the design and interpretation of the randomized control trial. Survey of 71 negative trials. N Engl J Med 1978;299:690–694.

8
Ethical Principles in Surgical Research

D.J. Roy, P. Black, and B. McPeek

"The surgical act is just too powerful and too dangerous to be loosed on an unsuspecting public in the hands of a surgeon who uses only his cerebellum." (1)

Judah Folkman, M.D.

Introduction

Research ethics is as integral a part of scientific judgment as clinical ethics is of clinical judgment (2). Many ethical issues in research arise from a failure to think as rigorously about the conditions for ethical consistency as about those for scientific validity. The ethical principles governing all surgical, clinical, and biomedical research with human subjects are fundamentally the same. They have been listed and discussed in numerous documents and countless publications over the past 40 years (3–10).

Although due regard must be maintained for the utility and necessity of institutional review boards, ethics committees, and participation of the general public in the ethical evaluation of protocols for research with human subjects, it is a mistake to view ethics as an external authoritarian imposition of regulations or constraints, perhaps even arbitrary in nature, on the process of clinical research. The design and the practice of research ethics should be primarily, though not exclusively, a matter of self-consistency and self-governance within clinical investigation.

Ethics and Research

Research ethics and scientific research pursue a common cognitive goal: to distinguish mere appearances from reality.

Scientific research, using measurement as its cardinal procedure, seeks to ascertain the actual relationships between phenomena. Uncritical reliance on initial observations, potentially distorted by bias, can lead to a systematic divergence from the truth (11). Rigorous research methods are devised precisely to counter the tendency to mistake a mere semblance of correlation for a judgment of fact.

Research ethics, a process of critical reflection and interdisciplinary collaboration, acts against the tendency to diverge systematically from what is right. As initial observations may fail to reveal true correlations, spontaneous desires or compulsions may not correspond to what we ought to do. What appears to be good in a limited perspective may contradict a greater and more commanding value. True values, like real correlations between phenomena, are not always immediately obvious. A spontaneous apparent good acquires the moral force of a value only upon passing through a process of critical reflection in which proposed courses of action and possible objects of choice are subjected to a series of questions that result in a value judgment. Value judgments, like judgments of fact and of truth, are governed by assent to sufficient evidence, not by submission to custom, convention, authority, brilliance, or emotion.

Working out the ethics of research requires the exercise of critical intelligence and judgment by a community of human beings engaged in the check and balance of attentive and mutually corrective discourse rather than in isolated monologues. The combination of interdisciplinary dialogue with the study of specific cases, whether of clinical practice or clinical research, acts as a counterforce to moral atomism, rampant relativism, and what Stephen Toulmin has called the tyranny of principles (12). *Principles, guidelines, and codes alone do not decide concrete cases.* Principles will fail to reveal their meaning—what they command, permit, and prohibit—until they are interpreted in the light of specific research situations.

This concept and method of ethics offer a basis for such organizations as institutional review boards (IRB's) or research ethics committees, without necessarily justifying their specific modes of operation. It must be emphasized, however, that ethical judgment is an integral component of clinical and scientific intelligence; clinical investigators are expected and entitled to perform as integrated human beings and professionals.

Controlled Clinical Research: An Ethical Imperative

)ral obligation to offer each pa-
.ilable treatment cannot be sep-
ical and ethical imperatives to
of treatment on the best avail-
ible evidence. The tension be-
dependent responsibilities of
.nd compassionate care, as well
sound and validated treatment,
ne practice of medicine today.
ises prior to, and as a moral real-
)m, any conflict of interests. It is not merely the expression of an individual physician–investigator's disordered intentions, but is a structural part of the medical profession's covenant with the human community.

Controlled clinical trials—randomized and multiply blinded, when randomization and blinding are feasible, ethically achievable, and scientifically appropriate—are an integral part of the ethical imperative that physicians and surgeons should *know* what they are doing when they intervene into the bodies, psyches, and lives of vulnerable, suffering human beings. The ethical requirement of precise and validated knowledge gathers force with the likelihood that clinical interventions will exert decisive and irreversible impacts on patients' futures and on future patients. Future patients have faces; they cannot be lumped together as part of society and set in opposition to patients occupying hospital beds today.

The standards of good medicine, determined by professional consensus based upon reliable methods of achieving validated knowledge, enter into the inner structure of the doctor-patient relationship. At the very least, this means "that what doctor and patient choose is not the untrammeled expression of the knowledge and values of each. It is limited by the professional norms that constrain the doctor's judgment and constrain it in the name of good medicine generally'' (13). Something more, though, is required. If the achievement of good medicine is an ethical imperative, this imperative must exert not only the *protective force* of a constraint on potentially misguided judgment and choice, but also the *constructive force* of an invocation to comprehending and voluntary collaboration in constantly redesigning the standards of good medicine. Professionally validated knowledge, without the collaboration of individual physicians and patients, would remain a utopian dream.

When there is uncertainty or definite doubt about the safety or efficacy of an innovative or established treatment, this position supports the strong view that there *is, not* simply *may be,* "a higher moral obligation to test it critically than to prescribe it year-in, year-out with the support of custom or of wishful thinking'' (14). When large numbers of innovative treatments are continuously introduced into clinical practice, as is the case today, rigorous testing is ethically mandatory both for the protection of individual patients and for the just use of limited resources. This holds true with even greater force in the light of evidence that many innovations show no advantage over existing treatments when they are subjected to properly controlled study (15). They may even be less effective, or harmful (16).

Conditions for the Ethical Conduct of Clinical Research

Conditional Ethics

If the practice of medicine is both morally mandatory and inherently experimental (17), controlled clinical trials cannot be inherently unethical. Clinical trials, whatever the tactics used to control for bias, will be unethical only to the extent that they fail to meet a set of necessary and interrelated conditions.

"Ethical justifiability" means consistency with the ethos and morality of the human community. Human communities vary from one culture and society to another, not only in their customs and art, but also in their governing perceptions and values regarding the body, health, disease, suffering, death and a host of other realities affecting the practice of medicine. The conditions for ethically justifiable research with human subjects arise from the requirements for consistency along each of these dimensions.

These conditions are structured. They range from fundamental principles of science, medicine, and philosophy across more specific norms, procedures, and regulations to encompass the tailored ethical judgments required for the unique characteristics and designs of individual clinical trials. The ethics of clinical research is open-ended, cumulative, and unfinished. A continual process of feedback is at work between tailored ethical judgments on specific trials and the principles, norms, procedures and regulations requisite for the ethical conduct of clinical research. Our knowledge of right and wrong is as subject to the process of evolution and cumulative growth as is our knowledge of fact and truth in science.

The concept of conditional ethics, so understood, implies that ethical justifiability is a graded, not a binary, characteristic of clinical trials. The rheostat rather than the on-off switch suggests an appropriate image.

Research Ethics and Cultural Diversity

Though science is largely transcultural, the human community has not yet developed a completely corresponding transcultural ethics. Differing views about what is normative in person–person, doctor–patient, and investigator–subject relationships may create the need for ethical compromise or accommodation in some multicentre trials, particularly when the collaborating centres are situated in different nations.

A Japanese physician–investigator may find it difficult to honour North American insistence on detailed disclosure to patients about the randomization process used to select treatment in a clinical trial for breast cancer or cancer of the prostate. Both physicians and patients in a culture that places great emphasis on trust in the physician as an integral part of the healing process may find an open admission of physician ignorance or uncertainty to be therapeutically damaging or even absurd.

North American culture emphasizes the value of individual autonomy. Chinese culture emphasizes the value of the family and the community. The approach to informed, comprehending, and voluntary consent may be quite different in each of these cultures. H. Tristam Engelhardt, Jr. has noted that in China the family and the community play a central role in resolving disputes and in obtaining a patient's consent in difficult situations.

"First, community social pressure is the first and usually very effective mode of obtaining agreement. Second, the family plays an important role in securing patient consent, even with adult patients. However, others, such as fellow-workers, are also involved." (18)

Sensitivity to the dominant values of other cultures should be an ethical requisite of international collaboration in multicentre trials. Accommodating cultural differences, even in ethnic groups within the pluralistic society of Western nations, will usually require a flexibility in procedures rather than the compromise of fundamental principles.

Scientific Adequacy

The Nuremberg Code and the Declaration of Helsinki have stated that research with human subjects must, as a general condition of ethical justifiability, conform to the canons of scientific methodology (19,20). Both insist on respect for accepted scientific principles, knowledge of the natural history of the disease or problem under study, adequate preliminary laboratory and animal experimentation, and the proper scientific and medical qualifications of investigators. This emphasis, though covering the basic preconditions for a valid and credible clinical trial, may sound like a quaint overemphasis of the obvious. However, the attempt in the early 1980's to treat two beta-thalassemic patients by modifying bone marrow with human beta-globin gene implants was widely criticized as premature and unethical, chiefly on two grounds. The treatment was tried without adequate preliminary experimentation with animal models of beta-thalassemia and without the solid foundation of adequate basic knowledge about the regulation of gene expression (21–25).

David R. Rutstein's maxim—"a poorly or improperly designed study involving human subjects . . . is by definition unethical" (26)—directs attention to the general rule of proportionality ethics. Inviting human beings to submit themselves to possibly heightened risk of discomfort, inconvenience, harm, or death, consuming scarce precious resources, and raising hopes, particularly in situations when hope is about all that patients have left, demand the balancing weight of a clinical trial that exhibits a high probability of achieving three objectives identified by David L. Sackett (27). They are: "validity (the results are true), generalizability (the results are widely applicable), and efficiency (the trial is affordable and resources are left over for patient care and for other health research)" (64).

Only reliable clinical knowledge merits widespread clinical application. The generalization of invalid clinical knowledge is inherently unethical and the extensive application of non-validated procedures is, at best, ethically dubious. In this context, randomization has gained wide recognition as one of the most effective tactics to control for selection bias, a major form of bias that leads to false conclusions about the safety, efficacy, or superiority of a given treatment.

Randomization has occupied center stage in scientific and ethical discussions of controlled clinical trials with human subjects. Though this emphasis has not been misplaced, a major shift of ethical attention is long overdue. The difficulties raised by the randomization process, already widely recognized and discussed in the literature, are no greater and may even be ethically less significant than the methodological confusion and deficiencies contributing to the generation of humanly costly and resource intensive randomized clinical trial results that are clinically implemented only in very limited ways.

The problem is not limited to the admitted need to translate the results of clinical trials into practice more effectively (28), nor can it be solved by technique alone or by more intensive and restricted focus on the careful blueprinting of randomization designs (29). Randomization, whatever its power, glorious achievements, limitations, or ethical challenges, is not the root of the basic problem of scientific adequacy as a condition for ethically justifiable clinical research with human subjects.

The problem is rooted in the current limitations of basic biomedical science. Meeting the demands of scientific adequacy, as a condition for the ethical justifiability of clinical research with human subjects, requires the development of what A. Feinstein has called the basic science of clinical practice. This requirement, as yet unfulfilled, is based on the fact that "the experiments of the laboratory and the bedside have major differences in scientific orientation, motivation, hypotheses, and values" (30).

A continuing failure to implement the consequences of these differences will exacerbate the ethical problems of clinical research, however great the increases in the number of publications and conferences on the meaning of respect for human dignity and the specifications of informed consent. Feinstein's suggested additional basic science of clinical practice would aim to bring cogent human information derived directly from the patient back into the boundaries of science. The goal of this science would be to give physicians and patients power over medical science and technology "by expanding it to include human data, by aiming it at human goals, and by making it respond to human aspirations" (31).

Clinical Research: A Human Relationship

Research with human subjects is ethically unjustifiable to the extent that it fails to honour four fundamental characteristics of an authentically human relationship. Charles Fried has identified these as: humanity, autonomy, lucidity and fidelity (13). These characteristics are essential qualifications of how physicians, clinical investigators, patients, and subjects should behave towards each other. Our attention, in this discussion, is understandably focussed on the behaviour of physicians and clinical investigators.

In a human relationship, a person is not treated simply as one of a class. The characteristic, humanity, stresses that each person is a unique individual with a correspondingly unique biology and individualized needs, weakness, strengths, and life plans. Humanity means attention to and respect for this "full human particularity" (13). Autonomy or self-determination implies the need and the capacity to deliberate about personal goals and the liberty to act accordingly. A relationship that fosters autonomy is notable for the absence of fraud, force, and the tendency to use another human being as a disposable resource.

Lucidity qualifies communication as honest, candid, and open to imparting all known information that is material to another's self-determination, deliberation, and choice of alternatives to realize individual life plans. This means sensitivity to another person's total life interests and capacities for comprehension. Lucidity is ill-served if clinical investigators look upon "obtaining informed consent" as some kind of legally imposed ritual. Clinical investigators sometimes speak as though consent is something *they* need for *their* research. They fail to grasp the reality that adequate information is primarily a need of the patient and a moral requirement of integrity in a human relationship.

Fidelity means faithfulness in responding to justified expectations that are integral components of a relationship. These expectations will vary from one kind of relationship to another. Patients enter into relationships with doctors justifiably expecting, however implicity, that their doctors are suitably qualified, are up-to-date with current standards of good medicine and skillful surgery, and are committed to restoring their patients to good health.

Informed, Comprehending, and Voluntary Consent

Physicians and clinical investigators have a primordial obligation to assure that their patients and volunteer subjects are adequately informed to enable them to consent comprehendingly and without coercion to the research procedures and interventions they are being invited to undergo. This condition for ethically justifiable research with human subjects, clearly established in the Nuremberg Code (19), has been subjected to relentless and detailed scrutiny over the past 30 years in over 4000 publications (32).

The ethical norm of informed, comprehending, and voluntary consent has its origin in the four characteristics of an authentic human relationship discussed earlier. Though each shapes the process of consent, humanity is the most difficult to respect. It is, nevertheless, singularly important in gauging the scope of disclosure of information in clinical practice and in clinical research.

The particularity of the patient's situation was a central issue in the Canadian Supreme Court case of Reibl versus Hughes. The Court's decision clarifies that, of three possible standards for determining the kinds of information that must be disclosed, that is, the professional, subjective patient, and objective patient standards, the latter is to be followed. If the professional standard would allow doctors and clinical investigators to set the threshold of disclosure "at a lower level than would serve the public interest and protection", the subjective patient standard would place physicians "at the mercy of the patient's bitter hindsight" (33).

The Court clarified that the objective or reasonable patient standard implies the need to match information to a patient's reasonably based particular concerns and preferences (34). This legally and ethically important case illustrates the essential moral difference between "obtaining" informed consent as a ritual kind of act, performed primarily to get treatment or research moving, and "educating" a patient or subject in an open searching conversation, carried out primarily to assure that the patient knows and understands everything required to make a free and reasonable decision.

This case also emphasizes that "informed consent" is part of a two-way transaction (33). The doctor also needs information if the patient is to be adequately informed. How can a physician or clinical investigator serve the life plans of a patient or subject if nothing is said about them in conversations about the treatment or the research? Doctors and clinical investigators are as much in need of knowing every essential of the life plans, concerns, and bodily situation of patients and subjects as the latter are in need of knowing every essential of the preferred treatments and proposed research procedures.

Physicians and clinical investigators bear primary responsibility for organizing consent conversations and making certain that this mutually informing process really takes place. Insecure and vulnerable patients and subjects may easily be cowed into silence, or even acquiescence, by the awesome environment of the hospital and the authority-laden image of the doctor (35). The hospital is the doctor's daily domain and home territory, which the patient enters as a frightened stranger. In these circumstances, voluntary consent doesn't come naturally. It requires sensitive perception and dedicated commitment on the part of physicians and clinical investigators if they are to serve the needs and goals of those who come to them for care and cure.

Clinical Research: A Therapeutic Relationship

Henry K. Beecher's statement, "Ordinary patients will not knowingly risk their health or their life for the sake of science" (36), is as true today as it was in 1966. Sick people come to doctors for care, relief, and cure. Though cure cannot be guaranteed and every intervention into the body carries its risk of harm, care encompasses the granting by patients, and the appropriating by doctors, "of some power over another so that the other will benefit" (37).

The expectation that doctors will help, and not harm, is the basis of the patient–doctor relationship, the primary content of the medical profession's societal mandate, and the guiding norm of one of medicine's most ancient ethical maxims (37). Fidelity to this expectation is an essential condition for ethically acceptable clinical research.

Claude Bernard gave precision to the meaning of this fidelity in his statement of a principle of medical and surgical morality:

"It is our duty and our right to perform an experiment on man whenever it can save his life, cure him, or gain him some personal benefit. The principle of medical and surgical morality, therefore consists in never performing an experiment which might be harmful to him to any extent, even though the result might be highly advantageous to science, that is to the health of others" (17).

This principle sets a basic right of patients, and a corresponding fundamental duty of doctors that takes precedence over any utilitarian calculus that would tolerate a sacrifice of the health or lives of individuals today for the putatively greater good of society or the patients of tomorrow.

This "Bernard" principle, though clearly essential for the ethical justifiability of clinical research with human subjects, is too pure and absolute in its Bernard wording to be realistic. Medicine is inherently experimental. It is clearly impossible, either in uncontrolled clinical practice or in controlled clinical trials, to abstain totally from interventions that might be harmful "to any extent". The factors of uncertainty and risk of harm, attendant upon any clinical intervention into the body, have to be accounted for in this principle of the primacy of the therapeutic obligation.

The therapeutic obligation in clinical practice, whether or not physician and patient are participants in a controlled clinical trial, has to be governed by proportionality ethics. Risks of harm or detriment have to be balanced by equal probability of benefit for the patient, that is weighty enough to compensate for any loss or injury that might occur. This principle complements the Nuremberg and Helsinki emphasis on the proportion to be maintained between the risks undertaken by subjects in clinical research and the scientific and humanitarian importance of the research objectives (19,20).

Harms and benefits are not totally susceptible to objective, generalizable measurement. They comprise both "hard" and "soft" data. The ethical implication is that it is impossible to determine that a proportion between harms and benefits holds for particular patients without giving due attention and weight to their personal interpretations of the total impact of a clinical intervention on their lives. This is the target of A. Feinstein's justified criticism of attempts to balance harms and benefits, or to judge a treatment's efficacy, on the basis of a dehumanized array of data. Such attempts fall short of their objective because they fail to assess the "total spectrum of a treatment's impact" (38).

The Therapeutic Relationship in Randomized Clinical Trials

One of the strongest recurrent ethical criticisms of randomized clinical trials is that they sin against the therapeutic relationship. Physician–investigators participating in such studies, so the critique runs, abandon fully individualized care of their patients and even subject some patients, via the randomization process, to inferior treatment. One assumption behind this criticism is that equipoise regarding safety and efficacy rarely exists between alternative treatments at the initiation of a controlled trial. There is usually some indication that one treatment is better than another, even if the indication falls short of a statistically rigorous demonstration. Even if equipoise does seem to hold at the initiation of a trial, secrecy about interim results when these favor one treatment over another means that some randomized patients, including both early and newly entered patients, will receive inferior treatment.

How can randomizing patients to inferior treatment, or maintaining them on inferior treatment until the trial reaches a certain minimum probability of error, be squared with the demands of the therapeutic relationship? This bottom-line question gathers force when patients suffer either death or serious deterioration of health as a consequence of the inferior treatment.

The foregoing criticism of randomized clinical trials does not sufficiently appreciate the proliferation of innovations and the attendant pervasiveness of uncertainty in medicine, the associated danger of using unvalidated procedures in clinical practice, and the intersection of goals in clinical therapy and interventional trials.

Surgical trials with human subjects are, with few exceptions, interventional rather than explicatory. Alvan Feinstein has identified the ethical significance of the differences between these two kinds of trials (39). In an *interventional* trial, the goal of the treatments employed is to change a patient's clinical course, not in a passing way to study some physiological variable, but in an enduring way and to enhance health and postpone death.

The goal of the therapeutic relationship—to care, relieve, and cure a suffering patient—is identical to the goal pursued by the physician–investigator in an interventional trial. The goal of the trial is to determine reliably whether the effects observed to follow upon a clinical intervention are due to the treatment, or whether one treatment is safer or more effective than its alternatives.

When there is no uncertainty about the safety, efficacy, or comparative worth of treatments, there is no need for an interventional trial. To the extent that such uncertainty does hold sway, it is impertinent to ask whether physician-investigators in an interventional trial are withholding known effective treatments from patients or are consigning patients to inferior treatment. That is precisely what is unknown, and can be reliably determined only by a properly designed trial. An interventional trial, assuming the fulfillment of essential scientific and ethical conditions, is more consistent with fidelity to the therapeutic relationship than unquestioning recommendation of one of several unvalidated treatments whose comparative worth is in dispute.

This position does not reject the principle of conscience. A physician, convinced of the superiority of a given treatment on the basis of available evidence, would be acting against his or her personal and professional conscience in participating in a randomization of patients to an alternative treatment that causes higher mortality or morbidity in the physician's opinion. It must be realized, however, that evidence sufficiently strong to constitute ethical grounds for an individual physician's refusal to participate in a randomized clinical trial may fall far short of a decisive argument against the ethical justifiability of the trial itself.

Clinical Trials and Surgical Research: Ethical Issues

To fit the reality of particular clinical trials, ethical decisions need two synchronized cutting edges: an upper blade of general ethical principles, and a continually re-shaped lower blade of definite answers to specific questions.

The Ethical Use of Animals in Surgical Research

It is generally and correctly assumed that the ethical justifiability of research with human subjects depends on adequate prior experimentation with animals. This does not mean that the use of animals in research requires no further justification. However, a comprehensive response to the question about whether we are morally justified "in imposing suffering on or taking the lives of other species solely for our own benefit" (40) would require an analysis of the expanding and unfinished debate on these issues (41–44). Since such an analysis would exceed the boundaries of this chapter, two major points have been selected for discussion.

First, differences between species do have moral significance. Ethical constraints on what we may impose on other animals to satisfy our own good and our own needs increase as the capacities and needs of the animals approach those of human beings. Second, the critical question is not whether, but under what conditions may we use animals in research?

Effective measures to assure the humane treatment of animals in research and to protect animals against wanton disregard of their needs and welfare are essential requirements of civilized scientific behavior. Fulfilling these requirements does not necessitate acceptance of either of the following positions:

- humans have no right to treat animals any differently than they would treat any member of their own species (45);
- animals should be used in research projects only when the results will directly benefit the animals themselves (45);
- there should be an immediate replacement of all animals used in experiments by alternative systems (43).

Sensitivity to the needs of animals and to their differential capacities for suffering from pain, constriction, and deprivation does necessitate careful attention to Lane Petter's five basic questions:

- Is the animal the best experimental system for the problem?
- Must the animal be conscious at any time during the experiment?
- Can the pain and discomfort associated with the experiment be lessened or eliminated?
- Could the number of animals involved be reduced?
- Is the problem under study worth solving (46,47)?

Necessity of experiment, humaneness of design, and a standard of pre- and post-operative care that is at least as good as that required for acceptable clinical veterinary practice (48) summarize the conditions for the ethical justifiability of using animals in research.

Standards in Surgical Research

There is no controversy about the desirability of high standards of evidence in surgical research. The well known division of opinion is about the kinds of design that are practicable and effective in producing such evidence (49–56). The rule governing such discussions should be: avoid fervent answers to global questions. Variations in the nature of the procedures under study, the clinical conditions to be treated, and different surgical specialties require differentiated judgments about the research design most appropriate for each research project.

The principle of differentiated judgment modifies, and is not a substitute for, the more general ethical rule: employ every possible tactic at the most opportune moment in the development of innovative surgical procedures to reduce the devastating effects of bias. Demanding that the standards of surgical research match the highest currently attainable in clinical investigation is not the same thing as insisting on identity of research design in surgical and medical trials. Methodological sophistication may indicate the need for research designs uniquely tailored for some surgical specialties (51,56–58).

Ethics and the Design of Surgical Research

The methodologically rigorous design of surgical trials poses several distinct and widely recognized difficulties (59,60), which have ethical implications.

First, it is generally impossible to achieve full blinding in surgical research. The extent of blinding achievable will vary depending on whether an operation is being compared with non-surgical treatment or the comparative safety and efficacy of two operations is the object of the trial. Though sham operations are ethically unjustifiable and would not be considered today, a measure of blinding may be possible when the physicians evaluating the patients' progress have not been involved in the trials (50,60–62).

Second, surgery has a powerful placebo effect that may exist independently of an operation's genuine efficacy. This fact, for which internal mammary artery ligation for the relief of angina offers some evidence, underscores the importance of blinding as a tactic in a methodologically rigorous trial in surgery. It is difficult to ethically justify the continued use of operations having little more than placebo efficacy (60)

Third, Francis D. Moore has observed that "the most remarkable and effective extensions of surgery have often not required elaborate statistical analysis for their establishment" (63). Though "often" is not equal to "regularly" or "generally", this observation invites a flexible attitude towards what H.A.F. Dudley has called the central dogma, namely "the concept of overriding need to prosecute controlled clinical trials as the only way of ensuring reliable knowledge" (64).

Fourth, there are situations where randomized clinical trials may be both impractical and ethically dubious. The advisability of a trial is open to serious questions when "thousands of patients must be treated to establish statistically significant, but very small, differences" (63).

Fifth, randomized clinical trials may be impossible when the course of treatment for a given condition is in a state of rapid evolution. For example, the arrival of coronary artery bypass grafting led to the abandonment of a randomized clinical trial of the Vineburg surgical procedure (57). Randomized clinical trials are perilous and dubious undertakings in situations where innovations are likely to be rapidly replaced by even better new procedures.

Sixth, the controversy over radial keratotomy, a surgical procedure to correct myopia, has emphasized once again how difficult it is to launch controlled studies of surgical innovations after they have become popular. The standard ethical objection to randomized trials in this situation is: how can one justify withholding a widely acclaimed procedure from a control group? The radial keratotomy controversy has added another objection: how can one justify withholding business from surgeons by concentrating use of the operation to those surgeons participating in a randomized clinical trial? The lawsuit launched in the United States against George O. Waring, an associate professor of ophthalmology, and against others involved in the "Prospective Evaluation of Radial Keratotomy" trial, has intensified and hardened divisions of opinion about how surgical innovations should be brought into the health care system (65).

Although a judgment on the justification of this particular lawsuit must be withheld, the wisdom of charging clinical researchers with conspiracy to monopolize an operation and with violation of antitrust laws when they undertake the evaluation of a new operation for safety and efficacy must be vigorously questioned. The good conscience of individual surgeons will never be an adequate substitute for methodologically rigorous evaluations of surgical innovations.

The goal of controlled clinical trials should not be confused with any set of methodological strategies or tactics. The goal is reliable knowledge. H.A.F. Dudley has emphasized that "there is a continuous rather than a discontinuous scale of reliability, not a quantum leap from none to near total reliability" (64). The role of randomized clinical trials should be gauged against that scale and in the light of the varying constraints of different clinical situations. We are coming to a more precise identification of the circumstances in which evaluations of efficacy cannot be made with randomized prospective studies (51,57,66). However, the recent results of the extracranial-intracranial bypass study should exercise a braking restraint on any latent enthusiasm for liberation from the rigors of controlled clinical trials (67).

Pre-Randomization Learning and Early Randomization

Thomas C. Chalmers has advanced methodological and ethical reasons for early randomization, indeed for the randomization of the first patient, in the evaluation of new medical treatments and surgical procedures (50,68) Succinctly, his position is: "Randomization from the beginning, with truly informed consent, is the only *ethical* way to begin the exploration of new therapies" (50).

Attention should be given to two methodological considerations, one supportive, the other critical of early randomization, before analyzing the ethical issue raised in the Chalmers position.

Pilot studies and pre-randomization learning periods followed by positive observational reports increase the likelihood that methodologically rigorous evaluations of new surgical procedures will be postponed unduly or simply never initiated. It becomes ethically difficult to randomize patients when one of the procedures under study has already won an enthusiastic constituency, however illusory the evidence for this enthusiasm may be (69,70). Early randomization, if practicable and successful, counters this tendency.

Early randomization may, however, be impossible or methodologically dubious in some surgical trials. Experience, technical skill, and masterful craftsmanship have to be acquired through practice. They cannot be taught and learned before an operation is actually performed. A new operation has little chance of being judged on its own merits until the surgeons performing it in a trial have acquired sufficient mastery of the procedures to permit a sufficient degree of standardization. Short of this, the same operation in the hands of different surgeons possessing quite variable levels of skill may well have quite divergent results (70). In such circumstances, a trial would more likely measure variances in surgical craftsmanship rather than the safety and effectiveness of the new operation. Indeed, with wide variations in surgical skill, the operations under study may not be the same. Moreover, potentially promising new operations for which "it takes years to reach optimum low risk and clinical benefit" (53) could be rejected, not on the basis of their real therapeutic merit, but because of initial high mortality rates due to surgeons' inexperience.

Chalmers recognizes the force of the methodological objection to very early randomization of patients in the evaluation of surgical innovations, particularly of technically difficult new operations. He has stated that "from the scientific standpoint alone, the technique should be fully developed before the randomized trial is begun" (50). Consonant with this observation, William Van den Linden has proposed a prerandomization practice period that "should last until the participants are fully conversant with every single detail of the new technique. It is not until then that a fair trial can be run" (62).

The Chalmer's position holds that running a fair trial can be in conflict with running an ethical trial. Though prerandomization practice periods would set the stage for a more reliable comparison of a new against an established operation, Chalmers observes that patients honestly informed about the potentially higher initial mortality or morbidity rates to be expected during this period would likely refuse to enter this surgical novitiate and demand the established operation (50). He argues that randomization from the beginning, with truly informed consent, is the only ethical way to evaluate new operations because patients are more likely to accept randomization if they are convinced that there is "an equal chance that the new operation might be better than the old from the beginning" (50).

The Chalmer's exclusive position on the ethical superiority of very early randomization is not convincing. The fact that a new operation has a good chance of being superior to an older established surgical treatment has to be modified by the word "eventually". The potential intrinsic merits of a new operation, once mastered, are not an antidote to the risks of potentially higher mortality or morbidity resulting from surgeons' underdeveloped skills in performing the new procedures. Lawrence Bonchek's observation and counter question is in order. "Randomization does not alter operative risk; it simply dictates that chance, not the patient, will determine exposure to the risk. Is such an arrangement more ethical (49)?"

Informing Patients About Randomization: Conflicting Views

Do the ethical principles requiring informed, comprehending, and voluntary consent necessitate telling patients how their treatments are selected in randomized clinical trials?

The ethical justifiability of randomization does not hinge only on physician "indifference" to the treatments. Equipoise of outcome of different treatments, whether only apparent at the beginning of a trial or increasingly evident as the trial progresses, does not justify the inference that patients will be, or ought to be, "indifferent" about the treatment they will receive (72). Physician-investigator uncertainty about the relative merits of alternative treatments does not mean that patient preference for one treatment over another is necessarily, or even generally, "capricious" (73). The treatments in a trial may exert significantly different impacts on patients' quality of life and life plans, whatever the initial state of knowledge or the eventual statistical results of the trial may be.

The management of breast cancer and cancer of the prostate are two clinical trial situations where the following conclusion is entirely appropriate: "It is not enough for the physician to have no reason to prefer one treatment over the other; in addition, there must be no reason for the patient to prefer one treatment" (74).

The harm–benefit ratio is a resultant of balancing multiple factors that must include effects that patients consider personally important. Reducing the ratio to the "hard" variables the trial is designed to measure can easily amount to a disregard of a patient's particular situation. Physician-investigators are not ethically justified in perceiving and treating patients exclusively as representatives of a given disease category. It is methodologically and ethically important that surgeon-investigators pay close attention to patient-subjects' unique personal differences. Good ethics and good science demand precisely that everybody *not* be treated alike in consent negotiations (75,76).

Lack of candor about randomization, and the associated additional concealments of information this would often entail, can be an act that bars patients from what they need to know to make the choices they consider most important for their lives. This is ethically unjustifiable in a trial that would otherwise be ethically acceptable. As a rule, patients should be informed about randomization. Justifiable exceptions will have to be justified. A generalization of such exceptions could arise when the differential impact on patients' lives are perceived, by patients and surgeons alike, as being just as important as the treatments' initial putative equality of outcome. In such situations, surgeons may be no less deterred from enrolling otherwise eligible candidates into a trial than the patients themselves are from participating.

The National Surgical Adjuvant Project for Breast and Bowel Cancer trial to compare the relative effectiveness of total and segmental mastectomy, with and without radiation, presents a challenging illustration of these difficulties (77). (See Section III, Chapter 4.)

Harmonizing a surgeon's responsibilities as physician with his or her duties as clinical investigator may be easier in word and in theory than it frequently is in act and in practice. The U.K. Cancer Research Campaign Working Party in Breast Conservation has noted: "It is one thing to admit doubt among one's colleagues, quite another to have to admit it to a patient" (35). At least equal to the difficulty of admitting uncertainty or ignorance is the need of confessing to patients that chance, not their surgeon, is in charge of selecting their treatment.

These admissions do require "mental gymnastics beyond the abilities of many" (77,79), surgeons as well as patients. Admittedly, this is not the way surgeons traditionally behave towards their patients in normal practice. Whether behavior in normal practice should be the norm for clinical research or vice-versa is a question meriting its own discussion.

Enrolling patients into randomized surgical trials without their knowledge and consent is not an answer to these and other difficulties surgeons experience with the process of randomization. Randomizing patients to treatment groups before initiating consent negotiations seems to alleviate the difficulty surgeons have when asking patients to participate in a trial without being able to tell them what treatment they will receive. Pre-randomization designs are less problematic ethically when all patient candidates, those assigned by chance to standard therapy and those similarly assigned to innovative therapy, are involved in consent negotiations. It is unethical to conduct a trial when some of the patient–subjects are totally unaware of the research process in which they have been enrolled and quite unaware of the alternative treatments they might have preferred.

However, involving all patient–subjects in consent negotiations does not directly guarantee that pre-randomization designs are ethically innocuous. Even if patients are told that their treatment has been selected by chance—and they should be told—the way in which the advantages and drawbacks of the alternative treatments are presented can amount to tender but real coercion (80). The voluntary, if not the informed, character of consent may be jeopardized by a linguistic tailoring of information that manipulates the patient's will without blinding the patient's intellect.

It should be emphasized that *this danger is not distinctive* to randomized clinical trials, whatever the randomization tactic may be. The danger is equal, if not greater, when a surgeon who is not participating in a trial convincingly presents one of several alternative treatments under study in a trial elsewhere as the best "in my judgment". This situation is the target of the U.K. Working Party's fifth practical proposal:

"Those doctors who treat patients with cancer but do not participate in randomized clinical trials should realize that they too have an obligation to discuss alternative forms of treatment with their patients. In our view the fact that they are not formally randomizing their patients does not reduce their obligation in this respect" (35).

This proposal suggests a return to the point mentioned earlier about norms of surgeon behavior towards patients in routine practice as contrasted with randomized surgical trials. Some respondents to the investigation of surgeons' reasons for not enrolling patients into the NSABP trial of treatments for breast cancer "believed that participating in a clinical trial would necessitate a major change in the traditional physician-patient interaction" (78). Some changes in that relationship, motivated or necessitated by participation in randomized surgical trials, may be highly desirable and merit introduction into routine surgical practice. Dropping the guise of sapiential authority, when the state of clinical knowledge offers no warrant for such an assumption of power, may advance the education of patient expectations, bolster patient autonomy, and, paradoxically, strengthen the trust of patients in their physicians.

Conclusion

The opening quotation was a surgeon's warning to fellow surgeons about the danger of acting without reflecting. A number of matters to which surgeon investigators should give primary attention in planning and conducting clinical trials have been discussed, but there are many other issues that are just as important.

The most prominent among these might be: the just distribution of burdens and benefits in the selection of patients as candidates for clinical trials; compensation for subjects injured in clinical trials; the requirements of clinical investigators' collaboration with institutional review boards or research ethics committees; the ethical conditions for terminating a controlled study; and the ethical dilemma of releasing interim results during the course of a randomized clinical trial.* The discussion of these matters would have required space far in excess of what could reasonably be allocated for this chapter. The principle adopted was to offer in-depth discussion of the questions distinctively important for surgical trials rather than attempt a more superficial treatment of many issues, however germane they may be to all clinical trials.

References

1. Folkman J. Surgical research: a contradiction in terms? J Surg Res 1984;36:298.
2. Pellegrino ED. The anatomy of clinical judgments: some notes on right reason and right action. In: Engelhardt H, Tristram Jr., Spicker SF, Towers B. Editors. Clinical judgment: a critical appraisal. Dordrecht-London-Boston: D. Reidel Publishing Company, 1979:169–195.
3. Bankowski Z, Howard-Jones N. Human experimentation and medical ethics. Geneva: CIOMS, 1982.
4. Beecher HK. Research and the individual. Boston: Little, Brown and Company, 1970.
5. Freund PA, editor. Experimentation with human subjects. New York: George Braziller, 1970.
6. Gray BH. Human subjects in medical experimentation. New York-Toronto: John Wiley & Sons, 1975.
7. Katz J. Experimentation with human beings. New York: Russel Sage Foundation, 1972.
8. Levine R. Ethics and regulation of clinical research. Baltimore-Munich: Urban & Schwarzenberg, 1981.
9. Shapiro SH, Louis TA. Editors. Clinical trials. New York: Marcel Dekker, Inc., 1983.
10. WHO and CIOMS. Proposed international guidelines for biomedical research involving human subjects. Geneva: CIOMS 1982.
11. Sackett DL. Bias in analytic research. J Chron Dis 1979;32:60.
12. Toulmin S. How medicine saved the life of ethics. Perspect Biol Med 1982;25:736–750.
13. Fried C. Medical experimentation. Amsterdam, Oxford: North Holland Publishing Co., 1974;151:101–104.
14. Green FHK. Quoted by Jackson DM. Moral responsibility in clinical research. Lancet, 1958;1:903. This reference comes from Feinstein AR. Clinical Biostatistics: XXVI. Medical ethics and the architecture of clinical research. Clin Pharmacol Ther, 1974;15:320.
15. Gilbert JP, McPeek B, Mosteller F. Statistics and ethics in surgery and anesthesia. Science 1977;198:684-689.
16. Silverman WA. The lesson of retrolental fibroplasia. Scientific American 1977;236:100–107.
17. Bernard C. An introduction to the study of experimental medicine. Translated by Greene HC. U.S.A.: Henry Schuman, Inc., 1949;101:1–261.
18. Engelhardt HT Jr. Bioethics in the Peoples Republic of China. Hast Cent Rpt 1980;10:8.

---

* See also Section I, Chapter 1.

19. The Nuremberg Code. Trials of war criminals before the Nuremberg military tribunals under control council law, no. 10, vol. 2 Washington, D.C.: U.S. Government Printing Office, 1949;181–182. Reprinted in Levine, Robert, Ethics and Regulation of Clinical Research, Appendix 3. (See reference 8 above); included as Appendix A in this textbook.
20. World Medical Association Declaration of Helsinki: Recommendations guiding medical doctors in biomedical research involving human subjects. Reprinted in Levine, Robert, Ethics and Regulation of Clinical Research, Appendix 4. (See reference 8 above).
21. Anderson WF, Fletcher JC. Gene therapy in human beings: when is it ethical to begin? N Engl J Med 1980;303:1293–1297.
22. Cline MJ, Mercola KE. The potential of inserting new genetic information. N Engl J Med 1980;303:1297–1300.
23. Editorial, Gene therapy: how ripe the time? Lancet 1981;I:196-197.
24. Grobstein C, Flower M. Gene therapy: proceed with caution. Hast Cent Rpt 1984;14:13–17.
25. Wade N, UCLA. Gene therapy racked by friendly fire. Science 1980;210:509–511.
26. Rutstein DD. The ethical design of human experiments. In Freund. Paul A, editor. Experimentation with human subjects, 383–401. (See Reference 5 above.)
27. Sackett DL. The competing objectives of randomized trials. N Engl J Med 1980;303:1059–1060.
28. Frederickson DS. Welcoming remarks, national conferences in clinical trials methodology. Clin Pharmacol Ther 1979;25:630–631.
29. Zelen M. A new design for randomized clinical trials. N Engl J Med 1979;300:1242–1245.
30. Feinstein AR. An additional basic science for clinical medicine: I. the constraining fundamental paradigms. Ann Int Med 1983;99:393–397.
31. Feinstein AR. An additional basic science for clinical medicine: IV. the development of clinimetrics. Ann Int Med 1983;99:843–848.
32. Woodward FP. Informed consent of volunteers: a direct measurement of comprehension and retention of information. Clin Res 1979;27:248–252.
33. Dickens BM. The modern law on informed consent. Modern Medicine of Canada 1982;37:706–710.
34. Reibl v. Hughes. 1980;2 S.C.R.:882.
35. Cancer research campaign working party on breast conservation, informed consent: ethical, legal, and medical implications for doctors and patients who participate in randomised clinical trials. Br Med J 1983;286:1117–1121.
36. Beecher HK. Ethics and clinical research. N Engl J Med 1966;274:1354–1360.
37. Jonsen AR. Do no harm. Ann Int Med 1978; 88:827–832.
38. Feinstein AR. Clinical biostatistics: XLI. hard science, soft data, and the challenges of choosing clinical variables in research. Clin Pharmacol Ther 1977;22:485–498.
39. Feinstein AR. Clinical biostatistics: XXVI. medical ethics and the architecture of clinical research. Clin Pharmacol Ther 1974;15:316–334.
40. Dresser R. Book Reviews: Dodds WJ, Barbara F, Orlans, editors. 1982, Scientific perspectives on animal welfare, Academic Press. New York: 131 pp. J Med Philos 1984;9:423–425.
41. Naverson J. Animal rights. Can J Phil 1977;VII:161–178.
42. Regan T, Singer P. Animal rights and human obligations. Englewood Cliffs: Prentice Hall, 1976.
43. Rowan AN, Rollin BE. Animal research--for and against: a philosophical, social, and historical perspective. Perspect Biol Med 1983;27:1–17.
44. Singer P. Animal liberation. New York: Random House, 1975.
45. McIntosh A. Animal rights and medical research. Future Health, Winter 1985:10–11.
46. Editorial. Animal experiments. Br Med J 1982; 284:368–369.
47. Lane-Petter W. The place and importance of the experimental animal in research. Proceedings of the Royal Society of Medicine 1972;65:343–344.
48. Russell JC, Secord DC. Holy dogs and the laboratory: some Canadian experiences with animal research. Perspect Biol Med 1985;28:374–381.
49. Broncheck LI. Are randomized trials appropriate for evaluating new operations? N Engl J Med 1979;301:44–45.
50. Chalmers TC. Randomized clinical trials in surgery. In Varco, RL, Delaney JP, editors. Controversy in surgery. Philadelphia: W.B. Saunders and Company, 1976:3–11.
51. Feinstein AR. The scientific and clinical tribulations of randomized clinical trials. Clin Res 1978;26:241–244.
52. Haines SJ. Randomized clinical trials in the evaluation of surgical innovation. J Neurosurg 1979;51:5–11.
53. Loop FD. A surgeon's view of randomized prospective studies. J Thorac Cariovasc Surg 1979;78:161–165.
54. Spodick DH. Randomized controlled clinical trials. The Behavioral Case. JAMA 1982; 247:2258–2260.
55. Spodick DH et al. Standards for surgical trials. Ann Thorac Surg 1979;27:284.
56. Van der Linden W. On the generalization of surgical trials results. Acta Chir Scand 1980;146:229–234.
57. Feinstein AR. An additional basic science for

clinical medicine. II. The limitations of randomized trials. Ann Int Med 1983;99:544–550.
58. Feinstein AR. An additional basic science for clincial medicine. III. The Challenges of comparison & measurements. Ann Int Med 1983;99:705–712.
59. Fisher LD, Kennedy JW. Randomized surgical clinical trials for treatment of coronary artery disease. Controlled Clinical Trials 1982;3:235–258.
60. Merlo G. Surgical trial: possibilities and objections. Eur surg Res 1984;16:1–4.
61. Editorial, Blindness in surgical trials. Lancet 1980;I:1229–1230.
62. Van der Linden W. Pitfalls in randomized surgical trials. Surgery 1980;87:258–262.
63. Moore FD. Perspectives, Surgery. Perspect Biol Med 1982;25:698–720.
64. Dudley HAF. The controlled clinical trial and the advance of reliable knowledge: an outsider looks in. Br Med J 1983; 237:957–960.
65. Norman C. Clinical trial stirs legal battles. Science 1985;227:1316–1318.
66. Fyfe IM. The randomized clinical trial: panacea or placebo? Can Med Assoc J 1984;131:1336–1339.
67. EC/IC Bypass Study Group. Failure of extracranial—intracranial arterial bypass to reduce the risk of ischemic stroke: results of an international randomized trial. N Engl J Med 1985;313:1191–1200.
68. Spodick DH. Randomize the first patient: scientific, ethical, and behavioral bases. Am J Cardiol 1983;51:916–917.
69. Editorial. Managing severe head injury--doing more and faring worse? Lancet 1980;I:1229.
70. McKinlay JB. From promising report to standard procedure: seven stages in the career of a medical innovation. Milbank Mem 1981;59:374–411.
71. Feilding LP, et al. Surgeon-related variables and the clinical trial. Lancet 1978;II:778–779.
72. Hill Sir Austin Bradford. Medical ethics and controlled trials. Br Med J 1963;1:1043–1049.
73. Eisenberg L. The social imperatives of medical research. Science 1977;198:1105–1110.
74. Angell M. Patients' preferences in randomized clinical trials. N Engl J Med 1984;310:1385–1387.
75. Brewin TB. Consent to randomized treatment. Lancet 1982; II:919–921.
76. Sade RM, Miller III, Clinton M. Letter. N Engl J Med 1983; 308:344.
77. Dudley HAF. Informed consent in surgical trials. Br Med J 1984;289:937–938.
78. Taylor K, Margolese RG, Soskolne CL. Physicians' reasons for not entering eligible patients in a randomized clinical trial of adjuvant surgery for breast cancer. N Engl J Med 1984; 310:1363–1367.
79. Editorial. Consent: how informed? Lancet 1984;I:1445–1447.
80. Ellenberg SS. Randomization designs in comparative clinical trials. N Engl J Med 1984;310:1404–1408.

SECTION III

Selected Strategies of Research

Introduction

No textbook could consider all the research strategies useful to an academic or clinician. This text only considers selective strategies. We have emphasized the arena of research in which the bridge scientist, a person who cares for patients, cares enough that he or she wishes to do more than is possible given the current state of our knowledge. We focus particularly on those strategies that will enable a clinician to have direct involvement in a research investigation without abandoning the operating theater or the wards.

The reader will note that relatively little space is devoted to strategies for laboratory research. Only three chapters in this section consider this realm. The knowledgeable reader is fully aware that the vast variety of opportunities, challenges, subjects, collaborative arrangements, and basic sciences that can be invoked in a research endeavor would require several textbooks for each one. The horizon of possibilities is so wide and the landscape is so heterogeneous that we have refrained from describing strategies in molecular, cellular, and pathophysiological research which, appropriately enough, are the burning interest of many academic surgeons. We acknowledge that the hypotheses generated in what is often called the "wet laboratory" are absolutely essential to the progress of science and of surgery. Ideas taken from hospital wards and operating rooms to the laboratory and brought back from the laboratory are the building blocks of clinical research as illustrated by Chiu and Mulder in Chapter 3.

Since we are clinicians and clinical methodologists, prominence is given to clinical research. We adhere arbitrarily to the definition of clinical research as investigation in which intact living human beings are the subjects. In contrast to basic research applied to clinical interests, where a challenging idea is the hallmark of excellence and the methods have generally been worked out, the ideas and related research questions in clinical and epidemiologic research are pedestrian. The challenge of clinical research is how to measure and how to design a study. The typical question may be as simple as "Does cigarette smoking cause cancer of the lung?" or, "Does use of drug A in conjunction with surgical intervention B improve the outcome for patients with disease C?". If the outcome is chest pain, or depression is a side effect, how does one measure such attributes? If it is impossible to find control groups in the hospital or in the community, how does one create comparable groups for comparison?

As written above, we editors are all clinicians responsible for the care of patients. If there is an imbalance in this book it is toward too much patient-oriented research. The principles of research are universal. They are as applicable to animal research as to clinical investigation. They work as well in the chemistry and the physiology laboratories as in the ward. As emphasized in several chapters our laboratory colleagues have their methods worked out rigorously and reliably. We clinical investigators lag behind in design, measurements and analysis. We hope this text will help redress some imbalances in accomplishment.

There are other common features that are shared by laboratory, clinical, and epidemiologic research. All strategies of potential use to clinicians require a certain degree of abstraction or the creation of artificial situations to permit the description of what exists, to relate cause and effect, or to assess the effectiveness of a particular intervention under controlled circumstances. The trick is to do all this in a manner that permits the drawing of conclusions that apply to the real world of patients or of nature. There is always a tension between the extent of the abstraction that must be done to render research feasible and the limit beyond which the research model would no longer reflect nature sufficiently to allow generalization of the results.

Clinical case studies are frequently done and reported. This is most appropriate. Consider the case in which a tumor was removed from the jaw of a patient at the Massachusetts General Hospital in 1846. The case report stated that a substance called ether was administered during the operation and that, after its conclusion, the patient reported that he had experienced no pain; Dr. John Cullens Warren performed the operation and Dr. William P.G. Morton, a Harvard medical student who was also a dental surgeon, administered the ether. This, the first properly recorded case report (1) of major surgery under general anesthesia, was a shot that was heard around the world. Case studies advance knowledge appreciably when the findings are dramatic. Another example of remarkable results in a series of case reports that required no controls arose from the discovery of penicillin. When the effects of interventions are not so dramatic, but subtle or even imperceptible, case studies and case series are not sufficient.

Clinicians, and particularly action-oriented surgeons, have a tendency to underestimate the importance of small gains in therapy or in knowledge. Nevertheless, small gains are the norm. Demonstrating them with scientific rigor so that they compound into an aggregate benefit of even a few percentage points of improved outcome for thousands or millions of people is central to clinical and surgical research today. Economists and bankers rest all their strategies on gaining a few percentage points that become significant when compounded over time and applied to large populations.

Despite the limitations on the inferences that can be drawn from case reports, descriptions of what happens or what exists are frequently the indispensable precursors of good controlled research. The observation and description of a side-effect, or an unexpected benefit usually come to our attention through case studies. Much progress in clinical research is attributable to the alert clinician who, though not a career scientist, is a sufficiently skillful observer and sophisticated consumer of research information to recognize the germ of a hypothesis and to write it up. Career scientists depend on career clinicians for pointers to a better future in medicine and surgery.

Case studies compel us to find out the frequency of occurrence of the phenomena we are interested in. That leads us to descriptive epidemiologic studies, such as a census (enumeration of an entire population), or the study of samples of a population where straightforward but important biostatistics help us to sample without bias. When the independent variable called "time" is important, we do longitudinal follow-up studies. Such studies are generally called cohort studies and are introduced in the chapter on statistics by Kramer (Section II, Chapter 3).

When we get to the elucidation of causes and effects, comparisons become essential. We can compare outcomes in two different cohorts (analytic cohort studies); contrast two sets of patients with different outcomes; evaluate exposures to therapy and risk factors in the past (case control or case referent studies); or do an experiment such as a randomized controlled clinical trial, the method most frequently used in clinical investigation nowadays. Our strongest, most reliable evidence for causation, for the effectiveness of a treatment, is the carefully performed randomized controlled trial. When nonbiological determinants of health and disease become important, or when we wish to study the efficiency rather than the effectiveness of interventions, we engage in health services research with the frequent collaboration of economists and social scientists. When manipulation of people as individuals in the aggregate becomes unethical or impractical, or we wish to look far into the future, we use simulation that may be computer-assisted.

In this section, Professors Lorenz and Troidl describe a unique experiment in which bridge scientists and bridge science successfully integrated laboratory investigation, clinical care and clinical research. Animal experimentation, as one of the essential precursors of good clinical research, is reviewed in the second chapter by Professors Isselhard and Kusche. Two full chapters are devoted to what might be considered the acme of surgical or other clinical investigation, the randomized controlled trial. Walters and Sackett give the rationale, the relevance, and the requirements for the evaluation of effectiveness. Margolese describes a collaborative multicenter controlled trial which met the requirement for large numbers of patients from different parts of the world. Schechter deals with investigative approaches for assessing the diagnostic process, Williams and Drucker present the main strategies in health services research and Spitzer introduces selected non-experimental designs.

We caution readers not to assume that they will have acquired adequate expertise in clinical investigation, statistics, epidemiology, or laboratory science as the result of simply having mastered this section. This is only a beginning. A second step can be accomplished through careful study of the material listed in the bibliographies. Expertise only comes after years of personal involvement.

References

1. Bigelow HJ. Insensibility during surgical operations produced by inhalation. Boston Medical and Surgical Journal 1846;35:309–317.

1

The Marburg Experiment

W. Lorenz and H. Troidl

Shortening the Communication Link—An Intellectual Challenge

The view that clinical research is always less "scientific", and therefore less valuable than biomedical research, reflects considerable prejudice. The fact that the clinician who takes care of patients cannot devote all his professional life to research is not, in itself, valid grounds for depreciating the quality of clinical science. Such value judgments based on any epistemiological model (1–4), are only valid and fair when the work of full-time investigators in clinical disciplines is compared with that of full-time basic research scientists.

Full-time research investigators in surgery, anaesthesia and intensive care suffer, however, from limited exposure to clinical practice. Life produces an infinite number of situations in which decisions have to be made. Clinicians need far more training to cope with them than it is possible to obtain in the ordinary five to six years of specialization. As a result, the sufficiently self-critical and responsible full-time research worker will never be able to feel safe in giving advice to individual patients. Basic research scientists who try to mimic clinical situations as closely as possible under experimental conditions, whether in controlled clinical trials, animal studies, cell biology experiments, or computer simulations of various clinical processes, have a similar problem.

The design and execution of original, methodologically reliable, and clinically relevant studies, require the close and continuing partnership of a full-time clinician and a full-time research worker, as a minimum. Some way has to be found to ensure an interaction between these two individuals that is characterized by complete and open communication. At the very least, it must result in better outcomes than either of them could achieve working completely on their own. At best, it will result in clinical trials that incorporate the most sophisticated strategies, basic science, and the most refined approaches to clinical practice.

The Marburg Experiment: One Approach to Closing the Gap Between the Clinic and the Research Laboratory

The Marburg experiment was designed to test one way of achieving close interaction between clinical surgery, basic sciences, and care of the surgical patient. It is neither the only, nor necessarily the best approach to solving the problem, but it does clearly illustrate what we are trying to do (5).

The Marburg Experiment began in 1970 when the Division of Experimental Surgery and Pathological Biochemistry was established at the Surgical Clinic of the University of Marburg. Professor H. Hamelmann, the Chairman of the Department of Surgery, supported both the concept and its implementation (5,6).

The experiment incorporated several assumptions that were not recognized at the time.

The "fat years" of a consumer society and poor communication between academic surgeons in Germany and their numerous partners in the period 1960–1970 caused the gulf that had developed between surgical research in the Western world and in Germany during the years of World War II, to open rather than close (5,7,8).

Investigators in Great Britain and in the United States had created the controlled clinical trial, case-control study, various methods of clinical decision-making, medical statistics that emphasized practical usefulness, and clinical studies with nearly 100% follow-up (6). These new approaches demanded far more information exchange and more complex organization than work with animals or retrospective surveys (9,10). Single, isolated cases no longer met the methodological demands of such rigorous studies (11).

Communication within the operational network illustrated by Fig. 1 was not effective for a variety of specific reasons that were more or less characteristic of West German society at this time. German academic surgeons had little contact with the English surgeons who were at the forefront in applying the new methodology to their clinical work, mainly because of the language barrier. The suppression and lack of interest in history that were prevalent after the Third Reich and World War II produced repetitive discovery of things that were "old hat". The academic surgeon saw less and less of his students and junior colleagues because of the massive flood of applicants, the aggressive behavior of student reformists, the introduction of impersonal examinations in the form of multiple-choice questionnaire that did not fit with the West German medical education system and the inflexible regulations of working hours. Communication with other disciplines, such as psychology and sociology, was obstructed by ideological differences, as was cooperation with basic scientists and statisticians by their increasingly specialized view-points and language (5,7,8).

"Continental" academic surgery appeared to have one advantage over the English system. In German-speaking countries, including Switzerland (12) general surgical training and clinical practice were regarded as being more useful in patient care than extreme specialization. Accordingly, the Marburg Experiment had to avoid the superspecialization of general surgeons and keep the time spent in research by the overworked clinician at an acceptable level, not only for a short period, but for many years during his professional life.

Our keyword was *integration* (Fig. 2), not just the frequently intended, but rarely experienced, cooperation. The academic surgeon makes not just one connection with the experimental or theoretical surgeon to collaborate in a series of experiments or the publication of a particular article; he combines almost all his scientific efforts with those of his personal, permanent

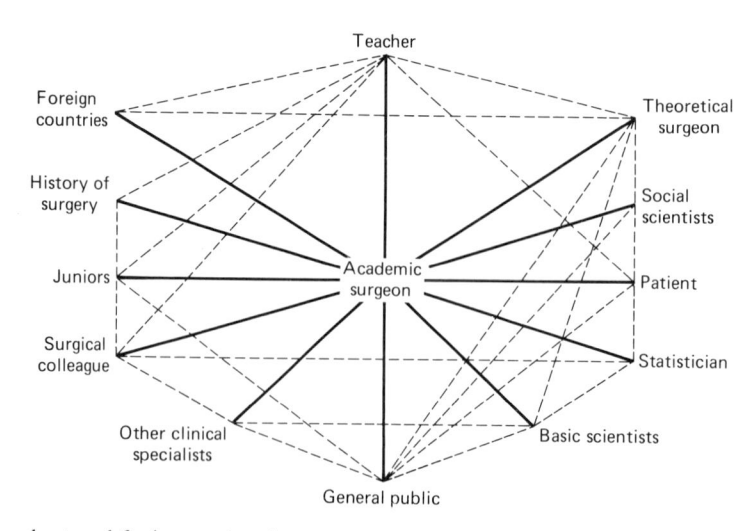

FIGURE 1. Operational network for interactions between an academic surgeon and his numerous communication partners. Solid lines: direct interactions; dotted model lines: indirect interactions by participating in connections between the various communicators. [From Lorenz and Röher (6); © Springer-Verlag, reprinted by permission.]

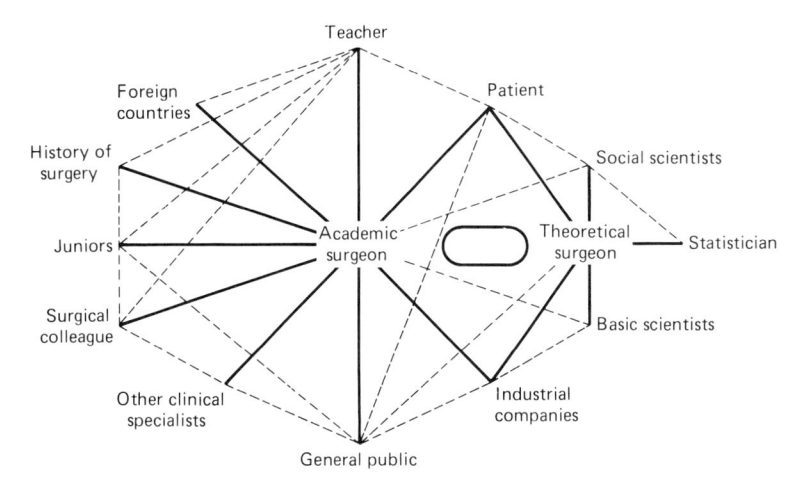

FIGURE 2. Operational network for interactions between academic surgeon and his numerous communication partners (integration concept of the Marburg experiment). [From Lorenz and Röher (6); © Springer-Verlag, reprinted by permission.]

partner in the basic sciences. Neither one nor the other, but only both, attempt to solve surgical research problems. The theoretical surgeon communicates with the basic scientists and brings the results back to the partnership (Fig. 2). The clinician enables the theoretical surgeon to contact his patients, to learn clinical science and to recognize the multiple dimensions of clinical problems. Only by these mutual, permanent interactions can the basic research scientist, usually called "experimental surgeon" become the theoretical surgeon who restricts his daily work in animals to spend most of his time thinking, observing, and formulating and testing hypotheses on various aspects of the care of the surgical patient. The resulting change in the Marburg Experiment over the years is reflected in the changing ratio of articles on human studies to those on animal studies (Fig. 3).

Characteristics of the Marburg Experiment

The Marburg experiment has been described in detail in two communications (5,6).

Theoretical surgery is interdisciplinary in its methods, but restricted in its objectives. Rather than being specialized, theoretical surgery is integrated with general surgery, surgical intensive care, and anesthesiology. It cooperates with the other disciplines according to the concept portrayed in Fig. 1.

Several new tasks were given to the theoretical surgeon (Table I) that are only effective, reasonable and useful if they are integrated with those of general surgery. They include contributions to surgical decision-making, methodological innovative clinical trials, and surgical science. "Contributions" denotes the requirement for the participation of the clinical partner whereas basic research in surgery can be carried

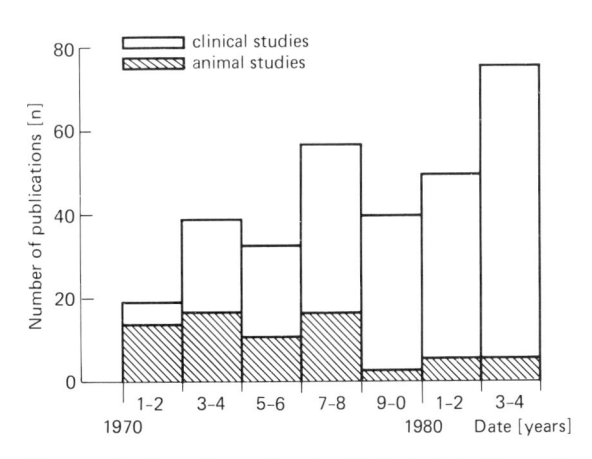

FIGURE 3. Quantity and ratio of clinical studies and animal work published in 1971–1984 in the Marburg experiment. Original articles and short communications taken from the file of the Department of Theoretical Surgery. Review articles and oral communications were excluded.

TABLE I. Tasks of the theoretical surgeon: Integration concept [from Lorenz and Röher (6); © Springer-Verlag, reprinted by permission].

Tasks	Examples
Contributions to surgical decision-making	Decision trees, computer-aided diagnosis and outcome analysis
Contributions to clinical trials	Design, coordination, and data analysis
Basic research in surgery	Application of methods and knowledge of basic science disciplines, with intention; therefore *planning* to be useful to surgery
Support in medical care	EDP in documentation, surgical audit
Contributions to the philosophy of surgery (metasurgery)	Long-lasting work on epistemiology, ethics, and social aspects of surgery

TABLE II. Organization of the small working teams (permanent teams) in the Marburg experiment [from Lorenz and Röher (6); © Springer-Verlag reprinted by permission].

Principle	Integration of clinical and theoretical research into a practical, long-lasting arrangement
Composition	1 senior and 1 junior clinician, 1 basic scientist, 1–2 technicians, 1–2 students
Functions	Research and specific medical care in a defined part of the clinical and research program of the two Departments
	Meeting at least once a week for about 2 h to coordinate and discuss
	Applying methods of medical decision-making to current problems
	Designing and conducting clinical trials and animal experiments
	Running a systematic follow-up
	Documenting records and literature in the specific field
Rooms and equipment	1 room for meetings (usually the basic scientist's office)
	1 laboratory with necessary equipment, access to all apparatus of both departments

out by either of the partners alone although it should not be for the reasons already given.

The intention of the Marburg Experiment was to create organizational structures that fostered both enthusiasm for and the ability to integrate research work. The organizational and spatial arrangements forced communication, especially when frustration and personal difficulties arose between the partners as human beings.

Small working teams were put together as permanent units (Table II) to interweave the staffs of the Departments of General and Theoretical Surgery. There are currently six such teams in Marburg; three have been in existence for fifteen years; three are fairly new.

A weekly colloquium is held by the two Departments. The clinical topics comprise reports, problems, controversies and recommendations from all of general surgery; the theoretical topics are illustrated by Tables IIIa and IIIb. Table IIIa lists the topics covered between 1971 and 1975; Table IIIb lists those on medical decision-making and clinical biostatistics from 1982 to 1983. Both the continuity and the changes within a period of ten years can be easily recognized.

Service functions are provided for the whole Centre of Operative Medicine by the Department of Theoretical Surgery (Table IV).

Basic scientists with full training in one theoretical discipline meet the needs for basic research expertise in the small working teams and communicate continuously with scientists with

TABLE IIIA. Topics on theoretical and basic research issues in the weekly colloquium for training in surgery and surgical research (1971–1975) [from Lorenz, Hamelmann and Troidl (5)].

Statistics	Sampling of attributes, randomization, parameters, histograms, comparison of relative frequencies (χ^2-test)
	Normal distribution (Student's *t*-test, *t*-test for paired data)
	Frequency distribution being significantly different from normal or being an unknown type of frequency distribution (Mann-Whitney test, Wilcoxon test)
Surgery	Controlled trials from all parts of surgery
	Basic knowledge in documentation
Clinical chemistry and biochemistry	Quality control
	Proteases
	Coagulation, fibrinolysis
	Complement system
Pharmacology	Technique for measuring blood pressure and blood flow
	Methods for determining oxygen tension in tissues
Pathology-Immunology	Mast cells
	Basic knowledge in allergy and immunology of transplantation

TABLE IIIB. Topics on medical decision-making (MDM) and clinical biostatistics in the weekly colloquium for training in surgery and surgical research (1982–1985) [from Lorenz and Röher (6); © Springer-Verlag, reprinted by permission].

Year	Topics of MDM and clinical biostatistics
1982	Construction of decision trees
	Utility analysis in surgical procedures
	Sample size in clinical *and* animal experimental studies
	The view of industry on conducting controlled clinical trials in surgery
1983	Computer-aided follow-up in patients with various types of carcinoma
	Computer-aided surveillance of patients with cardiac pace-makers
	Computer-aided diagnosis in acute abdominal pain
	Quality-adjusted life expectancy in tumour patients
	Calculation of risk rates in prospective (cohort) and retrospective trials

other theoretical disciplines who in other teams in work in the Department of Theoretical Surgery. At present, six theoretical disciplines are covered in the Department (Table V). All the basic scientists demonstrate their proficiency by publishing papers in peer-reviewed journals for their basic disciplines. The necessity of covering several basic research disciplines is illustrated by the causes of failure in clinical trials (Table VI). Poor statistics is only one reason.

The success of the Marburg experiment in coupling the clinic and the research laboratory is demonstrated by four examples (Table VII).

TABLE IV. Service functions of the Department of Theoretical Surgery in the Marburg experiment [from Lorenz and Röher (6); © Springer-Verlag, reprinted by permission].

Task	Examples
Advice	Designing clinical trials, statistics, computer applications
	Local ethical committee
	Purchase and maintenance of equipment
Service	Regional and supraregional information retrieval systems
	Central department of medical illustration
	Central animal laboratories
Surveillance	Radiation, data and animal protection
Teaching	Training of postgraduates and students in methods of theoretical surgery

This organizational structure refers both to the integration and co-operation concept.

TABLE V. Several basic research disciplines covered in the Marburg experiment.

Discipline	Scientists covering the field
(1) Statistics and information studies	1 mathematician (Ph.D. in mathematics, preclinical studies in medicine ("Physikum"))
	1 computer programmer
(2) Clinical pharmacology	1 physician (authorized to train pharmacologists)
(3) Clinical chemistry	1 clinical chemist (assistant professor in clinical chemistry)
(4) Biochemistry	2 chemists (Ph.D. in chemistry, preclinical and clinical studies in medicine) ("Praktisches Jahr")
(5) Laboratory animal science	1 veterinary surgeon
(6) Cell biology	1 biochemist (Ph.D. in the British system)

A qualification in medicine is attempted by most of the basic scientists. This official training facilitates work in a Department of Surgery (Centre of Operative Medicine) for many reasons, although it is not absolutely necessary. However, it helps to obtain a permanent and leading position in units of Theoretical Surgery or in German industry. From Lorenz and Röher (6); © Springer-Verlag, reprinted by permission.

Adverse Reactions to Anaesthetic Induction Agents

In 1968, Alfred Doenicke, Head of the Department of Anaesthesia, Surgical Outpatient Clinic of the University of Munich, observed life-threatening anaphylactoid reactions to intravenously administered propanidid. He suspected that kinin formation or histamine release were responsible for these reactions and established the first small working group to investigate this possibility. This group, of which one of us (W.L.) was a member, is still functioning seventeen years later.

TABLE VI. Reasons why controlled clinical trials fail other than poor statistics and ethics.

Relevant existing information has been neglected
Clinically unimportant end-points have been selected
Known prognostic factors have been omitted
Clinical pharmacology has been ignored
Methods of assessment are imprecise
Follow-up is incomplete
Medical audit and quality control are lacking or poor

Table constructed from items in Lorenz, Lancet (13).

TABLE VII. Short ways from the clinic to the laboratory and back—examples from work in the Marburg experiment.

	Clinical problem processing			Disciplines involved	
No.	Detection and definition	Investigation in laboratory	Solution and clinical application	Clinical	Basic research
1	Adverse reactions to anesthetics	Plasma histamine assay	Discarding drugs, prophylaxis	Anesthesiology	Clinical chemistry
2	Duodenal ulcer pathogenesis	Histamine assay in human biopsies	Prediction of therapeutic failures	Abdominal surgery	Biochemistry
3	Adverse reactions to plasma substitutes	Selection of animal species	Improvement of drugs	General surgery intensive care	Clinical pharmacology
4	Recurrent bleeding in upper GI tract haemorrhage	Computer-aided diagnosis (actuarial methods)	Monitoring system in ICU	Abdominal surgery, intensive care	Statistics

In the first series of experiments in human volunteers, gastric secretion and whole blood histamine were determined before and after the injection of propanidid since a reliable plasma histamine assay was not available then. In human subjects, gastric acid secretion was always augmented, but whole blood histamine remained constant in at least half of the persons tested (14). Since kinins did not stimulate gastric acid secretion, they were excluded as chemical factors causing the reactions, but histamine H_2-receptor antagonists had not yet been discovered as a means of identifying histamine.

The laboratory investigation (Table VII) began with the development of a fluorometric-fluoroenzymatic assay for plasma histamine (15) which, for the first time, was demonstrated to be sufficiently sensitive and specific to be of use in solving the problem (16,17). This was confirmed by several workers (18,19) who extended the studies to analgesics and muscle relaxants (20).

Using this assay, the small working team returned to studies in volunteers and patients (21,22). In other adverse reactions to propanidid, one of them with cardiac arrest (Fig. 4), a causal relationship between administration of the drug, release of histamine, and appearance of a histamine induced disease was shown for the first time (23). Thiopentone and methohexitone also caused histamine release (21,24), but etomidate was free from this side-effect (22). As a result, it was introduced into the market and enjoyed a good reputation for more than ten years (25). Propanidid and althesin, both of which were dissolved in the detergent and solubilizer cremophor El (21,22), were withdrawn from the market because of their ability to elicit anaphylactoid reactions. Two of the articles published on this subject have become citation classics (17,22).

In achieving all this, the small working team on perioperative risk research overcame the communication barriers described at the beginning of this chapter.

Duodenal Ulcer Pathogenesis and Histamine Storage and Metabolism

The etiology, pathogenesis, rational prophylaxis, and treatment of chronic peptic ulcer are not clearly understood. A series of chemical factors including hydrochloric acid, pepsin, gastrin, and acetylcholine released from the vagus nerve were suggested as chemical factors in the causation of this disease, but histamine was not implicated in chronic duodenal ulcer.

Following some typical animal studies with Heidenhain pouch dogs (26) and the first controlled clinical trial on the treatment of duodenal ulcer patients with different surgical procedures (27), the idea of combining the principles of modern analytical biochemistry with those of the controlled clinical trial to create a new type of a clinical study was done: the controlled biochemical trial. Work started, in 1973, with biopsies taken from patients with various gastric diseases during gastric endoscopy. Reliable assays for histamine and histamine methyltransferease activity were still not available for such small tissue samples and had to be developed at the beginning of studies.

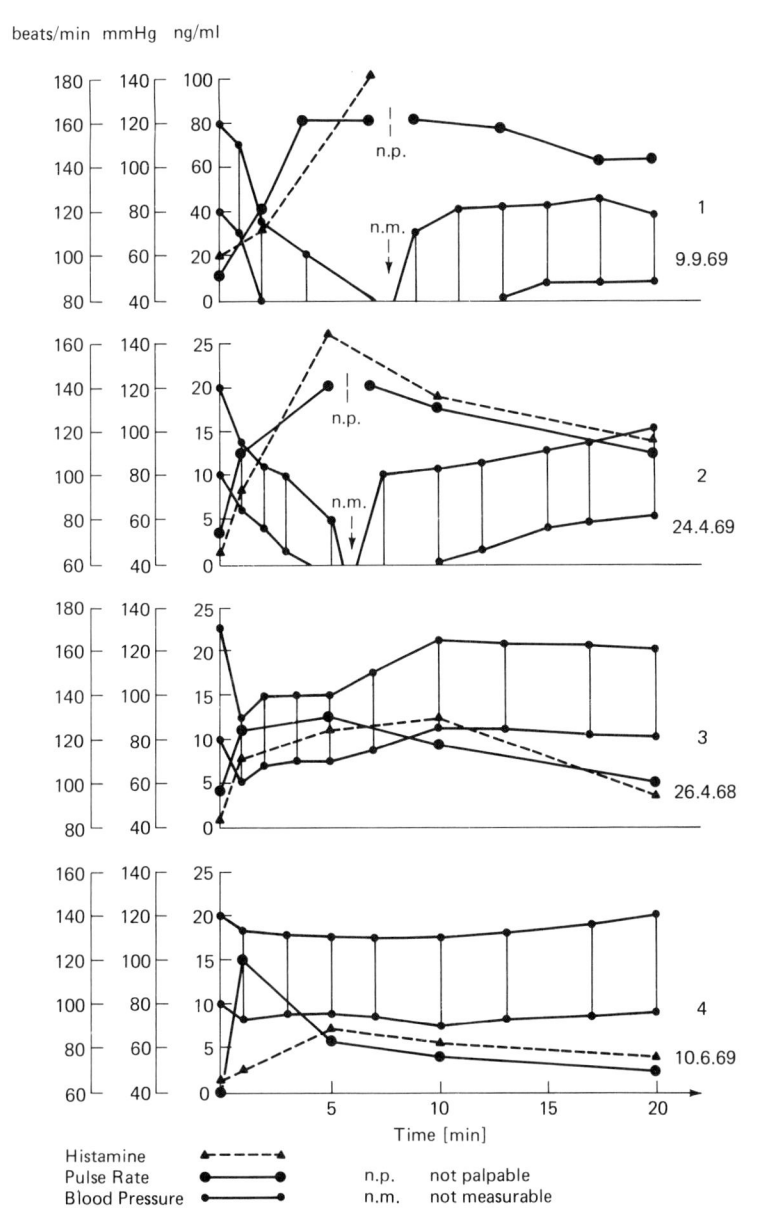

FIGURE 4. Correlation between plasma histamine levels, pulse rate and blood pressure in four cases of pseudoallergic reactions to propanidid (Epontol®). The first subject suffered from cardiac arrest. Reprinted by permission from Br J Anaesth 44 (1972) p 355, copyright Professional & Scientific Publications Ltd.

As soon as the assay methods became suitable (28), they were applied to the clinical problem and alterations in histamine storage (Fig. 5) and catabolism (Fig. 6) were specifically shown to be present in chronic duodenal ulcer disease in man (29,30). These changes were fully reversible after vagotomy (Fig. 7) (30,31). Since histamine H_2-receptor antagonists showed effects on histamine storage and metabolism that were similar to vagotomy (32,33), it was predicted that ulcer recurrences after taking the H_2-blockers, would not be successfully treated by vagotomy. This hypothesis was later supported by findings from clinical trials (34) and led to new strategies for treating and preventing duodenal ulcers by tablets and/or operations (35).

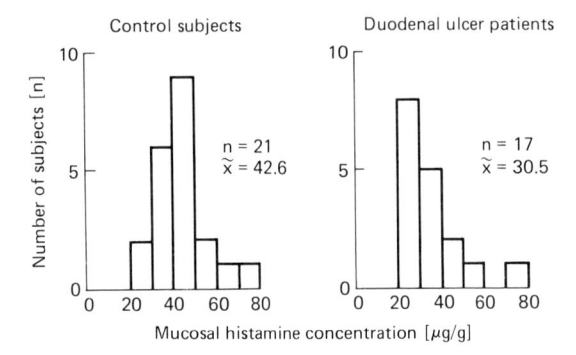

FIGURE 5. Histograms of histamine concentrations in human corpus mucosa of control subjects and duodenal ulcer patients. Only male subjects were included, x̃ = median. Statistical significance (Mann-Whitney test) $p < 0.025$. [From Troidl et al. (29).]

Adverse Reactions to Plasma Substitutes

Basic research often pays little attention to the selection of experimental animal and any new finding in any biological species is of interest to the life science disciplines. However, in surgical research and theoretical surgery, it is mandatory to select the animal species that is most similar to the sick human being with regard to the problem being investigated.

In the small working group on general perioperative risk, adverse reactions to plasma substitutes became a topic of major interest in the early 1970's (Table VII). These unwanted side-effects of drugs commonly used in anaesthesia and surgery were explained, in 1970, by suspecting kinin formation in adverse reactions to gelatin preparations (36) and to human albumin with the subsequent release of histamine from mast cells. These were the responses that were thought to occur when dextran was used clinically (37). These paradigms were based solely on studies with isolated rat peritoneal mast cells which did not react to polygeline and human albumin with histamine release (38), but very strongly to dextran in the presence of phosphatidyl serine (37).

Experiments in anaesthesized dogs produced a completely opposite picture (Fig. 8): gelatin preparations released histamine, but dextran did not (39). Studies in human volunteers and patients, undertaken immediately after the dog experiments (24,40), demonstrated that only the

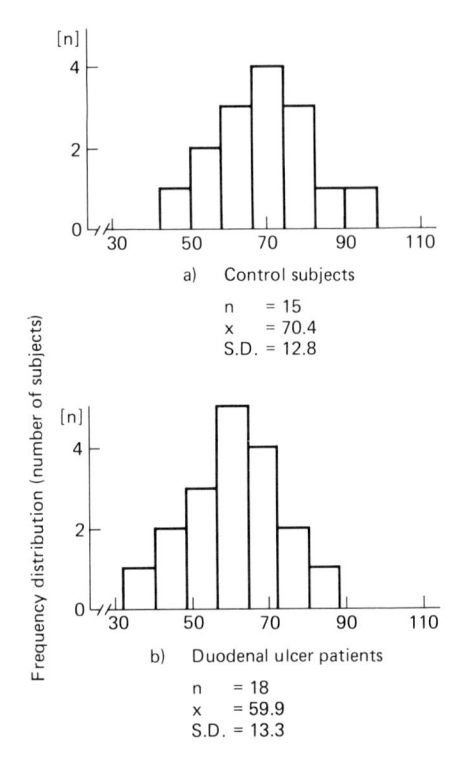

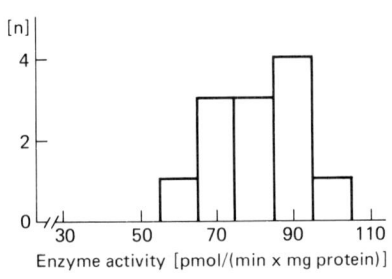

FIGURE 6. Histograms of histamine methyltransferase activity in corpus mucosa of male control subjects and duodenal ulcer patients before and after vagotomy. x̄ = mean values of the samples. SV = selective gastric vagotomy. [From Barth et al. (30), copyright Birkäuser Verlag Basel; reprinted by permission.]

dog model was clinically relevant. Accordingly, only this species was selected for extended work to improve the compatibility of plasma substitutes (41). It was then shown that an excess of the cross-linking material hexamethylene diisocyanate was responsible for the side-effects of the gelatin preparation polygeline (Haemaccel[R]). A new preparation, containing only a slight excess of the cross-linking material the amount

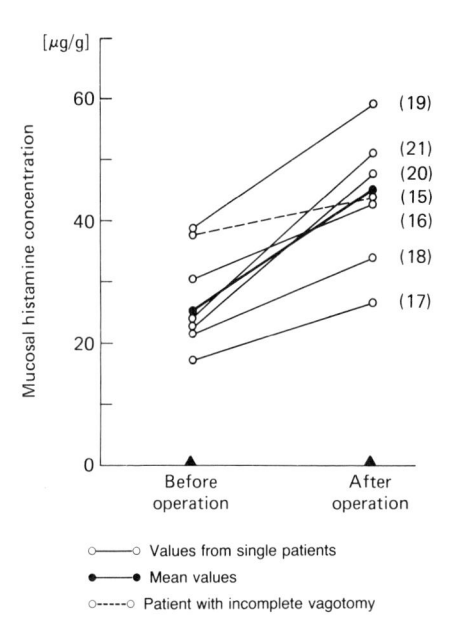

FIGURE 7. Histamine concentrations in the corpus mucosa of duodenal ulcer patients before and after selective gastric vagotomy with drainage. Numbers in parentheses = number of patients in the series. [From Troidl et al. (31), reprinted by permission of the publishers, Butterworth and Co.]

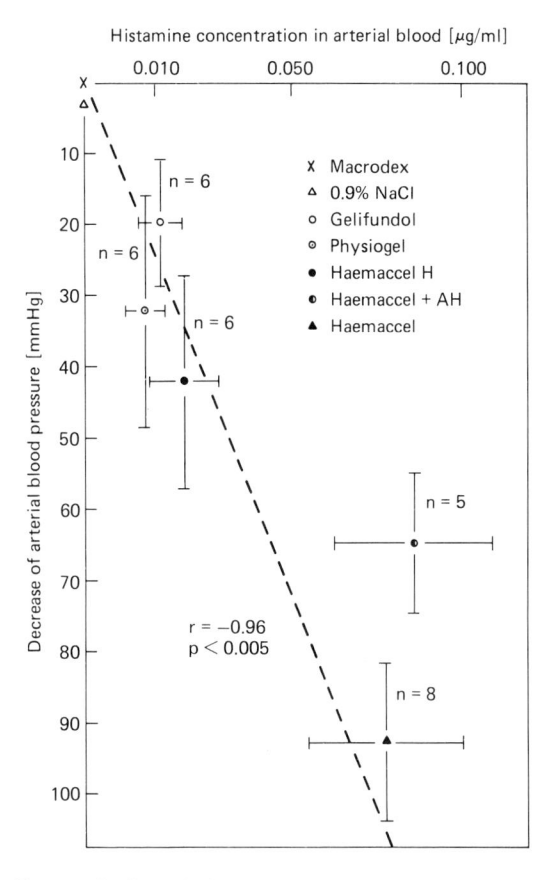

FIGURE 8. Correlation between maximum increase of blood histamine concentration and maximum hypotension in dogs undergoing isovolaemic haemodilution with several plasma substitutes. Mean values + S.E.M., Haemaccel H = high molecular weight polygeline. For further conditions see Messmer et al. (39).

stoichiometrically necessary, was produced by the company and tested in a controlled trial in dogs (41). This new preparation, Haemaccel-35, was well-tolerated in the animals.

Immediately after these tests in the laboratory, controlled clinical trials were conducted in human volunteers and patients. They showed, convincingly, that the side-effects of polygeline were drastically reduced and that Haemaccel-35 was as safe as human albumin and hydroxyethyl starch, the plasma substitutes with the lowest incidence of pseudoallergic reactions in man (41). This remarkable success of the clinic-laboratory partnership, Haemaccel-35, was used exclusively as the fluid for resuscitation in the Falkland Islands Campaign (42).

Recurrent Bleeding in Upper Gastrointestinal Tract Haemorrhage

The last of the four examples chosen (Table VII), is not related to histamine research, but to medical decision-making in upper gastrointestinal (GI) haemorrhage. It demonstrates that the Marburg experiment works in other fields and that the magic room of a mathematician and a computer scientist can be regarded as a laboratory. It is still mandatory, however, to maintain the close-coupling between the clinic and the laboratory.

Recurrent haemorrhage is one of the most serious prognostic signs in patients with upper GI bleeding (43). A study of the literature revealed that most authors either did not define recurrent bleeding or used inadequate definitions (44). Massive bleeding with haematemesis, fresh melaena, or shock is easily diagnosed without sophisticated definitions, but this type of haemorrhage occurs only in a minority of rebleeders and information about all types of rebleeding is required. The slow bleeding of small amounts over a longer period can have serious clinical consequences although it does not produce unique clinical signs and symptoms (45).

In a retrospective case-control study, patients with rebleeding and with no rebleeding after upper GI haemorrhage were investigated. Clinical variables (e.g., blood pressure, pulse rate, haemoglobin concentration, haematemesis, etc.), were analyzed for their ability to detect recurrent haemorrhage as early as possible using methods of medical decision-making [e.g., classification matrices and receiver operating characteristic (ROC) curves (45)].

No single diagnostic test for rebleeding, based on any of the clinical variables, showed a sensitivity of more than 60% together with a sufficiently high specificity. However, by using distinct combinations of diagnostic criteria, such as haematemesis and/or blood transfusion volume ≤ 1000 ml and/or falling haemoglobin concentration 2 g/100 ml the sensitivity of this diagnostic procedure for recurrent hemorrhage increased to 90% accompanied by a sufficiently high specificity (45) (Table VIII).

Immediately after the completion of these "laboratory tests", a monitoring system for the early detection of all types of rebleeding was introduced into the intensive care unit of the Department of General Surgery (46). The results of the first prospective validation study corresponded to those of the retrospective case-control study (Table IX). Although the system, at this moment, is far from being perfect, it may improve the patient's prognosis in upper GI bleeding. Further studies are needed to evaluate the impact of the system on the diagnostic strategy, the choice of treatment and the outcome of the disease.

TABLE IX. Comparison of the monitoring system for early diagnosis of recurrent bleeding with the clinical diagnosis obtained by emergency endoscopy and/or operation [from Ohmann et al. (46), reprinted by permission of Elsevier Science Publishers.]

Prospective Study (March 83–June 84)		Alarm of the monitoring system		
		yes	no	total
Recurrent Bleeding	yes	10	6	16
	no	9	55	64
	total	19	61	80

Conclusion

The Marburg experiment has been "on stream" now for fifteen years. We think it is one winning approach to ensuring *immediate* interaction and integration between clinical observation, decision-making, and basic research.

TABLE VIII. Sensitivity and specificity of combined diagnostic tests for recurrent bleeding in the upper GI-tract.

2 Diagnostic criteria	Sensitivity (%)	Specificity (%)
haematemesis and/or		
hypotension, syst. (mmHg) ≥ 20	64	95
tachycardia (b/min) ≥ 20	67	92
falling hemoglobin (g/dl) ≥ 2	69	94
blood transfusion (ml) ≥ 1000	71	93
3 Diagnostic criteria		
haematemesis and/or blood transfusion (ml) ≥ 1000 and/or	71	93
tachycardia (b/min) ≥ 20	83	87
hypotension, syst. (mmHg) ≥ 20	85	86
falling hemoglobin (g/dl) ≥ 2	91	78

A combined test was defined as positive if at least one of the criteria was present, and negative if none was present. For definition of sensitivity and specificity see Thon et al. (45).

References

1. Lakatos I, Musgrave A, Editors. Criticism and the growth of knowledge. Cambridge-London-New York: Cambridge University Press, 1975:1–282.
2. Stachowiak H. Medizin als handlungswissenschaft. In Gross R, editor. Modelle und realitaten in der medizin, schattauer verlag. Stuttgard-New York: 1983:7–22.
3. Stegmuller W. Theoriendynamik. Normale wissenschaft und wissenschaftliche revolutionen. Methodologie der forschungsprogramme oder epistemologische anarchie? In Probleme und resultate der wissenschaftstheorie und analytischen philosophie. Band II. Theorie und Erfahrung. Berlin-Heidelberg-New York: Springer Verlag, 1973:153–327.
4. Feyerabend PK. Wie wird man ein braver empirist? Ein aufruf zur toleranz in der erkenntnistheorie (how to be a good empiricist—a plea for tolerance in matters epidemiological). In Kruger L, editor. Erkenntnis-Probleme der Naturwis-

senschaften, Kiepenheuer—Witsch. Koln-Berlin: 1970:302–335.
5. Lorenz W, Hamelmann H, Troidl H. Marburg experiment on surgical research: a five-year experience on the cooperation between clinical and theoretical surgeons. Klin Wschr 1976;54:927–936.
6. Lorenz W, Roher HD. Fifteen years of the Marburg Experiment on surgical research. Part I: change from experimental to theoretical surgery. Theor Surg 1986;1:21–31.
7. Lorenz W. The progress of surgical science. Lancet II. 1983:1017–1017.
8. Lorenz W, Roher HD. Entwicklung wissenschaftlicher Aussagen. In Schreiber HW, Carstensen G, editors. Chirurgie im Wandel der Zeit 1945–1983. Berlin-Heidelberg: Springer Verlag, 1983:28–35.
9. Rohde H, Troidl H, Lorenz W. Systematic followup: a concept for evaluation of operative results in duodenal ulcer patients. Klin Wschr 1977;55:925–932.
10. Troidl H, Lorenz W, Rohde H, Fischer M, Vestweber KH, Hamelmann H. Trends in der chirurgie des chronischen ulces duodeni: eine prospektive kontrollierte aber noch immer nicht randomisierte studie. Chirurg 1979;50:285–290.
11. Lorenz W, Ohmann CH. Methodische Formen klinischer studien in der chirurgie: indikation und bewertung. Chirurg 1983;54:189–195.
12. Allgower M. Interdisziplinare zusammenarbeit in der chirurgie. Ther Umsch 1972;29:645.
13. Lorenz W. Attitudes to controlled clinical trials. Lancet I 1982:1460–1461.
14. Lorenz W, Doenicke A, Meyer R, et al. An improved method for the determination of histamine release in man: its application in studies with propanidid and thiopentone. Europ J Pharmacol 1972;19:180–190.
15. Lorenz W, Benesch L, Barth H, et al. Fluorometric assay of histamine in tissues and body fluids: choice of the purification procedure and identification in the nanogram range. Z Analyt Chem 1970;252:94–98.
16. Doenicke A, Lorenz W. Histaminfreisetzung und anaphylaktische reaktionen bei narkosen. Biochemische und Klinische Aspekte. Anaesthesist 1970;19:413–417.
17. Lorenz W, Reimann H-J, Barth H, et al. A sensitive and specific method for the determination of histamine in human whole blood and plasma. Hoppe-Seyler's Z Physiol Chem 1972;353:911–920.
18. Beaven MA, WoldeMussie E. Histamine in body fluids: its measurement in different clinical states. NER Allergy Proc 1984;5:300–310.
19. Moss J, Rosow CE, Savarese JJ, Philbin DM, Kniffen KJ. Role of histamine in the hypotensive action of d-tubocurarine in humans. Anesthesiology 1981;55:19–25.
20. Moss J, Rosow CE. Histamine release by narcotics and muscle relaxants in human. Anesthesiology 1983;59:330–338.
21. Lorenz W, Doenicke A, Meyer R, et al. Histamine release in man by propanidid and thiopentone: pharmacological effects and clinical consequences. Brit J Anaesth 1972;44:355–369.
22. Doenicke A, Lorenz W, Beigl R, et al. Histamine release after intravenous application of short-acting hypnotics: a comparison of etomidate, althesin (CT 1341) and Propanidid. Brit J Anaesth 1973;45:1097–1104.
23. Lorenz W, Roher HD, Doenicke A, Ohmann CH. Histamine release in anaesthesia and surgery: a new method to evaluate its clinical significance with several types of causal relationship. Clin anaesthesiol 1984;2:403–426.
24. Lorenz W, Seidel W, Doenicke A, et al. Elevated plasma histamine concentrations in surgery: causes and clinical significance. Klin Wschr 1974;52:419-425.
25. Watkins J. Etomidate: An "immunologically safe" anaesthetic agent. Anaesthesia 1983;38:34–38.
26. Troidl H, Lorenz W, Barth H, et al. Augmentation of pentagastrin stimulated gastric secretion in the Heidenhain pouch dog by amodiaquine: inhibition of histamine methyltransferase in vivo? Agents Actions 1973;3:157–167.
27. Seidel W, Troidl H, Lorenz W, et al. Eine prospektive, kontrollierte studie zur selektiven vagotomie beim chronischen duodenalulkus: fruhergebnisse mit einer standardisierten operationsauswahl u. operationstechnik. Klin Wschr 1973;51:477–486.
28. Rohde H, Lorenz W, Troidl H, Reimann H-J, Hafner G, Weber D. Histamine and peptic ulcer: influence of sample-taking on the precision and accuracy of fluorometric histamine assay in biopsies of human gastric mucosa. Agents Actions 1980;10:175–185.
29. Troidl H, Lorenz W, Rohde H, Hafner G, Ronzheimer M. Histamine and peptic ulcer: a prospective study of mucosal histamine concentrations in duodenal ulcer patients and in control subjects suffering from various gastrointestinal diseases. Klin Wschr 1976;54:947–956.
30. Barth H, Troidl H, Lorenz W, Rohde H, Glass R. Histamine and peptic ulcer disease: histamine methyltransferase activity in gastric mucosa of control subjects and duodenal ulcer patients before and after surgical treatment. Agents Actions 1977;7:75–79.
31. Troidl H, Rohde H, Lorenz W, Hafner G, Hamelmann H. Effect of selective gastric vagotomy on histamine concentration in gastric mucosa of

patients with duodenal ulcer. Brit J Surg 1978;65:101–16.
32. Man WK, Saunders JH, Ingoldby C, Spencer J. Effect of selective gastric vagotomy on histamine concentration in gastric mucosa of control subjects and duodenal ulcer patients before and after surgical treatment. Agents Actions 1977;7:75–79.
33. Lorenz W, Thon K, Barth H, Neugebauer E, Reimann H-J, Kuschej. Metabolism and function of gastric histamine in health and disease. J Clin Gastroenterol 1983;5(suppl. 1):37–56.
34. Hansen JH, Knigge U. Failure of proximal gastric vagotomy for duodenal ulcer resistant to cimetidine. Lancet 1984;II:84–86.
35. Lorenz W, Thon K, Ohmann CH, Roher HD. Symptomloses und kompliziertes ulcus pepticum als extreme erscheinungsformen der ulcuskrankheit: konsequenzen fur die wahl zwischen konservativer und chirurgischer therapie. Langenbecks Arch. Chir 1985;366:69–79.
36. Messmer K, Lorenz W, Haendle H, Klovekorn WP, Hutzel M. Acute hypotension and histamine liberation following rapid infusion of plasma substitutes in dogs. Europ Surg Res 1969;1:188–189.
37. Goth A. Histamine release by drugs and chemicals. In Histamine and antihistamines, International Encyclopedia of Pharmacology and Therapeutics, vol 1, Oxford-New York-Toronto-Sydney-Braunschweig: Pergamon Press, 1973:25–43.
38. Keller R. A study of the mastocytolytic effects of polycations in the presence of certain plasma substitutes. Bibl Haemat 1969;33:126–130.
39. Messmer K, Lorenz W, Sunder-Plassmann L, Kloevekorn WP, Hutzel M. Histamine release as cause of acute hypotension following rapid colloid infusion. Naunyn-Schmiedebergs Arch. Pharmak 1970;267:433–445.
40. Lorenz W, Doenicke A, Messmer K, et al. Histamine release in human subjects by modified gelatin (Haemaccel (R)) and dextran: an explanation for anaphylactoid reactions observed under clinical conditions? Brit J Anaesth 1976;48:151–165.
41. Lorenz W, Doenicke A, Schoning B, Karges H, Schmal A. Incidence and mechanisms of adverse reactions to polypeptides in man and dog. In Hennessen W, editor. Joint WHO/IABS symposium on the standardization of albumin, plasma substitutes and plasmapheresis, Geneva 1980. Develop. Biol. Standard. 48. Karger Verlag 1981:207–234.
42. Williams JG, Riley TRD, Moody RA. Resuscitation experience in the Falkland Islands Campaign. Brit Med J 1983;286:775–777.
43. Bennet JR, Dykes PW. Ulcerative disease of the stomach and the duodenum. In Dykes PW, Keighly MRB, editors. Gastrointestinal Haemorrhage, John Wright, Bristol. 1981:155–165.
44. DeDombal FT, Morgan AG, Staniland JR, Ohmann C. Clinical features computer analysis. In Dykes PW, Keighley MRB, editors. Gastrointestinal haemorrhage, John Wright Bristol. 1981:155–165.
45. Thon K, Ohmann CH, Stoltzing H, Lorenz W. Medical decision making in upper gastrointestinal bleeding: the impact of clinical criteria for the diagnosis of recurrent haemorrhage. Theor Sur 1986;1:32–39.
46. Ohmann CH, Thon K, Stoltzing H, Lorenz W. Medical decision making for monitoring patients with upper gastrointestinal bleeding. In van Bemmel JH, Gremy F, Zvarova J, editors. Medical decision making: Diagnostic strategies and experts systems. North-Holland: Elsevier Science Publishers B.V., 1985:136–139.

2

Animal Experimentation

W.H. Isselhard and J. Kusche

Introduction

Animal experimentation and research with animals is an integral part of clinical research, including surgery. The goal is to solve problems encountered in clinical practice and to develop new methods and approaches to the cure and alleviation of disease and disability. Animal experimentation is to be understood as research that will benefit both man and animals.

Scientific and biomedical research employing animals has a long, productive and exciting history. To pass over this history in a single paragraph does an injustice to many researchers and their innumerable accomplishments. The long list of names may be represented by John Hunter (1728–1793), the surgeon, anatomist and naturalist, and by Claude Bernard (1813–1878), the physiologist. Hunter introduced arterial ligation for treating aneuryisms, after the study of collateral circulation in the deer. He also conducted transplantation experiments in fowl, in the hope of establishing a technique for transplanting the human tooth. At the end of the Age of Enlightenment, he anticipated the value of research in animals for medical activities in man. Bernard elucidated functions of liver and pancreas and advocated the still modern concept of the "milieu interieur". At the threshold of modern natural sciences and medicine, he contributed to the development of medical sciences by insisting on the use of strict experimental methods in the study of biological problems. This history provides convincing proof that progress in clinical medicine is in large part linked to advances in other, "basic" sciences and that animal experimentation often was and still is the absolutely necessary key. A large body of facts and a remarkable knowledge of interactions in physiology, pathophysiology, biochemistry, microbiology as well as normal and pathological morphology stem from research in animals, the value of which cannot be overestimated. They provide the fundamental scientific basis for contemporary medicine and surgery.

The scientist working with animals as a scientific tool must be aware of and prepared for the fact that research with animals and animal experimentation give rise to scientific, ethical, legal and technical problems and controversies. These problems and their controversial discussions have existed for a long time. They change with times. To a large extent, they present themselves differently in different cultures and social communities. Especially in countries, where animal research has grown to huge dimensions, questions concerning animals and particularly concerning animal experimentation have attracted considerable public interest within the last decades. Unfortunately, the discussion of the totally oppositive views on and interests in animals has eventually become emotionalized. This is regrettable, because it makes a mutual consent nearly impossible and hinders the necessary elaboration of pragmatic solutions.

It is thus strongly recommended that every scientist working with animals be familiar with the problem of animal experimentation as well as local legal and ethical requirements for animal care. Animal experimentation demands the highest level of scientific and humane responsibility.

While it is not possible to provide the interested reader with a complete list of books, protocols and statements on animal experimentation, references 1–5 provide a comprehensive coverage of the more recent publications.

The Role of Animal Experimentation in Clinical Research

Animal experimentation has made it possible for surgery and most other disciplines of human and veterinary medicine to reach their present high standards. An enumeration of the achievements made in surgery, alone, with the help and sacrifice of animals is beyond the scope of this chapter; a catalogue of surgical developments accomplished without animal experimentation would be much shorter. Our relatively vast knowledge of facts and interactions in physiology, pathophysiology, biochemistry, and morphology is largely the result of research in animals and provides the roots of today's surgery. Careful and judicious research in animals of various species preceded the introduction, and accompanies the continuous amendment of surgical procedures and other therapeutic measures that are now taken for granted.

Only a few examples of the contributions such research has made can be given here, but they include: development of gastro-intestinal surgery including gastrectomy for the treatment of ulcers and malignancies; development of modern thoracic and pulmonary surgery; elaboration of essential components of our knowledge of peri-and postoperative pathophysiology and its consequences for prophylaxis and therapy; establishment of open-heart and coronary artery surgery, including development of the heart-lung-machine, hypothermia, induced cardiac arrest, and myocardial protection; advances in microsurgery; treatment of terminal renal insufficiency by dialysis or transplantation; transplantation of tissues and such life-supporting organs as the kidney, liver, heart, and pancreas; preservation of live tissues and organs being one of the prerequisites of transplantation on a large scale; development of neurosurgery; analysis and therapy of the various forms of shock; pilot preparation of the A.O.-techniques and other techniques of osteosynthesis; testing of artificial joints; and biological and synthetic replacement of bone defects.

Research involving animals will continue to be necessary in the future if we wish to enjoy the advantages of innovation and widening knowledge of biological processes, and the chance of being able to cure as yet incurable diseases and disorders.

Research in animals is usually the first step in attempts to make established operative interventions less cumbersome and stressful for patients. The development of endoscopy from a technique for direct inspection and diagnosis to a method for curative surgical intervention is an example. Many affected regions of the body can now be reached via natural apertures or small incisions, in comparison with earlier approaches that involved substantial disturbances to, or even destruction of, normal tissues. Similarly, animal experimentation has played an essential role in the development of the kidney-lithotripter and its routine application in patients with nephrolithiasis. Introduction of a similar method for the destruction of stones in the biliary system is only a question of time.

Work with and in animals is also an important constituent of teaching and learning prior to practice involving humans. The acquisition of medical and surgical skills, the avoidance of mistakes and wrong reactions that may have unfortunate consequences, and the development of sensitivity based on personal experience with extremely complex biological systems can only be achieved by means of intensive study of living organisms. Books, films, models, and modern audio-visual teaching methods are undoubtedly helpful in the teaching and learning processes, but they cannot completely replace work with living matter. The mandate and ethics of medicine require that the restoration and improvement of health be sought with the least possible risk to human patients. Lofty as this goal is, it does not absolve the investigator from a deep and continuing moral obligation to handle other than human life with care, responsibility, consideration, and respect.

The Differentiation of Living Matter

To appraise the importance, usefulness and the yield of experimentation in intact animals versus the use of alternative methods, it is worth devoting some discussion, in a very general way, to the differentiation of living matter.

All living matter is subject to very similar, if not identical, biological laws, i.e., all living matter functions according to very similar principles and mechanisms even though the degree of differentiation is extremely wide.

The cell is the smallest entity of self-supporting life. It may exist as a separate unicellular organism comprising all the attributes required to maintain its own existence and the continuation and evaluation of its species. Alternatively, the cell may be bound to the co-existence and co-functioning of many different cells whose number may be uncountable and whose potentialities for differentiation and performing different specific functions may be neither known nor understood definitively. The latter statement can be easily illustrated by a little reflection. What information and conclusions could a physician derive from a white blood cell count and a differential blood smear 30 years ago compared to the early hints the specialist now gets from alterations in cells in the blood for discriminating an early episode of rejection from a viral or bacterial infection after organ transplantation? Only one generation ago, the endothelium was assigned hardly any roles other than separating the blood from tissues and participating phyiologically in the blood-clotting processes and pathophysiologically in some vascular diseases and disorders. Today, biomedical science has started to realize that the endothelium has many differentiated physiological attributes like an organ, and may initiate or contribute to numerous pathologic processes.

Multicellular living systems originate from unicellular living matter. In its unicellular state, it already comprises all the species-specific characteristics of all the cells in the eventual whole multicellular organism. Multicellular living systems, however, are only able to exist independently and to continue the propagation and evolution of their species after they have reached a sufficiently differentiated multicellular state of ontogenesis, as determined by phylogenesis.

An increase in the differentiation of cells usually means an increase in abilities and the enhancement of specialized functions that accompanies the evolution of the special cells, tissues, organs, and organ systems that, with their multiple interdependencies, constitute the body of the organism. For most of the specialized cells and organs, differentiation implies the loss of certain properties, e.g., many differentiated cells totally lack any potential for regeneration. As a rule, more differentiated living systems are considered to be higher forms of animal life compared to less differentiated lower life forms. This view does not negate the fact that lower animal life has given rise to remarkable differentiations and capabilities. Human life can be rightfully regarded as the most differentiated living system.

Surgery is the art of palliative, curative or restorative intervention in highly differentiated organisms. It cannot be learned or taught, nor can it progress, without access to adequately differentiated living systems.

Alternatives to Animal Experimentation?

So-called alternative methods, as originally defined, are to be understood as alternatives to animal experimentation. Less radical and more realistic is the definition that classifies such methods and approaches as substitutes that will reduce animal experimentation (10,13,16,17). An animal experiment is defined as an intervention in, or treatment of, a living animal under strict scientific conditions. In the last few decades, the so-called alternative methods have been persistently propagated, often in an irrelevant way and usually on the basis of an over-valuation of their efficiency. The apparent aim of the protagonists is to represent animal experimentation as being useless and needless. The excessive zeal of antivivisectionists sometimes causes occupational and personal defamation and discrimination against the experimental investigator (18).

It must be appreciated that, for more than a century, biomedical research has taken advantage of experiments with living matter other than animals. It continuously improves these methods and designs new approaches. The scientific community distinguishes between *in vivo* studies in living animals and *in vitro* experiments with tissues or organs from sacrificed animals. The culturing of cells and the controlled growth of fetal organs, in whole or in part, are now established laboratory procedures, and studies in these preparations must be classified as *in vitro* experiments.

The important distinction between "schmerzfaehiger und nicht schmerzfaehiger Materie" (matter capable of suffering and not capable of suffering), is fully accepted by expert investigators (10) although it did not originate in the scientific community (15). An *in vivo* experiment with animals is an experiment with living matter capable of suffering, whereas an *in vitro* experiment makes use of living matter that is no longer capable of suffering.

Current biomedical and surgical research employs the following approaches, when they are appropriate:

1. experiments with surviving cells, tissues, organs, parts of organs, and organ systems,
2. experiments with cultured cells, tissues, and organs,
3. experiments with lower organisms,
4. work with non-biological materials,
5. calculations in immaterial models,
6. experiments involving a large variety of chemical, biochemical, molecular biological, microbiological, physical, and immunological methods of *in vitro* analysis.

It must be recognized, nevertheless, that cells, tissues and organs for *in vitro* studies have their origin in living animals. It should also be realized that numerous animal experiments are still needed for development, testing, quality control and comparative studies.

The prohibition of all animal experimentation and the exclusive use of alternative methods are not feasible, given the present state of scientific knowledge. This is particularly true for surgical research and experimental surgery. Problems like the care of the polytraumatized organism; the elaboration of more effective therapeutic approaches to different kinds of shock; management of multi-organ failure; the effect of rejection of organs, in whole or in part; tissue or organ substitution by biological or non-biological matter; the improvement of existing and the development of new devices like the heart–lung machine or the artificial heart; and the trial of new concepts of surgical interventions can only be studied in whole animals.

Results obtained in an *in vitro* study cannot always be transferred directly to the *in vivo* situation, e.g., an early cardioplegic agent (19) proved to be rather toxic in *in vitro* studies with isolated cells (20), but under *in vivo* conditions it was found to be only slightly inferior to more modern therapeutic agents (21,22). The scientific value of *in vitro* research must not, however, be underestimated. *In vitro* studies can reveal biological facts that may remain unrecognized in whole animal experiments due to their complexity. Even in surgical research, *in vitro* experiments may be of help in the solution of special problems, e.g., for the screening of cardioplegic and organ-protecting solutions and principles, and the determination of tolerances to various forms of deprivation, such as ischemia, anoxia, hypoxia, hypoperfusion, etc. Work with isolated or cultured cells, such as the preservation and transplantation of Langerhans'islets or the pre-operative "endothelialisation" of vascular prostheses is part of surgical research. The researcher has to be aware of the advantages, the disadvantages, and the limits of this scientific tool.

In 1959, *Russell* and *Burgch* (17) enunciated the 3 R's for research in animals: Replacement, Reduction, and Refinement. Replacement, as originally defined, refers:

"to a wide range of techniques in which animals were not required at all in the actual experiment or in which they were exposed to no distress. For example, a terminal experiment in which the animal is always under anesthesia until it is humanely killed would fall into the category of replacement. The use of tissue cultures and computer modeling represent the former category. The concept of Reduction focused on reducing the number of animals required by better experimental planning, statistical design, and statistical analysis. . . . The trial and error approach is less desirable than the hypothetico–deductive approach in which the researcher formulates a testable hypothesis. . . . Refinement dealt exclusively with experimentation in which the animal was subjected to some degree of stress during the investigation. The 3 R's principle thus centers mainly on the question of stress research."

Within the concept of the 3 R's "it is permissible to use an animal in research provided that the animal suffers no pain whatsoever" (16). *Rowan* (16) finds this concept to have changed its meaning "with the advent of the term 'alternatives' to laboratory animals". Now, "the main thrust is aimed at the total numbers of animals used, rather than at the question of stressful research. As a result, replacement and reduction refer solely to the number of animals used while refinement refers to the overall question of reducing the stress suffered by the laboratory animal. . . . An 'alternative' includes any system or method that covers one or more of the following:

1. replacing the use of laboratory animals altogether;
2. reducing the number of animals required;
3. refining an existing procedure or technique so as to minimize the level of stress or pain endured by the animal".

But, there is also the statement that "any 'alternative' must provide information or results which allow the investigator to draw the same conclusions with at least the same degree of confidence" (16,23) *Smyth* (13) has argued similarly.

It is important to know that not only the *in vitro* methods but also the commitment to humane *in vivo* experimentation with animals originated in the scientific community. Renowned scientific societies and science promotion societies have supported animal protection laws in various countries.

Animal Models

For clinical and surgical research, Wessler's definition of an animal model of human disease may be useful. An animal model is "a living organism with an inherited, naturally acquired or induced pathological process that in one or more respects closely resembles the same phenomenon in man"(24).

A more general definition covering all aspects of biomedical research was adapted from this definition by the Institute of Laboratory Animal Resources (ILAR) (25). An animal model might vary from a one-cell protozoan, the study of which can lead to a better understanding of cellular function, to the chimpanzee, one of the species phylogenetically closest to humans which may be the only species other than humans susceptible to a particular infectious agent (26). Animal models, according to Gill (27) are used mainly for three reasons:

1. to elucidate host defense mechanisms;
2. to point the way for subsequent studies in humans; and
3. to screen substances for effectiveness or toxicity.

There is no doubt that animal models have great merit in relation to points (1) and (2). An early example is the work of E. Jenner (1749–1823) who observed that milk maids affected by cowpox did not contract the malignant smallpox then epidemic in England. Another important example is the finding of Robert Koch that guinea pigs are highly susceptible to tuberculosis. He used it to establish the causal relationship between the tubercle bacillus and tuberculosis. Koch's postulates concerning infectious diseases cannot be fulfilled without a susceptible animal model. For further important historical animal models see the paper by Jones (28).

Point 3, above, is the subject of much debate, because it is doubtful whether animal experiments can accurately predict the toxicity of substances in humans, whether the current extent of animal experiments is necessary, and whether alternatives can replace animal experiments.

If animal models are used, they should be appropriate for the situation that is to be studied. For instance, a model of prostatic cancer that depends on a tumor growth that is insensitive to hormonal influence is not relevant to the clinical situation, as is an animal model of duodenal ulcer production that occurs without elevated acid output in the stomach.

There is probably no ideal model for any disease. The disease itself may be variable and may have many facets so that more than one animal model may be required. Although the ideal model may not exist, we should seek "its more modest cousin" (26), i.e., the most appropriate model available.

During a workshop on "Needs for New Animal Models", Leader and Padgett (29) listed nine criteria for a good animal model:

1. It should accurately reproduce the disease or lesions under study.
2. It should be available to multiple investigations. Sharing of animals and data among institutions has been an important factor in many research successes. It allows monitoring of the scientific validity of observations and stimulates further investigation.
3. It should be exportable.
4. If the disease under study is genetic, the species should be polytocous–producing multiple young at each birth.
5. The animal should be large enough for multiple biopsy samples.
6. It should fit into the available animal facilities of most laboratories. The accelerating costs of any changes in animal housing and care

standards make this criterion particularly relevant.
7. The animal should be easily handled by most investigators. However, convenience should not be the determinating factor in the selection of the model.
8. It should be available in multiple species.
9. The animals used in the model should survive long enough to be usable.

To ensure maximum comparability of results, another point should be added to the list of criteria. The animals for induced or spontaneous models of human disease should be genetically defined.

Although several populations of animals can be distinguished and their use has special advantages and disadvantages (27), it is difficult to say which is the most appropriate for mimicking a particular disease or effect of therapy in a human population.

1. Randomly-mating animal populations:

There are two types, those that are colony-bred and those found in the wild. The major use of the first type is testing the effects of drugs; the second type may be useful for developing studies relevant to human disease because it generates mutants and mimicks a disease process (27).

2. Outbred populations:

These animals are systematically bred to maintain maximal genetic heterogeneity and are useful for drug screening.

3. Inbred strains:

An inbred strain is defined as being the product of 20 generations of brother-sister matings. Inbreeding implies a genetic drift. When an inbred strain has been separated from its primary source for eight or more generations, it should be identified as a sub-line by giving it a laboratory designation that follows the strain name. For the mouse, a standardized nomenclature exists (30), but not for other species, such as the rat. The same rules for listing inbred strains should be used for species other than the mouse (31). The major use of inbred strains is the study of specific questions, such as drug effects on a tumor, in a genetically-defined population.

4. F_1 hybrids:

Two progenitor inbred strains are mated to form F_1 hybrids that are more resistant to environmental influences than the parent inbred strains. The F_1 hybrid provides a well-defined population with limited genetic diversity.

5. Coisogenic and congenic strains:

Two isogenic, i.e., genetically identical, strains that differ only at a single locus, the differential locus, are known as "coisogenic" strains. Such strains arise as a result of mutation within an inbred strain. Strains that approximate the coisogenic status can be developed by backcrossing a gene from a donor strain into an inbred strain (the background strain of the inbred partner). The resulting partially coisogenic strains that differ at the differential locus and an associated segment of chromosome, are known as "congenic" strains (30). The major use of these animals is to study the effects of one specific gene.

This chapter is not the place to describe the characteristics of the various animal models described in the literature. Bustad and coworkers (32) embarked on this task when they wrote a chapter in "The Future of Animals, Cells, Models and Systems in Research, Development, Education and Testing". When they exceeded 6000 references for animal models, they decided to publish their list as an appendix to the paper. We have limited ourselves to preparing Table I to give you some help in finding the animal model you need in a special situation. If you intend to study duodenal ulcer disease, for example, you can look for spontaneous animal models (33) or for an experimentally-induced model that was presented as a chemically-induced duodenal ulcer by Szabo (34,35). Even if your search does not produce the ideal animal model of this human disease, there are some models that come close to the human situation, e.g., the "Executive Monkey" (36), or resemble human duodenal ulcer disease in many ways, e.g. the cysteamine ulcer (37) (see Table II).

Remember, when a human disease is to be studied, you should reflect on the criteria for the appropriateness of an animal model, study the information that is available, and not leave animal models as a "neglected medical resource" (38).

TABLE I.

Animal Models of Thrombosis and Haemorrhagic Diseases	DHEW Publ. No. (NJH) 1976:76-382
Animal Models for Biomedical Research VI—Metabolic Disease	Fed Proc 1976;35:1992–1236
Naturally Occurring Animal Models of Disease	Appendix to the paper: of Human "Animal Models" by Bustad UK, Hegreberg GA, Padgett GA. In: The future of animals, cells, models and symptoms in research, development, education and testing. Washington, D.C.: Nat Acad of Sciences, 1975
Animal Models for Diabetes Mellitus: A Bibliography	ILAR News 1981;24:5–22
Animal Models and Hypoxia	Stefanovich V, editor. New York: Pergamon Press, 1981
Animal Models for Tumor Progression	Libovici J, Wolman M. Anticancer Res. 1984;4:165–168
Animal Models of Human Diseases	Cohen D. CRC-Press, 1985
Animal Models of Gastrointestinal Disease	Pfeiffer CJ. CRC-Press, 1985
Spontaneous Models of Human Disease	Andrews EJ, Ward EJ, Altman NH, editor. Academic Press, 1979
Animal Models of Human Disease	Handbook published by the registry of Comparative Pathology, Armed Forces Institute of Pathology, USA, continuing series of fascicles
Animal Quality and Models in Biomedical Research	Spiegel A, Ericksen S, Volleveld HA, editors. New York: S. Fischer Verlag; Stuttgart, 1980
Animal Models for Research on Aging	Washington, D.C.: National Academy Press, 1981
Bibliography of Naturally Occuring Animal Models of Disease	Hegreberg GA, Leathers C, editors. Pullman, Washington: Human Student Books Corp., 1982
Bibliography of Induced Animal Models of Human Disease	Hegreberg GA, Leathers C, editors. Pullman, Washington: Human Student Books Corp., 1982
Experimental Models of Chronic Inflammatory Disease	Glynn LE, Schlumberger HD, editors. Heidelberg, New York: Springer Verlag, 1977
Experimental Cardiovascular Diseases	Selge H, Heidelberg, New York: Springer Verlag, 1970

Quality Control

Quality of Experiments

In several studies, the quality of publications has been evaluated by reporting the frequency and accuracy of the statistical data and criteria published in them (3,40). In a similar exercise that focused on experimentation in animals, Juhr (41) investigated some volumes of "Laboratory Animal Science". The result of his study is shown in Table III. It provides a useful checklist of criteria that should be adhered to in a well-designed animal experiment. Control groups were described in only 14% of papers. Aspects of breeding, sex and age of the animals are frequently reported, but the conditions of animal care are rarely given. The environment and the handling of animals can have an important input on study parameters of interest. If these factors are not recognized and controlled, the validity of the research results may be questioned. For example, transportation of test animals affects such factors as total leucocyte counts and ACTH levels (42).

The principles of experimental design are discussed in Section III, but Table III shows that the calculation of sample sizes, or the choice of statistical tests, is not very different from those for clinical trials. Many people mistakenly assume that random allocation of animals is not necessary, because the animals represent a random sample taken from a well-defined population. Immich (43) has demonstrated that this technique is as necessary in animal experiments as it as in clinical trials.

Besides skillful design and presentation of the results, the optimum utilization of animal experiments includes attention to the possibility of reducing the number of animals necessary for each experiment. In every laboratory where several groups are performing animal experiments, information about planned studies should be exchanged to enable more than one research group to participate in a project. Sacrificing one rat today to obtain a colon sample, and another tomorrow to get a piece of muscle, is wasting animals. Every effort should be made to reduce the number of animals by such measures as using a two-step experimental design, a sequential trial, or the replacement of a time and animal consuming dose-response curve by the up and down method of Dixon (44) when the determination of an LD_{50} is required.

Lastly, but certainly not least, the quality of animal experiments depends on the correct handling and care of animals, and the proper use of anesthetics, analgesics and tranquilizers. If a procedure must be conducted without the use of an anesthetic, analgesic, or tranquilizer, because it would defeat the purpose of the experiment, the responsible investigator must personally supervise the procedure to ensure that it is carried out in accordance with institutional policies and local, state, or federal regulations. Muscle relaxants or paralytic drugs (e.g., succinylcholine or other curariform drugs) are not anesthetics, and they should not be used alone for surgical restraint.

Appropriate facilities and equipment should be available for surgical procedures. A facility intended for aseptic surgery should be maintained and used for that purpose only, and its cleanliness should be assured. Surgery on animals should only be performed by persons who are properly qualified by training and experience, and should be conducted in the same formal and respectful manner that characterizes the operating theater during surgery on humans.

Postsurgical care should include observation of the animal until it has recovered from anesthesia, administration of supportive fluids and drugs, care of surgical incisions, and regular monitoring to ensure the animal's physical comfort and optimal recovery. Appropriate medical records should be maintained.

Euthanasia should be performed by trained persons in accordance with institutional policies and applicable laws. The choice of method depends on the species of animal and the project in which the animal was used, e.g., it should not interfere with postmortem examinations. Procedures for euthanasia should follow approved guidelines, such as those already established by the American Veterinary Medical Association Panel on Euthanasia. Animals of most species can be killed quickly and humanely by the intravenous or intraperitoneal injection of a concentrated solution of barbiturate. Mice, rats, and hamsters can be killed by cervical dislocation, or by exposure to gaseous nitrogen or carbon dioxide in an uncrowded chamber. Ether and chloroform are effective, but their use is hazardous to personnel; ether is flammable and explosive, chloroform is toxic and possibly carcinogenic. If animals are killed by ether, special facilities and procedures are required for storage and disposal of carcasses. Storage in refrigeration equipment that is not explosion-proof, and disposal by incineration can cause serious explosions.

The environment and dietary regimen should

TABLE II. Comparison of chemically-induced duodenal ulcer with human duodenal ulcer [from Szabo (37)].

	Experimental duodenal ulcer	Human duodenal ulcer
Localization of the ulcer:	anterior & posterior wall	anterior & posterior wall
Tendency to perforate:	yes	yes
Penetration into the liver and/or pancreas:	yes	yes
Occurrence of "giant ulcer forms" & massive bleedings:	yes	yes
Presence of chronic healed and/or active ulcers:	yes	yes
Occurrence of pyloric ulcers with deformities of the pylorus	yes	yes
Accompanying adrenocortical necrosis:	frequent	rare(?)
Presence of functional and/or organic brain disorders:	±	+
Increased gastric acid output:	±	±
Elevated basal serum gastrin levels:	+	±
Supersensitivity of serum gastrin to food intake:	yes	yes
Response to		
Antacids	+	±
Antisecretory agents	+	+
H_2 receptor antagonists	+	+
Vagotomy	+	+
Availability to study pre-ulcerogenic and very early ulcerogenic functional and morphologic changes	yes	no

TABLE III. Frequency of items reported in papers involving animal experiments modified from Juhr (41).

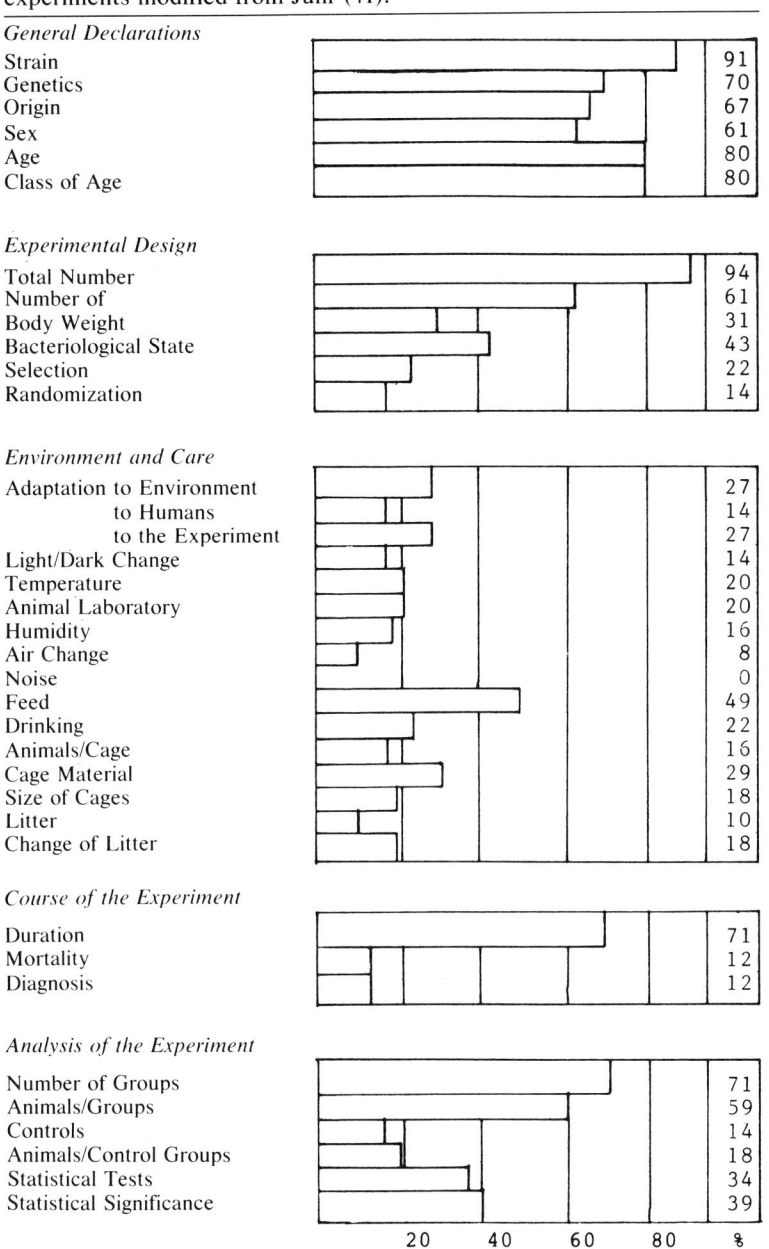

General Declarations

	%
Strain	91
Genetics	70
Origin	67
Sex	61
Age	80
Class of Age	80

Experimental Design

	%
Total Number	94
Number of	61
Body Weight	31
Bacteriological State	43
Selection	22
Randomization	14

Environment and Care

	%
Adaptation to Environment	27
to Humans	14
to the Experiment	27
Light/Dark Change	14
Temperature	20
Animal Laboratory	20
Humidity	16
Air Change	8
Noise	0
Feed	49
Drinking	22
Animals/Cage	16
Cage Material	29
Size of Cages	18
Litter	10
Change of Litter	18

Course of the Experiment

	%
Duration	71
Mortality	12
Diagnosis	12

Analysis of the Experiment

	%
Number of Groups	71
Animals/Groups	59
Controls	14
Animals/Control Groups	18
Statistical Tests	34
Statistical Significance	39

be suitable for each species. The components of the diet should be known and standardized and should be adapted to the age of the animals, when necessary. Young animals usually need a diet that is richer in protein than that given to adults. Information about normal values for the species used in an experiment can be very helpful in arriving at a first estimation of the reliability of your own measurements. Such data can be obtained from the textbooks listed in Appendix B.

Quality of Animals

A quality assurance program to adequately define and characterize research animals is important. Various commonly-occurring microorganisms cause subclinical infections in animals that may flare to produce high morbidity or mortality when the animals are stressed by an experiment. Such incidents frequently complicate the research results, invalidate the scientific data collected or their interpretation, and cause loss of money, time, and other research resources (41). Rodents, for example, should be free from sendai virus, mouse hepatitis virus, Reo 3 virus, lactic-dehydrogenase-elevating virus, lymphatic choriomeningitis virus, ectromelia, Salmonella, Hexamita, Pneumocystis, Haemobartonella, Eperythrozoon, Syphacia, Aspiculuris, Ectoparasites and the microorganisms listed in Table IV. When these pathogens infect and proliferate in animals, they cause subtle, long-term or short-term changes in organ and cell function, metabolism, and physiology, even though the animals appear to be clinically healthy. A sampling plan, for the microbiological or pathological monitoring of animals to detect the presence of diseased animals within adequate confidence limits, has been published by Hsu (45) along with a list of the pathogens and parasites that may be encountered.

All laboratory animals should be observed daily for clinical signs of illness, injury, or abnormal behaviour by a person trained to recognize such signs. All deviations from normal, and all deaths from unknown causes, should be reported promptly to the person responsible for animal disease control.

The most important link in a quality assurance program is probably the producer of the animals. The producers must insure proper breeding systems for both the inbred strains and outbred stocks to maintain their genetic integrity and characteristics. They should periodically perform health characterization and genetic monitoring of their animal colonies, and make their findings available at regular intervals or on request by those who purchase their animals. The methods used in genetic monitoring are listed in Table V. Research animals should always be obtained from a reliable vendor who consistently supplies high quality, genetically defined animals. Vendors should be periodically evaluated according to the management, economic, and other criteria listed in Table VI.

The aim of all these measures is to lower costs, reduce the number of animals necessary for an experiment, and improve the reliability of the results. The experimenter will feel better about a well-designed experiment when he has taken care to avoid any unneccessary injury to, and sacrifice of, whatever creatures have been involved.

Some Personal Comments

Learning to use animals in clinical and surgical research, recognizing the possibilities and limits of animal experimentation, and accepting the attendant responsibilities should be seen as privileges. Competence in animal experimentation has to be learned like any other skill. The fact that living matter is involved, whatever its place in the classification of living organisms, imposes a particular obligation on you, as the investigator.

The researcher and all co-workers—those involved directly in the experiment and those taking care of the animals in the animal quarters—ought to be aware that animals have their joys and feel discomfort, are sensitive, capable of suffering and enduring pain, can be afraid, and have memory. Members of the team who lack and cannot be taught respect, responsibility and

TABLE IV. Bacteria for which routine monitoring is recommended [modified from Hsu (45)].

Mice	Rats	Guinea pigs	Hamsters
Salmonella	Salmonella	Salmonella	Salmonella
Pseudomonas	Pasteurella	Streptococcus	Pasteurella
Corynebacterium	Diplococcus	Zooepidemicus	Bordetella
Pasteurella	Klebsiella	Bordetella	
Klebsiella	Pseudomonas	Klebsiella	
Bordetella bronchiseptica	Corynebacterium	Diplococcus	
Diplococcus pneumoniae	Bordetella		
Mycoplasma	Mycoplasma		

TABLE V. Methods for genetic monitoring modified from Hsu (45).

A. Breeding methods
B. *In vivo* histocompatibility testing
  1. Skin grafting
  2. Lymphoid tissue transplantation
  3. Tumor transplantation
C. *In vitro* histocompatibility testing
  1. Mixed lymphocyte reaction (MLR)
  2. Cell-mediated lympholysis (CML)
  3. Serology
D. Biochemical marker analysis
E. Embryo cryopreservation
F. Chromosomal banding
G. Mandible analysis

TABLE VI. Vendor evaluation modified by Hsu (45).

1. Type of practice (producer or dealer).
2. Type of facility (barrier or conventional).
3. Management and operation (accredited or not).
4. Professional and technical staff.
5. Availability of animal quality data.
6. Genetic uniformity and compatibility.
7. Methods of transportation.
8. Number, strain and species that can be supplied.
9. Reliability in meeting ordering specification.
10. Cost.
11. Quality of animals.

correct treatment of the animal as a fellow living being should not be allowed to use or handle animals.

You should go beyond the legal regulations in meticulously scrutinizing the scientific necessity, value, and mode of implementing each experiment (11). You bear ultimate moral responsibility for your actions and choices related to animal experimentation (46). There must always be a reasonable expectation that your study will contribute significantly to clinical knowledge and progress.

Experiments in animals should always be carefully thought out. A study of the literature relevant to the topic should precede the planning, and especially the implementation of any series of experiments. Helpful information can almost always be gained about the selection of relevant parameters, adequate methods of analysis, and appropriate animal model species. An animal species should not be used just because it is the one that is most readily available and most familiar to you. You should not find it repugnant to ask for advice and help. The animal is to be the surrogate of man!

The conception, planning, preparation, and performance of animal experiments is a major scientific responsibility. It requires time. It can rarely be discharged properly by adding it onto the end of a long day's work.

In vivo experiments and the sacrificing of animals without pain or fright at the end of experiments, or to obtain tissues or organs for *in vitro* experiments, must be performed by, or under the immediate and continuous supervision of, an appropriately qualified scientist. Experiments in animals should be performed with the assistance of a sufficient number of properly trained personnel; individual research has given ways to the team approach. Work on a do-it-yourself basis using self-taught techniques in a distant corner of a laboratory is contrary to the principles of experimentation in animals. Surgical research in animals should be confined to specialized and adequately equipped institutes, departments, or units.

The 3 R's—Replacement, Reduction, Refinement (17)—are important guides for research in animals. Animals should only be used after careful consideration has convinced you that no method other than an animal experiment can solve a problem, or provide the information that is needed. The scientific question should be formulated in such a way that a clear and valid answer can be reached with a minimum number of experiments. As many data as possible should be collected in each experiment, provided that over-instrumentation does not invalidate the model.

"The care and use of animals for experimental purposes should be based on the principle that pain and discomfort must be avoided. To this end, anesthetics and analgesic agents should be employed in an appropriate manner, unless specifically withheld as a requirement of the experiment. Pain-relieving drugs should be continued as long as necessary. Experiments in which pain and discomfort are an unavoidable consequence should be undertaken only when, on the basis of expert opinion, there are reasonable expectations that such studies will contribute to the ultimate enhancement of our knowledge of life. The degree of pain should never exceed that determined by the humanitarian importance of the problem to be solved by the experimental study'' (47). Surgical research and post-operative care, particularly in higher animals, should be conducted according to the same standards as surgery in humans.

The decision on the fate of an animal depends on the purpose of an experiment. The animal must either be sacrificed when the experiment is completed, or its subsequent life must be free from pain, grief and discomfort.

References

1. American Association of Pathologists: A workshop on needs for new animal models of human disease. Amer. J. Pathology 101, *No 3S, Suppl. to December 1980.*
2. Deutsche Forschungsgemeinschaft: Tierexperimentelle Forschung und Tierschutz Mitteilung III/ Kommission fuer Versuchstierforschung, 1981.
3. Gartner K, Hackbarth H, Stolte H, editors. Symposium on research animals and concepts of applicability to clinical medicine, Hannover FRG, 1981 Expl Biol Med Vol. 7, S. Karger, Basel, 1982.
4. Hoel DG. Animal experimentation and its relevance to man. Enviromental Health Perspectives 1980;32:25–30.
5. Hoff: Immoral and moral uses of animals. New Engl J Med 1980; 302:115–118.
6. IABS International 16th Congress for Biological Standardization, San Antonio/USA 1979: The standardization of animals to improve biomedical research. Basel: Production and Control S. Karger, 1980.
7. ILAR Symposium: The future of animals, cells, models and systems in research, development, education, and testing. Washington, D.C.: National Academy of Sciences, 1977.
8. Kubler K, editor. Der Tierversuch in der Arzneimittelforschung (interdisziplinaeres Fachgesprach im Bundesgesundheitsamt) BGA:-Berichte 1/1980.
9. McDaniel CG. Animal rights or human health? Med J Aust 1984; 855–857.
10. Merkenschlager M, Wilk W,: Gutachten ueber tierschutzgerechte Haltung von Versuchstieren. Gutachten ueber Tierversuche, Moeglichkeiten ihrer Einschraenkung und Ersetzbarkeit. Recommendations for the keeping of laboratory animals in accordance with animal protection principles. Parey-Berlin-Hamberg: Verlag Paul, 1979.
11. Riecker G. Aerztliche Ethik und Tierversuche Arzt und Krankenhaus 1984;11:306–312.
12. Sechzer JA, editor. The role of animals in biomedical research. Annals New York Academy of Sciences, 1983;406.
13. Smyth HD. Alternatives to animal experimentation. Solar Press, London: 1978. Alternativen zu tierversuchen. Ubersetzt aus dem englischen von A. Spiegel Fisher, Stuttgart, 1982.
14. Sontag KH. Der Tierversuch nach dem Stand der wissenschaftlichen Kenntnis. Pharm Ind 1982;44:4.
15. Weihe WH. Das Problem der Alternativen zum wissenschaftlichen Tierversuch. Fortschr Med 1982;100:2162–2166.
16. Rowan AN. The concept of the three R's, an introduction 16th IABS congress: the standardization of animals to improve biomedical research, production and control. San Antonio / USA 1979 Develop Biol Standard, Vol. 45, Karger S, Basel 1980;175–180.
17. Russell, WMS, Burch RL. The principle of humane experimental technique. Methuen U. Co, London: 1959.
18. Stiller H, Stiller M. Tierversuch und Tierexperimentator. F. Hirthammer Verlag, Muchen: 1977.
19. Kirsch U. Untersuchungen zum Eintritt der Totenstarre an ischamischen Meerschweinchenherzen in Normothermie Arzneim Forschung (Drug Research) 1970;20:1071–1074.
20. Carrentier S, Murawsky M, Carpentier A. Cytotoxicity of cardioplegic solutions: evaluation by tissue culture. Circulation 1981;64:(suppl. II),II:90—II 95.
21. Isselhard W, Schorn B, Huegel W, Uekermann U. Comparison of three methods of myocardial protection. Thorac Cardiovasc Surg 1963;28:329–126.
22. Huegel W, Lubbing H, Isselhard W, et al. Hemodynamics and metabolic status of the human heart after application of different forms of cardioplegic solutions. In: Isselhard W editor. Myocardial protection for cardiovascular surgery. Pharmazeutische Verlagsgesellschaft, Munchen: 1981.
23. Rowan AN. Laboratory animals and alternatives in the 80's. Int J Study Animal Problems 1980;1:162–169.
24. Wessler S. Introduction: what is a model? In: Animal models of thrombosis and hemorrhagic diseases. Bethesda, Maryland: Nat. Inst. Health, 1976:XI-XVI.
25. ILAR National Research Council committee on Animal Models for Research on Aging. Mammalian models for research on aging. Washington, D.C.: National Academy Press, 1981.
26. Held JR. Appropriate animal models. In: Sechzer JA editor. The role of amimal in biomedical research. Annals New York Academy of Sciences, 1983;406:13–19.
27. Gill THJ. The use of randomly bred and genetically defined animals in biomedical research. Am J Pathol 1981;100;21–32.
28. Jones TC. The value of animal models. Am J Pathol 1981;101:3–9.
29. Leader RW. Padgett GA: The genesis and validation of animal models. Am J Pathol 1981;101:11–17.
30. Festing FW. Inbred strains in biochemical research the MacMillen Press Ltd., London and Basingstoke, 1979.

31. Jay GE. Genetic strains and stocks. In: Durdette WJ, editor. Methodology in mammalian genetics. Holden-Day, San Francisco: 1963:83–126.
32. Bustad LK, Hegreberg GA, Padgett GA. Animal models. In: The future of animals, cells, models and systems in research development, education and testing. Nat. Academy of Sciences, 1977.
33. Andrews EJ, Ward BC, Altman NH, editors. Spontaneous models of human diseases. Academic Press, 1979.
34. Szabo S. Animal model of human disease: duodenal ucler disease. Animal model: cysteamine—induced acute and chronic duodenal ulcer in the rat. Amer J Pathol 1978;93,273–276.
35. Szabo S, Haith LR Jr, Reynolds ES. Pathogenesis of duodenal ulceration produced by cysteamine or proprionitrile: influence of vagotomy, sympathectomy, histamine depletion, H_2—receptor antagonists and hormones. Am J Dig Dis 1979;24,471–474.
36. Brady JV. Ulcers in "Executive" Monkeys. Sci Am 1958;199:99–100.
37. Szabo S. Discussion. Am J Pathol 1980;100:78–82.
38. Cornelius CE. Animal models: a neglected medical resource. N Engl J Med 1969;281:933–944.
39. McPeek B. Darstellung von Elementen des Designs und derer Analyse in klinischen Studien. In: Rohde H, Troidl H, editors. Das Margenkarzinom, 1984;35–39.
40. Pollock AV. Design and interpretation of clinical trials Br Med J 1985;290:243.
41. Juhr NC. Die Optimierung des Tierversuchs—Aufgabe einer Tierversuchskunde. In: Kuebler K editor. Der Tierversuch in der Arzneimittelforschung BGA berichte. 1981;1,57–62.
42. Held JR. Muhlbock memorial lecture: consideration in the provision and characterization of animal models. In: Spiegel A, Erichsen S, Solleveld HA, editors. Animal quality and models in biomedical research. Stuttgart, New York: G. Fischer Verlag, 1980;9–16.
43. Immich H. Medizinische Statistik F.K. Stuttgart, New York: Schattauer Verlag, 1974.
44. Dixon WJ. The up-and-down method for small samples Am. Statis. Assoc., 1965;60:967–978.
45. Hsu CK, New AW, Mayo JJ. Quality assurance of rodent models. 7th ICLAS Symp., Utrecht 1979 G. Fischer, Stuttgart, New York: 1979;17–28.
46. Bonnod J. Principles of ethics in animal experimentation. 16th IABS Congress: the standardization of animals to improve biomedical research, production and control. San Antonio 1979, Develop Biol Standard. S. Karger, Basel 1980;45:185–187.
47. Rowsell HC. The ethics of biomedical experimentation. In: the future of animals, cells, models and systems in research, development, education, and testing. Washington, D.C.: National Academy of Sciences, 1977.

3

A Case Study of the Evolution of a Surgical Research Project

R.C-J. Chiu and D.S. Mulder

In this book, a number of strategies on how to plan a research project, and how to organize a competent team of scientists to pursue such studies are discussed. The "Marburg Experiment" is an example of the "horizontal organization", in which a team of basic scientists are put together with clinicians to attack a problem. A similarly effective approach would be a "vertical organization", in which various collaborators of different expertise will be incorporated into the study, as the investigation progresses. In a complex project, this approach may prove cost-effective, as the specific collaborators are identified as the need for their particular expertise arises. The precondition for success with this approach is the availability of a wide variety of experts, and the establishment of superb communication within the research community. An example of such an approach in the North American context is described below to illustrate such a strategy. The project described is on an attempt to develop a new "biomechanically activated cardiac assist device", undertaken in our laboratory at McGill University.

The Clinical Problems to be Addressed

Research is undertaken to solve a surgical problem not amenable to current modes of therapy. Thus, the identification of such problems is the first step before they can be taken to the laboratory for possible solution. The problem to be addressed by our study concerns the vast number of patients who suffer from chronic heart failure, which is estimated to be approximately 2,300,000 patients in the U.S. alone. There are 400,000 new cases per year, with a five year survival of about 50%. For those patients who fall into the New York Heart Association Class IV functional category, the one year survival is only 50%; half of them suffer sudden death. It has been estimated that between 35,000 (NIH study) to 160,000 (Heart Failure study) patients per year may benefit from long-term cardiac assist devices. Currently, the most established and acceptable mode of therapy for many of those patients is cardiac transplantation. However, the most optimistic estimation of available cardiac donors in the United States for the forseeable future is less than 2,000 per year. The impact of this mode of therapy, therefore, will be limited. Furthermore, cyclosporin has not solved all the problems associated with allograft rejection, and continued monitoring with endomyocardial biopsies is required of all the patients. The alternative to such a *biological* approach is the use of *mechanical* artificial heart or cardiac assist devices. Current long-term devices, however, are still plagued by problems associated with thrombo-embolism and the external power source. Tubes or "tethers" connecting patients to the external power source not only limits the patients' mobility, but are constantly a potential source of infection. An alternate approach to cardiac assist, therefore, would be valuable if feasible.

The Conceptualization of a Hypothesis

We postulated that there would be many advantages if the patient's intrinsic energy sources, such as those generated by the skeletal muscle, could be used to power his cardiac assist device. The hypothesis to be tested is, therefore, whether the energy generated by the skeletal muscle can be harvested, and modified if necessary, to activate a totally implantable cardiac assist device, and achieve a significant hemodynamic improvement.

The Rationale

Using the patient's autogenous skeletal muscle as the power source would eliminate the need for donors, and for immunosuppression against allograft rejection. It also eliminates external power source as the device should be totally implantable. This would improve the patient's ambulation and eliminates the risk of infection through the tube or "tether". By selecting certain assist modes, one may also eliminate the more thrombogenic components in the present cardiac assist devices, such as the artificial valves. Thus, the advent of an effective skeletal muscle powered device should be a useful addition to the spectrum of cardiac assist devices currently under development (Table I).

Review of Literature and Identification of Specific Problems to be Solved

An extensive review of literature was undertaken, which indicated that the idea of utilizing skeletal muscle to assist the circulation goes back several decades. The approaches fall into two categories. One is to use skeletal muscle flap to replace a portion of damaged myocardium, or to enlarge a hypoplastic right or left ventricle. This approach to augment "regional" myocardial damage is termed cardiomyoplasty. The second approach is to use the skeletal muscle to activate a pump to augment the circulation, either in series or in parallel to the heart. Critical appraisal of previous work indicates that two major problems would have to be addressed before these techniques can become clinically applicable. The first is the problem of skeletal muscle fatigue, while the second is related to the pattern of skeletal muscle contraction which, in response to a single electrical impulse stimulation, generates contractions much shorter in duration and less in amplitude than those of the myocardium. However, we felt that recent advances in muscle physiology and electronics technology provided us with potential means to solve these problems. The first of such advances is the discovery by the muscle physiologists that the Type II, fast twitch skeletal muscle fibers can be transformed into Type I, slow fatigue resistant muscle fibers with electrical stimulation at 10 Hz for four to six weeks. This confers considerable fatigue resistance to the skeletal muscle and may solve the first problem. The second advance is the development of micro-chip and computer technology to allow the construction of miniaturized, implantable and programmable electronic stimulators.

We, next, set out the following research plan. In view of the considerable work done by Drs. Macoviak, Stephenson and their associates at the University of Pennsylvania in transforming the skeletal muscle to confer fatigue resistance, and the expertise of Dr. Salmons, a muscle physiologist at the University of Birmingham, in this area, we decided to learn the technique of muscle transformation from these investigators, and to adopt it for cardiac-assist, particularly for the augmentation of left ventricular

TABLE I. The "spectrum" of cardiac replacement and assist devices.

	Spectrum			
	Anatomical Replacement		Functional Replacement (Parallel)	Functional Augmentation (Series)
Biological	Orthotopic transplant	Heterotopic transplant		
Mechanical	Artificial heart	Biventricular assist	Left ventricular assist	Intraaortic balloon
Biomechanical			Myocardioplasty	Extraaortic counterpulsation

function. Parallel to this, we advanced the idea that a new stimulator which senses the R-wave of the heart, and processes the signal with appropriate delay followed by a burst of electrical "pulse train" stimuli, could produce summation of the skeletal muscle contraction, modulating it to match the duration and the amplitude of myocardial contractions. In order to be hemodynamically effective, such pulse train stimuli have to fall precisely into the selected segment of the cardiac cycle. To evaluate the feasibility of these ideas, we carried out the following preliminary studies.

Preliminary Studies and the Animal Model

First we consulted an electrical engineer and outlined the requirements for the new pulse train stimulator, capable of synchronizing with the R-waves of the electrocardiogram. Using a small grant from the Quebec Heart Foundation, we wired together a bulky Medtronic model 5837 generator available in the laboratory, to an Interstate Electronics Corporation stimulator in order to obtain the desired capabilities. We selected a canine model because of its size and availability. Using a rectus muscle pouch, we tested the new stimulator and found it produced the desired effects. We then proceeded to use this stimulator to augment left ventricular function using the cardiomyoplasty approach. The isometric left ventricular function measured by an intra-ventricular balloon during cardio-pulmonary bypass was assessed. with our pulse train stimulator turned on and off. Such as on-off "paired design" is advantageous, in reducing the sample size required for such studies. We published a preliminary report on the concept of pulse train stimulation timed to the cardiac cycle in 1980 (1) and the efficacy of synchronously stimulated skeletal muscle graft for myocardial repair in 1984 (2). In 1985, we described the feasibility of transforming a skeletal muscle to make it fatigue resistant for myocardial assist and for powering an accessory ventricle (3). Based on such experience and in order to obtain maximum muscle stretching prior to its contraction (to derive powerful contractile force according to Frank Starling's law), we then selected the extra-aortic balloon pump as the most feasible mode of the skeletal muscle powered assist devices. We achieved hemodynamically significant diastolic augmentation in a canine study and reported this in 1985 (4).

Progress and Interaction with other Disciplines

Throughout the progress of this project, we sought various experts related to the field of muscle physiology and electronic technology. A symposium held on this subject in Greece in June 1985 sponsored by the Neuroelectric Society, helped put together international groups of investigators and facilitated their interactions. In the area of muscle transformation, we benefitted from the expertise of Dr. Stanley Salmons, a muscle physiologist and a pioneer in this field. The team led by Dr. Larry Stephenson in Philadelphia as well as Dr. David Ianuzzo, an expert in muscle biochemistry at York University, Toronto worked with our team. With their input, we have confirmed that pulse train stimulator can induce muscle transformation in spite of the fact that its stimulation frequency is not a 10 Hz, as reported in the early studies. The possibility of "working transformation", that is, making the muscle generate hemodynamic work while inducing transformation of the muscle fibers to confer fatigue resistance at the same time, is currently under investigation. Simultaneous with these advances, we also worked with electronic and device engineers led by Dr. Aida Khalafalla, a biophysicist at Medtronics Incorporated in the United States. Medtronics is a leading pacemaker company with expertise in programmable pacemaker technology. The stimulator we devised was miniaturized and improved. An implantable device is being developed to facilitate chronic implantations. As the result of our preliminary studies, funding became available from the Medical Research Council of Canada, and to improve the implantable muscle powered assist device, we will collaborate with Novacor Corporation, a San Francisco based company in the forefront of developing electrically powered artifical hearts. Thus, we obtained the necessary expertise both from academic and industrial sources as the project progressed.

From the Bedside to the Laboratory, and Back Again

Now that the clinical problem has been taken to the laboratory for investigation and the efficacy of muscle powered cardiac-assist devices demonstrated, preliminary attempts are being made to bring them back to the patients. At the time of this writing, patients in Paris and in Pittsburgh have undergone cardiomyoplasty with the skeletal muscle flap stimulated in synchrony with the heart using a pulse train stimulator. These clinical attempts provide impetus for the further development of this new *mechanical* approach to cardiac assistance. When the pulse-train generators and the muscle powered assist devices become implantable in the near future, we will be looking forward to the clinical application of this technology in patients who suffer from global myocardial failure, in contrast to regional myocardial damage. Regional damage is more suited for cardiomyoplasty.

In conclusion, a surgical research project is initiated and guided by a principal investigator, who provides the direction and the coherence, while interacting and consulting freely with experts needed for the success of the project. This can be achieved either by "horizontal interaction", namely, the constitution of a research team, with various expertise from the outset, or by a process of "vertical interaction", in which necessary experts and collaborators are enticed as the project progresses. In a large project, both the horizontal and vertical interactions may take place simmultaneously. The ability to communicate and collaborate is a vital asset for a surgical investigator as science and technology become increasingly sophisticated.

References

1. Drinkwater DC, Chiu RC-J, Modry D, Wittnich C, Brown PR. Cardiac assist and myocardial repair with synchronously stimulated skeletal muscle. Surgical Forum 1980;31:271.
2. Dewar ML, Drinkwater DC, Wittnich C, Chiu RC-J. Synchronously stimulated skeletal muscle graft for myocardial repair: An experimental study. J Thorac & Cardiovasc Surg 1984;87:325.
3. Brister S, Fradet G, Dewar M, Wittnich C, Lough J, Chiu RC-J. Transforming skeletal muscle for myocardial assist: A feasibility study. Can J Surg 1985;28:341.
4. Neilson IR, Brister SJ, Khalafalls AS, Chiu RC-J. Left ventricular assist using a skeletal muscle powered device for diastolic augmentation: A canine study. J Heart Transplantation 1985;4:343.

4

Clinical Research

B. Walters and D.L. Sackett

Why Do Clinical Research?

This chapter and the two that follow are about *real* clinical research: posing and answering questions about the causes, diagnosis, prognosis, and management of surgical conditions in collaboration with human subjects. Let us begin by considering why clinicians should and do devote time and energy to clinical research.

First, why "clinical"? Because we *must* answer *clinical* questions. No matter how complete our knowledge of anatomy, physiology, pharmacology, and the like, each time we see a patient our thinking must go beyond these basic sciences as we decide whether to apply this or that diagnostic test; recommend operation *A*, operation *B*, or no operation at all; or prescribe drug *X*, drug *Y*, or nothing. Although the potential answers to these questions can originate in the laboratory, they will stand or fall on the basis of whether they do more good than harm to patients. The measurement of this good and harm, under circumstances that limit error, is a prerequisite to progress in patient care. Clinical research must must be carried out if clinical care is to improve, rather than simply change.

In succeeding chapters, the focus will be on clinical research into the diagnostic process and on large scale clinical trials; in this chapter, it is on two sorts of clinical questions:

1. Can we prevent or minimize the iatrogenic complications of a treatment already known to be efficacious?
2. Can we find a better treatment for this specific clinical problem?

To make our discussion of these questions easier to follow and more enjoyable, we shall employ a specific running example of each, i.e., "Can prophylactic antibiotics prevent iatrogenic CSF shunt infections?" and, "Is superficial temporal—middle cerebral artery anastomosis good for patients with symptomatic, surgically-inaccessible atherosclerosis of their internal carotid or middle cerebral arteries?".

But why carry out "research" to answer clinical questions? Can't we simply apply the operations and treatments our individual or combined experiences have shown us to be efficacious?

The problem is that it has been repeatedly shown that our uncontrolled experiences, however we may combine them, lead us into error. Those who doubt this should review the history of surgery for organ ptosis or constipation, the gastric freeze, and internal mammary ligation (1). Three of the reasons for ever falling into such error stand out (2).

1. Clinicians are more likely to recognize and remember favorable treatment responses in patients who comply with treatments and keep follow-up appointments. There are, however, five documented instances in which complaint patients in the *placebo* groups of randomized trials exhibited far more favorable outcomes, including survival, than their non-complaint companions (3-7). This demonstration of high compliance being a marker for better outcomes, even when a treatment is useless, illustrates how our uncontrolled clinical experiences can often cause us to

conclude that compliant patients must have been on efficacious therapy.
2. Unusual patterns of symptoms, e.g., transient ischemic attacks, or signs, e.g., high blood pressure levels, and extreme laboratory test results tend to return toward the more usual normal result when they are reassessed even a short time later (8). Given this universal tendency for "regression toward the mean", any treatment initiated in the interim will appear efficacious, regardless of its real efficacy.
3. Routine clinical practice is never "blind"; patients and their clinicians know when active treatment is underway. The "placebo effect", which has shown that angina pectoris can be relieved by the skin incision of a mock internal mammary ligation, (9) and the desire of patients and their clinicians to have treatments succeed can cause both parties to overestimate efficacy.

For the foregoing reasons, the "consensus" approach, based on uncontrolled clinical experience, risks precipitating the widespread application of treatments that are useless or that may even do more harm than good. The same treatments are much less likely to be judged efficacious in double-blind, randomized trials than in uncontrolled case-series or unblinded "open" comparisons with contemporaneous or historical series of patients. This fact of life is embodied in the maxim: "Therapeutic reports with controls have no enthusiasm, and reports with enthusiasm have no controls."

We must, therefore, answer our clinical questions in a manner that limits error and permits us to draw conclusions that will *not* vary about biologic and clinical phenomena that *do* vary. We use two methods to accomplish this:

1. *Design*—the way we assemble, manipulate, and make measurements on our patients. Proper design-inclusion criteria, random allocation, complete follow-up, objective outcome criteria, blinding, etc.—enables us to avoid systematic error or "bias", and
2. *Statistics*—the way we manipulate the data that arise from our clinical research. Proper statistics help us to limit non-systematic error or "noise".

Design is the primary focus of this chapter: statistics will only be discussed when necessary.

The emphasis throughout the chapter will be on *thinking*—"How might your answer be wrong", and "How can you safeguard against this?" rather than on such mindless *doing* or *cookbookery* as lists of do's and don'ts.

Finally, why should surgeons carry out clinical research on surgical problems rather than leaving it to some other group of clinicians or methodologists? There are at least three reasons. First, by reason of their training and experience, surgeons understand the questions that need to be asked about surgical conditions better than any other group of clinicians or methodologists. Second, surgeons can fuse clinical sense with good research design in a way that will generate results that are clinically credible as well as scientifically valid. Third, surgeons who seek academic careers face the difficult task of dividing their time between research and clinical surgery. When research takes place at a laboratory bench, it may be far removed from clinical practice; it may demand laboratory skills and basic science knowledge that are foreign to the practicing surgeon; and it may involve competition with full-time laboratory scientists with Ph.D's. Surgical scholars risk losing their grants if the time they spend in the lab is too little, and their surgical skills and credibility if it is too much.

Clinical research, in contrast, is generated, executed, and applied in the front lines of clinical practice; clinical research and clinical practice do not compete, they reinforce each other. This synergistic relationship has major implications for efficiency, productivity, and career satisfaction; the academic surgeon who wishes to live, as well as survive, should keep it in mind.

Translating a Clinical Problem into a Research Question

To translate a clinical problem into a research question, you must understand the biology and pathophysiology underlying the problem, define the clinical question you wish to pose and transform the clinical question into a scientific question that can be answered by "yes," "no," or a number.

Although the clinical care and outcome of many diseases have undergone major improvements in the absence of any profound understanding of their biology and pathophysiology, there is a consensus among biologists and clinicians that we are more likely to make advances in care if they arise as logical extrapolations based on the fundamental mechanisms of health and disease.

If your investigation is to be focused on an issue in therapy, the formulation of your clinical question will be influenced by the intended purpose of the answer since the questions posed can be of two different sorts (10–11). The first deals with explanation and asks such questions as "Can operation A reduce overnight acid secretion by the stomach?". The second deals with management and asks such questions as "Does offering operation A to patients with peptic ulcer do more good than harm?"

The two types of trial that result from the two types of question have contrasting attributes. The explanatory trial seeks to describe how a treatment produces its effects and to determine whether it can work under what are often ideal or restricted circumstances. The management trial seeks to determine all the consequences, both good and bad, of treating an illness in a certain way and whether the therapy works under clinical circumstances that are as close as possible to those usually encountered in practice. For sound scientific reason, the two types of trial may recruit study patients in quite different fashions. The explanatory trial may justifiably restrict admission to the patients who are most likely to consent to the particular operation and to respond to it. The management trial may, also justifiably, accept all comers, including patients with co-morbid conditions or poor compliance, to obtain a better estimate of the usefulness of starting down a particular treatment path. (some patients should be excluded from both sorts of trials, e.g., patients incorrectly diagnosed or subsequently shown, on blind adjudication, to violate the inclusion/exclusion criteria).

The experimental procedure may with good reason, be applied quite differently in the two sorts of trials. If an explanatory trial is an attempt to find out whether the operation *can* work in the best hands, the protocol may restrict it to the most experienced and gifted surgeons and may call for frequent follow-up examinations and other procedures that violate contemporaneous practice. The management trial, in contrast, usually strives to replicate current practice.

Finally, these two types of trial differ in the eligibility of the events used to determine the outcomes. The explanatory trial focuses on a restricted range of events and often seeks to exclude events that befall both experimental patients who have not received the experimental operation and control ("cross-over") patients who have, from analysis. In contrast, the management trial tends to encompass a wide range of events and usually includes all events that occur after randomization in order to assess the results of a decision to offer a particular operation.

When the question that is the essence of the trial is posed from the investigator's perspective, the issue of primary interest may be either explanation or management; when it is posed from the patient's perspective, the primary issue is management. In the latter case, for example, the fact and mode of dying are far more important than its cause, and all events are of interest.

For all the foregoing reasons, the specification of the clinical question deserves considerable thought, and always benefits from discussion and debate with one's colleagues.

The crucial third step is the conversion of the clinical question to a scientific one that can be answered by "yes," "no," or a number. The final product usually combines designation of the clinical condition, the intervention, and key clinical outcome. Your clinical question might state: "What is the role of extracranial-intracranial bypass in cerebrovascular disease?", but its lack of specificity is obvious. Such a clinical question must be converted into a scientific one before you can proceed to fashion the detailed protocol in an unambiguous way, e.g., "Among patients with symptomatic, surgically-inaccessible atherosclerosis of their internal carotid or middle cerebral arteries, will the performance of superficial temporal-middle cerebral artery anastomosis reduce the risk of subsequent fatal and non-fatal stroke?" Your colleagues can argue that the latter question is not the right one to ask, but they cannot say it is not specific.

Once your scientific question has been formulated, you can begin to fashion the study protocol, i.e., the document that describes the architecture of the investigation and details which patients will be assembled or excluded; who will do what to them and when and how; what measurements will be made upon them, by whom, when, and how; how the resulting data will be analyzed and interpreted; and what will be done about missing patients and data. Throughout the development of your protocol, you must repeatedly ask yourself the question that lies at the root of sound science, "How might my answer be wrong, and what can I do to protect against this?".

The next two sections describe the development of the protocols generated in response to the clinical questions presented at the beginning of this chapter. It is presented to illustrate key elements of proper study design, not as a set of knee-jerk reflexes to be mindlessly acted out for every study, but as a set of problem-solving responses to specific threats to the validity of the clinical investigations we were undertaking at the time. These sections are only an introduction to the development of study protocols and they should be supplemented by selective readings from the score of recent textbooks on clinical trials and, most important, from your personal experience in struggling to develop your own protocols.

Can We Find a Better Operation for This Clinical Problem?

Entire books have been devoted to the design of therapeutic trials. The information provided here will not suffice as a base from which to carry one out. However, it will accordingly raise, and hint at the answers to, the questions that will arise as you attempt such research. If you wish to proceed further, you must follow the questions and hints into the longer, more formal expositions of experimental research methods. Several of them are cited at the end of this chapter.

The trial we shall use for our example is the International Cooperative Study of Extracranial/Intracranial (EC/IC) Bypass, (12,13) in which one of us (DLS) was a co-investigator. It was designed and executed to answer the question, "Will anastomosis of the superficial temporal artery to the middle cerebral artery decrease the rate of stroke and stroke-related death among patients with symptomatic disease of the internal carotid and middle cerebral arteries?".

Which Patients Should Be Entered into the Trial?

Four issues have to be considered. The first is the establishment of a detailed description of the sort of patient who should be entered into the trial. Clearly, since we are testing the efficacy of an operation, we should enter those patients who are likely to benefit from the procedure. Moreover, the description, or "eligibility criteria", must be stated so clearly that clinicians who read the report of the trial will able to tell whether its results apply to specific patients in their practices. The description of EC/IC Bypass Trial patients read as follows [all subsequent excerpts are taken from the published protocol (12).]

To be eligible for the trial, patients have had to satisfy clinical, radiological, and exclusion criteria:

Clinical Inclusion Criteria

Patients had to have experienced, within 3 months prior to entry, one or both of the following: (i) transient ischemic attack(s) (TIA) in the carotid distribution [one or more episodes of distinct focal neurological dysfunction or monocular blindness (amaurosis fugax), the symptoms and signs of which cleared completely in less than 24 hours]; (ii) minor completed stroke(s) in the carotid distribution (one or more events of distinct focal neurologic dysfunction or amaurosis fugax, the signs of which persisted for more than 24 hours). Patients without useful residual function in the affected territory have not been entered.

Radiologic Inclusion Criteria

An angiogram demonstrating an atherosclerotic lesion in the appropriate territory has had to be submitted for central confirmation and adjudication by the principal neuroradiologist; bilateral common carotid arteriograms have been requested on all patients, and angiography of the vertebro-basilar circulation has been optional.

One or more of the following atherosclerotic lesions must have been demonstrated in vessels appropriate to the patient's symptoms: (i) stenosis or occlusion of the middle cerebral artery trunk; (ii) stenosis of the internal carotid artery at or above the C2 vertebral body (i.e. inaccessible to carotid endarterectomy); or (iii) internal carotid artery occlusion.

For radiological eligibility, stenosis has been defined as "any recognizable atherosclerotic lesion of the surgically inaccessible portion of the internal carotid artery or middle cerebral artery which, in the opinion of the attending neurosurgeon, might reasonably be expected to benefit from bypass surgery."

The second issue is the recurring question, "How could my answer be wrong?". In this step of the study, we would risk generating the wrong answer if we entered the wrong sorts of patients, specifically those who, because they are too ill or are suffering from co-morbid conditions, would not reasonably be expected to respond to, and benefit from, the operation. Such patients would have to be analyzed as treatment failures, and any attempts to remove them from analysis "after the fact" would damage the credibility of the study. It is far better to exclude them from the outset, and this is the purpose of "exclusion criteria":

Patients have been excluded from the study if they were unable to meet at least the following functional standards: (i) capability of self-care for most activities of daily living (may require some assistance); (ii) retention of some useful residual function in the affected arm or leg; (iii) comprehension intact with no evidence of Wernicke's receptive aphasia; (iv) no, or only mild, motor (expressive, Broca's) aphasia; (v) ability to handle their own oropharyngeal secretions.

Patients also have been excluded from the trail if any of the following pertained: inability to provide informed consent; evidence that the original stroke was due to cerebral hemorrhage; within 8 weeks of an acute cerebral ischemic event; exhibition of nonatherosclerotic conditions causing or likely to cause cerebral dysfunction (fibromuscular dysplasia, arteritis, blood dyscrasia, a cardiac source of cerebral emboli, chronic atrial fibrillation, complete heart block, significant valvular heart disease, cardiomyopathy, or nonatherosclerotic dissection); the presence of any morbid conditions(s) likely to lead to death within 5 years [cancer, renal failure (BUN> 50 mg%)], cardiomegaly [cardiothoracic ratio of >0.50(>0.55 in Japanese patients) (14–16) or any hepatic or pulmonary disease constituting an unacceptable anesthetic risk]; the occurrence of ischemic symptoms isolated to the vertebro-basilar circulation; prior participation in the study (regardless of the occurrence of new ischemic events or success or failure of previous therapy); myocardial infarction within the preceding 6 months; a fasting blood sugar of 300 mg% or more on the most recent assessment despite appropriate therapy; diastolic blood pressure >110 mm Hg (using disappearance of sounds for diastolic pressure) despite appropriate medical therapy. Once uncontrolled diabetes or hypertension were corrected, otherwise eligible patients could be entered.

The third issue is the inevitability that a mistake will be made in entering patients, regardless of good will and hard work. How should inappropriately entered patients be handled? Their removal at the end of the study, even though justified on scientific grounds, leaves the investigators open to criticism and damages the credibility of the result. It is far better to have the eligibility of all patients adjudicated shortly after entry by clinicians who are not only "blind" to the patient's treatment allocation, but also are not even entering patients into the study.

Every entry form has been reviewed by both the Central Office and the Methods Center. All angiograms have been reviewed (without knowledge of the treatment group to which the patient had been randomized) by the principal neuroradiologist at the Central Office. When this review has suggested that an ineligible patient had been entered, an external group of adjudicators (who were not real participants and were "blind" to the patient's allocation) has reviewed the entry data and angiograms and decided whether the patient should be excluded from the trial.

The fourth and final issue is the establishment and publication of explicit rules for dealing with the specific clinical situations that call for interpretation of, rather than mere adherence to, the study protocol.

Because cerebrovascular disease often involves multiple sites, guidelines for managing, and arbitrary rules for analyzing, specific clinical situations have been established. When "tandem lesions" (two lesions in the same vessel or sequence of vessels, one proximal to the other) have existed, and both lesions have fulfilled the entry criteria, the patient has been entered for the more distal lesion. If the proximal lesion has been amenable to endarterectomy, the decisions of whether to perform endarterectomy, and the selection of the initial site for surgery (i.e. endarterectomy or EC/IC bypass), have been left to the judgment of the participating surgeon. In patients judged to require external carotid endarterectomy as a preparation for bypass, it has been recommended that this be performed only after the patient has been randomized to the surgical group. If external carotid endarterectomy had been performed prior to randomization, then 30 days have had to elapse following endarterectomy before the patient could have been entered.

When contralateral carotid disease has existed and has been accessible to endarterectomy, the disease of whether and when to perform contralateral endarterectomy has again been left to the participating neurosurgeon. Once again, if contralateral endarterectomy has been carried out first, 30 days have had to elapse following contralateral endarterectomy before the patient could have been entered.

When eligible patients have had appropriate symptoms and angiographic lesions in both carotid distributions, the patient has been entered for the most recent clinically eligible event. If more than one TIA or stroke has occurred prior to entry, the most recent has served as the basis for enrollment.

In all of the above circumstances, if a 30-day waiting period has applied, the patient was still eligible for randomization, despite the passage of more than 3 months since the last episode of cerebral ischemia.

What Baseline Investigations Should Be Carried Out on Study Patients?

The study patients have already undergone several investigations to determine their eligibility for the trial. Why carry out any more? There are three reasons. First, when the clinical measure that will be used to determine whether surgery does more good than harm goes beyond mere mortality and involves the determination of symptoms, signs, or some level of function, it is important to make the initial measurement at the start of the trial. This insures that the measurement process is working properly, i.e. you can identify and correct problems in observer variation in making and interpreting the measurement; provides a baseline against which to identify differences within and between patients as the study proceeds; and provides key data for determining the comparability of the experimental and control groups at the start of the trial. The second reason for carrying out additional baseline measurements is to guide any ancillary therapy for disorders in either group during the study. The third reason is to obtain information for "prognostic stratification", as in the next section.

At entry, detailed neurological and medical histories and examinations have been carried out and recorded on standardized forms. The examination has included a 12-item functional status assessment in which the patient's ability to perform activities of daily living, such as eating, toileting, and ambulation, have been rated on a three-point scale: (1) able to perform task without difficulty; (2) able to perform task with difficulty; or, (3) unable to perform without mechanical or personal assistance. Additional historical data have been gathered about employment status, history of diabetes mellitus, hypertension, angina pectoris, myocardial infarction, intermittent claudication, cardiac surgery or other serious illness, current medications, and smoking habits. The patient's blood pressure, heart rate and rhythm, cardiac murmurs, and neck bruits have been recorded. Finally, the following baseline investigations have been carried out: hemoglobin; platelet count; prothrombin time; random blood glucose; blood urea nitrogen; cholesterol; electrocardiogram (for left ventricular hypertrophy, new or old myocardial infarction and rhythm); chest x-ray to estimate the cardiothoracic ratio; and, if available, a computerized tomographic (CT) scan of the head.

How Should Patients Be Allocated to Treatments?

How should we decide which patients will receive the experimental operation? The quick answer is randomize. The reasons for giving so unequivocal an answer are both historic (we have made such fools of ourselves when we have used other methods of determining efficacy) and scientific. The latter will be summarized with an example.

Suppose that a surgeon developed a new vascular bypass procedure to the point where it was ready for testing in humans. Because it was a lengthy procedure and not without risk, it was understandable that the surgeon carried out the first few bypasses on patients who were, for the most part, free of hypertension (even if it were controlled) or other extraneous disorders that increased their surgical risk. Suppose that the initial results were encouraging: all patients survived the procedure and their symptoms remained stable or even improved. In contrast, many of the poor-risk patients, who were rejected for surgery because of coexisting hypertension, either died or experienced progression of their symptoms. When the results are reported, a substantial segment of the profession might conclude that the bypass procedure is of obvious efficacy and ought to be performed on all good-risk, and even some poor-risk, patients.

The canny reader will have identified three properties of hypertension in this hypothetical example.

1. It is extraneous to the question posed. The efficacy of bypass surgery is at issue, not the biology of hypertension.
2. It is a determinant of the outcomes of interest. Hypertensives are more likely to experience progressive arterial disease and to die than normotensives.
3. It is unequally distributed among the treatment groups being compared and the inequality is marked. Very few hypertensives were bypassed; almost all were rejected for surgery.

In the technical jargon of causation, hypertension is a confounder, and the presence of such confounders has complicated the evaluation of the efficacy of almost all preventive, therapeutic, and rehabilitative maneouvres. Confounding leads to bias—the arrival at a conclusion that differs systematically from the truth—and examples abound in human research, whether experimental, where allocation to the manoeuvres under comparison occurs by random allocation, or subexperimental, where allocation occurs by any other process (17).

If confounding hampers the valid demonstration of efficacy and effectiveness, how can it be avoided? Briefly, seven strategies exist for preventing confounding; all of them attack the property of unequal distribution among treatment groups, but one is clearly superior to the rest. First, you could prevent confounding by restricting the criteria for inclusion, i.e., you could simply exclude hypertensives from either the operated or non-operated patients groups. Second, you could individually match, in both the sampling and analysis stages, operated and non-operated patients for their hypertension status. Third, you could carry out stratified sampling, i.e, create cohorts of operated and non-operated normotensives. Fifth, you could apply an adjustment or standardization procedure, analogous to age standardization, in the analysis. Six, you could establish a model for the risk of the outcome of interest that would include a correction factor for hypertension or could be expanded to include other possible confounders, such as symptomatic coronary heart disease and diabetes. Seventh and finally, you could randomly allocate appropriate patients to undergo or not undergo the new microvascular surgical techniques.

The final strategy, random allocation, has a profound advantage over the other six. Because random allocation prevents distortion by unknown as well as known confounders, it reduces bias from known confounders and from undiscovered potential confounders. This boon to validity places the true experiment, where allocation to the manoeuvres under comparison occurs by random allocation, above the sub-experiment, where allocation occurs by any other process, in determining the efficacy or effectiveness of any clinical manoeuvre or new technology. The true experiment is now the standard approach for determining the efficacy and effectiveness of chemotherapeutic agents and most other drugs and is increasingly used in evaluating surgical technology. The strategies can also be combined. For example, many trials involve randomization within prognostic strata, followed by adjustments for residual differences in the analysis. Such prognostic stratification ensures the baseline similarity of experimental and control groups for key attributes and contributes to the clinical credibility of the results:

If the patient has been judged eligible on clinical and radiographic grounds, informed consent has been requested. If obtained, a tentative date for surgery has been booked (to minimize the time interval between randomization and surgery) and the Methods Center has been contacted by telephone for registration and random allocation (for logistic reasons, a separate randomization center has been set up in Kyoto, Japan for patients from Japan and Taiwan). To ensure balance between the medical and surgical limbs of this trial, a stratified randomization has been carried out. The strata have been defined by the underlying vascular lesion (stenosis or occlusion of the middle cerebral or internal carotid artery), the presence or absence of a related neurologic deficit and, in the case of patients with internal carotic occlusion, whether related symptoms have occurred since its angiographic demonstration (some centers have joined the trial with a commitment to exclude patients with no symptoms since their internal carotic occlusions were demonstrated). Then, based on a computer-generated randomization scheme established at the Methods Center for each participating center and stratum, the patient has been assigned to either the medical or surgical limb of the trial.

A final remark on the timing of randomization is required. Because most methodologic purists, and journal editors, will insist on charging all event, including those occuring between randomization and operation, to their respective treatment groups, it is wise to have an early operative date already scheduled for a patient before he or she is randomized to cover the possibility of his or her being randomized to surgery.

How Should the Treatments Be Specified?

The experimental operation must be described in sufficient detail to accomplish two things. First, participating surgeons must have discussed and debated it in sufficient detail to have generated the precise operating room protocol that will be followed. Second, if the operation is found to do more good than harm, for those who read the trial report to replicate it precisely on their own patients.

Surgical trials must also take another issue into consideration at this stage of design. Which surgeons should do the experimental operations or, more precisely, how skilled and experienced should they be? The answer depends on the question being posed. If an explanatory trial is planned (i.e., can the operation work, under ideal circumstances?), only the best surgeons, with substantial experience and documented success in performing the operation, should participate and the quality of their work should be documented and assessed before and during the trial, as was done in the EC/IC Bypass Trial. If a management trial is planned (i.e., does the operation do more good than harm when performed under the circumstances of routine practice?), an equally sound case is made for having surgeons with average skill and experience take part.

Even random allocation and attention to the foregoing will not exclude all sources of bias, nor will it insure the validity and generalizability of the results of an experiment. First, the performance of additional therapeutic procedures on the experimental group should be avoided unless the same procedures are performed with equal vigor on the comparison group (17). For example, if experimental patients are seen more frequently than control patients, the additional opportunities for clinical evaluation and management may spuriously inflate the estimate of the benefit of the test therapy, or, by promoting the recognition of mild or transient side effects, inflate the estimate of harm. This problem is exaggerated in surgical trials, where it is usually impossible to use a major strategy for preventing co-intervention, i.e. the blinding of study patients and their clinicians to the experimental therapy through the use of placebo drugs and manoeuvres. Second, the trial that is most efficient insures that all experimental, but no control, subjects receive the test therapy. When members of the control group receive the test therapy—a major potential problem when "medical" patients "cross-over" and undergo the experimental surgery—the resulting contamination tends to systematically reduce any difference in outcomes between experimental and control subjects. The study architecture must recognize this danger and, if possible, participating clinicians must agree to protect against it, at least for some negotiated period of follow-up.

Patients randomized to the surgical limb have undergone microsurgical, end to side, anastomosis of the superficial temporal or occipital artery to a cortical branch of the middle cerebral artery. All participating surgeons have agreed to follow an identical procedure in the performance of the extra- to intracranial bypass, but minor variations in the surgical technique have been permitted and left to the individual surgeon's discretion.

Surgical patients have undergone postoperative angiography; the recommended timing has been 3 to 6 months following bypass. All the postoperative angiograms have been reviewed by the principal neuroradiologist at the Central Office. The success of the anastomosis has been assessed by the following features: the comparative size (smaller; same or larger) of the superficial temporal artery proximal to the anastomosis on preoperative and postoperative angiograms; the degree of retrograde flow in the middle cerebral circulation (none; slight; to the middle cerebral artery bifurcation; or to the internal carotid) and the number of branches of the middle cerebral artery filled. Overall flow through the bypass has been estimated as: none, slight, moderate, good, or excellent. Further follow-up angiograms have been recommended when the first postoperative angiogram has suggested poor bypass function.

A random sample of 20 preoperative and 20 postoperative angiograms have been reviewed a second time by the principal neuroradiologist (who had been blinded to his original report) to assess intraobserver agreement. Because previous randomized trials have established the efficacy of aspirin in patients with TIA and minor stroke (18), all patients (both medical and surgical) have been prescribed acetylsalicylic acid 325 mg. g.i.d. throughout the trial, unless contraindicated or not tolerated. Furthermore, the control of hypertension has been stressed and monitored in both medical and surgical patients; the treatment of other risk factors has been left to individual clinical judgment.

Patients who initially accepted their randomization to medical therapy but later underwent EC/IC bypass on the randomized side, or patients who accepted randomization to surgical therapy and then declined the operation were labeled "crossovers". Strokes occuring to such patients before their crossover are to be charged to the medical limb and the surgical limb, respectively, in the primary analysis. Those who had no events prior to the crossover were judged to have been randomized improperly and to have failed to give proper informed consent. They were considered as one of the exclusion categories.

What Sort of Follow-Up Should Be Carried Out?

Follow-up should be carried out with sufficient frequency and intensity to accomplish three things: identify important events; identify important side-effects; and keep track of the entire group of patients so that none are lost.

All patients, both medical and surgical, have been examined by a participating neurologist 6 weeks after randomization and at 3-month intervals thereafter; surgical patients have received an additional review approximately 30 days following surgery. At each visit, an interim history has been obtained and a detailed nerologic examination has been performed, including the functional status assessment. In addition, repeat assessments have been made of the patient's employment status, medical and smoking history, medications, blood pressure and cardiac status.

Other medical problems, medications and perioperative complications have been monitored to detect unexpected adverse effects of any medical and/or surgical treatment that patients have undergone during the trial.

What Should Be Done About Withdrawals?

The simple solution to the problem of withdrawals, to be pursued assiduously, but never achieved, is never to have any. They are the bane of all prospective clinical research because they bedevil the analysis should they be counted or not? What if we don't know what has become of them? Two rules of thumb may help. First, because a refusal to participate at entry to a trial, prior to randomization, can only detract from the generalizability of the result, whereas a refusal to continue to participate (i.e., a withdrawal) after randomization can also detract from the validity of the result, the former is always preferable. Consequently, it is wise to inform prospective subjects of all features of the study that might discourage their continuing cooperation. Second, withdrawal is a time for negotiation, not farewell. Attempts should be made to retain cooperation for at least certain portions of follow-up—if only by mail or telephone or through the patient's primary physician—so that it is at least possible to state whether withdrawn patients are alive at the conclusion of a trial.

Only patients who refused to continue under observation were to have been withdrawn from the trial; and others were to be retained. EC/IC surgery on the side opposite to the qualifying lesion and internal carotid endarterectomy on either side have been discouraged; however, patients who have undergone these additional procedures have not been withdrawn from the trial. A second EC/IC bypass on the same side has been permitted in a small number of surgical patients in whom it has appeared likely to improve bypass function; however, these surgical procedures have not, by themselves, constituted events, and such patients have not been withdrawn.

What Events Should Be Measured in the Trial, and How?

The events to be measured will follow from the question posed by the trial. They should be clinically important, highly reproducible measures of the success or failure of the experimental operation, including its complications. We will focus more on how to measure than on what is measured, and will once again consider, How might the answer be wrong?

Because many efficacious operations trade an immediate, small risk of death for later, larger benefits, it is important to measure the former and to continue long enough to capture the latter. Patients in the non-operated limb should receive equally-vigorous follow-up to render their events just as likely to be recognized and reported.

Surgical trials do not lend themselves to the bias-avoiding strategy of double-blindness. They can, nonetheless, use other strategy for limiting error. The clinical criteria for events can be made so "hard" and objective that they can be measured, this adjudication can sometimes be carried out on clinical records that have been "purged" of any mention of whether the study patient was in the operated group.

The main study events are the occurrence of fatal or nonfatal stroke following randomization. However, in order to include any excess perioperative risk, deaths from all causes have been included if they occurred between randomization and 30 days following EC/IC bypass among surgical patients and for a comparable duration among patients in the medical group.

Events have been identified and classified in one or more of three ways: First, participating neurologists have identified and reported them during routine patient follow-up. Second, the principal investigators at the Central Office have identified events during their Weekly Clinical Reviews of the follow-up data, supplemented when necessary by further communication with the participating neurologist. Third, a computer program at the Methods Center has identified possible events by comparing the functional status, signs and symptoms on each follow-up with those recorded on previous follow-up assessments.

The best current means for diagnosis (including CT scan where available) have been used to differentiate strokes due to infarction from those due to hemorrhage. The severity of the stroke, in terms of the impairment of functional status, has been rated on a 10-point scale, using information derived from the neurologic follow-up forms.

Transient ischemic attacks, other major cardiovascular morbidity and deaths from non-cerebrovascular causes have also been recorded but have not constituted main events. Thorough documentation has been sought for every death from any cause, including: autopsy findings, emergency room, operative and hospital discharge reports; death certificates; and the observations of any witnesses.

Adjudication of the cause of death and the occurrence and severity of strokes has been performed independently by a neurologist and a neurosurgeon who have not cared for patients in the study and have been blind both to the patients' treatments and to each other's judgments. Disagreement between the two adjudicators have been resolved by consensus. Disagreements between the adjudicators' consensus and the results of the Central Office's Weekly Clinical Reviews have been resolved through discussion with the principal clinical investigators.

How Should the Data Be Analyzed?

Neither the length nor the intent of this chapter permits a comprehensive discussion of the analysis of randomized trials. All we can do is state a few maxims:

1. Patient-centered research that is badly designed or badly analyzed is unethical, because it exposes humans to risks without guarding against bias and imprecision. The only solution is to involve competent biostatisticians as full collaborators from the very beginning of protocol development.
2. A clinical trial, like any other experiment, can answer only one or two questions, not more. Although the results of a trial should undergo as much sub-group and exploratory analysis, or "data-dredging", as time, budget, and energy allow, these explorations must be recognized as hypothesis-forming, not hypothesis-testing, exercise.
3. A trial should be stopped as soon as the better treatment is identified. This calls for interim analysis of the emerging results, and is another reason for obtaining biostatistical collaboration from the outset.

In order to discharge the ethical responsibility of stopping the trial as soon as a clear-cut conclusion is evident, the accumulating data have been analyzed at 6-month intervals. An "alerting" procedure has been developed and adopted that calls for the early stopping of the study to have been considered if two consecutive interim analyses have shown either that the surgically treated group are faring significantly better (at the $P = 0.02$ level) or that it has become very unlikely that any surgical benefit could have been demonstrated (19). The results of these interim analyses, known only to the principal epidemiologic investigator and chief biostatistician at the Methods Center, have been summarized and reported to the Monitoring Committee.

Appropriate allowance has been made for the statistical effect of these interim challenges of the data; if the trial has not been terminated early, a p-value of 0.04 or less would have constituted statistical significance in the final analysis.

How Many Patients Do We Need?

If the foregoing section failed to convince you of the need for early collaboration with a biostatistician, this one should. Investigators are unlikely to obtain clinical collaborators, and can almost never obtain outside research funds, without being able to explain how many patients they need in order to answer their study question. The bibliography at the end of this chapter lists sources of a full explanation of this issue.

Briefly, the four elements of any trial that, when specified, will determine the number of patients required for the study, are: (1) the expected rate of events in the control group; (2) the degree of reduction in the risk of these events that, if it occurred in the experimental group, would indicate that the operation was efficacious; (3) the risk the investigator is willing to run of drawing the false-positive conclusion that the operation is efficacious when, in truth, it is not; and (4) the risk the investigator is willing to run of drawing the false-negative conclusion that the operation is not efficacious when, in truth, it is.

The required sample size and duration of follow-up initially had been determined on the basis of data available when the protocol had been designed (February 1977). The following estimates and specifications have been employed.

1. For medically-treated patients: an expected combined stroke and stroke-death rate of 23.6% over 5 years (20–26).
2. For surgically-treated patients: an estimated 30-day perioperative stroke and death rate of 4% (21,24) followed by a 50% reduction in the subsequent rate of fatal and non-fatal stroke compared with medically-treated patients, for a net surgical benefit of 33% reduction in the 5-year risk of fatal and non-fatal stroke. It has been agreed that this degree of risk reduction constituted a clinically important surgical benefit which, if achieved in the trial, would justify advocating the EC/IC bypass procedure.
3. A risk of 5% of drawing the false-positive conclusion that surgery is no better than medical therapy when, in truth, surgery results in the clinically important benefit stated above (beta—0.10; power = 90%).

These considerations had required a sample size of 442 patients per treatment group, followed for an average of 5 years. Allowing for drop-outs, an initial total sample size target of 1,000 patients had been established.

By February 1981, 35% of trial patients had been entered with internal carotid artery occlusion without further ischemic symptoms since angiography. Because this group had been thought to be at a lower risk of subsequent stroke, it had been feared that large numbers of such cases might have obscured a surgical benefit to other patients. This situation was discussed by Executive Committee members who were blind with respect to events in both treatment groups, and they proposed to increase the total sample size target to 1,400 patients. This proposal was accepted by the Monitoring Committee and was implemented.

Adjustments to sample size calculations are available (25) for dropouts, crossovers and withdrawals. More important than these considerations, however, is the need to recognize that it is not enough simply to project estimates of the prevalence of the trial condition to the local population. Affected individuals must not only be around. They, and their referring clinicians, must be willing to participate; the experimental therapy and follow-up procedures must be acceptable to them; and they must satisfy the specific inclusion/exclusion criteria. Even when viewed through jaundiced eyes, the availability of suitable patients may still be overestimated, and safety margins of 100 to 400% have been suggested by scarred investigators.

When realistic estimates suggest that the required numbers of study patients may be hard to find, a number of strategies can be considered. First, you can rethink the issues of risk and responsiveness raised earlier and possibly increase the trial's efficiency. Second, you may wish to rethink the risks of false-positive and false-negative errors you are willing to take; when the restrictions are relaxed, the sample size requirements falls.

Third, you can attempt to reduce the noise in the measurement of events and outcomes by improving the precision of the measurements. The result will be higher values for the test statistic at any level of between-group differences. Where it is sensible, although impossible in most surgical trials, you can also benefit from the paired examination of treatment effects within individual study patients by performing crossover trials—this solution should have been explored when the basic architecture of your study was first considered. Finally, the local sample-size problem can be solved by converting to a multi-centre design, but this will incur substantial costs in administrative complexity and investigator effort (see Section III, Chapter 5).

Prerequisites for a Successful Surgical Research Project

The protocol for a clinical research study must not only be attractive to potential collaborators but must also set minimal performance criteria for continuing or abandoning the trial. Five elements of a protocol influence its attractiveness. First, there must be a convincing statement of the need for the trial. This statement must provide the basis on which clinicians can justify, to themselves, their colleagues and their patients, the special conditions and efforts required to insure the success of the trial. Second, the experimental manoeuvre must not only be clinically sensible and applicable, but also able to withstand close scrutiny so that the clinicians can defend it against its critics. For example, if a surgical operation is involved, the expertise with which it is executed may vary considerably and a biologically valuable manoeuvre may be made to appear useless or even harmful when it is performed with less than adequate skill. The credibility of the trial can be protected by invoking current specifications on clinical competency (e.g., surgical mortality and graft patency) as criteria that must be met prior to joining a trial in addition to a pledge to monitor performance during the trial. If, despite these precautions, the level of expertise is expected to change with time, it should be taken into account by balancing treatment allocations at several points during the trial and by using calendar time as a covariate in planning the analysis.

The third element in the attractiveness of the protocol to potential clinical collaborators is the specification of the minimum appropriate requirements for the documentation and follow-up of study patients. Clinical trials often gather far more data than are required to answer the question at hand. Investigators who feel burdened with excessive documentation of overly frequent follow-up visits may falter in their entry of new study patients. Fourth, the principal investigators must be perceived by their potential clinical collaborators as individuals who know what they are doing. Consequently, they must either possess or quickly establish their credibility in the relevant areas of clinical medicine, human biology, and research methods. Finally, each potential collaborator must be shown how participation in the trial will bring personal rewards, such as further education, additions to one's prestige and bibliography, and recognition as someone who has made a significant contribution to the generation of useful new knowledge.

The ultimate test of the feasibility a trial protocol is often provided by a brief pilot run in which only a small number of patients are entered. When you are considering whether to carry out a pilot study, you ought to bear its advantages and disadvantages in mind. A pilot study certainly can help you to identify and solve problems with definitions, data forms, and data flow and to "debug" the application of the study protocol. When study events are early and frequent, a pilot study can test, and possibly confirm your earlier sample size estimates. Finally, a pilot trial can, on rare occasions, provide definitive answers of efficacy when the test therapy is very, very good or very, very bad.

Against these potential advantages, you must consider the drawbacks and difficulties of such a pilot study. First, it will "consume" patients who would otherwise be in the formal trial. This happens because pilot studies are often executed in an unblinded mode and because they often lead to substantive changes in the protocol that make it impossible or inappropriate to include the subjects in later analysis. If study patients are in short supply, a pilot study could scuttle your trial. When study events are rare or late, a pilot study cannot provide a helpful commentary on your sample-size requirements and it may be difficult to interest potential clinical collaborators or funding agencies in committing themselves to a task with such meager short-term benefits. Finally, if your pilot study results are not going to be included in later analyses for efficacy, the ethics of including human subjects in it raises an additional problem.

Instead of adopting an all-or-none position on the need for a pilot study, you should define what you need to know prior to the formal execution of your protocol, and then consider alternative strategies for gaining this knowledge. For example, if the adequacy of forms, data flow, and definitions is at issue, they can be tested on "gram samples" of patients who, although they have the disorder of interest, are otherwise ineligible for the trial. Such patients can also be used to test the documentation and handling of events in order to telescope the long latent period that may occur in the trial proper. In this way, you can save eligible patients for the later, definitive trial and still do a pilot study by inviting ineligible patients to help you with the debugging of the study protocol.

When McFate Smith corresponded with the investigators in 12 large hypertension trials and asked them to identify their five worst problems, administrative problems led scientific problems by more than 2:1 (26). Although some were organizational problems of special pertinence to multi-centre trials, most were problems in the everyday management of the trial that could, if mishandled, destroy the credibility and validity of the trial. Accordingly, attention to administrative issues is the sixth and final prerequisite for a successful clinical trial.

The trial protocol, when translated into the working document for the trial (hereafter referred to as the study manual) should include all the study forms and the rules for their completion and submission. In addition, it is vitally important to include unambiguous rules in the study manual for following and reporting on study patients who refuse therapy, withdraw, fail to comply, suffer side-effects, drop out, or otherwise fail to adhere to the protocol, as well as precise and objective criteria for eligibility and events. The responsibilities for executing and documenting each step in the protocol need to be assigned, even to the point of writing job specifications where necessary.

Other key issues in the organization and administration of your trial may not appear in your study manual but they are, nonetheless, key factors in the success of your trial. Chief among these is the specification of the authority and responsibility of the clinical and methodologic investigators, who is to do what to whom, and "where the buck stops". Publication policies, especially those related to authorship, should be stated at the outset and should be accompanied by a pledge to present the results to your clinical collaborators first. The rules for monitoring trends in the data, often accomplished by forming committee of respected investigator who are outside the trial, and for halting the trial as soon as an unambiguous answer is apparent should be spelled out in advance.

The financial resources for the trial must be sufficient to support the staff and facilities required for the assessment and follow-up of both the study patients and the study data. A key requirement is the provision of sufficient funds for thoughtful secondary data analyses that can, in certain circumstances, provide important clues to the presentation, course, and prognosis of the disorder under study.

References

1. Bunker UP, Barnes BA, Mosteller F. Costs, risks and benefits of surgery. New York: Oxford University Press, 1977.
2. Sackett DL, Haynes RB, Tugwell P. Clinical epidemiology: a basic science for clinical medicine. Boston, Little, Brown, 1985.
3. Coronary Drug Project Research Group. Influence of adherence to treatment and response of cholesterol on mortality in the Coronary Drug Project. N Engl J Med 1980;303:1038–1041.
4. Asher WL, Harper HW. Effect of human chorionic gonadotropin on weight loss, hunger, and feeling of well-being. Amer J Clin Nutr 1973;26:211–218.
5. Hogarty GE, Goldberg. Drug and sociotherapy in the aftercare of schizophrenic patients,. Arch Gen Psychiatr 1973;28:54–64.
6. Fuller R, Roth H, Long S. Compliance with disulfiram treatment of alcoholism. J Chron Dis 1983;36:161–170.
7. Pizzo PA, Robichaud KJ, Edwards BK, Schumaker C, Kramer BS, Johnson A. Oral antibiotic prophylaxis in patients with cancer; a double-blind randomized placebo-controlled trial. J Pediatr 1983;102:125–133.
8. Sackett DL. Rules of evidence and clinical recommendations on the use of anti-thrombotic agents. Chest 1986; in press.
9. Cobb LA, Thomas GI, Dillard DH, Merendino KA, Bruce RA. An evaluation of internal-mammary-artery ligation by a double-blind technique. N Engl J Med 1959;260:1115–1118.
10. Schwartz D, Lellouch J. Explanatory and pragmatic attitudes in therapeutic trials. J Chron Dis 1967;20:637–648.
11. Sackett DL and Gent M. Controversy in counting and attributing events in clinical trials. N Engl J Med 1979;301:1410–1412.
12. EC/IC Bypass Study Group. International cooperative study of extracranial/intracranial arterial anastamosis (EC/IC) bypass study: methodology and entry characteristics. Stroke 1985;16:397–406.
13. EC/IC Bypass Study Group. Failure of extra cranial/intracranial arterial bypass to reduce the risk of ischemic stroke. N Engl J Med 1985;313:1191–1200.
14. Oberman A, Myers AR, Karunas TM, Epstein FH: Heart size of adults in a natural population— Tecumseh, Michigan: Variation by sex, age, height and weight. Circulation 1967;35:724.
15. Shibata H, Matsuzaki T, Shiohida K, Saito N. Study on usefulness of cardiothoracic ratio in the aged. Jpn J Geratrics 1976;13:406.
16. Yano K, Ueda S. Coronary heart disease in Hiroshima, Japan: analysis of the data at the initial examination, 1958–1960. Yale J Biol Med 1962-3;35;504.
17. Sackett DL. Bias in analytic research. J Chron Dis 1979;32:51–63.
18. Canadian Cooperative Study Group. A randomized trial of aspirin and sulfinpyrazone in threatened stroke. N Engl J Med 1978;299:53–59.
19. Taylor DW, Haynes RB, Sackett DL. Stopping rules for long-term clinical trials. (abstract) Controlled Clinical Trials 1980-;1:170.
20. Toole JF, Janeway R, Choi K, et al. Transient ischemic attacks due to atherosclerosis: a prospective study of 160 patients. Arch Neurol 1975;32:5–12.
21. Heyman A, Leviton A, Millikan CH, et al. Transient focal cerebral ischemia: epidemiologic and clinical aspects. Stroke 1974;5:277–287.
22. Matsumoto N, Whisnant JP, Kurland LT, Okazaki H. Natural history of stroke in Rochester, Minnesota, 1955 through 1969. Stroke 1973;4:20–29.
23. Fields WS, Maslenikov V, Meyer JS, Hass WK, Remington RD, MacDonald M. Joint study of extracranial arterial occlusion. V. Progress report of prognosis following surgery or nonsurgical treatment of transient cerebral ischemic attacks and cervical carotid artery lesions. JAMA 1970;211:1993–2003.
24. Delong WB. Microsurgical revascularization for cerebrovascular insufficiency. Stroke 1976;9:15–20.
25. Halperin M, Rogot E, Gurian J, Edener F. Sample sizes for medical trials with special reference to long-term therapy. J Chron Dis 1968;21:13–24.
26. Smith WM. Problems in long-term trials. In: mild hypertension: natural history and management. Gross F and Strasser T. editors. London: Pitman, 1979:244–253.

5

Multicentre Collaborative Clinical Trials in Surgical Research

R.G. Margolese

Introduction

The aim of basic research is to advance our understanding of physiological or pathological mechanisms and discover ways of improving treatments. The implementation of these advances is one of the concerns of clinical research. The difference between therapy and research in clinical treatment lies in the use of the scientific method to evaluate new ideas. In its simplest form, the question is: How do you know if what you are now doing is better than competing alternatives? Or: is the new approach better than the most accepted current methods?

The fathers of surgery studied the problems they faced, devised treatments and eventually published reviews of their experience to build a foundation of empirically-based knowledge. This approach, however, is no longer adequate for the complex problems being attacked in modern surgery. As treatments become more standardized and results more predictable, new ideas are likely to bring improvements that are incremental rather than revolutionary. Deciding whether changes in treatment represent true advances, and assessing the side-effects or toxicities of new therapies become very complex problems needing input from biostatisticians and clinically-sophisticated research methodologists.

The controlled clinical trial is the most rigorous method we have to evaluate and compare alternative treatments. During the last 2 or 3 decades, this procedure has been steadily replacing historical reviews or extensive personal experience as the basis for choosing treatment strategies.

The potential range of comparisons is vast, e.g., total versus partial mastectomy, antrectomy versus highly selective vagotomy for duodenal ulcer, duodenal ulcer surgery versus acid inhibitor treatment or coronary artery surgery versus medical treatment. Such studies require thoughtful preparation and design. The literature contains many examples of inadequately designed studies whose conclusions are not widely accepted and only generate further controversy.

Randomized Controlled Clinical Trials

The most exacting and most widely accepted design for clinical trials is the randomized controlled trial. The randomized clinical trial uses patients who will be accrued in the future rather than patients who have been treated and analyzed historically. Participating patients are assigned to treatments by random selection, rather than by any conscious decision, to insure the formation of a control group that differs from the treatment group only in the treatment being studied and in no other respect.

Without careful evaluation and control, expensive or dangerous treatments can be widely applied with little chance for benefit. The immediate acceptance of postoperative radiation therapy for breast cancer in the years following World War II is a good example. Improvement in equipment had made safe and effective radiation therapy available and it was widely assumed that radiation in addition to the then standard operation, radical mastectomy, would improve control and cure rates. This assumption went unquestioned for a long time, and radiation, although unproven as an adjunctive therapy, became standard treatment throughout North America.

By the late 1960's, the biology of cancer was better understood and randomized controlled clinical trials to evaluate the use of such radiotherapy were finally undertaken. The eventual result (1,2) was the discontinuance of the routine use of adjunctive radiation and a consequent reduction in morbidity and costs, without loss of survival benefit.

Evaluation of a therapy that is widely established is often difficult because of the need for a "no treatment" control arm, since it suggests the witholding of a putatively useful treatment. Evaluation of a new therapy before it is widely established is preferable because it can be compared to "standard therapy".

The difficulty in entering patients into a trial where treatment is determined by random selection has prompted investigators, for a long time, to search for other methods of choosing control groups, but no better method than randomization has yet been found.

Historical Controls

Historical controls remain a popular alternative to randomized controls. In this approach, a group of patients treated in the past is selected to serve as a control for a group currently receiving a new treatment. Patients can be matched for such factors as age, sex, and extent of disease. Although it sounds useful, there are many problems with this method. The selection of patients from historical records is subject to both intentional and unintentional bias; the investigator or clerk pulling old records may decide to exclude some patients for various reasons. Even without such bias, other unknown factors may be significant. A group of gastric carcinoma patients from the early 1970's may differ from contemporary patients in ways that we do not recognize. The natural history of the disease may have changed and the impact of new medical treatments or diagnostic techniques may be important. Does the current, wide-spread use of colonoscopy mean that the mix of patients with colon carcinoma is different now than it was 15 years ago? Does it introduce the *lead-time bias* that occurs when a tumor is found earlier than it might have been but not enough earlier to change the outcome of treatment. A patient will still fail at the same time he or she would have, but the survival time appears to be longer because the diagnosis was made earlier. The effect of a longer perceived length of disease is a misleading impression that the treatment has been beneficial.

Another type of bias is called *length bias*. Screening procedures, such as colonoscopy or mammography, tend to identify a larger proportion of slow-growing tumors. Since rapidly growing tumors tend to show up spontaneously between screenings, they are not found as often during screenings. Comparison of a set of cases in a situation where screening is used with an apparently similar set in an earlier era when screening was not used, can produce misleading conclusions. If the impact of a new treatment is the object of the study, such comfounding issues may preclude valid conclusions.

Studies with historical controls tend to give positive results more frequently than those with contemporary controls; confirmatory studies with better design often fail to reproduce the results of historically controlled studies.

Staging

If staging methods change over a period of time, outcomes may appear to improve without any change in treatment. Clinical staging in breast cancer was traditional for many decades; patients without palpable axillary nodes were deemed to be stage I, those with palpable nodes were classified in stage II. Then, Haagensen began the practice of surgical biopsy of axillary nodes before definitive mastectomy. Some patients with clinically negative nodes are now found on biopsy to have microscopically positive nodes and are moved to stage II. Because their lymph node metastases are sub-clinical or microscopic, these patients have the most favorable prognosis of those in stage II. The pool of stage I patients is also made smaller and consists of a group of selected patients who will do better than the group chosen originally on purely clinical grounds. The dilution of the stage II pool of patients by the inclusion of patients with the minimal metastatic load has the effect of improving stage II outcomes. Thus, with no change in therapy and no change in overall outcome, the figures for both stage I and stage II will be better when pathological staging is compared with clinical (3).

The same kind of shift is seen with the trend toward more exact surgical staging of ovarian cancer patients. The extension of the staging procedure to include peritoneal washings, multiple positional and lymph node biopsies, and removal of omentum, increases the accuracy of staging and moves patients from stages with more favorable prognoses to those with poorer outlooks to produce the same effects as was seen in the breast cancer example. Obviously the use of historical or non-randomized controls would lead to inaccurate conclusions if staging methods changed while different treatments were being compared.

Selection

When historical controls are used, certain criteria for eligibility are used and all the patients whose records conform with these criteria are included. Many patients who meet the same criteria, however, may be excluded from the experimental group for a variety of other reasons. They may live too far away, decline to participate in the study, may appear so frail to the investigator that he or she decides to withhold the treatment, or may present problems in administering the treatment that require their exclusion, e.g., skin burns, neutropenia, poor venous access or intercurrent illness.

Since none of these exclusion criteria are applied to historical controls, there may be significant differences between the two groups that will make the results uninterpretable or misleading.

An investigator who is convinced of the merit of a new treatment may decide to offer it to all of his or her patients consecutively and then attempt to compare these results with those obtained in other centers with historical controls. Bias can enter for a variety of reasons. If one treatment appears to be more modern or exciting, it may appeal to a specific category of patients. Some patients will hear of their doctor's preference for heart surgery versus medical treatment and will seek out a doctor whose preference conforms with their own. Patients who seek a surgical treatment may be younger, stronger, or more alert to many factors including better general health care and may therefore, be better candidates for surgery. Patients not seeking surgical treatment may have the opposite characteristics, i.e., they may be less concerned and even somewhat indifferent to many aspects of medical care. Even if the two treatments are the same, the first group may do better for a variety of other reasons, e.g., they may present with earlier tumors, have better general medical care, and be less likely to have complications or to die from other diseases. As a result, an investigator could conclude that one treatment is superior when it is not.

There are additional sources of bias. If a surgeon is known to prefer limited surgery, e.g. partial versus total mastectomy or excision of a rectal tumor versus abdominal perineal resection—there may be a difference in referral patterns in his or her community. Referring doctors may send patients with small tumors to this doctor and patients with large tumors to other centers for more traditional or radical procedures. The results with the limited surgery may be very good and may lead the investigator to conclude that it is better for all patients when the survival figures are only good because they apply to a selected group of patients with good prognosis.

Concurrent randomized controlled trials offer the best way to avoid such biases.

Randomized Controlled Trials in Breast Cancer

The history of breast cancer surgery illustrates a number of things about randomized clinical trials.

Halsted developed the radical mastectomy in response to the widely held view, in the 1890's that cancer was a local and regional problem that spread through the lymphatics and not by blood born metastasis. Given this premise, the solution seemed logical: extend the scope of surgery beyond the obvious clinical extent of the tumor and remove the regional lymph nodes as an integral portion of the surgical specimen.

Halsted's results did produce dramatically better control of local recurrence but had no overall effect on long-term survival; local recurrence rates dropped from 85% to 27%, but the l0-year survival rate remained at 10–12% (4). Nevertheless, the operation was quickly accepted universally, because of the local control advantage. In later decades, survival figures improved because patients began to seek treatment at earlier stages of their disease and these better results were unwittingly identified with Halstead's operation.

Some surgeons, seeing little improvement in cure rates, concluded that the radical surgery was not radical enough and proposed extending the operation to include the internal mammary or supraclavicular nodes (5,6). To support their views, they produced evidence that was blemished by the kinds of problems discussed earlier and results that were not reproducible in other studies.

In the 1950's, a few surgeons who were dissatisfied with the results of the radical procedures produced anecdotal reports of their experience with less extensive surgery. Neither their reports nor several reports of similar treatment programs published during the next 20 years were widely accepted and no substantial change in surgical practice occured (see Table I). Most suffered from weaknesses in methodology and the advocates of classical radical mastectomy found it easy to attack and discredit them. The lack of appropriate control groups, patient selection methods, and randomization techniques—and even the total absence of randomization—made it impossible to interpret or apply the results, correctly. As a result, any discussion of the merits of the alternative treatments, was drowned in the attacks on the credibility of the studies. Twenty to thirty years were lost in useless debate about the alternative hypotheses before they were tested rationally—a powerful demonstration of the need to design and execute studies in a manner that will make their findings credible.

By 1971, understanding the biology of cancer had changed considerably and hematogenous spread was recognized as a major problem. The idea that extending the scope of lymph node surgery would be beneficial was considered illogical by some individuals and the National Surgical Adjuvant Breast Project (NSABP) developed the protocol for an randomized clinical trial to resolve the controversy (see Fig.1). For patients with clinically negative axillary nodes, the specific aims of the trial were to determine; (1) whether the outcome results with total mastectomy followed by postoperative regional irradiation were equivalent to those with radical mastectomy and (2) whether total mastectomy followed by delayed axillary dissection, was as effective as initial radical mastectomy or total mastectomy plus regional node irradiation. For patients with clinically positive nodes, the objective was to determine whether radical mastectomy or total mastectomy followed by radiation produced equivalent outcomes (see Fig. 2).

Methods Used in the Breast Cancer Randomized Controlled Trials

In 3 years, 1765 patients were enrolled in the NSABP trial. Patient eligibility in terms of age, tumor stage, clinical axillary stage and medical history were all clearly defined. The specifics of the operations were described and workshops were held to instruct participating surgeons in how to execute operative procedures that would

TABLE I.

Author	Country	Date	Treatment Groups	Reference
McWhirter	U.K.	1955	Simple mastectomy and radiotherapy	(16)
Kaae	Den.	1959	Simple mastectomy and radiotherapy vs. extended radical mastectomy	(6)
Peters	Can.	1967	Wedge resection and irradiation	(17, 25)
Crile	U.S.A.	1975	Wide local excision	(19)
Wise	U.S.A.	1971	Local excision and irradiation	(26)
Atkins	U.K.	1972	Wide local excision and partial radiation	(27)
Mustakallio	Fin.	1972	Wide local excision plus radiation	(20, 28)
Harris	U.S.A.	1978	Radiation following local excision	(29)
Calle	France	1978	Local excision and radiation	(21)

FIGURE 1.

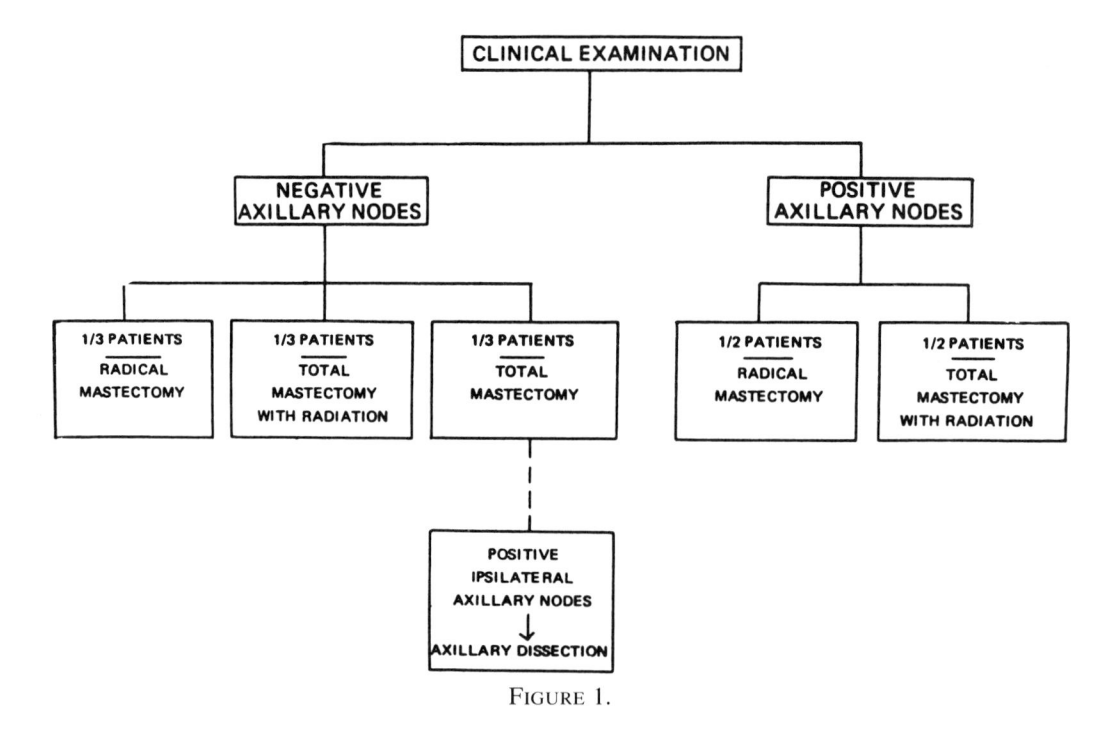

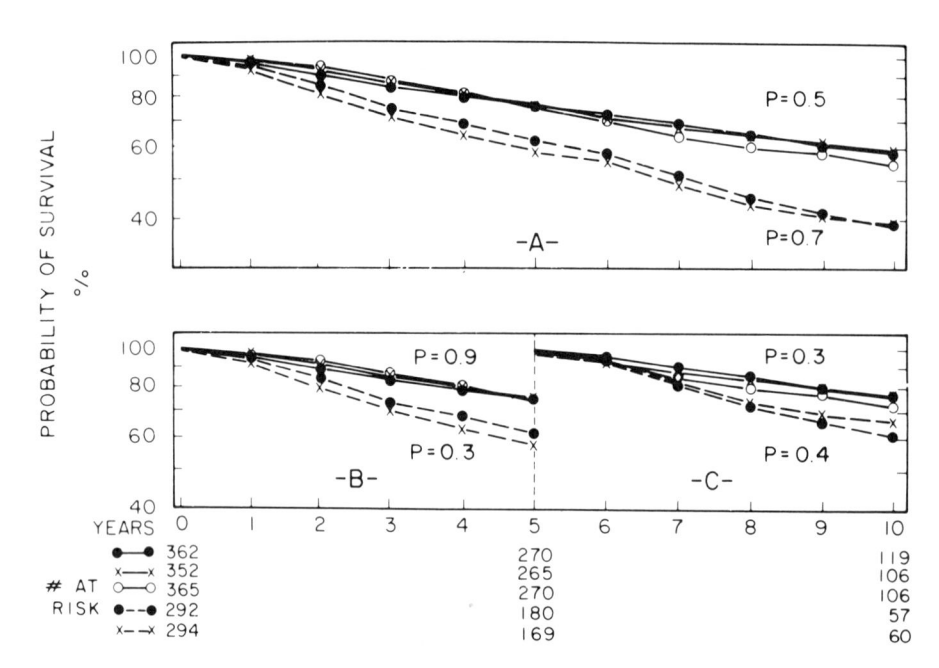

Survival through 10 Years (A), during the First 5 Years (B), and during the Second 5 Years for Patients Alive at the End of the 5th Year (C).

Patients were treated by radical mastectomy (solid circle), total mastectomy and radiation (x), or total mastectomy alone (open circle). There were no significant differences among the three groups of patients with clinically negative nodes (solid line) or between the two groups with positive nodes (broken line).

FIGURE 2.

be as uniform as possible. Similar processes were followed to ensure uniform pathological treatment of specimens and uniform radiation therapy.

Quality control was constantly maintained. At each institution, radiotherapy machine calibrations and techniques of treatment were examined and verified. To ensure that the operations were performed as intended, similar controls on operative reports and pathology techniques were maintained. For example, the average number of nodes found in radical mastectomy specimens on pathological examination was 15; in typical total mastectomy specimens it was zero. This result answers any criticism about the purity of the operative groups. All the factors that could possibly influence prognosis—age, race, endocrinine history, childbirth history, taking of contraceptive pills, etc.—were considered and compared to verify that the randomization process had distributed these covariates equally throughout the treatment arms.

The total patient enrollment goal was pre-determined from statistical analyses that indicated the sample size necessary to justify confidence in the results. Careful monitoring of the scientific methods was maintained from conception of the trial through to analysis of the results to insure scrupulous adherence to the protocol.

The methods of analysis used have been discussed in detail in the reports. Life table actuarial analyses were used extensively. A 5-year report was published in 1977 and a 10-year report, recently (7,8); both confirm the hypothesis that treatment of axillary lymph nodes does not influence the outcome. The findings also provide information on the biology of cancer.

The NSABP study illustrates the need for sound definition and understanding of the scientific problem under review. It is easy enough to pose a surgical question comparing treatment A to treatment B and have the statistician suggest an appropriate sample size, but selection of the individual treatments requires a great deal of thought and clinical judgment if the results are to be meaningful. A comparison of two minor surgical variants of a standard operation might meet all the statistical guidelines for a good study, but would hardly be worth doing because the question is unimportant.

The NSABP breast protocol was designed to confirm a fundamental change in biologic theory.

Although surgical removal was compared to irradiation of lymph nodes, a third arm of the study for negative node patients who were given no additional treatment provides insight into the biologic relevance of lymph nodes and the cancer process better. A simple comparison of surgical versus radiotherapy treatment of lymph nodes would have met the general methodologic guidelines, but would not have been as illuminating. If treating the lymph nodes does not improve prognosis, they are clearly not an intermediate station in the dissemination of cancer but merely one of the places to which cancer spreads when dissemination takes place. Positive nodes imply dissemination. Treatment of nodes alone cannot be useful. The study results made the need for systemic treatments clear and immediately prompted the generation of adjuvant chemotherapy studies.

Further Surgical Studies

The NSABP study also made it clear that evaluating surgery for local control was important and that it was now appropriate to ask the next question about the severity of surgical procedures. In the NSABP study using protocol B-04, just described, the outcome with simple mastectomy was shown to be equivalent to that with radical mastectomy. Protocol B-06 was then designed to compare simple mastectomy with partial mastectomy (or lumpectomy).

To justify the trial, The Protocol Design Committee had to consider two specific biologic questions and demonstrate the scientific and ethical merit of the trial with respect to them. The first concerned local recurrences; the second, the presence of multicentric tumor foci.

It could be expected that less extensive breast surgery might be followed by increased local recurrence rates. This increase could be important if local recurrences were shown to be associated with higher rates of metastatic disease and mortality from cancer. Accordingly, one question is, are local recurrences precursors of distant disease? Some evidence that local recurrence and distant disease appeared almost simultaneously in patients who relapsed (9) suggested that local recurrence is simply one of the places where metastatic disease appears rather than a source of it. If this is so, the premise that preventing local recurrence will improve survival figures is open to serious question.

Multicentric neoplasia is another important consideration in testing any limited surgical procedure. Many reports have indicated that patients with breast cancer have additional foci of non-invasive or minimally-invasive cancer in the affected breast. When serial sections are done, the incidence of multicentric disease ranges from 15 to 40 or 45% (10,11), but the true biologic significance of these foci is not known.

Biopsies of the other breast produce similar findings in 15 to 25% of women (12,13); if serial sections were done instead of biopsies, the incidence would probably approximate the 40 or 45% seen in the affected breast. In other words, the multicentric process is bilateral and diffuse. What happens in the opposite breasts of the thousands of women who have been treated by traditional unilateral mastectomy makes it clear that the subsequent incidence of contralateral cancer falls dramatically short of what would be expected if the positive microscopic findings were always associated with clinical cancer.

These arguments do not eliminate the possibility that local recurrence or multicentric disease might make partial mastectomy an inferior procedure. Genuine grounds for controversy exist since a clinical trial is required to clarify the biologic principles and the ultimate endpoints of the two treatments. The 3-arm study design used in the radical mastectomy protocol (B-04) would be appropriate for the new protocol (B-06). In B-04, the importance of lymph nodes was evluated by surgical treatment, by radiation, and by observation. In B-06, the breast parenchyma is being studied and the three treatments are surgical (total mastectomy), irradiation (segmental mastectomy and radiation therapy) and observation (segmental mastectomy without radiation therapy) (see Fig. 3).

Therefore, the 3 arm study design used in the radical mastectomy protocol (B-04) seems appropriate for the new protocol (B-06). In B-04 the importance of lymph nodes was evaluated by surgical treatment, by radiation, and by observation. In B-06 it is the breast parenchyma that is being studied and again, the 3 treatments are surgical (total mastectomy), irradiation (segmental mastectomy + radiation therapy) and observation (segmental mastectomy without radiation therapy). (see Fig. 4).

Protocol B-06 has been completed, and the first analysis confirms the hypothesis that the disease-free survival (DFS) and overall survival(S) rates are the same with the three methods of treatment (14). While B-06 was in progress, the Milan Group conducted a randomized con-

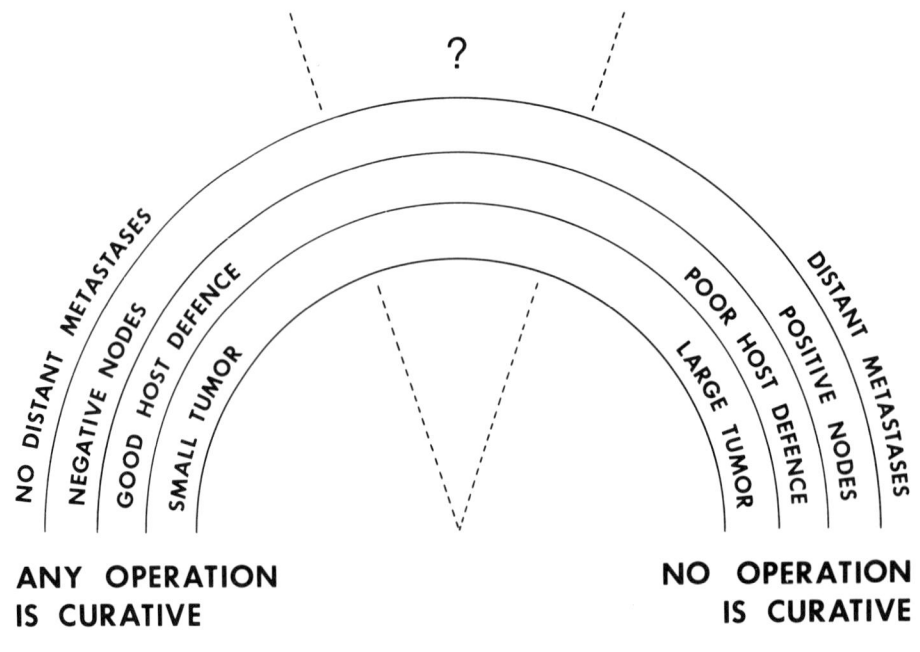

FIGURE 3.

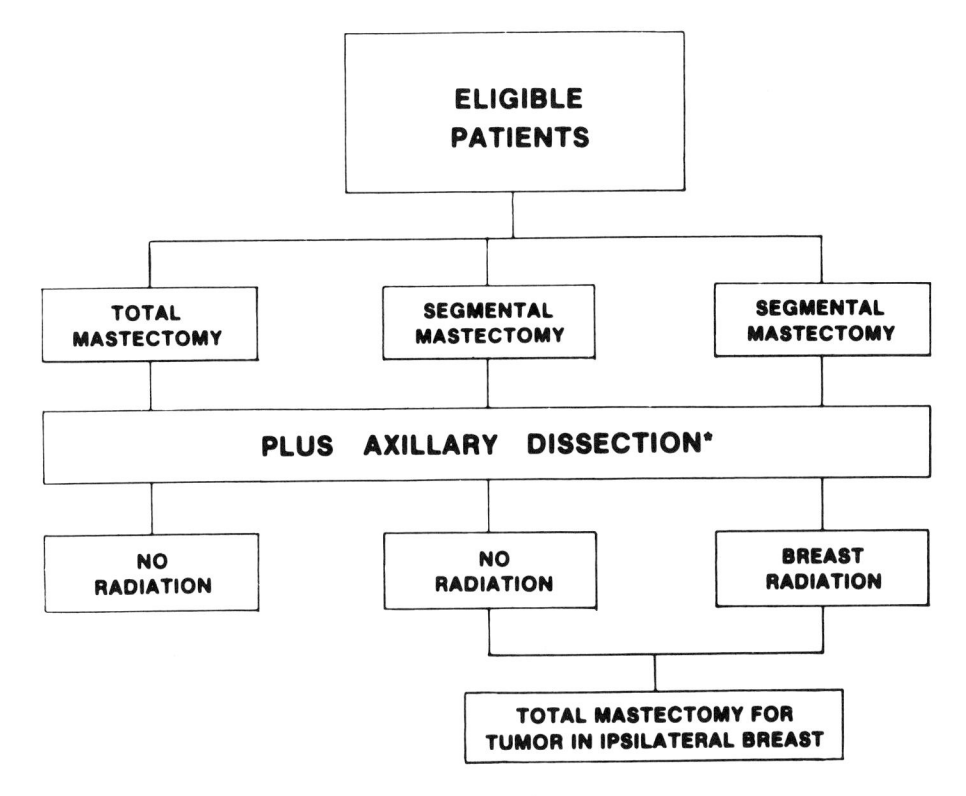

FIGURE 4.

trolled trial to compare quandrantectomy plus radiotherapy with radical mastectomy. Veronesi (15) has reported the DFS and S rates to be identical for both groups. The agreement in the findings of the only two contemporary randomized trials constitutes strong support for a major change in clinical practice (see Fig. 5).

It must be remembered that the results of B-06 apply only to the patients considered eligible for this trial, i.e., patients with tumors 4 cm or less in diameter and none of the grave signs of locally advanced disease. If the study had been done on patients with tumors 2 cm or less in diameter, the results would only apply to such

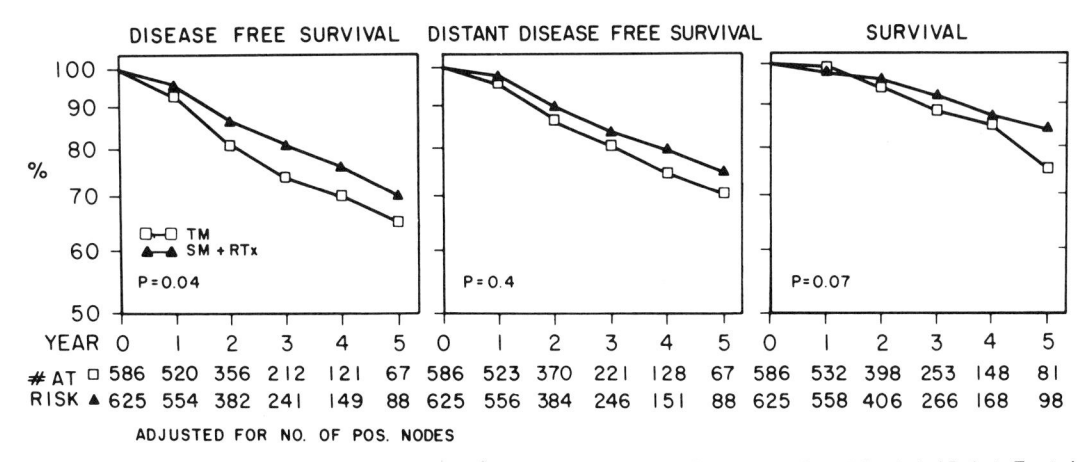

Life-Table Analysis Showing Disease-Free Survival, Distant-Disease-Free Survival, and Overall Survival of Patients Treated by Total Mastectomy (TM) or by Segmental Mastectomy plus Radiation (SM+RTx).

FIGURE 5.

patients and another study would be needed to determine whether patients with tumors larger than 2 cm could be considered for the same operation. Defining the patient population in a way that will make the results useful in clinical practice is an important consideration in study design.

The Significance of Randomized Controlled Surgical Trials

The NSABP and the Milan Group randomized clinical trials put biologic theories and surgical practices that had generated controversy for more than 50 years into perspective whereas the conclusions of other non-randomized clinical studies were not widely accepted (6,16,17) and contributed little, if anything to advancing our understanding and treatment of breast cancer. When protocol B-04 was begun, radical mastectomy accounted for 85% of the therapeutic procedures performed for primary breast cancer in the United States and Canada; it now accounts for less than 15%. (18)

Although a number of investigators in North America, England, France, and Finland pioneered into the concept of partial mastectomy and presented useful data, (17,19–21) only randomized controlled studies could generate sufficiently believable data to assure that partial mastectomy is an adequate operation for breast cancer patients.

Adjuvant Therapy

The randomized clinical trials based on protocols B-04 and B-06 were concerned with questions about the surgical treatment of breast cancer and they showed that making the surgery more radical was futile. Subsequently, it was hypothesized that when surgery failed, it was because micrometastases had already been established and that the number of metastatic cells in some patients might be small enough to be eliminated by doses of chemotherapy that would only palliate patients with gross metastatic disease. The need to evaluate systemic therapy as an adjunct to surgery was clearly evident.

Accordingly, the NSABP embarked on a test of the merit of adjuvant chemotherapy using a series of protocols with escalating drug regimens. The first protocol tested intermittent 5-day cycles on l-phenylanine mustard (L-Pam). When this was shown to have benefit, a second protocol comparing L-Pam against L-Pam plus 5-Fluorouracil (5-FU) was undertaken. This 2-drug combination was subsequently used as the standard for a series of 3-drug combinations (see Chart III) which have produced gains in D.F.S. and S rates for many subsets of patients.

Simultaneously, the Milan Group completed a successful randomized clinical trial evaluating cyclophosphamide, methotrexate, and 5-fluorouracil (CMF) in stage II patients. Taken together, these landmark studies (22–24) paved the way for a new generation of protocols for evaluating combinations of drugs and hormones in varying doses and schedules.

Advantages of Multicentre Collaboration Trials

Without the resources of collaborative groups, it would have been exceedingly difficult to allocate a small number of patients to so many drug choices and combinations. Within a period of 10 years, the NSABP has entered 10,000 patients into randomized clinical trials to assess the comparative value of using 1, 2 or 3 drugs and multi-modality combinations of immuno-, hormono-, and chemotherapies. The randomized clinical trials of the NSABP and other collaborative groups in Europe and North America, have contributed much to our knowledge of the biology of breast cancer in the process of pursuing improvement in DFS and S rates.

The same collaborative efforts have also demonstrated that breast cancer is not a single disease. Some subsets of patients respond well to some of therapy combinations while other subsets only respond to other combinations (a subset is a group of patients segregated by specific features, such as age, or particular disease characteristics).

Large numbers of patients for each protocol make it possible to stratify for important patient characteristics (see preceding chapter for detailed discussion of stratification). In an NSABP protocol for evaluating the efficacy of adding taxomifen to the standard 2-drug regimen, estrogen receptors (ER) and progesterone receptors (PR) were measured in all patients and recorded. A good response to taxomifen was seen in patients with high ER and PR levels and in older age groups. When subsequent studies were designed, pre-treatment determinations of ER and PR levels were used as a basis for assigning patients to different treatment groups to explore research questions, related to the different ER status.

If such studies had been attempted with only 150 patients in each arm, much of the information could not have been obtained. Splitting trial participants into groups that are large enough to be meaningful may require a total of 2000 patients. For example, if 1/2 the patients are premenopausal and 1/3 are ER positive, the pool of patients who fit both restrictions is only 333 out of 2000. Any further division, e.g., by lymph node class or cell type, will reduce the number of patients available for analysis even more. Since a busy urban hospital may only average about 100 new cases of primary breast cancer a year, it is obviously impractical to attempt a study requiring 2000 cases without some form of multicenter collaboration.

Many useful clinical trials are carried out in single centres but they are likely to be pilot studies or small studies using specific types of patient or treatment that would not lend themselves to a multi-institutional approach. Such studies frequently take a long time to accrue enough cases.

Most collaborative groups are composed of university, large urban, and smaller community hospitals to provide a more representative mix of patients than would be found in any single type of institution. As a result, the findings are more readily applicable to broad clinical practice. The necessity of having all participating hospitals comply with such special protocol requirements as immunochemical staining or high energy radiotherapeutic treatments may, however, exclude some of the institutions that would like to be involved. Such obstacles can often be surmounted by referral practices within the group. They do, however, require careful attention and should prompt efforts to design treatments that can be applied widely and to avoid treatments that are so esoteric they will never be practicable in a general way in the community.

Whatever the problems of collaborative studies may be, they are outweighed by the unique opportunities they afford for assembling adequate numbers of patients in a reasonably short period of time, to provide answers to specific questions that are more credible and more generalizable than could be obtained by smaller studies in highly specialized institutions.

Education and Technology Transfer

The need to standardize procedures in a multicentre clinical trial often requires the devotion of a great deal of energy to educating all the participating members. In NSABP protocol B-06, the segmental mastectomy operation was new to most surgeons in North America and early experience revealed unanticipated problems in its performance with respect to tumor control and cosmetic outcome. Several NSABP investigators who already had extensive experience with the operation proposed solutions that were discussed and refined in workshops of participating surgeons. the workshop concept was so successful that it was continued over the 8-year period of accrual for the protocol saving surgeons from having to learn the operation by repeating the same initial errors.

The involvement of community clinicians in routine group meetings of clinical trial organizations is an excellent way to promote the rapid transfer of ideas, techniques and knowledge. The discussion of new protocols and hypotheses is a valuable learning experience for all participants. Many people believe that involvement in clinical research and good clinical trial methodology lead to better clinical care for patients.

A collaborative multicentre randomized controlled trial is expensive, but the return on investment is worthwhile if the question it seeks to answer is clinically and socially important. Each participating institution needs money to maintain one or more secretarial data managers and to cover travel expenses for group meetings. The headquarters for a large project will need data managers, supervisors, biostatisticians, computer experts, and adequate computer resources. In addition large studies may require salaries for investigators as well. Even though the total outlay for such an entire apparatus may be large, a demonstration of the usefulness of some treatments and the desirability of abandoning others that are not, will result in reductions in morbidity and health care costs.

Many trials have been begun only to be abandoned for lack of adequate accrual of patients or lack of interest as years of slow accrual go by and other issues supplant the idea being tested. To avoid waste of funds, investigators have a responsibility to be sure that the treatments being studied are timely and meaningful and that the study can be done in a reasonable length of time.

The Organization and Management of Multicentre Collaborative Clinical Trials

The first part of this chapter dealt with the rationale for randomized clinical trials. Other areas of research could have been used to demonstrate the value of the randomized controlled trial, but the breast cancer story provides a special insight into some dramatic advances in surgery and chemotherapy, and the many facets that must be considered in designing and executing protocols. The chapter that precedes this one treats the design of clinical trials in some depth. This section provides a more general overview of some of the organizational points to be considered when setting up a single trial or a consortium of institutions to collaborate in clinical research.

The building of a collaborative group is best accomplished during the design phase of a trial. All the possible participants should be invited to meet at an early stage in the planning.

There should be a clear statement of the question to be addressed. It should include the relevant background material and the rationale for the proposed study. A concept sheet should rarely be longer than one page.

A *protocol design committee* is a suitable way to create the actual trial. The concept sheet is circulated and interested people with some experience in the area to be studied are asked to discuss the pros and cons of various aspects. The following should be included:

A definition of the surgery or other intervention to be performed. (A standard version of the operation is necessary. Any variations that are considered important or unimportant must be specified.)

Which types of patients are to be included in the study and which types are to be excluded.

Preliminary studies that need to be done before a patient is entered (e.g., kidney function tests if a renal-toxic drug is involved).

What special procedures need to be performed on the surgical specimen or the patient (e.g., receptor or immunofluorescent studies).

What pathological controls will be performed.

What follow-up intervals will be used; what observations will be made and recorded.

What records are to be kept. All protocols should have as a minimum:

1. On the study form--all vital information about the patient and the diagnosis. When a patient enters the study, the names and addresses of 3 relatives, who will always know the patient's whereabouts in the event he or she moves, should always be obtained. This information can be invaluable after several years of follow-up when a patient has suddenly moved away without leaving a forwarding address.

2. History--What pertinent data are required (e.g., in a breast cancer trial, information on birth control pills or estrogen replacement therapy might be recorded). For GI studies, dietary features might be documented.

3. Physical exam--items pertinent to the study should be specified, but be careful not to bog the study down with unnecessary details.

4. Progress forms--drug dose, toxicities and the status of the patient.

5. Follow-up--may include results of physical exam and laboratory and x-ray results.

A *principal investigator* should be identified at each participating institution. The principal investigator has overall responsibility for the conduct of the studies and the maintenance of the institution's level of activity and quality. He or she is the focal point for the dissemination of information about progress or changes in ongoing studies and the institution's representative in the collaborating group, especially for administrative and organizational aspects of the study.

A *study chairman* should be designated for each protocol. This person has responsibility for the ongoing conduct of the study. He or she can respond on an adhoc basis to unanticipated questions about patient eligibility for entry or about the conduct of the study. The chairman assumes responsibility for ensuring that data reports come in on time, that eligibility requirements are being met, and that no deviation occurs.

A *surgical monitoring committee* is a necessity in any surgical clinical investigation. The surgical operation should be clearly defined and a description of how it is to be performed should be provided in the protocol. The anatomic limits of the dissection and the anatomic structures to be preserved or removed should be clearly specified. For example, in NSABP colon studies, each type of segmental colon resection is clearly described, the vasculature to be divided is identified, and the scope of the operation report and compares it to the check-off data form to ensure that the surgical requirements are being met.

The *checklist* that is created for reviewing operative reports can be a part of the protocol documentation and it should be filled out by the operating surgeon following each operation. A second data form for such complications as an anastomotic leak or a seroma, should also be created so that a good statistical analysis can be performed at a later date.

A *pathology monitoring committee* is required to standardize the review of specimens. Many pathological features are difficult to quantify because they require personal interpretation, for example, histological grading. A pathology reference centre is the best way to assure standard diagnoses. A data form should be created to prompt the pathologist to provide answers to all relevant questions. This ensures good data control.

A *radiotherapy monitoring committee* should be created whenever radiotherapy is employed. If the effects of radiotherapy are being tested in a protocol, very careful attention to the planning and monitoring of the treatment is mandatory. All of the collaborating institutions should have their radiation therapy units calibrated, their methodology standardized, and their dose calculations reviewed centrally. Complications and toxicity should be monitored and recorded on data forms designed for this purpose.

A *chemotherapy monitoring committee* is needed to control adherence to the protocol and to monitor drug toxicities. A data form should be designed for easy supervision of any department from the stipulated schedules or doses, and for recording toxicities and any unanticipated problems.

All of these monitoring committees serve a two-fold purpose. One is to assure conformity to the protocol and to record and evaluate any deviations; the other is to monitor and document toxicity and alert investigators to serious problems that will require changes in the protocol when a patient's safety is concerned.

Such a quality control program strengthens confidence in the validity of the results. For example, a careful count of the number of positive axillary nodes and the total number of nodes examined is included in all NSABP protocols. This provided comforting reassurance when the segmental mastectomy with separate axillary dissection was introduced. It was easy to show that the number of positive nodes and the number of nodes obtained at operation did not differ from the number found with the modified radical mastectomy techniques, i.e., the separate axillary dissection provides the same accuracy for staging as the older procedure. The same assurance of accuracy in staging is particularly important, in chemotherapy protocols for Stage I patients. Any test of chemotherapy for negative-node patients would be weakened by the inclusion of inadequately or inaccurately staged patients who really belonged in stage II.

An *executive committee* should be created to make decisions and to oversee the continued functioning of the collaborating groups and their protocols. Ideally, this committee should comprise representatives from the various monitoring committees and the P.I. group.

A *quality control data management program* should be instituted at the group headquarters. It is one thing to define the data forms to be collected and the records to be kept, but another to ensure that they are accurate, complete, and punctual. Some form of infrequent audit will be needed to ensure that the data collected are correct. This is usually best done by a spot-check method in which the original hospital charts of randomly selected patients and certain predetermined data are examined, e.g., the accuracy of eligibility criteria and the consistency of drug administration. Pharmacology logs should also be examined and nursing notes correlated to make sure that the chemotherapy was given according to the protocol, and that the dose actually given corresponded with what was reported on the data forms.

A *data manager* should be set up for each institution that is accruing cases. This is a secretarial post with responsibility for maintaining and submitting accurately completed data forms on schedule. The data manager becomes involved with each patient at the time of consideration for entry into the protocol. To verify eligibility, perform the randomization, contact Headquarters to register the patient, and transmit the treatment assignment to the Investigator. The data manager will immediately assemble a dossier containing the required on study forms and will eventually keep a parallel protocol chart for each patient containing all the paperwork required by the protocol. A copy of every document sent to headquarters should be kept in the patient's protocol chart so that verification can be easily done on a moment's notice.

The data manager is also responsible for the scheduling of return visits for treatment or follow-up and for maintaining records on long-term scheduling. As patient numbers increase, it is very important to maintain complete follow-up and to ensure that no patient is lost to this process.

Data manager seminars at group meetings are an invaluable way of exchanging information and teaching the newer members of the organization the techniques of data management.

As the number of patients being followed increases, difficulties in tracking and scheduling can occur. For this reason, the Institutions at McGill Univerity have designed a computer-aided scheduling system (MPS-McGill Protocol System). This system contains master or template schedules for each protocol. Patients can be matched to a specific treatment program and a schedule can be generated at any time to show the data manager which patients are due for which treatments or tests in which time period. As dividends, patients can be given an individual copy of their schedules for the next time-frame and each participating laboratory can have advance lists of all the patients it will have to schedule in the coming weeks. This kind of system minimizes mistakes and assures the flow of good quality data.

Information dissemination becomes an important issue as the group grows and gains experience. Annual or semi-annual group meetings with a back-up system of mailings and updatings is one way to keep group communications current. Group meetings provide opportunities to disseminate information on the status of various studies, to discuss any problems, to explain any changes or clarifications in the conduct of the study, and to update participatnts on what has been learned so far.

Results will not be published until accrual targets are met, but toxicities can be discussed, and findings and correlations in ancillary areas can be presented. In one chemotherapy protocol, cytogenetic studies were done to learn more about the possibility of leukemia being caused by chemotherapy and the results were first presented at the group meeting.

The Group meetings also provide a forum for the exchange of information between participants and are an ideal way to stimulate and maintain interest in the study.

Workshops on such topics as the style and technique of informed consent have been very productive. The importance of workshops for surgeons, pathologists, chemotherapists and radiation therapists has been discussed earlier in this chapter. Workshops are an ideal approach to ensuring successful adherence to a protocol, especially when a new or non-standard treatment method is being used.

Decisions to close or abort a study or any portion of it should follow guidelines laid down in the protocol. The monitoring process, maintained by the executive committee, should provide information on when to close or abandon one arm of a study that is jeopardizing an otherwise good program. For example, in some aggressive chemotherapy programs, unexpected life-threatening toxicities may occur; if careful monitoring and evaluation will allow the study to be closed before too many patients are exposed to danger.

Probation and Suspension as a result of the monitoring of the performance of each participating center, it will sometimes become apparent that inadequate performance makes it necessary to place an institution on probation or to drop it completely from group membership. Rules and regulations should be spelled out when the group is organized so that this problem can be dealt with when the need arises. Such an event is very unfortunate and the existence of the monitoring process and of rules for dropping a center help to prevent it from happening.

Authorship: If a publication committee does not exist, there should be a clear decision at the outset regarding who will be responsible for writing the report. This ensures the completion of this task, helps in assigning appropriate credits for authorship and for participation in the study. The committee can also help to choose the journal for publication or the meeting at which the report will be presented.

Headquarters: One institution should act as the headquarters from which a full-time director and data manager(s) will supervise the day-to-day conduct of the trial.

Group statistician: Computer resources and personnel are discussed in Chapter 5 of Section II.

Ethics: In North America, the law requires the creation of Review Boards to consider the ethical aspects of research and patients' rights. The Ethics Review Board is usually made up of scientists not involved in the project, physicians who are not necessarily investigators, and members of the non-medical community, such as members of the clergy, and lawyers. The Board's role is to determine whether the proposed research is scientifically and ethically appropriate and whether the patients will receive adequate information about the choices presented to them. It is important that investigators cooperate with Review Boards to assure the proper conduct of the trial. Ethical principles in surgical research is the subject of Chapter 8 in Section II.

Conclusion

If you are considering a clinical trial, all of the points discussed in this chapter should be taken into account although some will be more important in some studies than in others. In practical terms, you should always design the ideal study and then make compromises necessary for feasibility. Setting down rules and guidelines at the beginning is the best way to proceed but unrealistic rigidity can be self-defeating. All rules or compromises should be considered in the light of how to anticipate and prevent adverse criticism about the conduct of the study or its outcome. The object is to do good clinical science and contribute to meaningful progress.

The randomized controlled clinical trial is the most reliable and useful investigative tool in clinical medicine. Despite its imperfections, it produces the most credible and generalizable results and has justifiably become and is likely to remain the mainstay of clinical research. It is doubtful that any clinical research program can now be developed without a good understanding of how randomized controlled trials are designed and implemented.

References

1. Butcher HR, Seaman WB, Eckert C, et al. Assessment of radical mastectomy and postoperative irradiation therapy in treatment of mammary cancer. Cancer 1964;17:480–485.
2. Paterson R, Russel MH. Clinical triasl in malignant disease—III breast cancer: evaluation of postoperative radiotherapy. J Fac Radiol 1959;10:175–180.
3. Feinstein AR, Sosin DM, Wells MPH. The Will Rogers phonemenon. Stage migration and new diagnostic techniques as a source of misleading statistics for survival in cancer. N Engl J Med 1985;213:1604–1608.
4. Lewis, Rhinecraft. A study of results—Johns Hopkins Hospital 1998-1931. Ann Surg 1932;25:336–400.
5. Urban JA, Baker HW. Radical mastectomy in continuity with en bloc resection of internal mammary lymph-node chain: new procedure for primary operable cancer of breast. Cancer 1951;5:992–1008.
6. Kaae S, Johansen H. Breast cancer: comparison of results of simple mastectomy with postoperative roentgen irradiation by McWhirter method with those of extended radical mastectomy. Acta Radio (Stockh) suppl. 1959;188:155–161.
7. Fisher B, Redmond C, Fisher E, et al. Ten year-results of a randomized clinical trail comparing radical mastectomy and total mastectomy wtih or without radiation . N Engl J Med 1985;312:674–681.
8. Fisher B, Montague E, Redmond C, et al. Comparison of radical mastectomy with alternative treatments for primary breast cancer. Cancer 1977;39:2827–2839.

9. Spratt JS. Locally recurrent cancer after radical mastecomy. Cancer 1967;20:1051–1053.
10. Morgenstern L, Kaufman PA, Friedman BN. Cast against tylectomy for carcinoma of breast—factor of multicentricity. Am J Surg 1975;130:251–258.
11. Rosen PP, Fracchia AA, Urban JA, Schottenfeld D, Robbins GF. Residual: mammary carcinoma following simulated partial mastectomy. year;volume:739–747.
12. Urban JA. Bilateral breast cancer. Cancer 1969;24:1310–1313.
13. Sandison AT. In: Crige G. Multicentric breast cancer: incidence of new cancers in homolateral breast after partial mastectomy. Cancer 1975;35:475–477.
14. Fisher B, Bauer M, Margolese R, et al. I. Five-year results of a randomized clinical trial comparing total mastectomy and segmental mastectomy with or without radiation in the treatment of breast cancer. N Engl J Med 1985;312:665–673.
15. Veronesi U, Saccozzi R, Del Vecchio M, et al. Comparing radical mastectomy with quadrantectomy, axillary dissection, and radiotherapy in patients with small cancers of the breast. N Engl J Med 1981;305:6–11.
16. McWhirter R. Simple mastectomy and radiotherapy in treatment of breast cancer. Br J Radiol 1955;28:128–139.
17. Peters MD. Cutting the "Gordian Knot" in early breast cancer. Ann R Coll Phys Surg Canada 1975;8:186–191.
18. Nemoto T, Vana J, Bedwani RN, Baker HW, McGregor FH, Murphy GP. Management and survival of female breast cancer: results of a national survey by the American College of Surgeons. Cancer 1975;35:2917–2924.
19. Crile G. Results of conservative treatment of breast cancer at 10 and 15 years. Ann Surg 1975;181:26–30.
20. Mustakallio S. Conservative treatment of breast carcinoma—review of 25 year, follow-up. Clin Radiol 1972;23:110–116.
21. Calle R, Pilleron JP, Schlienger P, et al. Conservative management of operable breast cancer: 10 years experience at the Foundation Curie. Cancer 1978;42:2045–2053.
22. Fisher B, Redmond C, Fisher E, et al. The contribution of recent NSABP clinical trials of primary breast cancer therapy to an understanding of tumor biology—an overview of findings. Cancer 1980;46:1009–1025.
23. Bonadonna G, Valagussa P. Adjuvant systemic therapy for resectable breast cancer. J Clin Oncol 1985;3:259–275.
24. Bonadonna G. Results of adjuvant therapy trial in breast cancer. Paper presented at White House conference on breast cancer, Bethesda MD, November 22, 1976.
25. Peters VM. Wedge resection and irradiation: effective treatment in early breast cancer. JAMA 1967;200:134–135.
26. Wise L, Mason AY, Ackerman LV. Local excision and irradiation: alternative method for treatment of early mammary cancer. Ann Surg 1971;174:393–401.
27. Atkins H, Hayward JL, Klugman DJ, Wayte AB. Treatment of early breast cancer: report after 10 years of clinical trial. Br Med J 1972;2:423–429.
28. Mustakallio S. Treatment of breast cancer by tumor extirpation and roentgen therapy instead of radical operation. J Fac Radiol 1953;6:23–26.

6

Evaluation of the Diagnostic Process

M.T. Schechter

Introduction

Yerushalmy's pioneering work (1) on observer variability in the interpretation of chest roentgenograms initiated a still-expanding interest in the evaluation of the diagnostic process. He introduced the terms *sensitivity* and *specificity* as measures of the validity of diagnostic tests and an entire methodology, including the concept of *predictive value* has developed in response to the geometric growth in and reliance on diagnostic testing in clinical practice.

Diagnostic Test Validity

Clinicians use diagnostic tests to ascertain whether a disease is present. For example, you can use a gallium scan to test for the presence or absence of an intra-abdominal abscess, or mammography to help you determine whether a palpable lump is malignant.

The disease state that a diagnostic test is meant to detect is sometimes referred to as the *target disease*. The *validity* of a diagnostic test refers simply to its ability to register an abnormal result for patients in whom the target disease is present and a normal result for patients in whom the target disease is absent. An ideal diagnostic test would exhibit both these behaviors, i.e., it would only register abnormal results for patients who have the target disease and only normal results for patients who are free of the target disease. Such a diagnostic test would be perfect in the sense that its results, would be perfectly predictive of the target disease state, i.e. absent or present. Unfortunately, most diagnostic tests do not perform this well and a number of concepts and techniques have been developed to gauge just how satisfactorily a given diagnostic test does perform.

If we are to judge how well a test performs in detecting a target disease in certain patients, we need some way of determining the truth about the presence or absence of the target disease in the same patients. To judge the capabilities of the gallium scan in diagnosing intra-abdominal abscess, for example, we need to know whether or not such abscesses are present in a group of patients and compare this information with the results obtained by means of the gallium scan. We could use the findings of laparotomy and subsequent pathological confirmation of an abscess as the determinant of the true target disease state. Similarly, we could use the results of laparotomy as the determinant for the presence of intra-peritoneal injury required to assess the performance of peritoneal lavage as a diagnostic manoevre. To assess mammography as a means of detecting malignant breast tumors, we could use pathological examination of the tumor as our determinant. The method one uses to confirm the presence or absence of the target disease in such determinations is known as the *gold standard*. In general, it should be the best clinical standard currently available for the particular target disease in question. When surgical exploration and pathological confirmation are available as part of the usual clinical management, they are obvious choices as gold standards; when they are not, other standards must be used. For example, to determine the validity of fibrinogen leg scanning as a diagnostic test for deep vein thrombosis

(D.V.T.) the best clinical standard currently available is venography. Consequently, the results of this radiological procedure are usually used as the gold standard for the presence or absence of DVT. Similarly, to check the validity of tests such as radionuclide angiography in the detection of coronary artery stenoses where surgical confirmation is only available in the relatively small number of patients who come to bypass surgery, coronary angiography is often used as the gold standard.

Figure 1 sets out the structure of a diagnostic test assessment in general terms. In essence, we merely compare the diagnostic test result (abnormal vs normal) against the gold standard result for the target disease (present vs absent). By convention, the test result is set out in the rows of a 2 × 2 table while the gold standard result is set out in the columns. Adoption of this arbitrary convention will help you to recall some of the definitions we will come to later. The upper left hand cell displays the number of patients who have the disease according to the gold standard and also have positive test results, i.e., the test correctly identifies them as having the target disease. Such patients are called *true positives (TP.)* The lower right hand cell displays the number of patients who do not have the disease and have negative test results, i.e., the *true negatives (TN)*. Taken together, the true positives and true negatives constitute all the patients in whom the diagnostic test is correct. The greater the proportion of patients that falls into these two groups is, the more accurate the diagnostic test.

The patients who fall into the two remaining cells give rise to whatever uncertainty there is. The number in the upper right hand cell represents the patients who do not have the disease but in whom the test results are erroneously positive. These patients are called *false positives (FP)*. The costs of this type of error are the unnecessary further investigations and treatments that might be undertaken and the effects of falsely labeling the patient. The number in the lower left hand cell represents the patients who have the disease but in whom the test results are erroneously negative i.e., the *false negatives (FN)*. The costs of this type of error are the morbidity and mortality associated with lack of immediate treatment. We have completed the table by adding the rows and columns (TP + FN, FP + TN, TP + FP, FN + TN).

Sensitivity is defined as the proportion of those with the disease who have a positive test result. This is sometimes shortened to "Positivity in disease". Sensitivity is a measure of how well the test performs at detecting the dis-

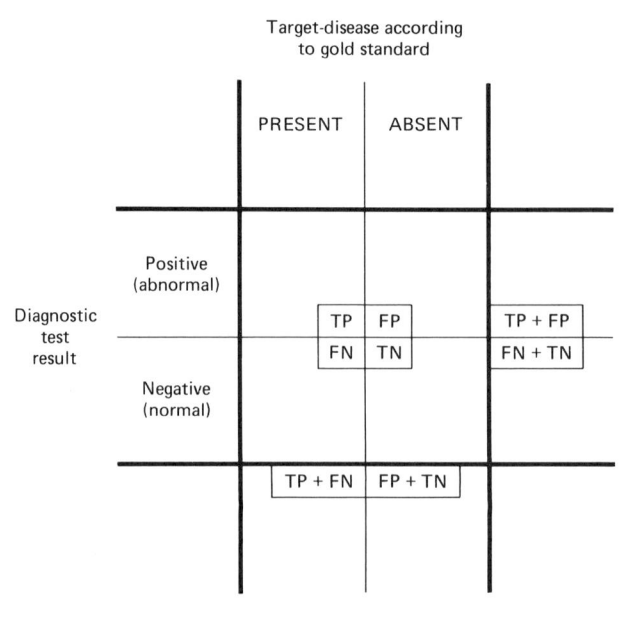

	PRESENT	ABSENT	
Positive (abnormal)	TP	FP	TP + FP
Negative (normal)	FN	TN	FN + TN
	TP + FN	FP + TN	

Target-disease according to gold standard / Diagnostic test result

FIGURE 1.

ease when it is present. It can be calculated from the first column of the table by the formula:

SENSITIVITY = TP / (TP + FN).

Specificity is defined as the proportion of those who do not have the disease who have negative test results -- sometimes referred to as "negativity in health". Specificity is a measure of how well the test performs at registering negative results when the target disease is absent. It can be computed from the second column of the table by the formula:

SPECIFICITY = TN / (TN + FP).

If you prefer the terminology of conditional probabilities, *sensitivity* is the conditional probability of a positive test given the presence of disease, and *specificity* is the conditional probability of a negative test given the absence of disease. These latter definitions are only included because you may encounter them in the literature.

Let us consider a diagnostic test assessment, adapted from Foti et al. (2), of a radioimmunoassay serum test for prostatic acid phosphatase (PAP) meant to detect prostatic carcinoma. Foti and his colleagues used 113 patients with prostatic carcinoma confirmed by the gold standard of surgical biopsy and 217 individuals free of prostatic cancer. The latter group consisted of normal individuals and patients with benign prostatic hyperplasia, previous prostatectomy, gastrointestinal disorders, or non-prostatic cancer. Sera from the 330 individuals were assessed by the assay for the presence of PAP and each specimen was characterized as positive (abnormal) or negative (normal). These results were then compared with the true prostatic cancer status of the 330 individuals to produce Fig. 2.

In the 113 patients with prostatic carcinoma, the PAP test was positive in 79, i.e., a *sensitivity* of 79/113 or 0.70. A *sensitivity* of 0.70 or 70% prompts the inference that, given 100 patients with prostatic carcinoma, the test will detect approximately 70 of them. This implies, in turn, that the test will miss about 30 of them. This latter figure, derived by subtracting the *sensitivity* as a percent from 100, is known as the *false negative rate*.

In the 217 patients who did not have prostatic carcinoma, the test was negative in 204, i.e., a *specificity* of 204/217 or 0.94. A *specificity* of 0.94 or 94% the inference that, given 100 patients without prostatic carcinoma, the test will be negative in about 94 of them and falsely positive in the remaining 6. The last figure, obtained by subtracting the specificity as a percent from 100, is known as the *false positive rate*.

	Prostatic carcinoma according to biopsy results		
Prostatic acid phosphatase result	PRESENT	ABSENT	
Positive (abnormal)	79 (TP)	13 (FP)	92 (TP + FP)
Negative (normal)	34 (FN)	204 (TN)	238 (FN + TN)
	113 (TP + FN)	217 (FP + TN)	330

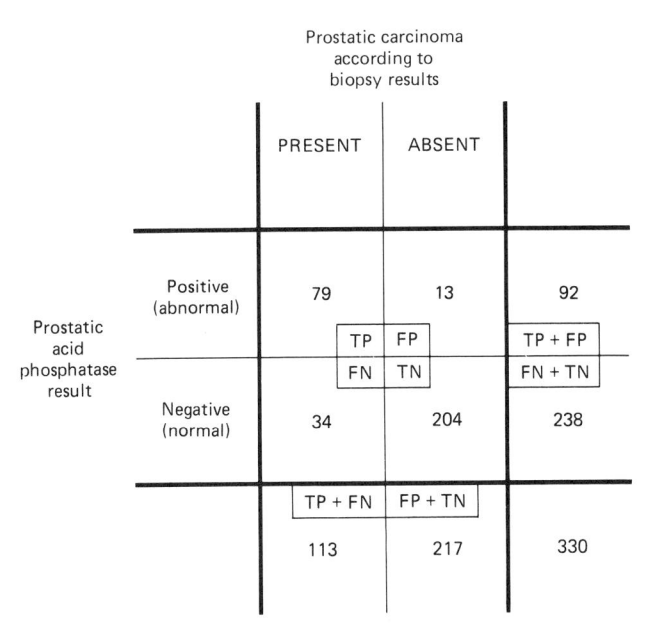

FIGURE 2.

Sensitivity and *specificity* are measures of a diagnostic test's validity; the higher these values are, the better the test is at detecting the presence and absence of disease, respectively. The higher the sensitivity is, the lower the false negative rate is, i.e., the lower the chances are of missing the target disease when it is present. The higher the specificity is, the lower the false positive rate is, i.e., the lower the chances are of obtaining a false positive result when the target disease is absent. In the PAP example with a sensitivity of 70% and a specificity of 94%, we have a test of high specificity but of only moderate sensitivity.

Diagnostic Test Utility (Usefulness)

To calculate sensitivity and specificity, you *must* know the true presence or absence of the target disease. This was illustrated earlier by a study that used 113 patients in whom biopsy had already established the actual presence of prostatic carcinoma. In many clinical situations, however we do not know whether the target disease is present or absent. If the results of a gold standard were available, there would be no need to use another diagnostic test.

In clinical practice, we are often confronted by additional problems when the presence of the target disease is uncertain. First, given that a patient has a positive test result, we need to know what the probability is that he or she has the target disease, i.e., the *positive predictive value* (PPV) of the test. The PPV reflects the degree of certainty we may have about the presence of the target disease in patients in whom the test is positive. Similarly, for patients with negative test results, we need to know the probability that the target disease is absent, i.e., the *negative predictive value* (NPV). The higher the PPV, the better the test is at "ruling in" the disease when the test result is positive; the higher the NPV, the better the test is at "ruling out" the disease when the test result is negative. Whereas sensitivity and specificity measure the test's intrinsic abilities to detect the presence and absence of the target disease, respectively, the predictive values measure the test's utility in clinical practice.

Let us consider a typical patient drawn at random from the entire group of 330 individuals in the study by Foti and his colleagues (Fig. 2). Suppose that, as would be true in clinical practice, we do not know whether the individual has prostatic carcinoma and we are going to rely on the PAP assay for the answers. Since 113 of the 330 individuals in the study have prostatic carcinoma, we know there is a probability of 113/330 or 34.2% that our randomly chosen individual has the disease. This measure of the proportion of diseased patients within the total population is known as the *prevalence* and is calculated using the formula:

PREVALENCE = (TP + FN) / (TP + FN + FP + TN).

The numerator, (TP + FN) is the total number of individuals with the disease, i.e., the sum of the cells in the left hand column of Fig. 2; the denominator is the total number of participants, i.e., the sum of all four cells in Fig. 2. Since there is a 34.2% chance that our typical patient, drawn at random from the sample, has prostatic cancer prior to undergoing the PAP test, the prevalence is also referred to as the *pre-test probability* or *pre-test likelihood* of the disease.

Let us now see how well the PAP performs at predicting the presence or absence of disease in our typical patient by supposing, first, that his test result is positive. Since there are 92 patients with positive test results, of whom 79 actually have prostatic cancer, there is a 79/92 or 85.9% chance that our patient has prostatic carcinoma. This is the PPV for this population (Fig. 2), i.e.,

PPV = TP / (TP + FP).

Since the PPV represents the probability of a patient having a given disease when the test result is positive, it is also referred to as the *post-test probability of a positive test* (PTL+). In this case, the PPV (or PTL+) is substantially higher (85.9%) than the pre-test probability of 34.2% and the test has performed very well at 'ruling in' prostatic carcinoma by markedly increasing the probability of its presence when the test is positive.

Now, suppose the PAP result in our randomly chosen individual is negative. Since there are 238 patients with negative test results, of whom 204 do not have the disease, there is a 204/238 or 85.7% chance that our subject is free of prostatic carcinoma. This is the negative predictive value (NPV) for this population (Fig. 2), i.e.,

$$NPV = TN / (FN + TN).$$

This NPV of 85.7% represents the probability of not having the disease when the PAP result is negative. If there is an 85.7% chance of not having the disease, there is a 14.3% chance of having it; subtracting the NPV from 100 gives the probability of having the disease even when the test is negative——the *post-test probability of a negative result*. As you might anticipate, the probability of having the disease after a negative test (14.3%) is lower than the pre-test probability of disease (34.2%). Consequently, the negative test result has contributed to 'ruling out' prostatic carcinoma by decreasing the probability of the presence of the disease from 34.2 to 14.3%.

The reader may have noticed an asymmetry. The *positive predictive value* (PPV) and the *post-test probability of a positive test* (PTL+) are synonymous, but the *negative predictive value* (NPV) and the *post-test probability of a negative test* (PTL−) are not. The NPV refers to the probability of the disease being absent in those with a negative result while the PTL−refers to the probability of the disease still being present in those with a negative result. Although the two quantities are clearly not the same, they are strictly related since they sum to 100% and one can be easily derived from the other.

The results of the PAP test in this particular population can be pictorially represented by a diagnostic tree diagram (Fig. 3). Such representations are very useful in the science of structuring clinical decisions known as 'clinical decision analysis'. The patient enters the test at the left of the diagram with a pre-test probability of prostatic carcinoma of 34.2%. If the test is positive, this probability rises to the post-test probability of a positive test (85.9%); if the test is negative, this probability falls to the post-test probability of a negative test (14.3%). The test appears, therefore, to provide some potentially useful information in this population. For patients with positive results, the probability of disease is sufficiently high (85.9%) to warrant biopsy and possible surgical exploration whereas for patients with negative results, the probability of disease is sufficiently low (14.3%) that the patient may be followed or given another noninvasive test if one is available.

On the basis of the sensitivity and specificity results of Foti and his colleagues, it was concluded in many quarters that the PAP radioimmunoassay could serve as an effective screening test for the early detection of prostatic cancer. Gittes stated, in an editorial that accompanied the report of Foti et al, "The grim finding has been that, overall, 90% of cases are first detected when they have already metastasized. The clear implication of the accompanying report is that mass screening on the basis of a blood test alone can reverse this gloomy experience" (3). The popular press reported a new blood test that promised to do for prostatic cancer what the Papanicolaou smear had accomplished for cancer of the cervix.

The utility of a test refers to its usefulness and its ability to affect patient care positively in a specific clinical situation. It can only be judged in relation to a *particular* clinical situation; a relatively good sensitivity and specificity, do *not* suffice to establish the clinical utility of a given test in *any* situation. Although sensitivity and specificity measure intrinsic qualities of a test's validity and may be assumed to remain relatively stable in different clinical situations, the predictive values and post-test probabilities can change drastically. Since the predictive values and post-test probabilities depend very heavily on the pre-test probability (prevalence), changes in prevalence can lead to marked changes in the predictive values and the clinical utility of a test. In other words, to adequately assess a diagnostic test for a specific clinical purpose, you must analyze it in relation to that particular purpose.

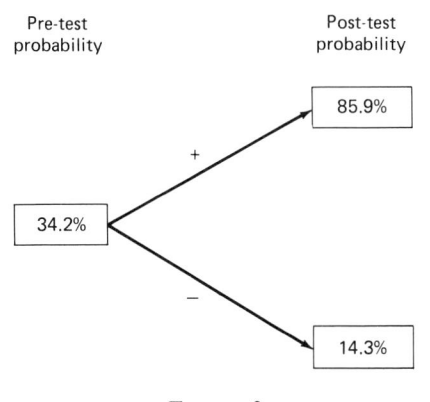

FIGURE 3.

Prostatic carcinoma

	Present	Absent	
Positive (abnormal)	TP	FP	TP + FP
Negative (normal)	FN	TN	FN + TN
	TP + FN	FP + TN	
	35	99,965	100,000

Prostatic carcinoma

	Present	Absent	
Positive (abnormal)	25		
	TP	FP	TP + FP
	FN	TN	FN + TN
Negative (normal)	10		
	TP + FN	FP + TN	
	35	99,965	100,000

Prostatic carcinoma

	Present	Absent	
Positive (abnormal)	25	5998	
	TP	FP	TP + FP
	FN	TN	FN + TN
Negative (normal)	10	93,967	
	TP + FN	FP + TN	
	35	99,965	100,000

FIGURE 4.

The original analysis of the PAP assay was carried out in a population of patients in whom the prevalence of prostatic cancer was 34.2%—hardly representative of the usual screening situation. Three years after the report of Foti et al, Watson and Tang presented their analysis of the PAP test as a screening test for prostatic cancer. On the basis of national data for the U.S.A. for the year 1964, these authors assumed that the prevalence of prostatic carcinoma among white American men was 35 cases per 100,000. They then used the PAP test's established sensitivity and specificity of 70% and 94%, respectively, to calculate its predictive values in the screening situation. To make these calculations, you begin by putting the hypothetical population of 100,000 as the total at the lower right hand corner of the 2 × 2 table (TP + FP + FN + TN) (Fig. 4a). Since there are an estimated 35 cases among this hypothetical group, the sum at the bottom of the left hand column (TP + FN) should read 35. It follows that the sum of the right hand column (FP + TN) should be 100,000 − 35 = 99,965 (Fig. 4a). Of the 35 men who have prostatic cancer, the test will be positive in about 70% (sensitivity), i.e., approximately 25, and this quantity can be entered in the TP cell (Fig. 4b). The remainder, 35 − 25 = 10, can be entered in the FN cell. Similarly, of the 99,965 men without prostatic carcinoma, the test will be negative in about 94% (specificity), i.e., approximately 93,967, and this quantity can be entered in the TN cell (Fig. 4c). The remainder, 99,965 − 93967 = 5,998, is entered in the FP cell (Fig. 4c). The table can be completed by simply adding the row totals (Fig. 5).

We can now calculate the predictive values and post-test probabilities for the screening situation. The positive predictive value (PPV) (or PTL+) is TP/(TP + FP) or 25/6023, i.e., 0.42%. The negative predictive value (NPV) is TN/(TN + FN) or 93967/93977, i.e., 99.99%. The post-test probability of a negative test, obtained by subtracting the NPV from 100% is therefore 0.01%. The probability of prostatic carcinoma prior to the test, (the pre-test likelihood or prevalence) was set at 35/100,000 or 0.035%.

Figure 6 is a diagnostic tree diagram that summarizes these results for the screening situation. The average asymptomatic man who would be screened by such a test approaches the test at the left of the diagram with a pre-test probability of prostatic cancer of 0.035%. (35 chances in 100,000). If his test is positive, the probability rises to only 0.42% (1 chance in 240). Thus, even with a positive test result, the chance of having prostatic cancer is still extremely slim and it would be hard to justify further invasive testing. Obviously the test is of little help, clin-

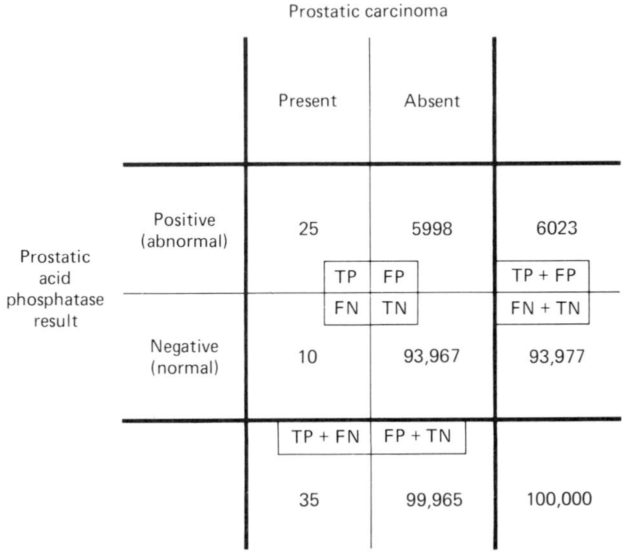

		Prostatic carcinoma		
		Present	Absent	
Prostatic acid phosphatase result	Positive (abnormal)	25 (TP)	5998 (FP)	6023 (TP + FP)
	Negative (normal)	10 (FN)	93,967 (TN)	93,977 (FN + TN)
		35 (TP + FN)	99,965 (FP + TN)	100,000

PPV = TP/(TP + FP) = 25/6023 = .0042 or 0.42%
NPV = TN/(TN + FN) = 93,967/93,977 = 0.9999 or 99.99%

FIGURE 5.

```
        Pre-test                    Post-test
       probability                 probability
                                  ┌────────┐
                              +   │ 0.42%  │
                          ╱       └────────┘
          ┌────────┐    ╱
          │ .035%  │ ──
          └────────┘    ╲
                          ╲   −   ┌────────┐
                                  │ 0.01%  │
                                  └────────┘
```

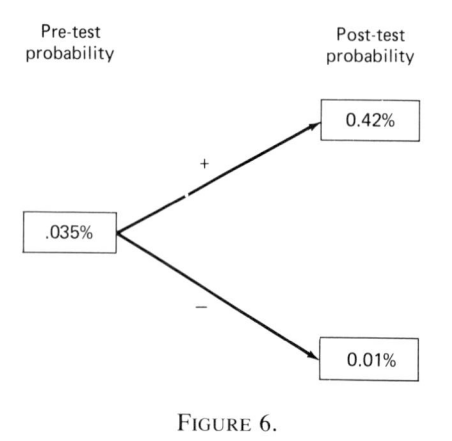

FIGURE 6.

ically, when it is positive in a screening situation. Moreover, since approximately 6% (6023/100,000) of all white American men would have positive PAP screening tests any policy of investigating positives further would involve the needless testing of significant numbers of healthy men. If the test is negative, the probability of disease falls to 0.01% (10/100,000). Although one could argue that the test is useful in the screening situation since it virtually rules out prostatic carcinoma when it is negative, this decreases in probability is of little benefit since the disease is exceptionally rare in the given population, anyway (35/100,000).

Our example illustrates the relationship between post-test likelihoods and pre-test likelihoods. In the diagnostic analysis carried out by Foti et al., the post-test likelihoods of a positive and negative test were relatively high (85.9% and 14.3%, respectively) because the pre-test likelihood was high (34.2%) prior to the test. In the screening analysis carried out by Watson and Tang, the post-test likelihoods of a positive and negative test were extremely low (0.42% and 0.01%, respectively) because the pre-test likelihood was very low (.035%) prior to the test. The pre-post-test likelihoods can be linked by a mathematical expression known as Bayes' Theorem. The following are two of many equivalent expressions for Bayes' Theorem:

$$PPV = \frac{P \cdot SENS}{(P \cdot SENS) + (1-P)(1-SPEC)}$$

where P, SENS, and SPEC represent the pre-test probability, sensitivity, and specificity, respectively, in decimal (e.g., 0.80) rather than percent (e.g., 80%) format. No matter which expression is used for Bayes' Theorem, they all have the common feature of expressing the post-test probabilities or predictive values in terms of the pre-test probability. They all demonstrate how dependent the former values are on the latter value, and provide a method for calculating post-test probabilities and predictive values for a given diagnostic test and a given pre-test probability. You are encouraged to calculate the predictive values for the PAP test in the screening situation by setting P at .00035, SENS at .70, and SPEC at 0.94, in the above formulas. You should derive the predictive values that were obtained before (except for possible slight differences due to rounding error). Clearly, these formulas provide an attractive alternative to the series of calculations and tables we went through before to derive the predictive values and post-test probabilities (Figs. 4a, 4b, 4c, and 5). Bayes' Theorem, in any of its different forms, is a relatively straightforward method of deriving the predictive values and post-test likelihoods that are central to the consideration of clinical utility. This type of analysis is sometimes referred to as "Bayesian analysis".

The PAP radioimmunoassay example illustrates several fundamental things about diagnostic tests. First, sensitivity and specificity measure the validity (accuracy) of a diagnostic test, but they have no direct bearing on its clinical utility. Second, the clinical utility of a test is best assessed by considering its predictive values and post-test probabilities in a specific clinical situation. Third, the predictive values and post-test probabilities depend very heavily on the pre-test probability (prevalence) of disease and, as a consequence, on both the clinical situation and the patient population in which a test is to be applied. This differs greatly from the popular misconceptions that test results are definitive (i.e., positive tests imply that patients are diseased and negative tests that they are not) and that the conclusions to be drawn from test results are independent of the patient who is tested.

The Assessment of Diagnostic Tests

New diagnostic tests and technologies are being developed at a constantly increasing rate, e.g., the prostatic acid phosphatase (PAP) test just discussed, positron emission tomography (PET), and magnetic resonance imaging (MRI). These new tests and techniques must obviously receive some form of evaluation before they enter into widespread clinical use and it is not surprising that the medical literature contains more and more articles about their "assessment".

Guidelines for the Assessment of New Tests or Techniques

The Purpose of the Diagnostic Test

Any proper assessment of a diagnostic test should begin with a clear statement of the proposed clinical purpose of the test. As we have just seen with the prostatic acid phosphatase radioimmunoassay test example, a clinical test may perform well in one situation e.g., diagnosis and fail in another, e.g., screening. The proposed clinical function dictates how the assessment itself should be carried out.

Clinical tests serve five different clinical functions: diagnosis, screening, staging, monitoring, and triage. *Diagnosis* is the "ruling in" or "ruling out" of a disease in a patient in whom the disease is clinically suspected (e.g., coronary angiography is a diagnositic technique for detecting coronary artery disease in a patient with angina). *Screening* refers to the presumptive detection of a disease in a group of individuals who are asymptomatic for a given disease and are not suspected of having it (e.g., mammography for the presumptive detection of breast cancer in middle aged women). *Staging* is the use of a clinical test to gauge how far a disease has advanced as a guide to treatment (e.g., mediastinoscopy to determine the resectability of a lung cancer). *Monitoring* uses a test to assess and adjust on-going therapy (e.g., prothrombin times to monitor the effect of anti-coagulant therapy). *Triage* refers to the use of a test to determine which patients should receive further invasive testing (e.g., Doppler studies to determine which patients should have cerebral angiography).

From the foregoing, it is clear that you should state the type of patient and the clinical setting in which you will use a test, and its purpose, before you embark on any assessment of it. The importance of this guideline will become more apparent as we continue.

The Spectrum and Number of Patients

When you are choosing the patients who will participate in a diagnostic test assessment, observe the rule: THE TYPE OF PATIENTS USED IN THE ASSESSMENT OF A TEST SHOULD REPLICATE THE TYPE OF PATIENTS FOR WHOM THE TEST IS INTENDED IN CLINICAL PRACTICE. Unfortunately, this rule is not always followed. To carry out an assessment, you require a population with the target disease to estimate sensitivity and a population free of the target disease to estimate specificity. You may be tempted, because of easy access, to use an already identified group with established, florid disease as the diseased group and a group of normal healthy controls as the non-diseased group. A moment's thought should convince you that such disparate groups would not challenge the clinical test with the wide spectrum of patients you and others will face in normal clinical practice. A test proposed for *diagnosis*, for example, should be assessed in a wide range of patients suspected of having the target disease and who may have other diseases that are often confused with the target disease. A *screening* test should be challenged with asymptomatic individuals like those it will be applied to in clinical practice.

The use of obviously diseased and healthy individuals as cases and controls will spuriously inflate both the sensitivity and specificity of the test since these individuals are most likely to have positive and negative tests, respectively. If you have started with a statement of the proposed function of the test, the proposed type of patient in whom it is to be used, and the proposed setting for its use, you merely need to assemble, consecutively, all the patients who match the specified profile seen in the appropriate setting(s) over a sufficient interval of time. The use of consecutive patients minimizes the possibility of introducing bias into the selection of patients and replicates the spectrum of patients the test will be applied to in its eventual clinical use.

If, for example, you wish to assess a new diagnostic test for DVT for use when patients first present themselves at the primary care level, you might consider using every consecutive patient who consults his or her family practitioner or arrives at his or her local emergency room with a swollen calf in whom DVT is suspected over a specified interval of time. Such a group will include patients who actually have DVT, in varying degrees of severity and some who have confusing disorders such as ruptured Baker's cysts or superficial thrombophlebitis. The performance of the test in such a group of patients will accurately reflect its performance in similar groups in similar primary care settings. If you propose to assess a *screening* test, for the early detection of prostatic carcinoma, you should state that the test is proposed for use in elderly men who are both asymptomatic and clinically normal, and then assess it in a large population of such individuals.

Too often, inadequate numbers of patients are used. For example, an investigator may assess a test in 25 diseased individuals, find that 20 of them have positive results, and conclude that the sensitivity is 80%. Technically, this is the best estimate for sensitivity based on the data but it should be noted that the 95% confidence limits around this estimate are very wide [64%,to 96%] (see Section II, Chapter 3). Although the investigator should take the conservative approach in such circumstances and use the lower limit (64%) as the estimate of sensitivity, more often than not sensitivity is simply stated as being 80%. The result is an overestimation of test validity. The only acceptable exception to the use of sufficient numbers of patients to ensure precise estimates occur when tests for rare target diseases are being assessed and the number of available patients is inescapably small.

The Gold Standard

The *gold standard* is the set of criteria used by investigators to determine which patients are truly diseased and which are not. Clearly, these criteria have a crucial impact on the 2 × 2 table and on determination of the sensitivity and specificity of the test. Gold standards may be definitive, e.g., histopathological results from biopsy, surgery, or autopsy, or may simply be the results of other diagnostic tests currently accepted as standards for the diagnosis of the target disease in question. In certain situations, the gold standard may be a complex of symptoms, signs, and test results, e.g., the classification systems for the diagnosis of rheumatoid arthritis, systemic lupus erythematosus, and rheumatic fever. In diagnostic test assessments, it is critically important that you use a gold standard that is well-defined, repeatable, and accepted as a current clinical standard for the diagnosis of the target disease. Anyone who reads your report on a diagnostic test assessment will want to know how the test will perform at detecting the presence or absence of the target disease in relation to the gold standard. If your gold standard is not well-defined or does not represent the current standard for diagnosis of the target disease, your assessment will be of little use because it will not be directly applicable to clinical practice. For example, since autopsy results or surgical findings are not usually available for patients with coronary artery disease (CAD), the results of coronary angiography are widely accepted as the clinical standard for diagnosis. Consequently if you wish to assess the performance of a new test in the diagnosis of CAD you might well utilize coronary angiography as your external gold standard for verifying the presence or absence of CAD in each patient; the angiographic criteria you use to establish the presence of CAD should be explicitly stated in your assessment report. Such explicit statements should include clear, repeatable criteria, such as "a stenosis of greater than 75% seen on independent review by two cardiologists" and avoid vague criteria, such as "any abnormality seen on angiography". The exact methods used to carry out the gold standard should also be described so that any reader can determine whether the gold standard, as used in your study corresponds with the one in use in his or her own clinical setting.

The Diagnostic Test

What has just been stated regarding the need for an exact, detailed description of your gold standard applies equally to the diagnostic test you are assessing, i.e., provide an explicit description of your test methodology, the conditions under which the test was performed, and how the patients were prepared. The detail you supply should be enough to enable the reader to perform the diagnostic test exactly as it was performed in your assessment.

When the test produces a quantitative result (e.g., the concentration of a serum constituent), you should assess its precision. The variability produced by the test technology can be assessed by comparing the results for several samples taken from the same patient at the same time; the intra-patient variability can be assessed by comparing the results for samples taken from the same patient at different times. The sensitivity, specificity, and predictive values should be calculated at several threshold values, e.g., the value that separates normal from abnormal results. When you choose a single threshold value, your choice should be justified.

If the test produces a qualitative result that requires interpretation (e.g., CT scans must be interpreted by a radiologist), clear and repeatable interpretation criteria must be given. In addition, you should assess both the inter and intra-observer variability in the interpretative component of the test by presenting the same consecutive panel of test results to two or more observers for independent review, and to a single observer for independent review on two or more separate occasions.

Independence

When each patient in your sample has undergone the diagnostic and gold standard tests, the results are compared in a 2 × 2 table (Fig. 2) to determine the test's validity and utility.

It is mandatory that the diagnostic test and the gold standard test be independent. Thus each patient must undergo both tests, i.e., the diagnostic test result must not influence the selection of who is to have the gold standard test. It also means that the process should be triple-blinded if possible, i.e., those who perform the tests, those who interpret them, and those who undergo them (the patients) should be kept 'blinded' until both tests have been performed and interpreted. The various individuals who perform, interpret, or undergo the diagnostic test, should be unaware of the gold standard results, if possible. Conversely, the various individuals who perform, interpret, or undergo the gold standard test, should be unaware of the diagnostic test results, if possible. If this independence is not maintained, expectation bias can occur and result in a spurious increase in the derived sensitivity, specificity, and predictive values. This is especially true when there is a significant subjective patient component or a significant interpretive component to the diagnostic test.

Assessment of Validity and Utility

When you have produced a 2 × 2 table; derived sensitivity, specificity, and predictive values; and concluded the test is useful if the values are reasonably high, you may think your job is finished. A proper assessment, however, should go on to consider the predictive values and post-test probabilities and their significance in the clinical situation proposed for the test. Since these values depend very heavily on the prevalence of the target disease in your patient sample (as determined by the gold standard), you must assess whether this prevalence is reasonably close to the true prevalence of the same disease in the proposed target population. It is virtually guaranteed that this will be so if you obeyed the principle of using all consecutive patients who are like those for whom the test is intended and who arrived at one or more settings similar to those in which use of the test is envisaged.

If, the prevalence in your patient sample is not a realistic estimate for the target population, you should recalculate the predictive values and post-test probabilities on the basis of a more realistic prevalence. This can be easily done using Baye's Theorem with the new prevalence value (P) and the derived sensitivity (SENS) and specificity (SPEC). Your assessment of clinical utility should center on whether the test provides enough information (on the basis of predictive values and post-test likelihoods) to cause a change in management. For example the radioimmunoassay test for PAP failed in the screening situation because the post-test likelihoods of a positive and negative test were not sufficiently different from the pre-test likelihood (prevalence) to affect any management decisions. A proper assessment, based on a realistic prevalence, could have demonstrated this in the initial analysis before any suggestions were made that the PAP should be utilized as a screening test.

When you assess clinical utility and the impact of the predictive values and post-test likelihood on clinical decisions, you must consider the consequences for false-positives and false-negatives. If the target disease is frequently fatal and a treatment exists that markedly alters the outcome (e.g., intra-abdominal bleeding, subdural hematoma, bacterial meningitis), false negatives are extremely undesirable and a high sensitivity is required. A high sensitivity value has the effect of markedly reducing the post-test likelihood of a negative test (i.e., the negative predictive value is raised) and provides reasonable certainty that the target disease is absent when the test is negative. If you are screening for a disease that is not immediately fatal if missed, for which no effective treatment is available, and/or for which the costs of labeling and further investigation of positives are high (e.g., cystic fibrosis in newborns), you will want to keep the number of false positives to a minimum and a high specificity will be required. A high specificity has the effect of markedly increasing the post-test likelihood of a positive test (i.e., the positive predictive value is raised) and provides reasonable certainty that the target disease is present when the test is positive.

In general, the impact of post-test likelihoods and predictive values on clinical decisions cannot be assessed without reference to the subsequent management of and consequences for positives and negatives.

References

1. Vershalmy J. Statistical problems in assessing methods of medical diagnosis with special reference to x-ray techniques. Public Health Rep 1947;62:1432–49.
2. Foti AG, Cooper JF, Hershman H, Malvaez RR. Detection of prostatic cancer by solid-shape radioimmunoassay of serum prostatic acid phosphatase. N Engl J Med 1977;297:1357–61.
3. Gittes R. Acid phosphatase reappraised. N Engl J Med 1977;297:1398–9.
4. Watson RA, Tang DB. The predictive value of prostatic acid phosphatase as a screening test for prostatic cancer. N Engl J Med 1980;303:497–9.
5. Bayes T. An essay toward solving a problem in the doctrine of chance. Philos Trans R Soc London 1763;53:370–418.

Additional Reading

1. Galen RS, Gambino SR. Beyond normality: the predictive value and efficiency of medical diagnoses. New York: John Wiley & Sons, 1975.
2. McNeil BJ, Keeler E, Adelstein SJ. Primer on certain elements of medical decision making. N Engl J Med 1975; 293:211–5.
3. Vecchio TJ. Predictive value of a single diagnostic test in unselected populations. N Engl J Med 1966;274:1171–3.
4. Department of Clinical Epidemiology and Biostatistics, McMaster University. How to read a clinical journal: II To learn about a diagnostic test. Can Med Assoc J 1981; 124:703–10.
5. Feinstein AR. On the sensitivity, specificity, and discrimination of diagnostic tests, in clinical biostatistics. St. Louis: CV Mosby Co., 1977:214–226.
6. Griner PF, Mayewski RJ, Mushlin AL, et al. Selection and interpretation of tests and procedures: principles and applications. Ann Int Med 1981;94:557–600.
7. Weinstein MC, Fineberg HV. Clinical decision analysis. Philadelphia: WB Sanunders Co., 1980.
8. Department of Clinical Epidemiology and Biostatistics, McMaster University: Interpretation of diagnostic data (six parts). Can Med Assoc J 1983;129:429–32, 559–64, 587, 705–10, 832–5, 947–54, 1093–9.
9. Sheps SB, Schechter MT. The assessment of diagnostic tests A survey of current medical research. JAMA 1984;252:2418%22.
10. Schechter MT, Sheps SB. Diagnostic testing revisited: pathways through uncertainty. Can Med Assoc J 1985;132:755–760.

7

Health Services Research: Focus on Surgery

J.I. Williams and W.R. Drucker

A Brief Overview of the Development of Health Services Research

Toward a Definition of the Field

Health services research is a field of study rather than a discipline. Investigators come from the health sciences (biostatistics, epidemiology, medicine and other health disciplines), management sciences (finance, management, marketing, organizational theory, and operations research), and the social sciences (anthropology, demography, economics, history, political science, psychology, and sociology). The mix of disciplines has shifted over time to meet changes in health policy, advances in research methods and technology, the availability of research funds, and the priorities of funding bodies.

A review of the literature reveals no one widely-accepted definition. Spitzer, Feinstein, Sackett (1) have defined health services research as the scientific investigation of alternate modes of service. It may focus on the providers, the structure of health manpower, and the organization of services; the health status and social and demographic characteristics of the population that determine utilization; the particular social and political milieu in which services are organized, the processes involved in the provision of care from the viewpoints of providers and consumers, and the outcomes for, or impact of health services on, patients, their families, and society at large. Alternatively, one can study the relationships between health status, the structure of services, the processes of service, and health outcomes.

In the Study on Surgical Services for the United States (SOSSUS) (2), undertaken by the American College of Surgeons and the American Surgical Association, focused on factors influencing patients, surgeons, and facilities. The factors influencing patients include patterns of disease, attitudes, socioeconomic status, and the availability and quality of care. With respect to surgeons, the study group focused on manpower supply, distribution, organization of practices, prevailing practices, workloads, and methods of remuneration. Ambulatory and inpatient facilities are related to patterns of payment, utilization, and various other factors that are internal and external to surgical services.

Classical epidemiologists have noted that the epidemiologic perspective should serve as the basic framework for health services research (3,4). At some point, health services have to be related to the numbers of individuals at risk, the incidence or prevalence of disease, and the determinants of disease, the natural history of the resulting health problems. While the cited definition includes the epidemiologic perspective, health services research requires data on the political context, organization, and functioning of services; the sociopersonal characteristics of individuals that determine the use of services; and the measures of functional status and quality of life used to assess the impact of health services. All these pieces of information are additional to the demographic and clinical data traditionally employed in epidemiologic research.

The goal of health services is to provide efficacious care to persons who can benefit from it in a manner that is acceptable to the providers, at an acceptable cost to the public-at-large. The purpose of health services research is to determine whether the goal has been achieved, in whole or in part, and to identify the factors that enhance or diminish the possibility of achieving it.

The Development of Health Services Research

Two major conferences have been held on health services research. The Health Services Research Study Section of the United States Public Health Service commissioned the first one, and a series of meetings were held, beginning in 1965. The *Milbank Memorial Fund Quarterly* published the proceedings in 1966. The United States Center for Health Services Research, sponsored the second conference in 1984, *Medical Care* published the results in 1985.

The Institute of Medicine of the National Academy of Sciences has reviewed health services research projects funded by the federal government in the United States, and published its report in 1979 (5). Georgopoulos (6) reviewed 1303 studies of hospital organization published between 1960 and 1969, (7) Flook and Sanazaro reviewed 1,293 studies through 1972. Culyer et al (8) have compiled a bibliography of health economics, articles written in English; Griffiths (9) has noted articles from Western European sources; and Van Eimeren and Kopke (10) have abstracted nearly 5000 health research studies from 27 countries. More recently Warner and Luce (11), completed a major review of studies of cost-benefit analysis of health interventions.

While health services research projects are reported from countries around the world, most of the research is carried out by investigators from the United States. In addition to the research funds provided by the National Center for Health Services Research, the National Institutes of Health gives grants for research and training. The Office of Technology Assessment of the Congress of the United States commissions reviews of major new health technologies. Major private foundations also study health services directly or fund research projects. In the 1970's, the United States provided federal funds to establish university centers for health services research. A large number of university and private research firms now compete for contracts.

In Canada, the federal and provincial governments have commissioned major health service inquiries, both before and after the introduction of universal, public medical care insurance. The federal and provincial governments have also established foundations or government organizations to review and fund proposals for health services research.

In Great Britain, the government has commissioned major studies on the National Health System and research proposals by independent investigators are also funded. The World Health Organization has sponsored internal comparisons of Health Services.

In Canada, Great Britain and the United States, researchers are generally located in university departments of their basic disciplines or in multidisciplinary departments in schools of medicine. In the United States, researchers may also be concentrated in schools of public health.

Research studies reflect shifts in health policy over the past 20 years. Twenty years ago, the major issues were the availability of, and access to health resources and financial coverage of the costs of health services. The most striking change, noted by Neuhauser (12) is the shift in focus from the internal dynamics of medical care to its costs and effects.

Relatively few of the health services studies focus on surgery. In this chapter, we highlight the major research issues that have emerged in relation to surgical services.

The terms encountered most commonly in published articles are *organization of health services, financing of health services, availability, accessibility, utilization, health manpower, health status, need, demand, supply, mode of practice, method of payment, patient-provider relationships, health beliefs, health promotion, information systems, technology assessment, clinical decision-making, monitoring, quality assurance, risk management, efficacy, effectiveness, benefit and evaluation.*

Availability, Accessibility, and Acceptability of Surgical Services

Although the issue is not settled, there is a growing consensus that there is a surplus of medical doctors in North America. Governments are decreasing the number of approved post-graduate training positions, and some states and provinces are beginning to reduce the size of medical school classes. There are also concerns about the total number of physicians, their distribution by region and their types of practice. Health service researchers are focusing on physician: population ratios (availability), the accessibility of physicians to the public, and patterns of utilization.

Availability

Availability relates to the *supply* of health resources. Inventories of health manpower, hospitals and other services are now rather common place. The numbers of physicians and hospital beds, by specialty and region, are given. Rates are derived to show either physicians (specialists) or hospital beds per 10,000 or 100,000 population, or the number of persons per physician. Marked variations are evident between countries and within countries in resource-population ratios, particularly for surgical specialties (13,14).

There is little agreement on optimal surgeon: population ratios. The SOSSUS group concluded that there were too many surgeons, low workloads, and a wide spread in their distribution (15), after studying the surgery performed, in 1970, in four diverse geographical areas. Surgical services were weighted in terms of time and complexity, using California Relative Values, and workload estimates were derived for the physicians performing surgery in the areas studied. Williams (16) used the same procedures to study surgical services in Rhode Island, in 1977, and compared the results to the 1970 findings. He found that the trends had continued, in spite of the recommendations from SOSSUS.

The SOSSUS conclusions cannot be extended to other jurisdictions. In Canada, almost 50% of graduating physicians become general practitioners and family physicians; the percentage is now 70% in some provinces. Current concerns are about recruiting physicians into specialty residency training programs and placing specialists in the more rural and remote regions.

In most industrialized countries, the rural and remote regions have less favourable physician-population ratios, even in communities with hospitals equipped to provide surgical services. Various placement and incentive systems are used to achieve a more equitable distribution, but best, they offer only short-term solutions; no system has achieved the goal of long-term placement of health manpower in underserviced areas.

Mortality rates for some diseases have declined, particularly heart diseases, but the rates for other diseases, including most cancers, have not. Verbugge (17) has examined age-specific mortality after age 45 in the United States, and has attempted to determine whether the declines are due to reductions in incidence and prevalence, or increases in survival rates for persons with disease. Since no notable declines are evident in the incidence or prevalence of major diseases, the inescapable conclusion is that individuals in the United States will live longer, but in worsening states of health. Consequently, as individuals born during the post-war baby boom age, the need and demand for all health services will outstrip current supplies (18).

In Canada, Lefebvre, Zsigmond, and Devereaux (19) studied the potential impact of an aging population on hospital beds (1979). By applying the 1975 rates of hospital admissions and average lengths of stay to various projections of the age-sex composition of Canadian society, they estimated that demand would outstrip the availability of hospital beds in the 1990's. Using similar projections, a task force in Ontario (20) has projected that the demand for physicians' services will outstrip the supply by 2001.

Detsky (21) has outlined the mechanisms used by the state to regulate the supply of physicians:

1. funds for medical schools based on the number of students,
2. financial aid to students,
3. control of the number of residency training positions,
4. setting of size and composition of the medical student body, and
5. regulating the flow of foreign medical graduates.

Governments vary in the extent to which they regulate physician supply, in toto or by speciality. One can anticipate that governments will monitor the supply of health resources and projected levels of demand, and search for less costly ways of meeting the requirements.

Accessibility

In the 1960's and 1970's, there was concern about basic inequities in access to health care related to age, place of residence, race, and ability to pay. Respondents selected in large probability samples were used to study the determinants of health services accessibility to the population at large. The major health surveys conducted in the home included those by the National Center for Health Studies, the Centre for Health Administration Studies at the University of Chicago (22,23), the Internal Comparison of Medical Care Utilization of the World Health Organization (24) conducted in eight countries, and Cartwright and others in England (25,26).

By comparing the self-reports of symptoms, disability and other health problems with health services used by respondents, investigators have attempted to measure unmet need (27). There is now a consensus that needs are the principal reasons for using health services, and that inequities in access have been reduced over time. The changes are related to increases in the health insurance coverage of the populations surveyed.

Although the surveys ask about outpatient and hospitals services, surgical services have not been a major focus of any of the studies. Andersen, Lion, and Anderson (22) noted an increase in the use of surgical services over two decades in the United States. They only report an increase in rates of 5 surgical services per 100 person-years in 1963 to 6 per 100 person-years in 1970.

Some surgical services, such as abortion, tubal ligation, vasectomy (fertility control), plastic or reconstructive surgery for basically cosmetic reasons and elective repairs of joints damaged by arthritis or injury are driven by consumer demand. Other procedures have become popular or fashionable and are provided, in part, in response to demand. The effect of demand on utilization of surgical services has not been studied extensively.

Surgery is largely performed to correct specific health problems, referred to surgeons by other physicians. Cunsumers may have a perception of the availability of surgeons in their areas, but it is unlikely that they identify their unmet needs and the required level of access to relevant surgical services.

Acceptability

Beyond the study of availability and accessibility of health services, researchers have focused on acceptability, in terms of patient satisfaction. Patients have been asked questions about the timing involved in obtaining primary care, the facilities, the costs involved, the competence of the clinician, and the quality of the doctor-patient relationships. The best summary of the literature has been written by Ware and Associates (28).

Most of the measures were developed for the study of community-based ambulatory care. Research on doctor–patient communication and compliance tend to focus on medical care and regimes that require doctor–patient interactions over a period of time. Because the surgeon–patient relationship is immediate and ends relatively soon after treatment, its character and quality differ fundamentally from that with the physician who provides comprehensive and continuous care.

Patient complaints, claims of damage, and malpractice suits have become matters of concern. In some jurisdictions, the increase in medical liability insurance fees has become sufficiently large to force changes in the ways surgeons practice.

Few studies have examined which patients are most likely to initiate legal action or the characteristics of the physicians against whom the action is taken. Some evidence suggests that patients are more likely to sue if their physicians have not taken time to communicate and establish an adequately therapeutic relationship with the patient.

When dissatisfaction leads to a formal complaint and legal action, the insurance industry and the legal sector play key roles in the process, but health service researchers have been slow to initiate studies in these areas.

Utilization

Data forms for the administration and financial reimbursement of health services rendered have become major sources of information on those who provide and consume health services. Hospital discharge summaries, such as those submitted to PAS in the United States or the HMRI in Canada, and billing statements of physicians provide basic information about the specialties of physicians, diagnoses, and services rendered, as well as the age, sex, and residence of patients. Hospital discharge summaries tend to be more complete and available for secondary analysis than outpatient data.

Depending on the political jurisdiction, data

on inpatient services are likely to be more available and more informative than those on outpatient services. Outpatient data are only collected if third party payment is involved, and the governments or insurance companies who gather them tend to use unique formats and processing systems. The lack of availability of information on outpatient surgical services becomes more important as the proportion of surgical services performed on an outpatient basis increases.

Most comparisons of surgical services focus on in-hospital procedures. Studies have looked at surgical utilization rates over time, or at national or international variations occurring at the same time. While there are variations in all surgical procedures, most of the studies focus on elective procedures, such as tonsillectomy/adenoidectomy, hysterectomy, excision of varicose veins, and coronary bypass. Given the lack of agreement in defining need, diagnosis and clinical decision-making, non-medical factors may play a major role in determining how many elective surgical services are performed.

McCathy, Finkel and Reichlin (29) have noted that, in the United States, the rates of surgical services remained relatively constant between 1940 and 1970, but rose 24% between 1970 and 1978. While some surgical services, such as operations on the knee, cataracts, and prostate increased 70.3, 46.9, and 43.5%, respectively, appendectomies and T/A's declined by 6 and 43.3%, respectively. More recently, concern has been expressed about the steady increase in the number of coronary bypass procedures. Although it was only introduced in the early 1970's by 1981 it had become the most commonly performed major surgical procedure (160,000 procedures) in the United States (30).

Some health economists, such as Evans (31) in Canada, believe that physicians hold a monopoly over medical services and can create a demand for them. These economists hold that the increase in surgical procedures is a direct reflection of the increasing number of surgeons performing them.

McCarthy and Finkel (32) considered other reasons, such as changes in diagnostic coding procedures, improvements in technology, and increased consumer demand arising from coverage of costs by health insurance. Improvements in technology have improved the benefits of surgery while reducing the risks. Some increase in demand also arises from the increased coverage of the population by health insurance. The research question now is what is the relative importance of the various factors in explaining variations and changes in the rates of surgical services?

McPherson, Wennberg, Hovind and Clifford (14) have studied variations in surgical rates in New England, England and Norway; McPherson, Strong, Epstein, and Jones (13) have studied variations in England and Wales, Canada, and the United States; and, Stockwell and Vayda (33) made earlier comparisons between Canada, England, and Wales. At the risk of over-generalization, two sets of conclusions can be drawn from these studies. The utilization rates of surgical services are highest in the United States and Canada, lowest in England and Wales, and midway in Norway. Secondly, the within-country variations were greatest in Canada, followed by the United States, Norway, England and Wales, in that order. The differences appear to be related to variations in the availability of surgical services.

Some studies, such as those by Wennberg (34) in New England, Vayda and his associates in Ontario (35), and Roos, Roos et al (36), in Manitoba, have focused on variations within countries. Essentially, they all found large variations in the rates for elective surgery that cannot be explained by differences in demographic characteristics, indicators of health status, or other characteristics. Depending on the elective procedure under review, the variations seem to depend on the availability of surgical resources, be they hospital services or surgeons.

Wennberg and Gittelson (37) and Wennberg (38) are proponents of small area analysis of utilization, i.e., discrete hospital market areas of between 10,000 and 200,000 residents. It is a supply-side model in which analysis focuses on the relationship between hospital beds, personnel, modes of practice, and utilization rates. Census data on demographic and economic characteristics are used to describe the population; utilization rates can be adjusted for age, sex, and other confounding variables. Special purpose household health interviews may also be used to define patterns of consumer behavior in the areas.

The surveys conducted to assess access, availability, and satisfaction with service have been based on a model developed by Andersen

(39). This epidemiologic model of consumer behaviour describes predisposing factors, enabling factors, and need as the primary determinants of utilization, with need as the most important Hulka and Wheat, (40)

Wennberg (38) favours the supply model over the needs model, for two reasons. Firstly, Roos and Roos (41) have demonstrated that, for the aged in Manitoba, variations in surgical rates are not related to the health needs or status of the elderly; rates of surgical use were higher among the more highly educated elderly and this suggests that the difference may be due to demand. Wennberg's study (38) confirmed the lack of relationship between variations in surgical rates and apparent need. Secondly, Wennberg would rather focus on factors that can be changed by health policy; health status cannot be so changed.

Roos and her associates (42) have extended their studies to look at patterns of hospital admission and readmission of patients of family practitioners, internists, general surgeons or obstetrician/gynecologists, when they were the unique providers of hospital care. Again there were marked variations in hospital admissions and readmissions which could not be explained by the health or sociodemographic characteristics of the patients. Physicians who were high users had 27% of the patients, and they accounted for 42% of the hospital days. The high users tended to be rural physicians in areas with high bed-to-population ratios and hospitals with low occupancy rates. The patterns did not vary significantly by the specialty of the physician providing hospital care.

Utilization reviews and studies of local hospital markets have their problems. Studies, such as those just described, have focused on elective procedures for conditions where medical uncertainty is supposedly high and the role of nonmedical factors can be assessed. It would be interesting to see if the same patterns hold for surgery driven by demand, such as plastic surgery for cosmetic purposes, and for surgery that is required or urgent. In the studies of cardiovascular or even breast surgery for cancer, there are large elements of uncertainty, and nonmedical factors may play an important role in decision-making.

Local hospital markets may also be served by secondary or tertiary hospitals in other regions or areas. When patients in one area go to another area for specific procedures, it is not clear how important the factors in the local hospital market are.

Measures of functioning, disease, and disability that are suitable for household interviews or drawing epidemiologic profiles may be such crude measures of need that important variations in the requirements for surgical services can and may be missed. Since models are lacking for research to demonstrate how changes in modes of practices or clinical decision-making are related to supply factors, it is not clear how health policy could be altered to effect the desired changes in surgeons' clinical decisions.

The marked variations are not characterized either in terms of "over "or "under" utilization. Appropriate utilization can only be judged by relating the expected benefits to specific needs. Beyond need, there is the consideration of demand. At some point, consumer demands and preferences have to be taken into account, but this has not been done yet in surgical services research.

There is little question that surgeons are influenced by nonmedical factors when they make surgical decisions. Eisenberg (43) believes that physicians' personal desires and interests, motives when acting for patients, and concerns for social good are among these factors. Personal desires include income, style of practice, practice setting, and the desired role in clinical leadership. Physicians also take account of patients' ability to pay, desire for quality clinical care in the face of uncertainty, and other demands, including defensive medicine and convenience. The tradeoffs in decision-making become more complex when the constraints of societal resources are added to the balance between the physician's personal desires and the patient's well-being.

Outcomes

Since the goal is to provide health services to those whom it may benefit, researchers have studied the impact of medical and surgical care on the lives of patients and have developed measures for determining the effects of interventions on health status. The highest priority outcome is avoidance of death, the second is prevention of disability, and the third is reduction of morbidity from disease and interventions. Functional status and quality of life are related, but independent, concerns. Ideally, if the first three goals are achieved, the last two will follow, but not necessarily so. Interventions may be made when death or disability are inescapable, and the health professional is striving to improve the functional status or the quality of the life that remains. A discussion of specific measures of outcome is provided in Section II, Chapter 2.

Surgeons are free to introduce technical innovations or change surgical procedures at will; their efficacy or effectiveness need not be demonstrated. Once styles of practice are established, surgeons have no reason to change unless they come under the scrutiny of discipline reviews or legal proceedings.

If surgeons deem certain innovations or changes in procedures to be beneficial, they may report them as case studies or as outcomes in a cohort of patients over time. In teaching and research institutions, the experiences of patients receiving new surgical services can be compared with those of patients receiving conventional therapy. Observational or non-experimental studies have their advantages and limitations, and their value can be determined by how well controlled they are in design, execution, and analysis.

Ideally, a given surgical intervention only takes place after its efficacy and effectiveness have been established in well designed studies. A treatment's efficacy is defined as the outcome observed in a specific population of patients who receive a defined treatment—usually in the context of a controlled trial of the treatment. In the real world surgeons vary, e.g., in skill and techniques, hospitals vary, and patients vary, e.g., in compliance.

Effectiveness is defined as the outcomes likely to be achieved when a treatment is introduced into clinical practice. In general, the effects achieved in real life are less than the optimal effects obtained in a controlled trial. A treatment found to be efficacious in the relatively artificial conditions of a controlled trial often proves to be relatively less effective when introduced into widespread clinical practice.

In summary, efficacy deals with the question, "*can* an intervention work?" Effectiveness, in contrast, answers "*does* it work" in the real world.

Although controversies about the efficacy of various surgical procedures abound, there have been relatively few clinical trials as noted by Chalmers (44). Nevertheless, there have been a few noteworthy trials, such as those undertaken since 1971 by the National Surgical Adjuvant Breast Project Group to assess alternative forms of surgical, chemical, and radiation treatments for cancer of the breast (see Section III, Chapter 4). For specific types of breast cancer, it is now established that a combination of segmental mastectomy, breast irridation and chemotherapy provide the best effects over five years. In earlier research, the NSABP showed that the same effects could be achieved with simple as with total mastectomy.

Randomized controlled trials by the Veterans' Administration (45), the European Coronary Surgery Study Group (46), and the Coronary Artery Surgery Study (47,48) have established the short term efficacy and long term effectiveness of coronary artery bypass surgery, for patients with impaired left ventricular function in terms of survival and quality of life. The improvements have not extended to employment or recreational activities. The same studies have established that medical management is preferable for patients with angina or clogged vessels who do have impaired left ventricular function. In the latter group, surgical treatment reduces angina and pain, and improves the quality of life, but does not reduce mortality.

Although these results have been accepted scientifically, appropriate changes in surgical practice for cancer of the breast (49) and coronary artery disease in the United States (30) have been slow to follow. Each year, thousands of patients, who are inappropriate candidates according to the criteria established by the three cited studies, have coronary bypass operations.

The major randomized trial reported most recently is the one on extracranial-intracranial (EC/IC) arterial bypass by the EC/IC Bypass Study Group (50,51). Patients with symptomatic atherosclerotic disease of the internal carotid artery were randomly assigned to the best medical care currently possible or to medical care with bypass surgery. During the period of follow-up, which averaged 56 months, the bypass patients demonstrated a lack of benefits with respect to mortality, morbidity, and disability, when compared to the medically-treated patients. No subgroup of patients benefited specifically from the procedures. It will be interesting to see what impact the study has on the subsequent incidences of EC/IC bypass procedures.

It is harder to evaluate surgical procedures than medical care by means of randomized clinical trials. In medical care, specifically drug trials, patients who meet the eligibility criteria can be randomly assigned to a therapy and be placed on standard protocols while keeping both the physicians and patients blind to the assignments.

In surgical care, the surgeon and patient are unavoidably aware of the assigned treatment arm. Moreover, since surgeons vary in skill and make minor modifications in their techniques, the treatment itself can never be completely standardized. Surgeons have confidence in their professional skills and patients have faith that the procedure selected by their surgeon is the best one for them. Since neither the surgeons nor the patients are blind to the procedures used, the assessments of outcomes by either groups is likely to be biased (52).

At one point, the National Surgical Adjuvant Project for Breast and Bowel Cancers faced the difficulty of having participating physicians accruing eligible patients to a trial. The informed consent protocol involved having the participating physicians explain the treatment options to the patients, and then specifying the treatment procedure after consent had been obtained. It was difficult for the surgeons to discuss the uncertainty of treatment, when they themselves had successfully performed the procedures and would be expected to do so again once the patients had been assigned (53). The problem was resolved by making assignments to the treatment arm before obtaining consent. Subsequently, the accrual rates increased to acceptable levels because the surgeons found they could comfortably discuss a particular procedure with the patients, and then ask them to participate.

The scientific and ethical issues of randomized trials are intensified if the effects of the experimental therapeutic maneouver can not be reversed. Generally speaking, the risk of this occuring is greater for trials for surgical interventions than medical interventions. There is no question about the randomized, controlled trial being the optimal design for the evaluation of clinical interventions. As Rudicel and Esdaile (55) suggest, there are times when scientific and ethical issues dictate that other designs should be employed in surgical trials. Finding the best design for a trial is a constant challenge to the clinician and methodologist alike.

Trials of modes of delivering and paying for health services can be organized (56). In patient care trials, like those just cited, the goal is to assess the effect of a specific treatment intervention on clinical outcomes. In health services trials, the goal may be the assessment of i) different modes of payment and insurance (Health Insurance Experiment Study by the Rand Corporation) (54); ii) a new type of health professional (e.g., Burlington randomized trial of nurse practitioners)(55), facility, or practice (e.g., outpatient surgery versus inpatient surgery); or iii) the introduction of new arrangements for health care (e.g., reorganization of emergency medical services and introduction of paramedic services into Kings County, Washington) (56).

Depending on the kind of health service under study, the experimental unit may comprise providers, practices, hospitals, geographical areas, or insurance plans. Ideally, the unit of analysis should be the same as the unit of assignment; if it is not (e.g., if communities or neighborhoods are assigned to a new or a conventional organization of services, but the responses of individuals in the community are used as the unit of analysis), difficulties will be encountered in the design of the trial.

Trials of new services present a number of problems. While you may randomly assign experimental units to different modes of delivering health services, everyone concerned will be aware of the assignments and will react accordingly. For example, once a trial is set, those involved in providing service in a traditional mode may strive to show that their services are as good or better than the new ones, and may succeed in doing so by working harder than usual. Another problem arises if the new mode is evaluated during the introductory period when organizational problems are common and those delivering the service have not had a chance to achieve an operating level of efficiency. Lastly, individuals involved in the conventional mode of delivering services may lobby or maneuver to protect their interests if the new mode is perceived as a threat. The health services trial must be carefully designed and implemented if the new mode of delivery is to receive a fair and objective testing.

Cost Analysis

Given the current emphasis on cost containment and the rationing of health services, it is not surprising that economic analysis of medical care is a major part of health services research. The cost of health care includes service costs, out-of-pocket expenses paid by patients and their families, and indirect costs. The service costs include the fees or salaries of the health care providers, the cost of technical services, and the fraction of overhead and administrative costs allocated to each service. Patients and their families may pay supplemental costs for drugs, appliances, travel expenses, and other goods and services directly related to treatment. Service costs and out-of-pocket expenses can be referred to as direct costs.

Indirect costs include time lost from work and the burden imposed by uncertainty, pain and suffering on patients and their families, but the assignment of dollars values to the indirect costs is controversial (31). More detailed information on this topic is provided by Drummond (57) and by Stoddart and Drummond (58,59).

The four types of cost analysis are: cost-efficiency, cost-effectiveness, cost benefit and cost-utility. Cost-efficiency analysis is the simplest. It focuses on the cost per unit of service produced, without regard to the effects. Generally, it is assumed that the effects of the two modes of health service delivery (e.g., surgical care in an outpatient center versus in hospital) are equivalent and acceptable. Costs are analyzed, usually from the perspective of the provider, and a judgment is made concerning the relative efficiency of the two modes of health service delivery.

Cost-effectiveness analysis involves relating marginal differences in cost per unit of service to marginal differences in effects or outcomes. Pineault and his associates (60) compared costs, clinical outcomes, and patient satisfaction for patients who received tubal ligations, hernia repairs or meniscectomies on an inpatient versus on outpatient basis. The clinical outcomes were comparable, but the efficiency of outpatient surgery produced savings of $86.00 for each tubal ligation and $115.00 for each hernia repair. The outpatient cost of each meniscectomy was $173.00 higher for outpatients than for inpatients. Aside from the costs, the outpatients thought that the length of care they received was too short and clearly preferred inpatient care, particularly the meniscectomy patients. Although the indirect costs identified by the consumers were not put into dollar terms, it is clear that they have to be taken into account.

A major problem in cost-effectiveness analyses is deciding how to equate the different outcomes. In the study just described the clinical outcomes were judged to be equivalent, but the consumers preferred inpatient services and it is not clear how these preferences should be weighted in the results.

Cost-benefit analysis tries to translate all the effects or outcomes of importance into economic terms, i.e. in dollars or other monetary units. The calculations include the costs of treatment over time, lifetime earnings, and external costs and benefits encountered by patients and then families, such as the impact on family life and opportunities forgone by one or more family members. Money loses value over time through inflation, and interest or dividends could be earned by investing it rather than expending it on health care. Consequently, the costs saved over time or the benefits gained in the future, have to be discounted and expressed in terms of their monetary value when the medical care is delivered. A number of assumptions and value judgments have to be made about the economic values to be attached to the effects of care over time and the discount rate to be applied (31).

For example, patients with stable angina may undergo coronary bypass surgery and experience symptomatic relief, but the other effects and benefits would be the same if they received medical care, instead. Hemenway and associates (61) estimate that the cost of care over three years is four times higher for surgical than for medical patients. The challenge is how to state the benefits of relief from angina and other complaints in monetary terms so that the reduction in psychic costs achieved by surgery can be compared to the increase in the cost of care incurred by surgery.

Boyle and Torrance (62) recommend cost utility analysis as an alternative to cost benefit analysis. Once the effects of health care are known, the health status of the individual can be described in terms of the key dimensions of functioning. Respondents are then asked to rate each discrete health state on a continuum of 0 (the same as death) to 1 (normal health and functioning). The mean utility value for a given health state is then used to estimate the value of the care. It takes the place of benefits expressed in economic terms in the analysis.

In an economic evaluation of a neo-natal intensive care unit, Boyle, Torrance et al. (63,64) used cost-effectiveness, cost-benefit analyses, and cost-utility analysis to assess the impact of intensive care on very low birthweight infants. Some health states were given negative utility values, i.e., severe mental or physical disability was rated as being worse than death. Although some infants weighing < 1000 grams survived, their health states were such that the value of intensive care for then could be questioned in terms of cost-utility or cost-benefit. This is a new approach to economic analysis, and clinicians and researchers, alike, are debating its merit.

Warner and Luce (11) reviewed cost-benefit and cost-effectiveness studies and found that relatively few economic evaluations of surgical services were published prior to 1980. Most are included in a book on "Costs, Risks, and Benefits of Surgery," edited by Bunker, Barnes, and Mosteller (65).

Organization and Financing of Medical Care

Alternate strategies for rationing health care (66) and cost-containment are controversial topics. In the United States and England, and to a lesser extent in Canada, the relative merits of private and public control of health resources (67) are debated and considerable attention is now devoted to the effects of alternative modes of payment and organization on the costs and quality of health care. This section will be limited to brief discussions of a second opinion for elective surgery, alternative organizations for surgical centers, and modes of payment for health care.

Second Opinion for Elective Surgery

Various states in the United States have set up programs that require patients receiving public assistance for medical expenses to obtain a second medical opinion before payment can be authorized for designated elective surgical procedures. The goal is to contain costs by curtailing unnecessary surgery. McCarthy and Finkel (68,29) have reviewed and summarized a number of studies of the outcomes and cost savings associated with such programs. Two or three years after surgery was originally recommended and a second opinion had been obtained on the need for it 11.1% had had neither medical nor surgical care. The savings more than offset the costs of the second opinion (69).

Finkel and Associates (70) also noted that 25% of the patients for whom the first and second physicians agreed that surgery was necessary did not have it. It is not known what the consequences were for the health of the patients.

Alternative Organization of Surgical Centers

In the United States, profit and non-profit corporations, such as the Health Maintenance Organization, large groups of physicians in practice, and multihospital systems are reorganizing health services. One result of studies documenting the cost efficiency of performing selected procedures on an outpatient basis, is the formation of Free-standing Ambulatory Surgery Centers (FASC). Ermann and Gabel (71) have provided an overview of their activities. In 1983, over 370,000 operations were performed in about 250 FASCs. The same authors estimate that, by 1986, 900,000 operations will be performed in 270 FASCs.

Although it is easy to understand how substantial cost savings can be achieved, the case-mix and severity of cases may not be the same in FASCs as it is in hospitals, and cost savings relate only to the costs of providing care, without considering the direct and indirect costs paid by patients. The few studies of outcomes in FASCs reveal small numbers of surgically related deaths and post-operative complications, but this may be the result of careful screening of patients prior to surgery (72).

So far, no data system in the United States has uniform information on all surgical patients. Davis (73) has recommended that such a system be put in place and that the following classification be used to define the levels of surgical care provided:

Level 1. Minor ambulatory surgery—Surgery on patients who are neither hospitalized nor held for observation following surgery.

Level 2. Minor ambulatory surgery—outpatient surgery where a period of post-operative care is provided.

Level 3. Inhospital surgery.

If hospitals provide care for patients with more serious surgical and other health problems, and FASC provide care for young, healthy patients, FASC should be more efficient when only operating costs are compared. Any research study must control for the differences in case-mix, and then compare the FASC with hospitals in complete cost-effectiveness analysis.

Mode of Payment

Patients in Health Maintenance Organizations have lower rates of hospitalization due, in part, to the range of services provided in HMOs and in part, to a more conservative philosophy about hospital care. LoGerfo and colleagues (74) compared the rate of surgical intervention for patients in an HMO with that for patients in a large independent practice in the same area. They concluded that part of the difference in rates was due to the fee-for-service incentives present in the private practice but not in the HMO.

There is concern that the cost-containment push in the United States and elsewhere could lead to a lowering of the quality of, and access to, health care for the poor (75). Ermann and Gabel (76) recommend that studies on the impact of reorganization of services address the issues of quality and access as well as cost.

Monitoring, Quality Assurance, and Information Systems

Studies of interventions follow a pattern. The development of the intervention occurs first and clinical trials of it take place later. Ideally, its efficacy and effectiveness are established through well controlled trials, and its marginal effects and benefits yield acceptable cost ratios vis-à-vis other interventions. The next step is to make sure that, in a large scale implementation, the intervention is effectively and efficiently (quality assurance) provided to the patients in the community who need it. The last steps are to assess the impact of the intervention in terms of the public good, and to determine what changes, if any, should be made.

Monitoring, quality assurance, and information systems are required to determine whether efficacious and effective surgical services are being efficiently provided to the patients who can benefit from them. Monitoring can be simply a review of the rates of delivery of specific surgical services to detect outliers. For example, Luft (77,78) studied the relation between hospital size and case mortality rates. The hospital discharge summaries of > 800,000 surgical patients taken from the PAS files for 1974 and 1975 were grouped by patients' age and sex and the presence of single or multiple diagnoses. For each of the 20 patient groups so established, Luft compared the specific surgical case fatality rates for hospitals grouped according to the frequency with which they provided the same specific surgical services. For open heart, coronary artery bypass, vascular, and transurethral prostatic surgery, case fatality rates consistently dropped as the number of such operations increased in any given hospital. For a second set of operations, the case fatality rates were highest in hospitals where the operations were relatively infrequently and lower in hospitals where they were performed a basic number times each year; and no further decline in fatality rates occurred in hospitals where more than the same basic number of operations were performed. Case fatality rates for the third set of surgical procedures were not related to the surgical activity levels of the hospitals. On the basis of these results, Luft suggested that specific sets of operations should be regionalized so that the hospitals providing them could do so often enough to minimize case mortality rates. Luft recognized, however, that the linkage between frequency of operations and reduction of case mortality rates cannot be specified.

Farber, Kaiser, and Wenzel (79) reviewed 25,000 surgical operations in the state of Virginia and came to similar conclusions about the frequency of operations and infection rates. Infection rates in appendectomy, herniorrhaphy, cholecystectomy, colon resection, and abdominal hysterectomy cases were inversely related to the logarithm of the number of such operations.

The Government of Saskatchewan expressed its concern about the increasing number of hysterectomies being performed by appointing a professional monitoring commission. The subsequent dramatic drop in the number of hysterectomies was attributed to this surveillance (80). But a similar experiment with a medical care review organization did not alter patterns of medical care in New Mexico (81).

Quality assurance systems go one step further. They review the entire spectrum of providers' practice activities to identify questionable areas and to pinpoint specific providers whose practices require change. In the United States and Canada, hospitals must have active quality assurance programs to maintain their accreditation.

Donabedian (82,83) and Williamson et al (84,85) have written definitive treatises on the design and implementation of quality assurance programs. Such programs should include measures of structure, process, and outcome, and their standards and criteria should reflect the findings of evaluative studies in health care. However, it is not yet possible to describe the systems currently being put into place nor to discern what cost effective improvements they have produced in the provision of health care.

The current lack of appropriate information constrains, and impedes the activities of health service researchers and clinical investigators. The revolutions in computer design and data management systems offer some hope that adequate informational data bases will eventually become realities, but it is beyond the scope of this chapter to discuss how they could be designed to overcome the constraints that researchers face.

Conclusion

Health services research has developed very rapidly during the past 20 years, and the issues that dominate the field relate to cost containment, outcomes, and quality of care. There is, however, no direct relation between health services management, health policy decision-making and the availability of information from health services research. Because studies have to be focused on specific places, persons, and events within a given time period, the results may not be applicable to other settings. Even studies in the same area may yield findings that are contradictory, in whole or in part. Decision-makers are understandably slow to adopt controversial findings, unless they predisposed to believe them. When the information obtained is consistent over a series of studies, it can be sufficiently persuasive that providers, the public, and policy makers have to pay attention. This is when health services research is most likely to have its greatest impact.

Despite the contemporary limitations of health services research, some issues require systematic study to assess the impact of health services on society. For example, millions of dollars and extensive efforts by the health professions, hospitals and government have been directed into the establishment of regional trauma programs in the United States. According to the Emergency Medical Services System legislation of 1973 and 1976, 303 nationally-designed, geographic EMS areas with the following characteristics (86) were to be formed:

1. Rapid notification of injury (one emergency telephone number, 911, and coordinated communication between police, fire, and ambulance services).
2. Immediate provision of basic and advanced life support by ambulance services.
3. Designated regional hospitals with trauma teams and definitive trauma services; and,
4. Triage protocols and transfer agreements between hospitals.

The respective roles and responsibilities of ambulance personnel, physicians in the emergency room, the organization of hospital services for trauma victims; and what technologies to employ at the accident or injury site, in the ambulance, in the emergency room, and in the hospital have been topics of considerable debate.

Surgeons in the United States have established the American Trauma Association as a forum for debates about the organization of EMSs and a stimulator of research on the impact of such services. Surgeons are also involved in such related associations as the American Association of Automotive Medicine. Numerous clinical and some regional studies have attempted to evaluate the outcomes of trauma care. Measures of the severity if different injuries have been developed to estimate the expected mortality and morbidity; their precision and predictive power are being evaluated in clinical and methodological studies. Attempts are also being made to establish a national trauma registry.

Although widespread improvements have occurred in emergency services, the shape and character of trauma services varies from region to region. In Canada, provinces are being pressed to upgrade emergency medical services and to introduce regional trauma programs, but there is considerable controversy about which policies should be pursued.

Given the improvements made in the health sector during the last 20 years, it is not clear what potential effects or benefits can be expected from specific recommendations or changes. Because most of the innovations and changes in the United States were not evaluated in well controlled studies, so the relative contributions made by various components of the EMS cannot be specified. Well designed studies in clinical and health services research could provide important information. The active participation of surgeons in research on surgical services is essential.

References

1. Spitzer WO, Feinstein AR, Sackett DL. What is a health care trial. JAMA 1975:233;161–163.
2. Study of Surgical Services for the United States. Surgery in the United States. American College of American Surgeons Association 1976.
3. Morris JN. Uses of Epidemiology 2nd ed. London: E&S Livingstone, 1964.
4. Buck C. The role of epidemiology in health care research. pp 37–43 (ed) Larsen DE, Love EJ. Health Care Research: A symposium Calgary: University of Calgary.
5. Institute Of Medicine. Report of A Study, Health Services Research. National Academy of Sciences, Washington, D.C. 1979;1–102.
6. Georgopoulos B. Hospital organization research: review and source book. Philadelphia WB Saunders 1975.
7. Flook EE, Sanazaro PJ. Health services research and R&D in perspective. Ann Arbor: Health Administration Press, 1973.
8. Culyer AJ, Wiseman J, Walker A. An annotated bibliography of health economics: English language sources. New York: St. Martin's Press 1977.
9. Griffiths DAT, Rigoni R, Tacier P, et al. An annoted bibliography of health economics: Western European sources. New York: St. Martin's Press, 1980.
10. Van Eimeren W, Kopcke W. Bestandsaufnahime: Gesundheitsystemforschung (State of the art report: health services research). Muchen Institut Fur Medizinische Informationsrerarbeitung, Statistik und Beomathematik 1979.
11. Warner KE, Luce BR. Cost-Benefit and Cost-Effectiveness Analysis in Health Care: Principles, Practice, and Potential. Ann Arbor: Health Administration Press, 1982.
12. Neuhauser, D. Health services research, 1984. Medical Care 1985;23:739–742.
13. McPherson K, Strong PM, Epstein A. et al. Regional variations in the use of common surgical procedures: within and between England and Wales, Canada and the United States of America. Social Science and Medicine 1981;15: 273–288.
14. McPherson K, Wennberg JE, Hovind OB, Clifford P. Small area variations in use of common surgical procedures. An interaction comparison of New England, England and Norway. NEJM 1982;307:1310–1314.
15. Nickerson RJ, Colton T, Peterson OL, Bloom BS, Hauch WWJr. Doctors who perform operations. A study on in hospital surgery in 4 diverse geographic areas. NEJM Part I 1976;295:921–926. Part II 1976;295:982–989.
16. Williams DC. Surgeons and Surgery in Rhode Island 1970 and 1977. NEJM 1982;305:1319–1323.
17. Verbugge LM. Longer Life but Worsening Health? Trends in Health and Mortality of Middle aged and Older Persons. Milbank Memorial Fund Quarterly Health and Society. 1984;62:475–516.
18. Rice DP, Feldman JJ. Living Longer in the United States: Demographic changes and Health Needs of the Elderly. Milbank Memorial Fund Quarterly Health and Society. 1983;61:362–396.
19. Lefebvre LA, Zsigmond Z, Devereaux MS. A prognosis for Hospitals: The effects of population change on the need for hospital space. Ottawa: Statistics Canada, 1979.
20. Medical Manpower for Ontario. Toronto: Ontario Council of Health, 1983.
21. Detsky AS. The Economic Foundations of National Health Policy. Cambridge Massachusetts: Ballinger Publishing Co., 1978.
22. Andersen R, Lion J, Anderson OW. Two decades of health services: social survey trends in use and expenditure. Cambridge, Mass: Ballinger Publishing Co. 1976.
23. Aday LA, Andersen R, Fleming GV. Health Care in the U.S. Equitable for Whom? Beverly Hills: Sage Publications, 1980.
24. Kohn R, White KL (eds). Health Care: An International Study. New York: Oxford University Press, 1976.
25. Cartwright A. Patients and their doctors: A Study of General Practice. London: Routledge & Kegan Paul, 1967.
26. Hannay DR. The Symptom Iceberg: A Study of Community Health. London: Routledge & Kegan Paul, 1979.

27. Aday LA, Andersen R. Development of Indices of Access to Medical Care. Ann Arbor, Michigan: Health Administration Press, 1975.
28. Ware JE Jr, et al. The measurement and meaning of patient satisfaction. Health and Medical Care Services Review 1978;1:1–16.
29. McCarthy EG, Eugene C, Finkel, Ruchlin, HS. Second Opinion Elective Surgery. Boston: Auburn House Publishing Co., 1981.
30. Braunwald E. Effects of Coronary-Artery Bypass Grafting on Survival: Implications of the Randomized Coronary-Artery Surgery Study. NEJM 1983;309:1181–1184.
31. Evans RG. Strained Mercy: The Economics of Canadian Health Care. Toronto: Butterworth, 1984.
32. McCarthy EG, Finkel ML. Second Opinion Elective Surgery Programs: Outcome, Status, Overtime. Medical Care 1978;16:984–994.
33. Stockwell H, Vayda E. Variations in Surgery in Ontario. Medical Care 1979;17:390–395.
34. Wennberg JE. Factors governing utilization of hospital services. Hosp Prac 1979;14:110–27.
35. Vayda E, Mindell WR. Variations in operative rates, what do they mean? Surgical Clinics in North America 1982;62:627–639.
36. Roos LL Jr, Roos NP. What are we learning about surgery? An update on the Manitoba study of common surgical procedures pp341–365 in Boan JA (ed) Proceedings of the Second Canadian Conference on Health Economics. Regina: The University of Regina, 1984.
37. Wennberg J, Gittlesohn A. Variations in medical care among small areas. Scientific American 1982;246(4)120–134.
38. Wennberg JE. On Patient Need, Equity, Supplier-induced Demand, and the Need to Assess the Outcome of Common Medical Practices. Med. Care 1985;23(5)512–520.
39. Andersen R. A Behavioral Model of Families Use of Health Services. Chicago: University of Chicago Center for Health Administration Studies No.25, 1968.
40. Hulka BS, Wheat JR. Patterns of utilization: The Patient Perspective. Medical Care 1985;23:438–460.
41. Roos NP, Roos LL Jr. Surgical Rate Variations: Do they Reflect Health on Socioeconomic Characteristics of the Population. Medical Care 1982;20:945.
42. Roos NP, Flowerdew G, Wajda A. Variations in hospital practices: A population based study in Manitoba, Canada. American J of Public Health 1986;76:45–51.
43. Eisenberg JM. Physician Utilization: The State of Research About Physicians' Practice Patterns. Med Care 1985;23(5):461–483.
44. Chalmers TC. Randomized clinical trails in surgery. pp 3–12 in Varco RL and Delaney (Eds) Controversy in Surgery. Philadelphia: WB Saunders, 1976.
45. Murphy ML, Hultgren HN, Detre K, et al. Treatment of chronic stable angina: a preliminary report of survival data of the randomized Veteran's Administration Cooperative Study. NEJM 1977;297:621–627.
46. European Coronary Study Group. Long term results of prospective randomized trial of coronary artery bypass surgery in stable angina pectoris. Lancet 1982;2:1173–1180.
47. CASS Principal Investigators. Coronary Artery Surgery Study Group (CASS): A randomized trial of coronary bypass surgery: quality of life in randomized subjects. Circulation 1983;68:951–960.
48. CASS Principal Investigators. Coronary Artery Surgery Study Group (CASS): A randomized trial of coronary artery surgery: survival data. Circulation 1983;68:939–950.
49. Kleinman JC, Machlin SR, Modaris J, Makuc D, Feldman JJ. Changing Practice in the Surgical Treatment of Breast Cancer. Medical Care 1983;21:1232–1242.
50. EC/IC Bypass Study Group. The international study of extracranial/intracranial Arterial Anastomis (EC/IC Bypass Study): Methodology and entry characteristics. Stroke 1985;16:397–406.
51. EC/IC Bypass Study Group. Failure of Extracranial-intracranial arterial bypass to reduce the risk of ischemic stroke: results of a randomized trial. NEJM 1985:313:1191–1200.
52. Rudicel S, Esdaile J. The randomized trial in orthopaedics: Obligation or Option? Bone Joint Surg 1985;67A:1284–1293.
53. Taylor KM, Margolese RG, Soskolne CL. Physicians' reasons for not entering eligible patients in a randomized clinical trial of surgery for breast cancer. NEJM 1984;310:1363–1367.
54. Brook RH, Ware JE Jr, Rogers WH et al. Does free care improve adults' health? Results from a randomized controlled trial. NEJM 1983;309:1426–14434
55. Spitzer WO, Sackett DL, Sibley JC et al. Burlington randomized trial of the nurse practitioner. New England Journal of Medicine 1974;290:251–256.
56. Eisenberg MS, Hallstrom AP, Copass MK, et al. Treatment of ventricular fibrillation emergency medical technician defibrillation and paramedic services. JAMA 1984;251:1723–1726.
57. Drummond MF. Principles of Economic Appraisal in Health Care. New York, Oxford University Press, 1980.
58. Stoddard GL, Drummond MF. How to read clinical journals; VII To understand an economic

evaluation (part A) CMAJ 1984;130:1428–1433.
59. Stoddart GL, Drummond MF. How to read clinical journals: VII To understand an economic evaluation (part B) CMAJ 1984;130:1542–1549.
60. Pineault R, Contandriopoulos AP, Valois M. et al. Randomized Clinical Trial of One-day Surgery: Patient Satisfaction, Clinical Outcomes, and Costs. Med Care 1985;(23)2:171–182.
61. Hemenway D, Sherman H, Mudge GH Jr et al. Comparative costs versus symptomatic and employment benefits of medical and surgical treatment of stable angina pectoris. Medical Care, 1985;23:133–141.
62. Boyle MH, Torrance GW. Developing multiattribute health indexes. Medical Care 1984:22:1045–1057.
63. Boyle MH, Torrance GW, Sinclair JC, Horwood SP. Economic evaluation of neonatal intensive care of very-low-birth-weight infants. NEJM 1983;308:1330–1337.
64. Harwood SP, Boyle MH, Torrance GW, Sinclair JC. Mortality and morbidity of 500- to 1499- gram birth weight infants live-born to residents of a defined geographic region before and after neonatal intensive care. Pediatrics 1982;69:613–620
65. Bunker JP, Barnes BA, Mosteller F (eds) Costs, Risks and Benefits of Surgery. New York, Oxford University Press, 1977.
66. Aaron HJ, Schwartz WB. The Painful Percription. Washington DC: Brookings Institute, 1984.
67. McLachlin G, Maynard A (eds). The Public/Private Mix for Health: The Relevance and Effects of Change. London: The Nuffield Provincial Hospital Trust, 1982.
68. McCarthy EG, Finkel ML. Surgical utilization in the USA. Medical Care 1980;18:883–891.
69. Ruchlin HS, Finkel ML, McCarthy EG. Efficacy of Second Opinion Consultation Program: A Cost Benefit Program. Medical Care 1982;20:3–20.
70. Finkel ML, Ruchlin HS, Parsons SK. Eight Years Experience with Second Opinion Elective Surgery Program: Utilization and Economic Analyses. Washington DC: US Department of Health and Human Services, Health Care Financing Administration, 1981.
71. Ermann D, Gabel J. The Changing Face of American Health Care: Multihospital Systems, Emergency Centers and Surgery Centers. Medical Care 1985;23:401–420.
72. Natof H. Complications associated with ambulatory surgical centers. JAMA 1980;244:92.
73. Davis JE. The Need to Redefine Levels of Surgical Care. JAMA 1984;251:2527–2528.
74. Martin SG, Schwartz M, Cooper D, et al. Health Care Financing Grants and Contract Reports: The Effect of a Mandatory Second Opinion Program on Medical Surgery Rates - An Analysis of the Massacheusetts Consultation Program for Elective Surgery. Washington DC: U.S. Department of Health and Human Services 1980.
75. Mechanic D. Cost containment and the quality of medical care: Rationing strategies in an era of constrained resources. Milbank Memorial Fund Quarterly Health and Society 1985;63:453–475.
76. Ermann D, Gabel J. The changing face of American health care: Multihispital systems, emergency centers, and surgery centers. Med Care 1985;23:401–420.
77. Luft HS, Bunker JP, Enthoven AC. Should Operations be Regionalized: The Emperical Relationship between Surgical Volume and Mortality. NEJM 1979;301:1364–1369.
78. Luft HS. The relationship between surgical volume and mortality. An exploration of causal factors and alternative models. Medical Care 1980;18:940–959.
79. Farber BF, Kaiser DL, Wenzel RP. Relation between surgical volume and incidence of post-operative wound infection. NEJM 1981;305:200–204.
80. Dyck FJ, Murphy FA, Murphy JK et al. Effect of surveillance on the number of hysterectomies in the province of Saskatchewan. NEJM 1977;296:1326–1328.
81. Brook RH, Williams KA, Rolph JE. Controlling the use and cost of medical service. The New Mexico Experimental Care Review Organization: A Four Year Case Study. Medical Care 1978;16:Supplement 9:1–76.
82. Donabedian A. Explorations in Quality Assurance and Monitoring Vol I The Definition of Quality and Approaches to its Assessment. Ann Arbor: Health Administration Press, 1980.
83. Donabedian A. Explorations in Quality Assurance and Monitoring Vol II The Criteria and Standards of Quality. Ann Arbor: Health Administration Press, 1980.
84. Williamson JW, Hudson JI, Nevins MM. Principles of Quality Assurance and Cost Containment in Health Care: A Guide for Medical Students, Residents, and other Health Professionals. San Francisco: Jossey Bass Publications, 1982.
85. Williamson JW, Barr DM, Fee E, et al. Teaching Quality Assurance and Cost Containment in Health Care: A Faculty Guide. San Francisco: Jossey Bass 1982.
86. Boyd DR. Comprehensive regional trauma and emergency medical service delivery systems: a goal of the 1980's. Critical Care Quarterly 1982;1–21.

8

Selected Non-Experimental Methods: An Orientation

W.O. Spitzer

Introduction

Clinical investigators and members of interdisciplinary research teams will be interested in some strategies characteristically used by epidemiologists and biostatisticians. Such research is best conducted in close alliance with clinicians if the questions are about patient care. Clinicians formally trained in epidemiologic methods will have spent several years mastering the theoretical basis for this research and acquiring experience in field work which is often as challenging as the theory.

We intend this chapter as an orientation to those who seek meaningful and knowledgeable partnership in clinical and epidemiologic research. The designs presented are used less frequently than the controlled trials in surgical research. The bibliography will permit those who wish to pursue understanding of strategies presented here in overview to do so in considerable depth.

Allusion has been made in various chapters in this textbook to uncontrolled case studies and case series. Such efforts are indispensable precursors to good clinical and epidemiological research. However, the role of such work should be restricted strictly to *hypothesis generation* except when findings are dramatic. For instance, the discovery that penicillin could cure hitherto consistently incurable disorders, was so striking that controlled studies and inferential statistics became unnecessary. However, such dramatic advances in any field of medicine are the exception rather than the rule. Characteristically, advances in clinical science are small, and progress is incremental. Improvements can be subtle enough that the changes must be demonstrated carefully with the best attainable rigor of design and the highest sophistication of appropriate statistics. Admissible rules of scientific logic must be followed. *One of the key rules is that research questions or hypotheses are tested only after they have been set forth in advance*, not through fishing expeditions in existing data or even data-dredging of information we may have gathered ourselves. It is important to generate hypotheses, but it is essential to test them following an explicit protocol written and diffused in advance.

Experimental Versus Non-Experimental Designs

An experimental design is one in which one group of eligible subjects or patients exposed to an intervention or a maneuver is compared to one or more control groups comparable to the intervention groups in all respects, save for the intervention or maneuver of interest. *The essential characteristic of an experiment is that the intervention or the maneuver is assigned by the investigator to the exposed group and that the comparison interventions or maneuvers (e.g., placebo or the best accepted current therapy) is also assigned by the investigator to the control group or control groups. To express it another way, the assignment of the maneuvers is under control of the investigator.*

Generally an investigator in such circumstances chooses to randomly assign subjects to the intervention or the control group. However, it is possible to have controlled studies that do not use random assignment or allocation of subjects to treatment groups, but are still experimental. The assignment may be done in an systematic fashion by other preselected means, (e.g., by alternate assignment rules, by odd-and-even hospital file numbers) or, conceivably, on a judgmental basis. In our current understanding of clinical science, the experiment which is a randomized controlled trial (RCT) is the "gold standard" of research. See Section III, Chapter 3 where Walters and Sackett discuss in detail the advantages of the randomized and controlled approach for the assessment of effectiveness.

I prefer to call designs in which the investigator does not control the assignment of study subjects to "treated" versus "untreated" groups by the term *non-experimental*. There are several equivalent words which one finds in the literature for non-experimental designs. These include; *subexperimental* (used by Walters and Sackett), *quasi-experimental* (a term which I do not accept, a design does or does not meet the criteria to be deemed experimental), or *observational,* (which is also unacceptable because the word incorrectly suggests that experimental designs do not involve observation of phenomena).

The balance of this chapter will introduce the reader to some types of non-experimental research. The list is not exhaustive. It will cover "before and after" approaches, cohort designs, cross-sectional designs (with particular attention to the case-referent or case-control method) and a brief discussion of historical controls. The orientation will only provide a road map for parts of quite a territory of research methodology.Many of the details for sub-sections of the territory, can be found in Section 2, Chapter 3 by Kramer and Troidl, in the chapter on clinical research by Walters and Sackett (Section III, Chapter 4) and in Margolese's review of multi-centre RCT's (Section III, Chapter 5) and in the chapters by Schechter (Section III, Chapter 6, Section II, Chapter 7). Uncontrolled series have already been referred to in the introduction and will not be considered further.

Cohorts

The word *cohort,* from the Latin, is a Roman military term. It referred to a group of soldiers of a certain category. It could have been 100 or 500 infantrymen, 500 cavalry warriors, etc. Its first and most important use in clinical and epidemiologic research, is to designate a number of persons (patients or healthy individuals) who share common attributes considered relevant to the research questions at issue. It could be 500 persons aged 20–49, experiencing a first incidence of low back pain, who have no clinically objective signs of neurological deficit. The cohort could be 10,000 diabetics aged 50–79, eligible for inclusion by definite criteria and unaffected by peripheral vascular complications. It could be 25 one-week survivors of liver transplants, aged 13 months to 60 months.

Sometimes the only intervention or manoeuvre of interest in studying a cohort is the passage of time. Thus, for the diabetics unaffected by peripheral vascular complications, one might wish to discover how many complications affect that *population* of diabetics over a five year period, stratified by age in half-decades. Or, a new drug to delay or prevent peripheral vascular complications may have introduced into the market. A study might then determine the rate of development of such complications in a cohort of persons using the drug.

For any cohort, it is important to decide in advance what the dependent variable or the target outcome will be. The outcome events become the numerators for rates calculated in cohort studies (such as incidence). For survivors of liver transplants, the dependent variable or target outcome might be death. For a cohort of patients with osteosarcoma, it might be length of disability-free survival. For a cohort of women with indwelling urinary catheters it might be new infections in the post-operative period. The fundamental characteristic of the cohort is that the study subjects are identified and delineated by explicit criteria *before* the declared target outcome or dependent variable of interest is manifest among the same subjects. Cohorts are denominators for target outcomes. The target outcomes or dependent variables are the numerators. *In cohort studies, the denominators are always identified and delineated before the dependent variables are observed.* That is why cohort studies are sometimes called follow-up studies.

Cohorts may be followed in time as a single group without making any comparisons with any other group. Such work is referred to as descriptive, or more specifically, a single cohort study or an uncontrolled cohort study. Sometimes it is possible to compare two or more cohorts and follow them simultaneously. For instance, it may be possible to assemble 20,000 men who became exposed and continue to be exposed to occupationally-related radiation in nuclear plants starting in 1971 and follow them to determine the total number of any new cancers detected through 1995. This could be done at the same time as one follows another 20,000 men in other energy-related industries, similar in most respects to nuclear power generating plants, except for the exposure to measured levels of radiation in the workplace. This second cohort of 20,000 men assembled in 1971 would also be followed through 1995. Note why this is not an experimental design. The investigator did not assign the men to be or to not be exposed to radiation or to be or not to be in one type of industry or other. *The men self-selected themselves.* (However, it can and should be established that the two self-selected cohorts are sufficiently comparable to follow them forward in time and compare the rate of development of new cancers between two groups.) With two or more groups, we have a cohort analytic study or a cohort comparison study. It is worth emphasizing that all 40,000 men, the 20,000 exposed and the 20,000 not exposed were all free of the target outcome of interest (cancer) *at the time the cohort was assembled in 1971.*

The main disadvantages of cohort studies are that they generally require very large number of subjects in the denominator so that meaningful numerators can emerge as dependent variables. That is not true in certain clinically-oriented studies (e.g., liver transplant studies where the outcomes of interest are not rare). The precision of the answers depends greatly on the size of the numerator. Also, cohort studies sometimes require long followup with all the consequent problems of logistics, the most important one being losses to followup.

Cross-Sectional Designs

Cross-sectional designs are those in which de nominators are delineated at the same time that numerator events are measured. Thus one might establish all victims of motorcycle accidents who are within a particular city of 500,000 persons and designate those motorcycle victims as the denominator of interest. For the target outcome in the numerator, one might measure the extent of physical disability of the motorcycle victims. This will have been established *at the same time* as the eligible study subjects were included in the denominator. A more rigorous approach is a cross-sectional study where comparisons are made among groups of people. For instance, one might study all motorcycle victims in one city of 500,000 and compare them with motorcycle victims of another city of 500,000 in a neighboring state. The difference is, that in the first city, use of helmets is not mandatory by law, whereas in the second city, it is. In both cities, a quantitative assessment of the extent of disability among the victims is done using a new "disability index" where 0 is death and 100 is freedom from disability. Suppose that in city A, one measures an average "disability index" of 68 points and in city B, the mean "disability index" is 48 points. One would tend to conclude from such a cross-sectional study that city B is better off than city A. One would also tend to impute the benefit to the law on helmet use. This example was chosen to show the pitfalls which cross-sectional designs could create and to illustrate how cohort studies are superior when feasible because they are not as vulnerable to biases and misinterpretation. It is easy to see that community A could actually be better off than community B simply by virtue of having had lower mortality. Community B may have had higher mortality with the surviving victims having less disability. If one had started with a cohort approach which would have identified all motorcycle *riders* in both communities *before* introduction of the law and followed both groups forward in time starting at some point close to the introduction of the new law in the second city, then the confusion between survival and residual disability would not occur. However, very often, due to reasons of budget, unavailability of data, unavailability of time or ethical constraints, a cohort study cannot be done, and all that one can do is a cross-sectional study. It is important to stress that when data emerge only from cross-sectional studies, one can only reach tentative conclusions that a particular exposure factor or a particular intervention is *associated* with a particular target outcome or dependent variable.

Case-Referent or Case-Control Studies

A special case of the cross-sectional approach in which target outcomes are measured at the same time that one identifies study subjects is the *case-referent* study. It has been most frequently designated in the literature as a *case control* study. Tactically, the distinct feature of the case-referent study is that the two groups compared, the group of *cases* and the *subjects from the referent group* are identified with reference to the presence or absence of the target outcome of interest. One then determines in each of the two groups of patients compared, how frequently an exposure of interest occurred. For instance, one might take 400 neonates with meningomyelocoele from among a group of university childrens' hospitals and compare them to a second reference group of 400 very young children, matched by age who were referred to the same hospitals for management of severe trauma. The question of such a project is whether exposure to a particular garden herbicide of the mother during pregnancy might be associated with development of meningomyelocoele. One would interview the mothers of both groups of children to determine the proportion of exposure of each group during the corresponding pregnancies. Suppose that 32% of the mothers of children with meningomyelocoele report being exposed to the chemical herbicide and that only 8% of the mothers of children with multiple trauma report such exposure. One would then conclude children whose mothers were exposed to the herbicide are approximately five and a half times as likely to be born with meningomyelocoele. In statistical or epidemiologic terms one would say that the odds ratio is about five.

In case-referent research, if one obtains odds ratios that are high, like 6 or 11 or 20 (meaning that a target outcome is 6 times more likely or 11 times more likely or 20 times more likely to occur in the presence of a suspected risk factor as compared to the absence of the risk factor) then one has evidence of *association* between the target outcome and the risk factor, and the strength of the association, as reflected in the high odds ratios *would suggest but not prove causality* of the risk factor with respect to the target outcome. Findings from case-referent studies can seldom be taken as conclusive evidence of cause, no matter how high the odds ratios. Moreover, odds ratios from case-referent studies are often only in the order or 1.3 or 1.8 or about 2. In such cases, (assuming that statistical significance has been attained) the evidence of association can be invoked to draw causal inferences only at great peril. There are specific ground rules about diagnosing causality from association. These were first introduced by Bradford Hill in his classical textbook of medical statistics (see bibliography) and discussed further in the next section.

The terminology readers will encounter about the statistics in the methodology of case referent studies include words for estimates of association frequently used. They include in addition to *odds ratio, relative risk, risk ratio and relative odds*. In recent years, Miettinen has developed the theory underlining case referent studies which permitted substantial advances in the understanding of this strategy. He introduced the concept of *study base* as the hypothetical conceptual denominator of relevance for these types of studies (see bibliography). Clinicians participating with methodologists in case-referent studies should make a serious attempt to master both the theory and the logistical challenges of the case-referent approach. The theoretical and practical difficulties can be formidable despite the advantages of smaller sample sizes and much shorter study periods.

The key disadvantages to the case-referent method are vulnerability to bias (see Ibrahim and Spitzer, bibliography) and the difficulty in judicious choice of reference groups for comparison. The advantages include smaller numbers of patients and shorter followup. In the case of a rare disease, the case-referent method is often the only feasible way of evaluating association between a risk factor and a clinical outcome.

Association Is Not Necessarily Causation

All clinicians must constantly remind themselves that association does not mean causation. Ordinarily we can develop truly convincing evidence for causation only through experimental approaches. The strongest, most reliable evidence for cause and effect is the randomized controlled trial. Without such trials, sometimes an association is a causal one. Sir Austin Bradford Hill suggests nine features one might consider in looking at associations between factors and outcomes when the evidence is derived from non-experimental methods. If many of these features are present, we are more secure in postulating causation.

Hill put the *strength of the association* first on the list. If the exposed population shows the outcome variable in a very marked degree, we are much more comfortable in inferring causation. High odds ratios mean a strong association. Of course, we are sometimes misled. A very strong association between two factors may be just that, a strong association and not cause and effect at all.

Next on Hill's list of features to be considered in attributing causation, he placed *consistency of the observed association*. The connection between smoking and lung cancer has been repeatedly observed by different workers in different countries using quite different populations over many years. Hill places great weight on similar results reached from quite different designs. He finds this much more convincing than similar results from a collection of similarly designed studies. We all know in medicine and surgery that very weakly designed studies all pointing in the same direction have frequently misled us into believing causation when in fact the same mistake was simple repeated.

Hill's third characteristic is the *specificity of the association*. If the association is unusual, if it is limited to specifically exposed persons who develop unusual outcomes, this is a strong argument in favor of causation. The peculiar form of deformity produced by exposure of pregnant women to thalidomide and the association between acquired immune deficiency syndrome and very rare Kaposi sarcoma are recent examples of this characteristic.

The fourth factor Hill considers is the *temporal relationship of the observed association*. An inference of causation is severely undermined when the effects appears before the cause. In the epidemics of Minamata disease seen in several parts of the world a few years ago, the emission of organic mercury toxic wastes preceded the great increase of reported cases of the neurological disorder.

As a fifth factor Hill looks for an association that reveals a *dose-response curve or biological gradients*. For example, those who smoked more cigarettes have a higher death rate from smoking than both non-smokers and those who smoke but a few cigarettes. A reverse gradient, such as a decreasing incidence of cancer of the lung among ex-smokers is particularly persuasive.

The sixth feature Hill looks for is *biological plausibility*. If the association seems to make no sense at all, as in a relationship between the number of Presbyterian ministers in Scotland and the increasing population of Chicago, Hill suggests that we should be cautious in inferring causation. At the same time we learn more and more about biology. When Professor Oliver Wendell Holmes of the Harvard medical school in 1847 drew attention to the association between the hand-washing habits of obstetrical surgeons and the incidence of puerperal fever among the mothers then attended, no one paid much attention because they could see no biological plausibility in the association. Twenty years later, after the work of Pasteur and Lister, the association seemed to have biological plausibility.

Hill's seventh factor is *coherence of the evidence*. Hill says that a cause and effect interpretation of an association should not seriously conflict with the generally known facts of the natural history and biology of the disease studied. Hill points out that the association of lung cancer and cigarette smoking is coherent with the increase in smoking among men that took place between 1910 and 1920 and the later increase among women. The isolation of carcinogenic factors from cigarette smoke and the histopathologic evidence of irritation of the airway epithelium of heavy smokers lends further evidence of coherence.

For his eighth factor, Hill asks if the *association is reversible*. When the government withdrew the suspect pharmaceutical from the market, did reported cases of phocomelia fall? When smokers stop using cigarettes, does the rate at which they develop lung cancer fall? We call this evidence of reversibility.

Finally, as a ninth factor Hill suggests we look for *analogies*. After having discovered a drug effect of thalidomide on fetuses, we are much more ready to accept somewhat similar evidence that another drug might cause fetal defects.

Clearly none of these nine factors brings indisputable evidence for or against a cause and effect hypothesis. Yet, at the same time they do with greater or lesser strength suggest instances when an association may be one of causation.

For causation we prefer to have the evidence of a soundly conceived and executed experiment—one that employs the appropriate strengthening factors of random allocation to treatment, appropriate varieties of blindness on the part of the experimenter, the patient, the evaluator of the outcome, and perhaps the statistician who analyzes the data. Employing strengthening factors such as random allocation and blindness is no more an aspersion on the honesty of experiments than requiring rubber gloves is a comment on the personal hygiene of the surgeon.

Ascribing causation is serious business. The best advice one could give about drawing conclusions on cause from non-experimental designs is to study Bradford Hill's criteria very carefully.

Before-and-After Studies

One common non-experimental design is the uncontrolled "before and after" design. In a sense, if study subjects are assembled properly at the outset, it is a special case of the single cohort study. There are times when one cannot institute a comparative study with two or more cohorts for ethical or other reasons. One is then left with a single group of comparable persons that one can follow forward in time. Consider all eligible drivers in the state of Victoria, Australia as a cohort. Consider an intervention of interest, the introduction of compulsory use of seatbelts while driving. Given that it is possible to determine the number of accidents entailing death or physical injury to drivers and passengers per 100,000 persons "exposed to automobile transport" one can then effect a "before and after study". For instance, for the full year prior to royal assent of the new law, determinations of accidents can be made of the exposed citizens of that state after stratification by age. One might then repeat the determinations one full year after the law is in effect and see if there was any difference in rates. If the change (presumably a drop) is truly dramatic, one may not need comparison cohorts or concurrent experimental trials of any kind.

When before and after studies must be done, the design is strengthened by having several sequential measurements before the event or "independent variable" of interest and several measures after. In the example we are discussing, assume now that measures had been taken for odd numbers of years for a decade before the introduction of the law and that the rates of accidents classified and measured identically had been stable. If one had then done the same ascertainments for a decade *after* introduction of the new law in odd years, and there were a stable *sustained* new lower level, the conclusions about the relationship between the new law and prevention of accidents and death would be greatly strengthened. If one is doing before and after studies, one should seek every opportunity to have at least two measures before and two measures after. A "step down" or "step up" of the measurement in the dependent variables coinciding with the "treatment" or exposure to the independent variable becomes a much stronger set of data upon which to base conclusions on association.

If a "before and after" study does not give convincing evidence of change, then one should be very cautious in interpreting the results even if one has several determinations before and after. Other things (confounders or effect modifiers) could have been operating at the same time. For instance, the price of gasoline might have changed, or driving habits might have altered. Other laws might have affected the rate of accidents (such as lower speed limits). It then becomes important to attempt additional before and after studies, historically or concurrently, in other jurisdictions. The replications can be helpful in teasing out the confounding or effect-modifying impact of unrelated factors.

Historical Controls

A fairly popular approach in research is to compare the results of a treatment or prevention or rehabilitation among current patients eligible for such interventions with results obtained in the past. It could be the recent past, or it could be the cumulative experience over several years, even decades. Some investigators examine the results of current innovations with earlier results of their own hospitals or all hospitals and clinics in their own university. Historical controls are also assembled through evaluation of reports in the literature from the past. This type of strategy combines some elements of the "before and after" methods and some aspects of case-series reports. My opinion is that unless changes are dramatic, such as the improvement in outcome with surgical treatment of mitral stenosis compared to the experience before introduction of that operation, they should never be considered conclusive. If the results are equivocal or the gains marginal, then comparisons of current new therapy with the experience of historical controls should be limited to hypothesis generation. Happily for surgeons involved in clinical research, major advances in outcome of patients treated with surgical innovations have been relatively more frequent than has been the case for clinical investigators studying new medical interventions. However, one should always approach research dependent on historical controls with a great deal of constructive skepticism. Some of the reasons for the caution include the fact that clinical science advances in general. Thus, it is easy to attribute improvement to an intervention at issue when the benefit could very well be due to the entire array of accompanying interventions employed in the total management of a particular type of patient. Secondly, changes could be merely those of improved record-keeping of an investigator committed to a new treatment. Purpose-gathered current records are generally better than those gathered routinely for other needs, especially in the very distant past. Thirdly, clinical classifications for diagnoses and even for interventions change and one can never be sure among historical controls that one has the same category of eligible subjects as one does in the concurrent treatment group. That is especially true if they are not from the same institution.

Descriptive Studies

Non-experimental studies include assembling data about large numbers of patients or subjects for descriptive purposes. This goes somewhat beyond the case series in that it may involve an attempt to confine eligibility of subjects to certain geographic boundaries, or to a particular time frame. For instance, we may wish to identify patterns of illness and health among those diagnosed with Parkinson's Disease in all countries within certain latitudes north and south of the equator from 1961 to 1980. One may also wish to describe the patterns of disease in countries beyond those latitudes south and north if one suspects climactic factors as a risk in the disease. Or one may wish to characterize the morphologic nature of vessel disease in the heart among all subjects admitted to all hospitals of a given city with any disorder falling under the general rubric of ischaemic heart disease. Such descriptive work can be highly important and relevant. It helps focus the process of hypothesis generation and of hypothesis testing in other types of research, including health services research. It provides data that enables a scientifically sound choice of strategy of research approch for a given problem. It helps establish the feasibility of certain projects.

Summary

Clinical and epidemiologic investigation can be considered to have three broad purposes, the *description of what is*, *prediction of what could happen* in the future and *establishing cause and effect* in etiologic and therapeutic investigation.

The experiment is by far the strongest evidence that can be invoked to diagnose causality from association. It is the gold standard of clinical, epidemiologic and health care research. It should be used whenever it is ethically and practically feasible. In only a few instances of the history of medicine has the non-experimental design led to firm conclusions in any one study about cause and effect. If one is unable to do experiments, there are a series of non-experimental strategies that can be considered. With respect to establishing a causal significance from an association, the hierarchy of rigor of evidence goes from the cohort analytic study, to the well-designed case-referent study, to the uncontrolled cohort with a before and after design. Only when striking findings show major changes, should case studies be invoked to establish cause and effect relationships. Generally, if not an experiment, no one single study should be used as conclusive evidence about any one question. It is important to seek a profile of several non-experimental studies. If most of them tend to point in the same direction, especially if they have been planned and designed in different countries at different time by different investigators with different kinds of patients, then causality might become a tenable verdict. It is worth emphasizing that other important rules of admissibility of scientific evidence are summarized in Bradford Hill's criteria cited above.

Prediction of the future depends in part on the faithfulness with which interventions assessed through experimental and non-experimental methods reflect current and future realities. One must have some sense of the extent of circumstances surrounding a treatment, such as competing medical treatments, the milieu of health service organizations of the country concerned, and the basic nature of the population for which predictions are made to conform with the characteristics described and studied in a particular project. Mathematical modelling based in part on empirical evidence gathered through experimental and non-experimental studies can have an important role in predicting the future. This text has not dealt with such modelling nor with laboratory simulation except through passing, reference. A balanced overview of selected strategies requires mention of modelling and simulation.

Some investigators scorn the use of anything less than the gold standard in clinical and epidemiologic research. While we believe that the highest feasible level of rigor should always be attempted, we also feel that some data is always better than no data. We feel that when legitimate real world constraints do not permit randomized controlled trials, every other avenue of pursuit of new knowledge should be followed as far as one can and as carefully as one can.

Given the substantial compromises that must be made at the broad strategy level in non-experimental research, one must exert much care in the choice of all patients or study subjects, in the validity and reliability of data-gathering and in the selection of the best possible statistical techniques to avoid errors of interpretation.

Bibliography

1. Bradford-Hill A. Principles of medical statistics. Chapter XXIV 9th ed. New York: Oxford University Press, 1971.
2. Campbell DT, Stanley JC. Experimental and quasi-experimental designs for research. Chicago: McNally & Co., 1963.
3. Cook TD, Campbell DT. Quasi-experimentation. Chicago: Rand McNally, 1979.
4. Feinstein AR. Clinical epidemiology: the architecture of clinical research. Philadelphia: W.B. Saunders, 1985.
5. Fletcher RH, Fletcher SW, Wagner EH. Clinical epidemiology: the essentials. Baltimore: Williams & Williams, 1982.
6. Friedman GD. Primer of epidemiology. 2nd ed. New York: McGraw-Hill, 1980.
7. Ibrahim M, Spitzer WO. The case-control study: consensus and controversy. J Chron Dis 1979;32:1–190.
8. Kleinbaum DG, Kupper LL, Morgenstern H. Epidemiologic research. Belmont, CA: Lifetime Learning Publications, 1982.
9. Lilienfeld AM, Lilienfeld DE. Foundations of epidemiology. 2nd ed. Oxford: Oxford University Press, 1980.
10. Miettinen OS. Theoretical epidemiology: principles of occurrence research in medicine. New York: John Wiley and Sons, 1985.
11. Sackett DL, Haynes RB, Tugwell P. Clinical epidemiology: a basic science for clinical medicine. Boston: Little Brown, 1985.
12. Schlesselman JJ. Case-control studies. Oxford: Oxford University Press, 1982.
13. Swinscow, TDV. Statistics at square one. London: British Medical Association, 1976.

Section IV

Reporting Your Work

Introduction

Even when research has been well designed, responsibly conducted, and judiciously analyzed, it is all a sterile exercise if the results fail to reach the target audience. Many scientists who are brilliant in the conception of ideas or the execution of research never receive the recognition they deserve because of problems in communication. This section has been written to help you avoid or surmount such problems. You will find helpful suggestions about writing abstracts, presenting short reports, writing and submitting articles to peer-reviewed scientific journals, preparing audio-visual aids, chairing panels, and acquiring other communication skills that are increasingly essential components of success in any research endeavour. Reading about them is not enough; you can only develop skill in communicating by communicating.

1
Writing an Effective Abstract

B.A. Pruitt, Jr. and A.D. Mason, Jr.

An abstract should be a concise distillate or synopsis of the work which is being reported and as such must emphasize what was done, how it was done, the results obtained, and the author's interpretation of the results. In most instances, the organization or publication to which the abstract is submitted defines its length (usually one standard size double-spaced typewritten page, i.e., approximately 200 to 250 words) and that limit is inviolable. This required brevity necessitates that the abstract be free of all extraneous material.

Mechanical and technical factors as well as presentation and content determine the strength and reviewer attractiveness of an abstract. If the source of the abstract is to be "blinded" to the reviewer, the originating institution should not be surreptitiously identified in the body of the abstract. Although they are becoming more popular, abstracts prepared on dot matrix printers are often not welcomed by reviewers, who find a typed abstract easier to read. A grammatically correct abstract, free of typographical errors, jargon and colloquialisms will be viewed with favor but requires meticulous proofreading of each successive draft—capricious word processors have been known to drop out words, phrases, and even entire sentences. Acronyms should be used sparingly (never in the title) and only if widely accepted. Each acronym must be presented in parentheses after its first citation in the abstract. Data tables should be easily read, with entries kept to the essential minimum, units of measurement defined, the number of entries or observations stated, and levels of statistical significance defined and indicated by conventional symbols.

The format of an abstract is usually that of a scientific report or presentation, i.e., title, introduction, materials and methods, results, discussion, and conclusions. An interesting or even clever title can enhance attractiveness, but cuteness is to be avoided at all costs. It is sometimes appropriate for the title to be presented as the question addressed by the reported research, thus reducing or even eliminating the need for an introduction. In general, the introduction should be limited to a sentence or, at the most, two sentences that establish the importance of the problem addressed and the rationale for the study.

The abstract should emphasize results and materials and methods, in that order of importance. Materials and methods should be described in generic or categorical terms, with specific details of data processing, experimental procedure, and fine points of technology or technique left for the presentation or publication. Control or comparison groups or proposed models should also be described in general terms but with sufficient detail to verify relevance and appropriateness. All of the information contained in these two sections must, of course, be covered in the presentation and the final publication. The abstract itself must focus upon the results of greatest importance and widest applicability and provide the basis for any conclusions drawn. The materials and methods and results sections of an abstract are customarily written in the past tense, but in the other sections the present tense can be used as appropriate (1).

The discussion should focus upon the present study and explain in concise fashion the applicability of the results to the problem addressed, omitting needless reference to the work of others or even the author's previous work in that field. The word "significant" should be applied only when a difference has been statistically verified.

The conclusions section should consist of one or, at the most, two sentences and should be confined to the work being reported. In the conclusions, hypotheses should be clearly separated from facts (2) and one should not unwarrantedly extrapolate the findings beyond the point supported by the data presented. In the case of a clinical study, the conclusions should make clear how the results influence patient management or outcome. In the case of a laboratory study, the conclusions should explain the importance of the findings to understanding of biologic processes and disease mechanisms or, if relevant, clinical application.

It is obvious that the potential quality of an abstract is directly related to the quality of the study being reported. Any clinical or laboratory study should be conducted according to an experimental design that will permit appropriate statistical assay and answer the question being asked. *A priori* statistical comparisons reported in the abstract must be those comparisons that were planned before the study began; *a posteriori* comparisons should be clearly identified. Serial comparisons of multiple non-independent test groups by means of *t*-tests without appropriate adjustment is considered a fatal flaw by many reviewers. The attribution of a trend to data that approach but do not reach a level of statistical significance is apt to be regarded by reviewers as wading by the "no swimming" sign. In the preparation of an abstract reporting a chronologically lenghty series of cases, one should keep in mind improvements in general care and changes in treatment modalities that have occurred across time and stratify patients within appropriate time segments.

The acceptability of an abstract will be enhanced if the abstract topic is related to the subject of the meeting, conforms to the interests of the membership of the sponsoring organization, and deals with a subject which has not been featured at recent meetings of the organization to which it is being submitted. Topics of clinical relevance and significance will be most favorably considered for programs in which clinical medicine is emphasized. Similarly, laboratory studies will be most favorably reviewed for programs in which research and the understanding of disease processes is emphasized. An abstract addressing a non-existent, archaic, or even a recently well covered problem or one that could be perceived as a reinvention of the wheel will elicit little enthusiasm on the part of reviewers. Single case reports are similarly lightly regarded unless the information presented illustrates a general principle or reports a spectacular result of importance to an entire class of patients. Negative studies will, in general, receive little consideration unless they refute established dogma, break icons, gore oxen, or dispel myths.

There are certain features of an abstract that are likely to dampen the enthusiasm of all but the most inexperienced of reviewers (3). Although brevity is the essence of an abstract, it should not read like a telegram. The abstract should not represent merely a review of the work of others or address a self-created strawman. In the introduction, one should avoid sentences that begin with "The following experiment was performed to. . .," since it should be obvious from the introduction and body of the abstract why the experiment was performed. In the discussion section, space should not be devoted to things "not done" or "not found" and one should consider only the data that were generated in the study being reported. There should be no surprise endings with conclusions unrelated to the information provided in the abstract or not supported by the data presented. The conclusions can usually be stated without a preamble, such as "The results of this study showed. . ."

The abstract should not intermix materials and methods with results or conclusions; the integrity of each section should be maintained. The abstract should not promise any answer that is not provided and the authors should not request a carte blanche for "work in progress" or "to be done." Vague generalizations regarding data to be presented, results to be discussed, experience to be reviewed, or techniques to be described should be avoided. References to a nondescript "extensive experience" or self-denigrating comments regarding a "limited" or "modest" experience will not excite the enthusiasm of reviewers. It goes without saying that the abstract should contain only information at hand, since subsequently generated data may significantly alter the results and interpretation of the research and necessitate an embarrassing withdrawal of an accepted paper. Important research results are not so perishable that one cannot delay submission until the research is completed.

It is much more difficult to describe the key aspects of a study as an abstract than to write the paper for publication. A first draft is never submittable and even the final draft should be reviewed by each co-author as well as selected peers. Even in these anti-paternalistic times, it is a courtesy to offer the department chairman the opportunity to review the abstract, particularly if he will have to answer to his colleagues for the results and conclusions. Good abstracts are made better by rewriting and the need for this "aging" process speaks against writing the abstract the night before the submission deadline. Though robust results often speak for themselves, even the best are enhanced by an outstanding presentation; the fate of a report of more fragile results frequently hinges on the quality of the abstract.

References

1. Warren R. The abstract. Arch Surg 1976;111:635–636.
2. Baue AE. Writing a good abstract is not abstract writing. Arch Surg 1979;114:11–12.
3. Pruitt BA Jr. Improve your next abstract. Presented at the Seventh Annual Meeting of the American Burn Association, Denver, Colorado, March 20–22, 1975.

2

The Ten-Minute Presentation

M. Evans and A.V. Pollock

"Begin with an arresting sentence; close with a strong summary; in between speak simply, clearly, and always to the point; and above all be brief."

William J. Mayo

Sir Austin Bradford Hill's aphorism (1) applies equally to scientific papers and 10-minute presentations: "Why did you start, what did you do, what answer did you get, and what does it mean anyway?" Sir Hugh Casson, past president of the Royal Academy and famous lecturer and after-dinner speaker, indicated the amount of work required when he said during an interview that the secret of his success was that for each minute of speaking he did an hour of preparation.

As the speaker, you have to distill what is probably about two years' work. You must include some background, a brief description of your methods and results, and a succinct explanation of where they fit in the realm of current knowledge.

Collection and Preparation of Data

Let us assume that you are presenting the results of a controlled clinical trial, and that the data are stored on floppy discs or in some equally easily retrievable form. The first step is to produce a large comparability table; the headings will be the events being studied and the important variables will be listed down the left hand margin (Table I). From this, you can spot important differences and test their statistical significance.

Submission Of Abstract

This is the appropriate stage at which to write an abstract which is usually restricted to 200 words. It should state the aim of the trial (in one sentence), the number of patients in each arm of the study (whole numbers, not percentages), the number of events in each arm, the statistical significance of differences and (again in one sentence) the conclusions to be drawn.

You draft the paper when the abstract has been accepted for presentation. This will bring to mind the finer points that you may have forgotten in the (often long) interval between submission and acceptance of the abstract.

TABLE I. Table of comparability.

	Group A		Group B	
	total number	wound infection (%)	total number	wound infection (%)
Male				
Female				
Age < 60				
60–64				
65+				
Organ incised:				
stomach and duodenum				
gall bladder and ducts				
small bowel				
large bowel				
Contamination:				
clean				
potential				
light				
heavy				
etc.				

Planning Of Slides

The next steps are the design and preparation of slides. They must be simple (one idea, one slide) and it is sensible to incorporate salient numbers; in the excitement of making your presentation, you may find it difficult to remember exact figures.

Bad slides evoke more criticism than any other component of a presentation. If you have a medical art department you are lucky, but do not wait until the last minute and then present the staff with reams of information to be squashed onto a few slides (the "if I'd wanted them tomorrow I'd have asked for them tomorrow" syndrome). Take your ideas, in good time, and ask the artist for advice on how the material can be presented to best advantage.

If you have no medical art department, you will have to construct your own slides but there are simple rules to take you through it step by step (2, 3) so do not despair. It will be difficult the first time, before you learn the little tricks and short cuts, but it will mean that you will not be dependent on other people and, as time goes by and you become more experienced, you will get a lot of pleasure out of developing a style of your own.

Technique of Presentation

There is a fundamental difference between the written and the spoken word (4). It is essential to remember that in the 10-minute presentation you are talking to people, and the vocabulary should be that of a conversation, not an editorial. Speak slowly and clearly, and vary pace and pitch for emphasis. Try to communicate your enthusiasm for the subject; you are giving one of perhaps twenty 10-minute papers at the particular meeting, and "a person who desires to make an impression must stand out in some way from the masses"(5).

There is controversy about whether or not a speaker should take notes or a manuscript onto the platform. Some fear that as soon as someone has even written headings in front of him, he may become stilted and afraid of drying up if he loses his place. A master speaker who has no prompts of any kind, and who forgets what comes next, can conceal his predicament by requesting the next slide while he collects his thoughts, instead of shifting through sheaves of paper with rising panic. Indeed, the rules of the Surgical Research Society in Great Britain forbid reading from a manuscript. British practice holds that a paper should only be read if it is being given in a foreign language. Yet, in North America, the almost universal practice is for a ten minute paper to be read from a manuscript. The editors found themselves divided on this issue and nearly came to fisticuffs. Those who read argue that only master speakers can successfully carry off the "no-notes" style, that a manuscript ensures you deliver your material in the allotted time. Conversely, a fear that one who reads will overrun his time is cited by advocates of the European "no-notes" school. When presenting a ten minute talk at a meeting in another country, one may wish to enquire about local custom.

It is, nevertheless, important to rehearse in order to get the timing right. It is more than bad manners to exceed the allotted time; accurate timekeeping is essential to the success of any meeting, particularly when there are parallel sessions. It is embarrassing to both you and your audience if you have to be asked to finish. A 10-minute presentation should run for about 8 minutes in rehearsal; it always takes longer on the day and it is better to finish early rather than late, thereby leaving more time for discussion.

One should always examine one's slides on a big screen. Defects that are not apparent with even the best of small projectors have a nasty habit of making themselves obvious in a lecture hall. Using a hand projector, or laying the slides out on a portable X-ray screen, is not enough although the latter is a good way of putting the presentation together in the first place.

When you have rehearsed once or twice, it is wise to discard your notes and make a list of slides in their correct sequence. This is all you need as a prompt. If you miss out something important during the presentation, you can usually correct the omission when you are answering questions.

Personal Appearance

There is no place for eccentricity of apparel in a speaker. Impressions are important; people unconsciously associate an untidy person with slovenly work. If you are in doubt about how to dress (particularly at a foreign meeting), be formal rather than informal. Dress neatly and plainly, and make sure that your shoes are clean and your hair is tidy. There is no place for loud ties or frilly dresses—you only have 10 minutes to get your message across and you want to focus the audience's attention on your work, not your appearance.

Attitude

STAND STILL. Keep your hands resting on the lectern, not in your pockets. Do not use the pointer unless it is absolutely necessary and, if it is electric, make sure that it is turned off when not in use so that it does not dart madly all over the lecture hall and divert the attention of the audience. Do not use it at all unless your hand is steady, otherwise you will merely draw attention to your own nervous state rather than to the point you are trying to make. If you know the chairman, address him by name; otherwise Mr. (or Madam) Chairman is quite correct. "Chairperson" may be accurate, but it sounds rather silly. Do have an introductory sentence, however short. "Mr. Chairman, ladies and gentlemen, first slide please" is a slovenly way to start. Throughout your presentation speak to the audience, not to the screen. It is your listeners who will judge you and who will lose interest if you are discourteous.

Resist the temptation to try to be funny. Senior men may regard it as impertinent coming from a junior. Even an experienced speaker can misjudge his audience to such an extent that a badly-placed joke may fall embarrassingly flat, or offend a section of the audience.

Remember that however well you speak, the words "finally" or "in conclusion" will rivet the attention of your audience. Do not waste the opportunity (6). The speaker who says "finally" several times raises false hopes and is as irritating as the one who reads all his slides, implying that the audience is illiterate.

Question time can frighten the inexperienced speaker. Always be polite, even if a member of the audience tries to vex you. If someone is rude, or is merely trying to present his own results, thank him for his comments; do not get involved in a wrangle.

It is useful to take a small pad and pen onto the platform with you so that you can jot down questions; it is always embarrassing to have to ask someone to repeat a question because you have forgotten it. If someone asks a question to which you do not know the answer, say so; nobody is an encyclopedia. It is far better to acknowledge ignorance than to make a fool of yourself trying to conceal it.

Attention to Detail

Before you start, make sure that you have inspected the lectern and know the functions of all the switches. If you are giving a paper on behalf of several people, introduce yourself to your chairman beforehand so that he is sure of your name and position when he introduces you. Always check and clean your slides before putting them in the carousel; slides can slip in the mounts during transit. It is wise to take a few spare mounts with you in case any get broken. If you are traveling by air, never let your slides leave your side; checked baggage goes astray too often to be sure that you and your slides will arrive at the same destination at the same time.

Make yourself known to the projectionist, especially if you have special instructions or requests (for example, a blank slide to separate sections can cause consternation if it is unexpected).

Speaking to an International Audience

If you are speaking to an audience whose first language is not your own, it is better to err on the side of speaking too slowly. If most members of the audience are foreign, it is courteous to have your key slides translated into their language. You can then use dual projection to enable those less familiar with your tongue to get the gist of your presentation. If dual projection facilities are not available, a summary slide in the appropriate foreign language will suffice.

It is important when making a presentation to an international audience to keep the use of abbreviations to a minimum and to explain, carefully, those that you do use. An accepted list has been published (7) but even these are not familiar to everyone. It is not only abbreviations that cause misunderstanding. Certain colloquial figures of speech may also not be understood by your audience.

Conclusions

Burkhart (8) presented the following picture of an inept lecturer: ". . . verbosity overtakes conciseness; disorganized presentation overtakes clear thinking and careful preparation; mumbles overtake articulateness; and, worst of all, you can't read the slides beyond the third row."

It is sensible to take the advice of experts (6, 9, 10) about what not to do on a platform. It is, however, vital that any instructions about speaking should be few, short and positive. They can be summarized as:

–stand still
–speak up
–do not read
–learn your first and last sentences but, for the rest, tell the audience about your work as you would a friend.

A good speaker does not wander about the platform as if searching for the exit; he does not wave his arms, or the pointer, for emphasis; he chats—rather than lectures or reads; and he establishes rapport with the audience by referring, for instance, to a previous speaker's comments, and by being enthusiastic about his subject. His slides will be easily read by people in the back row and his talk will have a beginning, a middle and an end.

Although a speaker who follows all these maxims makes it look easy, you can be sure that he has taken a lot of trouble to get his slides correct, has rehearsed with his slides in front of a critical audience of colleagues and has usually changed the order of his slides several times; he will not have memorized his speech.

It is as important to present your work in a polished form as it is to conduct your research carefully. It is a stimulating exercise and must be considered an integral part of any research project.

References

1. Hill AB. The reasons for writing. Brit Med J 1965;iv:870–871.
2. Dudley HAF. The Presentation of original work in medicine and biology. Edinburgh: Churchill Livingstone, 1977.
3. Evans M. Use slides. How to do it. In Lock SP, editor. 2nd ed. London: British Medical Association, 1985.
4. Howard P. The State of the language. English observed. London; Hamish Hamilton, 1984.
5. Hopkins C. Scientific advertising. London: McGibbon and Kee, 1968.
6. Meadow R. Speaking at medical meetings. Lancet 1969; ii:631–633.
7. International Steering Committee of Medical Editors. Uniform requirements for manuscripts submitted to biomedical Journals. Brit Med J 1979;i:532–535.
8. Burkhardt S. Do as I say, not as I do? Brit Med J 1983; 287:893.
9. Hawkins CF. Speaking and writing in medicine. Thomas, Springfield, 1967.
10. Calnan J, Barabas A. Speaking at medical meetings—a practical guide. London: Heinemann Medical Books Ltd., 1972.

3

The Longer Talk

B. McPeek and C. Herfarth

A good friend and colleague has invited you to come to London and present the results of your research. You are, of course, honored and flattered at the invitation. But what do you do? How do you respond?

First, consider the invitation. A wise and gracious host will tell you about the audience and the occasion. He will tell you what he has in mind, the purpose of the talk, and any suggestions he may have regarding the topic. Pay close attention to these three issues. If you are contacted by letter, it is a good idea to telephone your host to be certain you understand the audience and occasion, the specific purpose of the talk, and your host's ideas about the subject. If the invitation comes in person or by telephone, be sure the discussion does not end until you are certain you understand the setting, purpose, and proposed subject.

A good talk not only reflects your interests and enthusiasm but also the interests, concerns, and limitations of the audience who will hear it. In order to speak *to*, rather than *at*, any group you must analyze the audience. From your host, you will learn about the expected size of the audience; its composition in terms of age, sex, and professional or educational status; and the scope of its interest in and knowledge of your subject. Analyze the occasion also. In what setting and what circumstance will you speak? What will precede and follow your talk? What rules or customs prevail? What is the room or auditorium like? How is it equipped?

What is your host looking for in the talk? Is it a detailed presentation for specialists familiar with your work in the field, or are you to introduce new concepts to a younger audience? Is a presentation for scientists or clinicians from other fields intended? Should it be specific and concrete, or more general? Should you stress the clinical aspects or the more theoretical scientific applications? Is your host committed to a specific subject, or have you been given a more general invitation to "come and tell us about your latest work".

You will want to give great attention to selecting your subject. The audience and occasion ordinarily determine the purpose of the talk, and the purpose will influence your subject.

If you are lucky, you know your subject and have recently spoken on it. You may have a talk almost ready to deliver. You know what has worked well in the recent past, with what kinds of audiences and occasions, and you have appropriate visual aids prepared. Only a little refining is necessary. Perhaps you will want to make some new slides, or cite fresh examples keyed to the new audience.

Frequently, there is more to do. Your knowledge of the subject may be sound and up to date, but you have not given the talk before. If several years have passed since you last talked on the subject, you will need to gather additional information to bring your talk up to date.

A rare unhappy soul finds that a research job must be done after he has committed himself to speak on a subject.

Before you accept the invitation, be brutally realistic about the request. Do not let your pleasure at being asked to speak, or the honor of the occasion carry you away. Only you know the other demands on your time. Your host may have an overly optimistic view of your knowledge. Consider what you know about the topic and how much preparation will be required before you can speak on it. Be prepared to suggest an alternative topic or topics, suitable to the audience and occasion and congruent with your host's purpose for the speech. Remember, only *you* know what you can do with the material and time you have available. Many speakers prefer not to respond to an invitation immediately, but to take a day to be sure they are not being asked to agree to something they cannot carry off well and comfortably.

The longer talk differs from a written paper or a ten-minute presentation of research. If readers start to read a paper in a journal, they can leave it if they do not like it. A ten-minute oral presentation may be painful to some in the audience, but it will be over in a short time.

The longer talk has a captive audience. Much as we may be tempted, most of us are shy about getting up and walking out. You and your host have a serious obligation to select a topic that will interest the audience and be suitable to the occasion. For this reason, be cautious about selecting too narrow a subject for a longer talk. A narrowly focused subject may be appropriate for a written paper or a brief ten-minute talk, but the longer talk generally draws a more diverse audience, and usually requires a more general topic.

After you have agreed to speak on a specific subject, you must construct your talk. Many speakers start by carrying a notebook around with them and as ideas occur, perhaps at random, they jot them down. Make sure you note down all ideas. Things may occur while you are getting up in the morning, at lunch, or as you are going to bed at night. Many of these ideas will be good, but most of them will be lost if you don't write them down as soon as they occur to you.

Next, you will want to rank your ideas in terms of their importance and start to develop an outline. Then assemble the available materials from your own previous work or from the work of others in the field. Perhaps, you need a library search to make sure you have not missed a recent paper. You may want to telephone colleagues you know are working in the same area. They may know of new work you have missed, or may have a fresh suggestion you can incorporate. You will, of course, want to graciously acknowledge their assistance when you give your talk. At this time, make a preliminary list of the ideas to be included, and indicate their arrangement. Wait until you have gathered necessary supporting material before making a complete outline or final speech plan. Keep the plan flexible and continue to make adjustments as you go along. Only when you are sure you have the basic material in hand do you arrange the points you expect to make in their final order.

A talk generally has an opening or introduction, a main body, and an ending or closing. Most speakers start by working on the body of the talk.

Remember, you want the audience to grasp and be able to recall important data and ideas about the subject. A talk is not the opportunity to parade your own knowledge, nor should you try to see how much ground you can cover in a given time. Rather, your efforts should be focused on securing your listeners' understanding and on presenting material in such a way that it will be recalled.

Speakers should consider the following guidelines:

1. Keep the principal ideas few in number. If masses of data are given too rapidly, your audience will become bewildered and will catch only an occasional point here and there. In particular, when you are discussing a new or complex topic, do not try to deal with too many major ideas or to pass over any of them too quickly. Select the data and the concepts that are essential to understanding your subject. Then, through the use of appropriate visual aids or supporting material, hold each topic in the minds of your audience until you are sure it has been absorbed.
2. Define unusual terms. Frequently in science, there is a specific meaning for a word that has a different or more general meaning in ordinary use. Stop to define a strange or ambiguous term before you go ahead. Sometimes the meaning of a word is clarified by telling the audience what it does not mean.
3. Present information at an appropriate rate. Pace your delivery so that the talk keeps moving forward at a speed calculated to insure understanding but avoid boredom.
4. Wherever possible use concrete illustrations. Don't be too abstract. The famous statistician, Frederick Mosteller (1), reports that he

learned an important idea for presenting new material from a friend, Professor E. K. Rourke. Rourke calls his idea, "P–G–P". The letters stand for *particular, general, particular*. Rourke believes that a difficult concept is best presented by a *particular* example to motivate the listener and clarify the technique. The *general* refers to a general treatment of the technique you present. It is necessarily more abstract. Rourke then drives the whole thing home with a second *particular* example. The point of your effort is to have the information retained after the talk.

5. Clarity is almost as important as accuracy of detail. Try to present statistics in round numbers: say "about half", rather than "48.92%". Be honest, but try to avoid explanations that are so extensively qualified that the central point is lost in a mass of details. Visual aids help with data presentation. After a mass of data has been presented, a slide can sometimes drive home the major point.

6. Relate new material to something the audience already knows. Listeners want to put new information in context. Help them by showing how your work developed from previous work. For example, in speaking about a new or innovative treatment, compare the new treatment to standard practice.

7. Be easy to follow. Make transitions explicit. As you pass from one point to another, make clear to the audience that you are leaving one aspect and moving to another. Let them know where you are going and how your new point relates to the preceding one.

Once you have the body of the talk in hand, think about the beginning and the closing. First and last impressions are important. We are likely to make up our mind about a speaker on our first impression though we may change our opinion later. Yet, we generally carry away from a talk, and remember for some time, the last things the speaker says.

The beginning of a talk requires special consideration as it sets the stage for what follows. It may be impossible to cancel the bad impression made by a poor beginning. The introduction of a talk depends in part on the occasion and the audience. Speakers need to win the attention of the audience and to prepare them for the ideas they are to hear. You may wish to refer to the occasion, to extend a greeting to the chairman of the meeting, and to thank your host. You want to make clear the specific topic you are going to discuss, and to lead the audience easily and naturally into it. Some speakers ask a rhetorical question, cite a vivid example, or offer a startling opinion. Speakers should attempt to tie their own experience or interests to those of the listeners.

Absolutely the last thing you will do is begin by undermining the audience's confidence in your ability. Don't begin by saying, "I'm not quite sure why I was asked to speak on this topic" or, "I wish I were a better speaker". If you aren't worth listening to, the audience will quickly discover it.

The ending of a talk should be both a finish and a summing up. You want to focus the thoughts of the audience on your central theme. You want to bring your important points together in a condensed and unified form to sum up their overall significance. Tie your talk together so that the pattern of your presentation comes to an end. Deliver a strong concluding sentence and then stop.

After you have a final outline in hand, develop the wording of your talk. Either speak it through or write it out. Generally, it is best to start by reading the detailed outline to fix major ideas in your mind. Then, "give" the talk to an empty room several times. Word your sentences in different ways until you discover the most effective way to state them. The first several times you will need to hold the outline, but put it aside as soon as you can.

This is a repetitive process. With each repetition, you become increasingly sure of yourself. Don't try to fix the exact words you will use at the time of your final delivery. Just now you want to master the ideas, not the language.

After you have finished wording the speech, you will want to practice for fluency. Deliver the speech to an empty room aloud several times from beginning to end. If you plan to show slides, introduce them at this point. If you plan to use a blackboard, have a blackboard in your room and write or draw on the board the way you will at the time you actually speak. Have a friend listen and time you so that you know how long you take.

After you have practiced awhile, use a tape

recorder to record the talk exactly as you hope to say it. Remember, *don't read* it, *speak* it. Using the recording, you can make a typescript of the talk.

Some speakers like to use a typescript at the time they give the talk. For an important talk, we use a triple-spaced typescript in a looseleaf binder. We can mark the appropriate points for slides or other visual aids on the typescript in pencil. Almost no one today reads a talk verbatim from the manuscript, other than heads of state or those speaking for great institutions. No one but a polished actor should try to commit a talk to memory and recite it like a part in a play.

Many speakers don't like to have a manuscript with them. They prefer to speak from the outline or from a set of notes, perhaps on small cards. The authors fear they might stumble on the way up to the lectern, drop the cards on the floor, and scramble their thoughts, their talk, and their self-control.

By now, you have your talk pretty well in hand. You have a manuscript, or an outline, and will be comfortable about speaking it.

At this point, step back. Look the talk over carefully with a cold eye. Rank order your individual points to see exactly which part of the talk is the central one. If you had to shorten the talk drastically, say to 15 minutes from your expected hour, what points would you really try to make to the audience? Occasionally, there are last minute changes in a schedule, and you will want to be able to react to these. To shorten a talk, the only thing you can do is to omit whole sections of it. Do not even think about trying to speak faster. An attempt to go through and delete extraneous sentences will not gain you more than a few minutes. Lay out a careful plan as to how you would shorten the talk if you had to. This exercise is worthwhile.

Lengthening a talk is no problem. In the first place, audiences are always pleased when a speaker does not take quite as long as they expect. How many times can you remember that ever having happened? If you do find that you have a great deal more time available than you have material for, restrain yourself. Do not add extraneous filler. Don't take up time with long-winded stories, simply move ahead and give the talk you have, crisply and carefully. Audiences almost always like more time for questions, and when good questions come along you can expand on the points they raise.

Again, practice with your tape recorder. The greatest value of a tape recorder is to help you appreciate weaknesses you might otherwise miss. Use the tape recorder systematically, not like a toy. Play the recorded talk back. Do this once or twice to get the overall sound of it, then take a paper and pencil in hand while you play it back again. This time, look for monotony of voice and note the places where it was most noticeable. Now, replay it again and look for repetitions or for hemming and hawing—note them. By this repetitive process of playing and replaying the talk over and over, each time listening for a single fault, you can completely transform an average talk and improve it out of all recognition.

If you really want to become a master speaker, look to an even newer method. Technologic advancements have brought the cost of small television cameras and video cassette recorders low enough that they are increasingly available in universities and hospitals as well as the homes of individuals. The newer cameras and video recorders are reliable and easy to use. Many universities and scientific societies offer workshops that allow faculty to video record themselves while giving a lecture. Most speakers, even well known lecturers, are appalled when they first see and hear themselves on the television monitor. Yet, by looking at themselves, by seeing and listening, they uncover weaknesses in delivery and, of course, identifying weaknesses is the first step toward fixing them. Speakers who want to improve platform performance use the camera and video cassette recorder repeatedly, employing much the same tactics as those just recommended for the microphone and tape recorder. The visual image, however, has much greater impact then sound alone. Speakers study and modify dress, body stance, bizarre bobbing and weaving movements, facial expression, and the use of gestures. With remarkably little effort, a wooden, toneless, monotonous delivery soon becomes lively and interesting. Bad habits melt away, replaced by an effective platform manner. Both excellent and poor speakers routinely find this technique helpful.

Remember that, as a speaker, your appearance is important. Consider carefully what you wear. Inquire beforehand about the degree of formality expected. If anything, dress a bit on the conservative side. This will almost never offend your audience whereas if you err on the side of informality, the effectiveness of your message is undermined.

Stage fright affects us all to a greater or a lesser degree. Many years ago, the famous surgeon, Professor Edward D. Churchill, gave his personal treatment for stage fright. (Churchill was well known as an effective speaker.) Each time he got up in an auditorium he would stand silently for a few seconds in front of the podium and do two things. First, he remembered that he was the speaker and was in charge of the occasion. Second, he looked out over the assembly and, in his minds' eye, tried to visualize the members of the audience dressed only in their underwear. He reported that the technique never failed and that the second step was particularly effective when facing a front row of distinguished professors.

At the time you agreed to speak, you learned something about the room or auditorium to be used from your host. Now that the talk is almost prepared, telephone your host and confirm the program. Make sure that you understand what facilities are available, what the room is like, where the speaker stands, and where the audience sits. After all, things might have changed.

At this time, with a week or so to go, develop a strategy for handling disasters. What will you do if the projector gives out in the middle of the talk? Think about your slides. What do they really show? If you had to select only two or three, which are the crucial ones? What are their main points? Could a blackboard sketch substitute in a pinch. Don't scare yourself silly, but think in advance how you could repair a variety of problems.

When traveling a distance, it is a good idea to have a copy of your talk and an extra set of slides in another piece of luggage. Sometimes, airlines lose bags and you would not want the world's only copy of your talk and slides to be mislaid.

The day of the talk, arrive at the room you are going to use early so you have a chance to look over the auditorium for yourself. Usually the podium is fixed, but sometimes you can move the lectern to one side so that you can more easily see the slides and use a pointer without turning your back on your audience.

In giving talks, you must be prepared for the possibility of surprises. Perhaps there is no chalk, or no eraser, or maybe not even the expected blackboard. Try out everything in the room. See that you can turn the lights on and off. If there is a projector, have someone plug it in to make sure that it works and your slides fit. Focus it. Make sure there is enough light at the lectern for you to see your notes. Locate the pointer. If there is a microphone, try it out. Find out how far you should stand from it. Have some water near by in case your throat dries up. You may feel embarrassed about all these preparations and a lecturer testing a microphone always feels silly, but you will look even sillier fumbling around during the talk. Strange things happen, be ready for them.

Professor Frederick Mosteller (1) offers the following suggestions:

1. You find the door locked or the room occupied. Relax. Let your host work it out. Introduce yourself to people waiting around and chat with them. Don't complain.
2. The room is too small. Already you are a great success. Don't apologize. Say how happy you are to see such a large audience.
3. Sometimes only two or three people show up. Go ahead with your talk as though you hadn't noticed. See it as an opportunity to share your work with those who are really interested. You may decide to turn the talk into a seminar with a lot of audience participation.
4. Sometimes at the last minute, the schedule must be changed. Perhaps a previous speaker ran over his time limit and used some of your time. Your talk is now too long. If you have prepared your speech as described above, you know exactly which 20 minutes of your talk are the most important. Tell the audience what is important, then stop for questions. Try not to let anyone suspect that you had expected to have more time.

Finally, don't feel bad when some of these things happen. They happen everywhere. Someday you will be host and it will happen to one of your guests.

Of course, the truth is, you will be a great success. You have purposely and systematically set about preparing and delivering a great talk. You have selected a good topic, gathered the material, and rehearsed thoroughly.

After the talk is over, you are pleased that your planning and forethought have paid off so handsomely. The delivery and the audience's response were just as you had hoped. Nothing went wrong, but you knew that you were prepared to cope with the unexpected, and this only added to your poise and confidence. You felt good up there. Your host is delighted and so are you.

References

1. Mosteller F. Classroom and platform performance. Am Statistician 1980;34:11–17.

4

Presenting Your Work at International Meetings

T. Aoki and J-H. Alexandre

The Advantages of International Exchange in Science

Scholars, particularly those near the beginning of their research careers, find that presenting their research results personally at international academic and research meetings imparts a special impetus to learning how to communicate their findings concisely, lucidly and effectively to their peers. Such presentations provide on-the-spot opportunities for substantial and stimulating discussions of the significance and implications of your work.

If you are a young investigator, preparing to make the results of your research public, you should take part in repeated discussions of your work at academic and research meetings with the leaders in your field before you publish it. Such discussions serve to clarify the procedural and analytical methods of your study, the pertinency of your conclusions and their relation to other related and future issues. If the points generated from these discussions can be included in your subsequent published article, it will likely receive a higher evaluation than material submitted before adequate deliberation.

The basic purpose for presenting research at meetings is the same for domestic and international gatherings. "Free paper sessions" have increased recently because conference hosts would like to see an increased number of participants and the researchers do not want to participate in discussions unless they are given the opportunity to present their own research. When these free paper sessions do not provide enough time for discussion because of overcrowding, the clarifying and defining function of an effective scientific exchange are frustrated.

When problems in the management of the meeting result in inadequate time for discussions, be prepared to shorten your presentation, if it is necessary to do so for the sake of having a full discussion.

International meetings obviously provide more opportunity for discussion from a global perspective than domestic meetings. Non-native speakers of the language used at international meetings must give careful thought to the words they select to express scientific facts. This exercise often leads to new insights, and realizations that were previously only vaguely understood or grasped by the author in his mother tongue. The greatest disadvantage of international meetings is the language barrier. There is a real possibility that adequate discussion of your paper will not be possible after you have presented it. Try to prearrange some discussion to "break the ice". There is a possibility that errors may arise in the understanding of scientific "facts" as the result of misinterpretations of your presentation or your answers to questions during the discussion period caused by language problems. Discussion slides prepared in advance to answer questions you anticipate can help prevent this problem.

Extra effort is required to exploit the advantages gained from international exchange. It is particularly important for young researchers to learn to reach out across the language barrier for these rewards.

The accurate expression of facts presupposes

our recognition that language, itself, is a science. Our deepest understanding of science is realized in the context of its translation into foreign languages, the meanings of each of their words, and the nuances behind their usage. The scientific element of research is heightened when the researcher gives careful thought to what kind of facts should be expressed under what circumstances and with which words. This helps us experience the common language of all researchers which is science itself in a much richer way.

One significant benefit of attending international meetings is the stimulus it gives to mastering the multilingual approach to thinking—the approach that ultimately trains your mind to think in the scientific mode. Young scientists are advised to seek language education aggressively in order to acquire the minimal level of language ability needed for the communication of basic facts.

Suggestions for Speakers

Presenting a paper at an international meeting calls for strict discipline in facing many handicaps, meeting specific requirements and analyzing what is appropriate for a given situation.

The Subject

Most often, ideas, personal experiences or the results of advanced research are presented and are likely to be compared to the ideas and results of related team research in other countries. More and more meetings focus on very precise themes so you may find that your paper is almost identical to the presentation that precedes or follows it. Don't let this destabilize you. Compliment the other speaker, and proceed. Emphasize, if you can, the details which make your research methods, approach, perspective or future studies different from the others.

The Speaker

An international gathering eagerly awaits you. If you are famous, the audience will want to attach a face to your name; if you are unknown, you have an opportunity to contribute your new information or perspective to what has been published. You must take advantage of this chance to gain the interest of an international audience. Speaking with ease, clarity and conviction will add more weight to the information you have come to present.

The International Audience

Because they are accustomed to attending similar conferences, many members of your audience will be very demanding as far as style, content and adherence to time restrictions are concerned. For some, the language of your presentation will be a problem. English is now the most commonly used language at international meetings; Spanish, French, German and Japanese are used less often. When the program indicates the possibility of simultaneous translation, appropriate preparation is required. A few specific cases merit consideration.

English as the Only Language

If English is your mother tongue, you must remember to speak slowly, pronounce each word clearly and pause frequently for your Japanese, French, German and Spanish listeners. If at all possible, use bilingual slides with English on the left side and the language of the host country on the right.

If you are asked to make a presentation in English and your mother tongue is German, French, Japanese or Spanish, etc., your preparation may be long and difficult. You will have to rehearse your presentation a number of times in front of a critical audience or with a tape recorder to be sure that you will remain within your time limit (10 or 15 minutes). Under no circumstances should you expect an extension of the allotted time because of the language difficulties. You must prepare a short two page manuscript, typed with double spaces, in sections of 5 minutes each, from which you can read the introduction and the conclusion of your paper. Your slides, which are best committed to memory, must parallel the talk and contain a maximum of 20 clearly visible words. If speaking in English is a struggle for you and you have complex slides to present, it is accepted practice to all that you read your presentation. You must, however, read slowly, take time to face your audience, look straight at a third or fourth row listener, and frequently scan the room.

Simultaneous Translation

When simultaneous translation is available, your presentation will have to be slow-paced to give the translator a chance to keep up with you. Pause when you are presenting visual material, and be sure to provide the translator with a copy of the manuscript and a translation well in advance. If possible, visit the auditorium ahead of time to assess where you will be in relation to your audience, the chairman, the moderator and the projection screens. If two projectors are available, you may be able to judge which material would be best projected on the right or on the left.

On Stage

Before you begin to speak, sit down in the front of the room near the podium so that you will not have to run to the stage, trip over a wire on the way, or have to catch your breath when you get there. Be sure to note how close the microphone is and to face your listeners—you must not turn your back to them, you must remain standing without waving your arms or walking about. Keep an eye on the time.

Four important points to remember are:

take a big breath before you start to talk;
speak slowly and loudly;
enunciate clearly, and
be confident in yourself.

When you and your presentation are well prepared, your audience will be hanging on your every word.

As the timer goes off, you must finish the sentence you are in and then go directly to your concluding three sentences. By then your information has surely been conveyed and everyone knows that you cannot say everything in so short a time. The discussion period will allow some time for relevant questions and the hallways are there for the exchanges of addresses and references. Your extra effort to make a clear, concise presentation will help your own research, and will win the respect of your international colleagues.

5

Chairing Panels, Seminars and Consensus Conferences

M.F. McKneally, B. McPeek, D.S. Mulder, W.O. Spitzer, and H. Troidl*

Introduction

Scholars are frequently called upon to chair panel discussions, to moderate or conduct seminars involving large numbers of peers, or guide the deliberations of consensus conferences. The success and productivity of any of these meetings depend on the expertise, tact, and wisdom of the chairperson, the specialized knowledge and communications skills of the principal participants, and the care and thought put into the planning and organization of the meeting.

The Choice and Function of the Moderator

The moderator is the key to any successful joint discussion. The qualities needed to chair a panel or any other discussion are the same as those desired in the individual who will chair any committee. He, or she, should be a good speaker and be able to intervene in a firm and positive manner, maintain reasonable discipline, and adhere to an agreed timetable and agenda. Although the person chairing a meeting should possess a good overall knowledge of the subject under discussion, familiarity with its more abstruse aspects is not necessary.

The individual chosen may be an authority in some part of the field under discussion and may be well-known as a strong protagonist of certain controversial beliefs. It must be stressed, however that the moderator must control the expression of personal convictions, and allow and encourage the expression of contrary views. Finding someone who will behave in this way is sometimes easier said than done. The difficulty is the same as that found in legal circles where a person who has been an outstanding advocate may find it hard, on being elevated to a judgeship, to assume the impartial attitude appropriate to that office. Adequate knowledge of the personalities of those being considered as possible moderators and their previous performance in similar situations is helpful in avoiding the selection of someone who might otherwise seem suitable. In contrast, some individuals have rightly earned reputations as superb moderators and are widely sought after for this role.

At the end of any panel discussion, the speakers and the audience should feel that, although you, as moderator have exercised firm control, you have maintained a reasonably objective stance throughout the meeting and have given all members of the panel a fair deal. This will not happen, however, simply as a matter of good luck or even of the considerable skill the moderator may exercise during the meeting itself.

To ensure the kind of success just described, you, in your role as moderator, will need to get in touch with the speakers before the meeting to define the limits of their discussion very clearly and to obtain outlines of what they intend to say.

You can facilitate discipline through certain "dirty tricks", such as using a gavel; placing a samurai sword, water-pistol or rose on the table in front of you and leaving their intended use to each speaker's imagination; or announcing that

---

*With the advice of J.C. Goligher.

at the end of the time allocated, that a trap-door will open under the speaker. You can deal with the speaker who is particularly long-winded and uncontrollable, by standing up, walking to the podium, eventually, yet gently, taking the microphone, sharing the problem of time-pressure with the speaker and the audience, and inviting the speaker to continue the discussion during some subsequent part of the program that may never materialize.

Be sure to have two people available for sorting questions. For foreign guests, use translated slides and movies and try to avoid inviting guests who have a language problem to be panel members. If it is absolutely necessary to use such an expert guest from another country, try to have him give a separate presentation and minimize his participation in the discussion. You must know his communication skills. If it is appropriate to engage him in the panel discussion, a translator should be available to communicate the nuances of questions and answers.

You can enliven boring questions by simply changing the age or setting of the clinical problem presented by the questioner. Turning off the microphone is a very effective way to deal with questioners from the audience who take advantage of the opportunity to present long-winded statements or arguments instead of questions.

One of your duties is to bring out the strong points of each member of the panel by skillful questioning so that his or her strengths are shown to best advantage. This is best done in an atmosphere of cordiality and good humour. Knowing your panelists well, personally, and knowing their communication skills and clinical experience will help you to foster such an atmosphere. At the close of a panel discussion, it is useful to have a closing statement that you have worked up during the course of the panel discussion.

The Choice of Speakers

Choose speakers, or panelists for their special knowledge and for their abilities to express their opinions. The speaker you select for a symposium may differ somewhat from one who would be ideal for a panel discussion where you want to avoid the possibility of uneven coverage and too many speakers being assigned to relatively esoteric topics. For a panel discussion, you must have adequate though not superfluous coverage of all the major aspects of the topic being examined. In particular, ensure that both sides of any controversial issue are fairly represented. The people you choose specifically for a panel discussion will usually be accepted authorities who are accustomed to participating in such events and are expert at expounding their ideas and engaging in debate.

When symposia or panel discussions are held at international meetings, it is usually in the interest of good relations between countries to choose a group of speakers of mixed nationality. For a panel discussion, this custom creates a real problem in regard to language since it can seriously frustrate the success of the effort. No entirely satisfactory solution exists. One way of dealing with this difficulty is to conduct the discussion entirely in one language, which usually means English. Although many doctors whose native language is not English have a good command of English, relatively few of them are up to the "rough and tumble" of a brisk, hard-hitting panel discussion in a language that is not their mother tongue. One of the things that is most difficult to transmit across the language barrier is humour, since it so often depends on subtle nuances in the meaning of words that are difficult for anyone except a real language expert to appreciate. As a consequence, panel discussions in English with multi-national participants tend to be rather humourless affairs in sharp contrast to the spirit that pervades a really first class panel discussion in which an element of humour is an important if not indispensable ingredient.

The alternative plan is to use several languages during the discussion according to the nationalities of the various speakers and to rely on simultaneous translation to make it intelligible. However, despite the immense skill displayed by the most experienced interpreters at major international conferences in translating quite complex ideas extemporaneously and with astonishing rapidity and accuracy, simultaneous translation inevitably slows and occasionally confuses the process of discussion. It also tends to suppress attempts to enliven the proceedings.

Panel Discussion

Panel discussions have been particularly popular and successful in the U.S.A. for some years, but they are now widely used in most other countries as well. They tend to follow two formats. One is used in connection with a formal symposium on a broad subject or during formal research presentations when it is decided that, instead of the usual 10-minute discussion after each paper, there will be a combined one-half hour discussion period involving all of the speakers at the end of the formal presentations. The moderator will frequently ask for participation from the audience through written questions or by having the discussant come to a floor microphone in the auditorium. The other format is a true panel discussion in which the panel takes its place on the platform, the moderator offers some brief introductory remarks, and each of the speakers, in turn, speaks for not more than 5 to 8 minutes on a particular aspect of the main theme in which he or she has special expertise or interest. An open discussion follows. The aim of any discussion is to further illuminate what the speakers have said by allowing the various points made during their set talks to be expanded, challenged, and defended. A panel discussion has the same objective, but usually achieves it in a more authoritative and emphatic way because of the presence on the panel of several experts who are able to offer well-based opinions on any issue that may be raised. Properly handled by the moderator, such a group can provide a very lively, informative and entertaining exposition of the subject under consideration.

Another variation is for the moderator to pick a controversial clinical problem and have each speaker present his or her views on the optimal management of such a clinical problem in a short formal illustrative talk. The moderator then presents a typical clinical question to the panel and usually reveals the key investigative studies when they are requested by a member of the panel or prompted by a question from the audience. Surgeons with opposing views are often asked to defend their positions in relation to the particular problem that has been presented. This often leads to a stimulating discussion in which the audience can participate by written or spoken questions.

Audiences like panel discussions because of the opportunity it gives them to interact through questions and brief comments, to observe more than one speaker, and to hear different points of view. Each format has its advantages when it comes to getting an interchange going among panel members with different experiences, backgrounds, and views. The panel format can be thought of as a small seminar conducted by a panel in front of a large audience that listens and has only a limited opportunity to contribute to the discussion through questions and invited comments.

Prediscussion Planning

Choice of Topics for Formal Presentation by Speakers

The moderator must clearly outline the topic or problem to be discussed during the course of the panel discussion, and then assign a precise topic to each of the selected speakers for presentation in a 5- to 8- minute talk. The moderator should carefully study the assigned subjects and determine whether there are obvious defects in the overall coverage of the main theme that might have to be remedied during the discussion. A carefully-written mandate to individual speakers from the moderator, well in advance of the panel discussion, is the only effective method of preventing duplication and ensuring adequate coverage of the chosen topic.

Briefing by Preliminary Meeting and/ or Correspondence

Most successful moderators hold a preliminary meeting with their panelists the day or morning before the discussion is to take place. If you have been chosen to act as moderator, you should use this occasion to explain your thoughts on how the discussion should go and to briefly review the presentation of each speaker. At this meeting, you can refine the general strategy, change the order of the talks to make them more effective, and deal with other minor technical problems to ensure that the formal presentation will go smoothly.

The panel members will frequently discuss potential questions and suggest who might be best-equipped to handle particular questions from the audience. You can also discuss any questions you have prepared in a general or specific way to lay the groundwork for a lively debate. Occasionally, it is impossible to arrange a preliminary meeting of this kind and you may have to rely on the second best arrangement, correspondence with the panelists.

Course of the Actual Discussion

The moderator usually introduces the topic of the panel discussion and briefly introduces the panelists just prior to their formal 5- to 8-minute presentations. The classic method of securing participation by the audience is to invite them to submit written questions. Small sheets of paper should be available for this purpose so that members of the audience can write down any questions that occur to them during the formal presentations or even during the discussion period. These sheets are collected by assistants who stroll the aisles. There is often a break for coffee between the portion of the symposium allocated to the presentation of papers and the subsequent period assigned to the panel discussion. This convenient interval is automatically available to you to look through the first batch of questions, before the discussion begins. In a separate panel discussion, the sorting of questions is more difficult, because it has to be done during the short pre-discussion talks or even between some of the answers to other questions. The alternate way of obtaining questions from the audience is to allow people to come to microphones strategically placed about the conference room to put their queries orally. In some centers, this method is preferred because it seems to provide more spontaneous and direct contact between the audience and the speakers, but it suffers from several disadvantages. Some people are inhibited by having to make their way to a microphone or summon one. There may be delays if insufficient microphones are available, but with an adequate number this need not be a major problem.

The most serious objection to oral questioning is that it largely denies you control of the discussion, as the moderator, because you do not know what questions are going to come up. Unless you interrupt the process to put queries of your own, you cannot direct the discussion to cover the issues you consider to be the most important. A further possible drawback is that once some speakers have reached a microphone, they lose any inhibitions they might have about being verbose and take a lot of precious time airing their own personal views.

One important and controversial matter is how much you wish to involve the audience in the discussion process. If you are prepared to leave the questioning largely to the audience and to let it take its own course, it is entirely optional to you whether you allow only written or oral questions, or both. If you prefer to control the evolution of the discussion yourself——which we consider to be much the better policy for most panel discussions—you can only do so by restricting the audience to written questions to give you a chance to scrutinize them and decide which of them you wish to use. You can often control the discussion most effectively by grouping the submitted questions into topic areas that fall within the realm of expertise of particular members of the panel.

Seminars

Seminars are usually small group presentations. The seminar leader may function almost as a lecturer or teacher, or the seminar, particularly if it is small, may function almost like a group discussion. Ordinarily there is a great deal of audience participation. Speakers at seminars sometimes give a lecture, but more often, they give a few remarks and are interrupted by questions from the audience. A discussion may ensue, and then the speaker goes on to cover another topic, again punctuated by discussion and interruption.

Several of the points made about the organization of a panel discussion, such as the choice of chairman and speakers and the way the discussion is conducted, also apply to a lesser extent to a seminar since it is a much less elaborate affair. The key note is informality. Since a seminar is usually held in a smaller room with a more limited audience, written questions would be inappropriate and all the questioning is done orally. Microphones are usually quite unnecessary. The object of the exercise is to create a relaxed atmosphere in which a ready exchange of ideas and opinions can take place and people's doubts can be either confirmed or laid to rest.

Consensus Conferences

A consensus conference is quite different from a panel discussion or seminar. It is a formalized way of seeking advice (1). A consensus conference is usually called by a policy maker, such as the Director of the National Institutes of Health, or the Minister of Health, or of Science and Technology.

The convening authority seeks the advice of the consensus conference members. Usually a consensus conference is called only to deal with a major unresolved scientific, medical, or social problem when the convening authority wishes advice about the best possible course of action, given the state of scientific knowledge at the time of the conference.

A consensus conference usually makes specific recommendations about policy. Sometimes, the policy recommendations relate to the treatment of particular groups of patients by physicians. Sometimes, the recommendations call for specific actions on the part of institutional or governmental authorities. A consensus conference almost always attempts to reach an agreement among the experts as to exactly what is known about the specified topic, what issues are settled, and what issues are still open to debate. It usually tries to focus the attention of the convening authority on areas of potentially fruitful research.

Participation in a consensus conference is almost invariably by invitation only. Considerable effort on the part of the convening authority is put into getting the best possible experts in the field. The convening authority not only wants the best possible advice but ordinarily is most anxious to have advice that cannot be successfully assailed later. For this reason, members of consensus conferences are sought from a wide spectrum of scientific backgrounds and a special effort is frequently made to ensure the representation of groups that might otherwise be inclined to attack the findings of the conference. In North America, representatives of minorities, of women, or of particular political groups, or sometimes of those who have a vested interest in one side or the other of an issue are deliberately included. This is an attempt to ensure that the whole process can be seen by observers as being thorough, complete, inclusive, and very carefully and honestly executed.

Consensus conferences have proven to be a useful mechanism for translating evidence from a number of clinical research studies into clinical applicability and professional policy. A consensus conference gives attention not only to scientific evidence, but also to the admissibility of such evidence. The personal, unsupported opinions of panel members, no matter how senior or prestigious they be, or perceive themselves to be, should carry less weight. The National Institutes of Health in the U.S.A. have used consensus conferences to integrate the considered opinions of recognized experts in various controversial areas, such as burn therapy, immune modulation of cancer patients, and the management of the multiply-injured patient.

If you are asked to chair such a conference, seek the support of a very high calibre scientific secretary who will not only keep good notes during the deliberations, but write a good account of what has happened so that the report of the discussion will reflect the true consensus, faithfully. It is extremely difficult to chair a meeting effectively and take notes at the same time. With a scientific secretary, it will also be easier for you to end up with a report that avoids introducing your own biases more heavily than is warranted.

Courtesy

As the moderator of a panel discussion, seminar or consensus conference you should be firm and keep control of the deliberations but observe scrupulous courtesy. This should be directed toward your audience and your peers. The same high standards should be fostered and upheld among all those present in the audience or at the conference table.

References

1. Hoaglin D, Light R, McPeek B, et al. Data for decisions: information strategies for policy makers. Cambridge, Mass.: Abt. Press, 1982.

6

The Poster Session, Audio Visual Aids

Y. Reid and K-H. Vestweber

Audio-Visual Aids

Experienced speakers follow the advice given in the old adage:

"Tell them what you're going to tell them.
Tell them.
Tell them what you've told them."

That clever summary neglects to mention a crucial dimension. It's important to not only "tell" your audience what you're going to tell them, but to "show" them. A key element in a successful presentation is the effective use of audio-visual aids, such as slides, overhead transparencies, films, videotapes, and models. A good audio-visual aid will enhance your presentation and increase your audience's comprehension.

Unfortunately, a poorly chosen or designed audio-visual aid can detract from an otherwise excellent talk. The time and attention devoted to the selection and preparation of audio-visual aids should equal that devoted to the talk itself. Your presentation needs should guide you as you choose the most suitable audio-visual medium for your purpose.

Slides and overhead transparencies will be the most easily available, convenient, and appropriate choices for many speakers, while film or videotape may be ideal for the surgeon who wishes to demonstrate a procedure to a larger audience. Whichever medium you choose, there are a few general guidelines that apply to all visuals.

First, when you're developing your materials, KISS . . . *K*eep *I*t *S*imple and *S*uccinct. As you revise your speech from its more formal written style to a less verbose and more conversational style, you should shift your thinking from words to pictures. Try to imagine creative ways to represent your message visually, as well as verbally. Remember that the eye reacts to color, brightness, contrast, size, and blank space. Try to use these parameters to best advantage as you plan your visual aids.

One way to learn the techniques of good visual design is to cultivate a close working relationship with your art and/or audio-visual department. Many universities and medical centers employ experienced artists, photographers, and technicians who can assist you with your program, suggest effective ways to deliver your message, and work with you to produce professional quality materials. If you do not have access to such a department, contact local free-lancing medical, dental, or general photographers or a mail order facility.

Slides

Slides come in many shapes and sizes . . . from the $3\frac{1}{4} \times 4$ inch glass lantern slides to the popular 2×2 inch 35mm film slides in paper or plastic mounts.

In any format, good slides can be valuable adjuncts to your verbal presentation; bad slides can distract—and detract—from it. A slide that is sloppily made, illegible, or too complex or confusing reflects poorly on the lecturer. Apologies offered for the crowded slide, "Well, I doubt if you can see this . . ." or "I'm sorry about this busy slide . . .", impress the audience only with the speaker's lack of communication skills, not with his profundity.

You should only use slides in your presentations if they add information, are clear and comprehensible, and are legible to your entire audience, including viewers at the back of the room.

A few do's and don'ts for making and presenting slides:

Format may vary to suit the projection equipment available. The most prevalent slide projector is the Carousel with an 80 slide tray. Because thick plastic mounts may get stuck and not drop well, thin plastic or paper mounts are preferable. However, if carbon arc or other high intensity and extremely hot projection lamps are used, glass mounting is essential to prevent slides from burning or melting even as you are speaking about them.

The viewing portion of slides is rectangular, in a ratio of 2:3. It's best if your slides are all aligned in one direction, horizontally or vertically. Otherwise, when a projector is set so that horizontal slides fill the screen, the rare vertical slide will extend beyond the top and bottom of the screen and a disruptive adjustment will be required. Another advantage of horizontal slides is that their dimensions correspond to those of a TV screen.

Content. Slides should supplement your text, not echo it word for word. A good slide gives your audience a visual representation of the concept you're presenting or adds new information. At the same time, avoid total slide-text dissociation.

In a similar vein, reading your slides to the audience is unnecessary and insulting and it should be discouraged. Viewers can absorb the information more quickly than you can read it aloud.

An average slide may require only 15 seconds of reading time, but it may be necessary to display a more complex slide for up to a minute to permit adequate audience comprehension.

To ensure clear, comprehensible slides, you should present only one thought or idea per slide, and never more than two. To give more information, make two slides.

Use as few words as possible.

Use 5 words or less for the title. Title lettering should be larger than the body lettering—suggest 36 points (½ inch).

Use no more than 7 lines per slide.

Each line should have no more than 7 words.

Use large lettering or type. Lettering in the body of the slide should be no smaller than 18 points (¼ inch). A 2 × 2 inch slide should be legible when held 14 inches from your eye. If you can't read it, your audience won't be able to either.

To begin preparing your material, review the sequence of your presentation and develop a series of handwritten or roughly sketched 5 by 8 cards to represent your visuals. This rough script is called a storyboard—or visual outline— and can help you organize your thoughts and make early revisions before you spend time and resources on the final product.

Lettering. Many options are available for lettering. Handwriting, stencils, dry transfer, typewriters, and computers have all been used to produce acceptable letters, numbers, and symbols. Your choice will depend on your designs, funds, available staff, and equipment.

Hand lettering onto sturdy bond paper without watermarks can be done with or without a stencil. Draw a guide line in pencil to align your letters and erase it prior to production. Another option is to light your work table from below and use a separate, lined, guide sheet that becomes visible under your copy. If you use a stencil, trace the outline of each letter with a fine-tipped, carbon-ink pen, then fill in the letter with a uniformly-colored ink.

Art supply stores can supply you with transfer letters of various types along with instructions for their use. Some may necessitate your making a photocopy of your "master" before the slide can be produced.

Typewriter lettering can often be inadequate. A ball or typing element that is worn or imperfect can result in print that looks smudged or uneven when blown up by projection. Before you use a typewriter, you must be sure that the typing face is clean, and that it provides crisp, clear type.

You should preferably use a 10 space/inch typewriter (pica). Some slidemakers prefer acetate-ink rather than carbon-ink ribbons to avoid the fine spraying of ink that may show up with negative wash and diazo processing. Others recommend mylar or unused carbon fabric ribbon.

Double space all typing, and use a maximum of 45 typing spaces per line. Use sanserif type, not serif; the letters appear more discrete. For large audiences, type in uppercase letters with an ORATOR ball if one is available.

Mechanical lettering resources are available from production studios and supply outlets. Prices vary with the equipment and services required.

Computer lettering and design are burgeoning. Many user-friendly programs that provide extensive graphics design cability are available for most business and some home computers. In addition, special printing systems allow production of professionally acceptable finished "masters" in a variety of styles and colors. Contact your computer department or retail outlet for further information. Many commercial photography and film production houses now use computer technology for slide design and manufacture.

Charts and Graphs. Copying machines can enlarge or reduce tables and illustrations from books and journals and allow their production as slides. Don't yield to this temptation! An illustration that is well suited to the reader who has the time and opportunity to repeatedly refer to it and return to the text for clarification may be ill-suited to the viewer who must capture the information in less then a minute.

Consequently, you should develop new visuals that are targeted specifically at your audience. Digest and simplify the information and parcel it out among several slides instead of just one. For example, most tables tend to contain too much data for easy immediate comprehension. It is better to demonstrate each point you wish to stress through a line graph, bar chart, or pie chart. If you do use tables, remember to limit yourself to 1 point per slide, 7 words per line, and 7 lines per slide. Center your title, align your columns, and leave a clear margin for contrast. Use large type for listings and headings, and round off numbers, if possible. It is best to save complex tables and graphs for handouts.

A linear graph may present data trends more clearly than a table. When you are drawing line graphs, space your coordinates widely and label them clearly in large type with rounded units. Avoid including too many details in your diagram. You should have no more than 2 lines per slide; each should be at least ⅛ inch thick, clearly labeled, and different in appearance from the other (solid vs. hatched). Label points with large circles, triangles, and squares, and draw line breaks at intersections.

When small differences in values occur, they may be less difficult to perceive if they are demonstrated by a bar graph (histogram). The bars, especially if colored differently, are ideal for showing contrasts. You should decide which format, i.e. horizontal or vertical bars, shows your results best. Draw the bars wide, with a maximum of 7 bars per slide. Keep lettering outside the bars, and don't crowd the columns. Separating the bars may make the graph less confusing.

Pie charts are excellent when you have wide variances in your results. The circle should nearly fill the slide and contain no more than 7 slices. Use color for contrast. Put numbers inside the pie, words outside. Be sure your percentage figures add up to 100%.

You can give appropriate credit for borrowed illustrations on the slides, or in you talk to avoid picture "clutter".

X-rays. Most X-ray films make poor slides. Even a relatively sharp roentgenogram may produce a confusing, out-of-focus slide. If you do use them, be sure your slides are clear and sharp, and that the area in question is shown well. When you are making the slide, zoom in on the area of interest, put it on one half of the slide, and label it clearly. The other half of the slide should show a corresponding line drawing to assist with identification. Drawings should be simple, in black and white, and avoid shades of gray.

Pathological specimens. Photographing unusual specimens can be difficult. A properly lighted specimen stand that reduces reflection and provides a non-distracting background is often necessary. You should include views of both the surface of a specimen and of a cut section of it on one orientation slide. Inclusion of a centimeter ruler in the same photograph can assist in estimating size. Specimens should be rinsed clean, unless the presence of blood is necessary for demonstration purposes.

Microscope slides often transfer poorly to film. The slide should be well stained to bring out contrast and detail. Use the minimum magnification necessary to show the features you wish. A higher magnification may make it more difficult to obtain clear pictures. Focus down on the area of interest, and take the picture from the center of the field to avoid perimetric distortion. The finished slide should have a focus dot to assist the projectionist or, even better, add labels to indicate the areas of interest on one side of the slide, or an adjacent line drawing.

Color. Many color options are available. Your choice will depend on your needs for emphasis. One of the most popular and most restful to the eyes is the diazo—the blue background with white letters. Newer methods can now produce longer-lasting backgrounds in many colors, but some are more translucent than others. The transparency of the slide is important when you consider room lighting and your audience's need to take notes easily. White print on a dark background is better in lighted rooms, whereas dark print on a light background is better in dark rooms. White on black negatives are hard to read at a distance and in partially lit rooms.

Avoid jumping from colored slides to slides with black letters on a bare white background; the brightness can be disturbing. For audience comfort, it's a good idea to maintain a constant level of light coming through your slides.

Graphs, charts, and lettering can be colored to enhance contrast, during production or postproduction, with color gels available from your art supplier. It's best to do linear graphs as positives, i.e., dark lines on a light background. Despite the temptation, use color with caution. It is most effective when it has a purpose.

Style should be uniform and consistent, unless a change is needed for emphasis. Too many variations can be jarring or distracting.

You and your art director can decide on a style that best suits your needs. Some speakers prefer slides with titles and bullets of information, others choose a series of graphs and charts. Occasionally, an artist can produce a symbol or cartoon theme to add a touch of variety or humor.

Avoid the use of abbreviations and ditto marks. Many slidemakers suggest the omission of dates on slides; a superfluous date many render a good slide obsolete.

After you're done, check and double-check for spelling errors. A slide sent for production with misspellings will no doubt be well produced—with misspellings.

When you receive your slides, recheck them for accuracy, content, and quality. Be sure they are properly framed in their holders, i.e., without white borders, and that their holders are sealed and unwarped.

Touch up any blemishes with special paint (available from Kodak).

Wipe off fingerprints.

Label your slides as noted below, and store in a slide album or tray.

View your slides with colleagues for rehearsal and critical review. Examples of good slides or surgical subjects are included in the appendix to this chapter, kindly provided by the Society of Thoracic Surgeons.

For the speech, rehearse, rehearse, rehearse. Though most conferences provide projection equipment, consider bringing your own projector with a spare bulb to provide a back-up if the need arises.

Load your slide tray in advance. Hold the slide so that you can read it, number it on the bottom right corner, and put a marker dot on the bottom left corner. For proper positioning for front projection, put your slides in the slot by holding the bottom right corner and flipping the side over into slot. If the slide is properly in the tray, the dot will be at the top right. Then, put the locking top on the tray to avoid an accidental spill. Note, rear projection will require you to flip the slide to make the writing look "backward" before you place it in the tray.

Use opaque slides for pauses, and at the beginning and end. The sudden flash of a white screen blinds, and irritates the audience.

Start your tray with a "focus" slide. Your projectionist can use this slide to focus without displaying the first slide for your talk.

Do not ask the operator to return to a previous slide. If you need to refer to a slide shown earlier, make a duplicate copy, and insert it in the appropriate position.

Talk to the projectionist at least 10–15 minutes prior to your speech. Review procedures for advancing the slide, i.e., whether you or the projectionist will do it, and agree on the appropriate cues. If you have a written text for your talk, provide the projectionist with a copy, preferably with the slide changes noted on it.

Adjust the projector so that the screen is filled

by the slide, i.e., the projected image of the slide should be as large as possible.

If possible, run the slides through to make sure they are in good condition and in proper order. A run through will also help to warm the slides to avoid buckling of the film and distortion at the edges.

Once you have begun, remember to talk to your audience, and not to your slides. Your slides should be well-labeled, but you may wish to use a pointer occasionally. If you do, focus it to a sharp spot or arrow, and point it directly at your target. Do not wave the pointer about or in circles, and don't point it at the audience. If you are not using it, turn it off.

Transparencies

Transparencies, shown with an overhead projector, are an easy and inexpensive audio-visual tool for the lecturer. They can be made quickly, and can be corrected or adjusted at the lecture site. They are an ideal aid for the lecturer who does not have time to prepare slides for a presentation to a small audience.

The principles governing good transparency production are the same as those for slides—KISS (*K*eep *I*t *S*imple, *S*uccinct). Your pre-production thinking and planning should follow the same lines, only the production will differ. Once you have your text or design, it can be processed through a transparency-making machine in about one minute. Your cell is dry and ready to use. You can add color for emphasis and contrast directly onto the transparency with a felt tip pen or highlighter.

Here are a few other tips about transparencies. The lettering options are the same as those listed under slides, but heat-resistant compounds, such as carbon-based ink or soft pencil, must be used. Otherwise, make a photocopy of your original material and use it to make the transparency.

Although they will not look as professional as they would with artwork or transfer lettering, transparencies can be hand-lettered with felt-tip pens or wax pencils. Do not press too hard on the wax pencil, however, or you will spray the wax and leave "crumb" trails.

Follow the rules noted above for content, style, size and legibility, etc. Remember to leave at least a one-inch margin free of writing or printing. Do not copy illustrations or tables from books without first assessing their communication value as visuals.

If the transparency is oriented so that you can read it as you face the audience, it's the right way up for projection onto the screen. This enables you to look at your audience and your transparency without having to look at the screen. You can point with your finger or a pencil onto the transparency instead of using a pointer on the screen. Sometimes, you can jot lightly-penciled notes, on your transparency, that are invisible to your audience to assist you during your talk.

Be sure to inspect the projector and to adjust it so that your transparency fills the screen. When you transfer sheets, try to do it smoothly without leaving an open space between cells. The sudden brightness between darker cells may be disturbing to your audience.

Videotape and Film

The "moving media" are ideally suited to demonstrating the techniques and procedures of an operation to a larger audience. Each medium has certain advantages and some speakers use a combination of videotape and film. Although color brightness and picture clarity may be slightly better with film, its drawbacks include cost, processing-time, complicated editing requirements, and the lack of an immediate print for feedback. Some film makers will videorecord, simultaneously, to have a tape for on-site review as a guarantee for their film shots.

Videotape is relatively inexpensive and easy to use. The lighting requirements are not as exacting as they are for film, and the sound is recorded directly onto the tape. The result is immediately viewable, and an unsuccessful scene can be quickly erased and reshot. Editing is best left to an expert, but the process is not difficult; the desired pieces of tape are transferred to a new master tape in the appropriate sequence.

For both film and videotape, certain basic principles must be followed to ensure a successful production. The most important is "advance planning".

First, discuss your needs with your audio-visual department. What would you like to demonstrate in you production? The AV staff can assist you by suggesting the most effective way to capture a technique or skill on film or tape.

Next, run through the procedure with your crew and staff. Describe the location you must use, the numbers of people around the operating table (and in the way of the camera), the room available for equipment use and storage, and the basics of the operation, including the time and temperature limitations imposed by the welfare of your patient. Develop an "outline" of the session with your medical and audio-visual personnel.

Decide on equipment and format. Most videotaping should be done with 3/4 inch U-matic (professional Beta) tape. One-inch tape will give you a better copy, but is more expensive.

Select your patient and get a signed release for taping or filming for educational use. The patient should be lean; operative field exposure and anatomic details are often poor with obese patients.

If possible, rehearse with your crew and staff prior to the actual operation. Even with the benefit of such rehearsals, count on taking at least twice the normal time for the actual operation.

The camera eye should record from the surgeon's "point of view". The surgeon should therefore stand slightly to the side of his/her normal position during filming. Be sure that what the camera sees is what you want to show; close-ups and zoom-shots can focus in on the area of interest.

Though bleeding is unavoidable, it's better to reduce bloody scenes, unless they are instructive. Stop the film or tape, clean the field, and reshoot. Gloves should be rinsed or changed, and instruments should be wiped. An extra, sterile gown should be available to cover a soiled one. Drapes, pads, and sponges in the field should be replaced with clean ones, but avoid white or very light-colored drapes and keep white sponges to a minimum. Cover retractors to avoid light reflections.

After the operation, view the processed film or videotape with an editor, and develop your program. Edit ruthlessly, the fewer unnecessary pictures you retain, the more direct will be the effect.

Once your "master" is completed, make copies for review to safeguard the master from scratching or other damage.

To show videotape at a lecture, be sure that your equipment is functioning properly. Unless you have a large-screen TV, it is best to have several sets scattered throughout the hall to make sure the audience can see your presentation clearly. Before the talk, play some of the tape, and check the visibility from all the seats. Then, cue-up the tape to the point where you would like to begin.

Film, and the projector, should be inspected prior to the lecture, and should be threaded and cued onto the machine. Run the film a bit to ensure its proper alignment and to adjust the sound level. Then, back it up to a point just before the title, just at the end of the countdown clock.

An experienced operator should always be present to deal with such malfunctions as a blown bulb, film misalignment, or break in the film. Be prepared to draw your audience's attention away from the operator with standby material, or the next part of your talk, until the trouble is corrected.

Videodiscs

Videodiscs are a new technology with tremendous potential for the future. The current cost of producing and pressing discs, however, make them impractical for the average producer and even the consumer of health information. In brief, videodiscs are not a practical choice for doctors right now.

Models

Given the small size of most models, they are most effectively used with a small audience or on a table display at a poster session. Care should be taken with any model, small or large, to present it only when it is needed. Otherwise, it will be a distraction for your audience during the rest of your talk.

The Poster Session

The poster session is becoming more prevalent as a means of communicating information, because it allows direct interchange between the presenter and the interested observer.

You may be asked to provide an abstract for distribution with the program for the meeting. Follow the same format you use for journal submissions.

You will also be given a time and a space allocation. Check with the Program Committee to determine how much space you will be given and what equipment will be provided. Typically, you will be provided with a 4 × 8 foot mounting area or bulletin board and, occasionally, a display table.

Print the title of your poster session in a continuous strip with letters at least 1 inch high. You should also list the name(s) of the author(s) and the number of the abstract.

Follow your printed presentation format. List the abstract, objectives, methods and materials, results, and conclusions in smaller type. Keep your summaries of each category succinct, and supplement them with visual aids. Arrange the categories sequentially, and use arrows or ribbons to guide your viewers' eyes around the board. A variety of styles, shades, and colors of type may be effective in enhancing contrast or attracting attention.

Visuals are crucial to the presentation. Photographs should be mounted on a backing that is heavy enough to prevent curling. To reduce glare, avoid glossy photos or the use of plastic sleeves.

When you design your visuals, use the guidelines cited above for slide preparation. Emphasis on schematic drawings and charts, instead of on words and complicated tables, will ensure a successful presentation. Complex data and detailed graphs can be given to observers in supplementary handouts and referred to in one-on-one discussions or in follow-up communications.

Though the environment of the poster session will allow for more detailed discussion and explanation of confusing or complicated points, your visual aids should be developed according to the same communication principles as you would use for a larger lecture. Effective interchange of information will depend on your remembering a simple word—KISS. *K*eep *I*t *S*imple and *S*uccinct.

Further Reading

1. American College of Surgeons. Principles of preparing and using slides. Society of Thoracic Surgeons. Newport Press Inc., 1982.
2. McCormick WD. Present your papers to listeners not readers: tips on talks. Can Med Assoc J 1979;121(9):1304–12.
3. Finlayson M. Let's keep the audience awake. J Audiov Media Med 1983;(3):107–8.
4. Shambaugh GE Jr. How to write (and publish) a medical paper and how to deliver it. Laryngoscope 1982;(5):494–6.
5. Zollinger R, Pace W, Kienzle G. A practical outline for preparing medical talks and papers. New York: Macmillan, 1961.
6. Bowers WF. Techniques in medical communication. Springfield, Ill: Charles Thomas, 1963.
7. Hawkins C. Speaking and writing in medicine: the art of communication. Springfield, Ill: Charles Thomas, 1967.
8. Tilly D. Preparing graphics for visual presentation. Dent Clin North Am 1983;27(1):75–94.
9. Tribe H. Selecting and preparing illustrations for publication and presentation. Dent Clin North Am 1983;27(1):95–107.
10. Hawkins CF, Hammerley DP. Speaking at meetings. Med Biol Illus 1966;16:229–234.
11. Lane A. Multiple slide presentation. J Audiov Media Med 1981;(4):66.
12. Essex-Lopresti M. Illuminating an address: a guide for speakers at medical meetings. Med Educ 1980;(1):8–11.
13. Bodenkammer DJ, et al. Producing slides of radiographs, J Biol Photogr Assoc 1979;(3):117–21.
14. Gore EM. Using color to design effective projected transparencies. J Biocommun 1980;(2):2–3.
15. Williams PC. Suggestions for speakers and standards for slides. J Inst Biol 1965;12(2):65–70.
16. Soderstrom RM. Slides: making or breaking your speech, J Reprod Med 1981;6(2):57–64.
17. Lloyd WC, III. Rapid preparation of lecture slides using the computer. Ophthal Surg 1984;(8):678–9.
18. Hoexter B, et al. Essentials of audiovisual presentations: Is your audience listening or sleeping. Dis Colon Rect 1984;(1):55–9.

19. Greenberg S. New materials and methods for producing coloured teaching slides. J Audiov Media Med 1984;(3):114–5.
20. McPheeters V. Writing for audiovisual media. J Audiov Media Med 1981;(4):94.
21. Evans M. The use of slides in teaching—a practical guide, Med Educ 1981;(3):186–91.
22. Jeffries J, Bates J. The executive's guide to meetings, conferences, and audiovisual presentations. New York: McGraw-Hill, 1983.

The Society of Thoracic Surgeons

Presenting Slides at the Society of Thoracic Surgeons Meeting

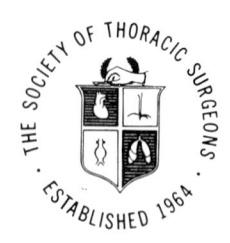

**The Society of Thoracic Surgeons
111 E. Wacker Dr.
Chicago, IL 60601**

Congratulations! You have been selected to present your paper before the annual meeting of the Society of Thoracic Surgeons. Whether your presentation is a resounding triumph or a complete disaster will depend as much on its style and quality as on the content of your paper. Whether your presentation is effective in communicating your thoughts may rest largely on your visual aids.

You will be giving your paper to an audience of well over 1,000 people in a **large** room with a low ceiling (Fig. 1). The projection screen will likely be too small for the room because the ceiling will limit its vertical height. How then do you prepare slides that can be read and understood by the person sitting in the last row? — By including a limited amount of material on each slide and by making the lettering large enough to be read anywhere in the auditorium.

If lettering, for example, is to be clearly recognized from a projected picture, it must be visible within the minimally acceptable viewing angle of the remotest member of the audience. This angle is 10° arc. Calculations show that to see a capital letter from this distance, the letter must be **at least** 3% of the height of the entire picture or peice of artwork. The thickness of the letter should be between 15-20% of the letter height (Fig. 2). If the material on a slide can be read **easily** when the slide is viewed with the naked eye against the light, it will probably be satisfactory. The motto is KISS (Keep It Simple, Sir).

The area of a horizontal 35mm slide will fill the screen. The vertical position should not be used if at all possible. At the same magnification as a horizontal slide, the vertically positioned slide will spill off the top and bottom of the screen.

The following are examples, both good and bad, of the typical kinds of slides shown at the Society meeting.

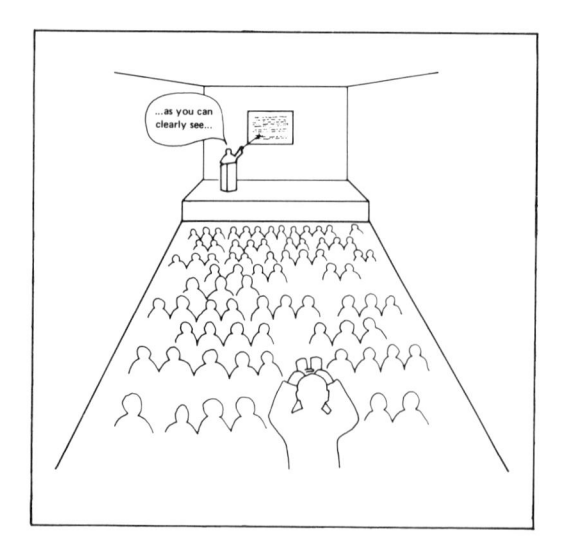

Figure 1. At the Society meeting.

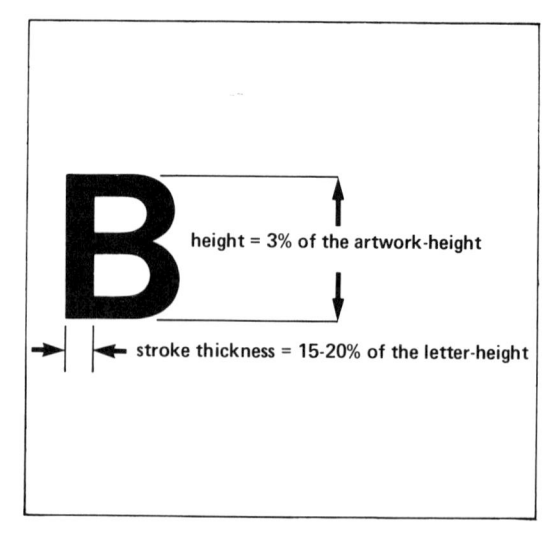

Figure 2. Correct sizing of letters.

I. Tables or Lists

Each slide should convey a single message in **no more** than 5-6 lines, with no more than 4-5 words or numbers in a line. Bold type style should be used. Hand lettering or Prestype is far superior to typewriting. The slide must transmit a large amount of projected light. The room will be in semidarkness only and the intensity of the light projected through the slide drops off inversely as the square of the distance from the projector to screen, usually the length of the room. Color should be used for emphasis, not decoration (Figs. 3A, 3B).

Composition of Cardioplegic Solution

NaCl	24 Meq/L
KCl	20 Meq/L
MgSO4	6 Meq/L
THAM	4 Meq/L
Glucose	50 g/Litre
Temperature	4° C
Osmolality	340 mOsm/Litre
pH	8.1

Figure 3. (A) Good example: Table.

Figure 3. (B) Poor example: Table.

II. Artwork

Simple, well-done black and white line drawings will project much better than complicated or intricate drawings attempting to present a great detail. Avoid the use of grays for shading and artistic effect. While appropriate for an art museum or gallery where there is time to contemplate a work of art, in the context of a rapidly moving medical presentation, it subverts quick, easy comprehension of the message and distracts the viewer from listening to the simultaneous oral presentation (Figs. 4A, 4B).

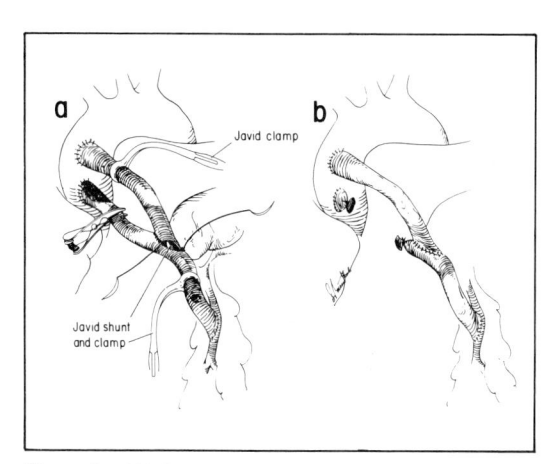

Figure 4. (A) Good example: Line drawing.

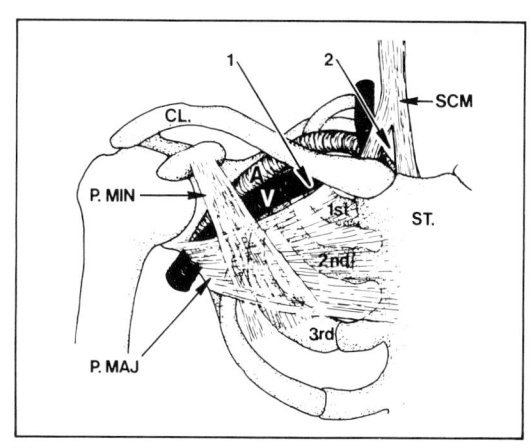

Figure 4. (B) Poor example: Line drawing.

III. Photomicrographs

The components of a photomicrograph or electron micrograph should show up very clearly. Sharp focus and good contrast between light and dark areas are essential, especially when several different kinds of structures appear in the same print. Magnification should be high enough to clearly demonstrate all of the features mentioned. (Figs. 5A, 5B)

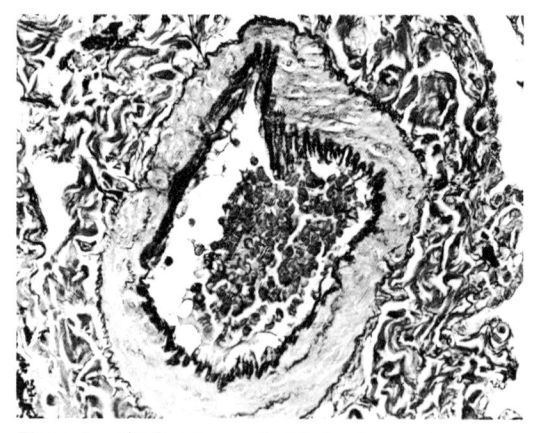

Figure 5. (A) Good example: Photomicrograph.

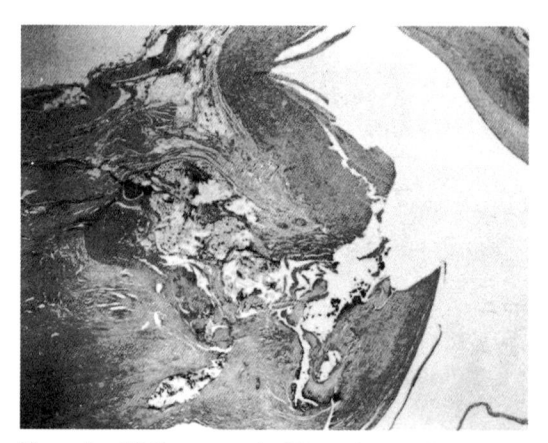

Figure 5. (B) Poor example: Photomicrograph.

IV. Anatomical Specimens and Intraoperative Photographs

Photographs of operative specimens are usually poor. If a photograph of an operation is necessary to make a point, be sure only the essential elements are in the slide. Do not show retractors, tubes, blood-stained drapes, etc.

The specimen should fill most of the 35mm format and should be in color. The background should enhance the specimen and **not** be blood-stained. A centimeter rule should be used as a scale. Carefully placed lettering and arrows can prove helpful. Be sure the entire depth of the specimen is in focus (Figs. 6A, 6B)

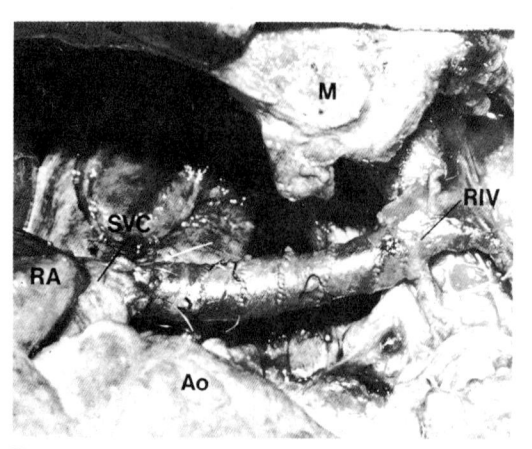

Figure 6. (A) Good example: Anatomical specimen.

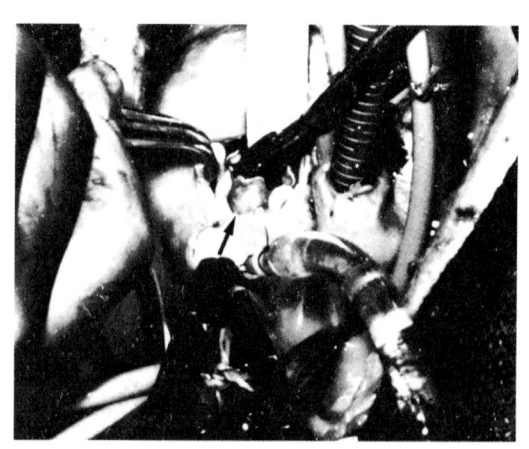

Figure 6. (B) Poor example: Anatomical specimen.

V. Graphs

Histogram (bar graph). A histogram should present no more than 5-6 bars. Bars should be solid and broad and if two or more sets of information appear on each bar, they should be clearly discernible from one another (Figs. 7A, 7B).

Line graph. Line graphs should not have more than three separate lines. If the lines overlap very much, a different design should be used for each line. Lines should be heavy enough for easy identification. Multiple numbers and symbols on the graph often contribute to confusion rather than allay it. (Figs. 7C, 7D)

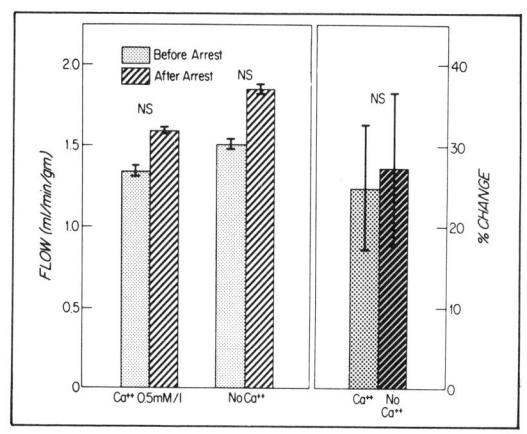

Figure 7. (A) Good example: Histogram.

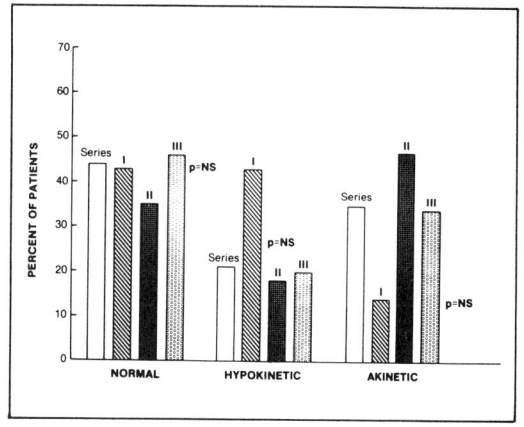

Figure 7. (B) Poor example: Histogram.

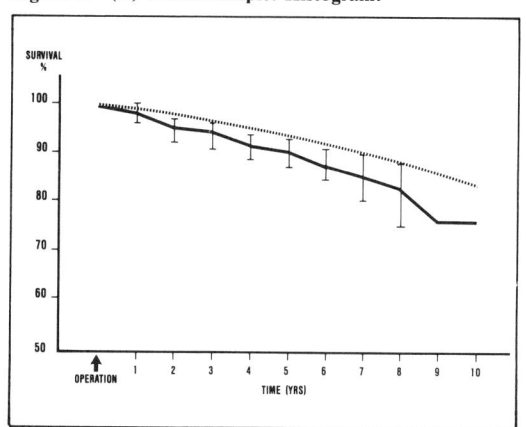

Figure 7. (C) Good example: Line graph.

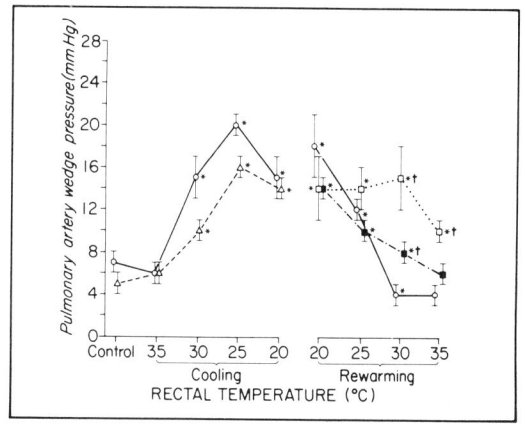

Figure 7. (D) Poor example: Line graph.

VI. Surgical Instruments

Photographs of instruments should contain no more than 3-4 objects per slide. There should be a clear contrast between the background and the instruments. Groups of instruments should be arranged in an orderly fashion. Centimeter rules are often helpful (Figs. 8A, 8B).

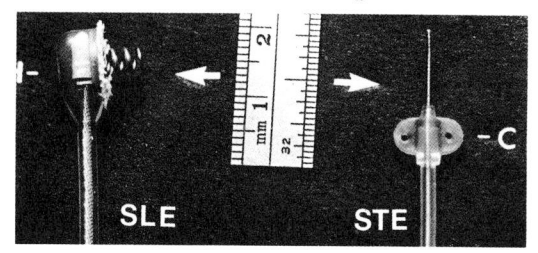

Figure 8. (A) Good example: Surgical instruments.

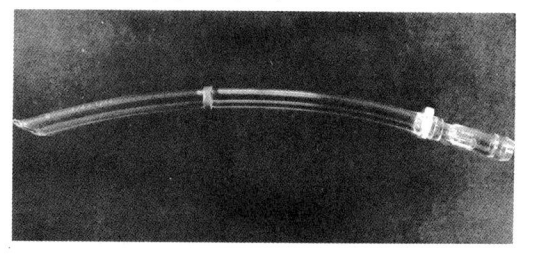

Figure 8. (B) Poor example: Surgical instruments.

VII. Valves

Photographs of valves are often projected to illustrate damage or other kinds of problems that have occured. A sharply focused photograph with sufficient depth of field to include the height of the valve should be prepared. The background should contrast sharply with the valve; white or black usually work well. The valve should be placed to demonstrate the area of interest clearly (Figs. 9A, 9B).

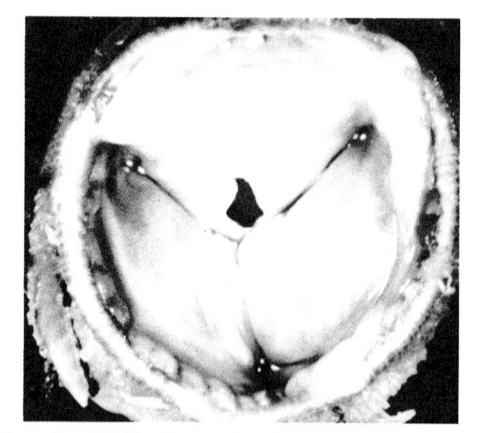

Figure 9. (A) Good example: Valve.

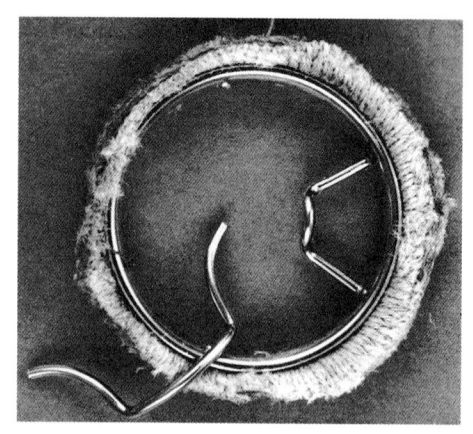

Figure 9. (B) Poor example: Valve.

VIII. Studies with Accompanying Drawings

Frequently, a study (angiogram, arteriogram, tomogram) will not demonstrate a point clearly, but will be the only alternative available. Having a line interpretation of what is shown in the study drawn in close proportion and presented alongside of the study can alleviate this problem (Figs. 10A, 10B).

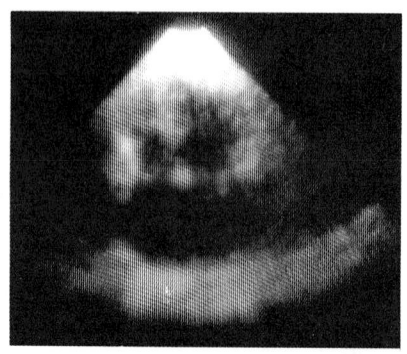

Figure 10. (A) Two dimensional echocardiogram with (B) line interpretation.

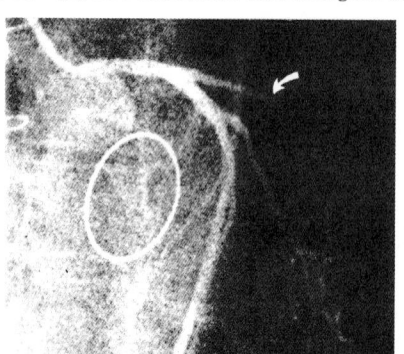

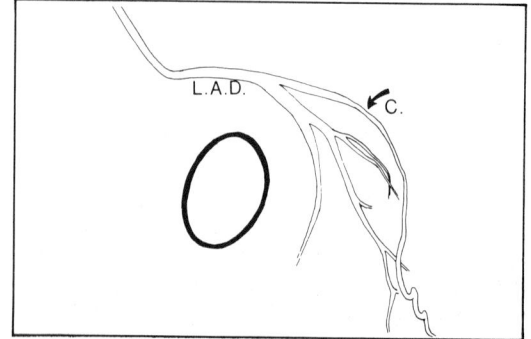

Figure 10. (C) Coronary arteriogram with (D) line interpretation.

IX. Roentgenograms and Angiograms

Roentgenograms. No more than two roentgenograms should appear on a slide, for example, an anteroposterior and a lateral. The reproduction should be clear and there should be sharp contrast between light and dark areas. As much as possible, only the area of essential pathology and anatomical orientation should be shown (Figs. 11A, 11B).

Angiograms. Fuzzy angiograms are a waste of time. Aim for as much clarity and good contrast between light and dark areas as possible. A small amount of retouching is often advisable. The contrast medium used should appear white on dark background (Figs. 11C, 11D).

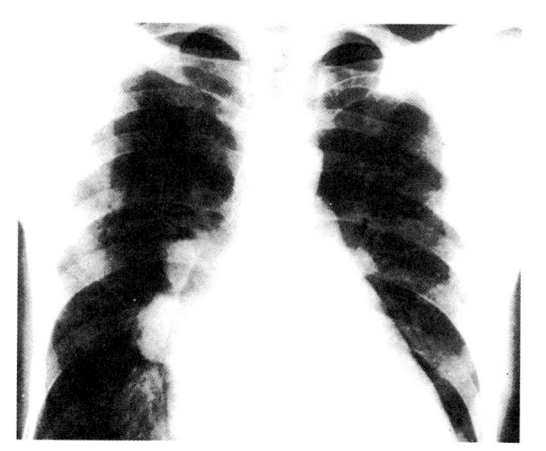

Figure 11. (A) Good example: Chest roentgenogram.

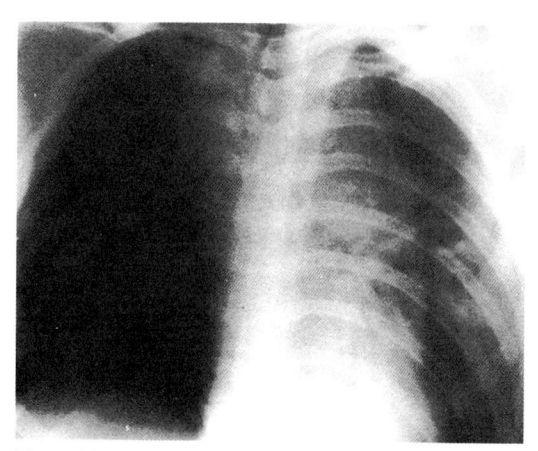

Figure 11. (B) Poor example: Chest roentgenogram.

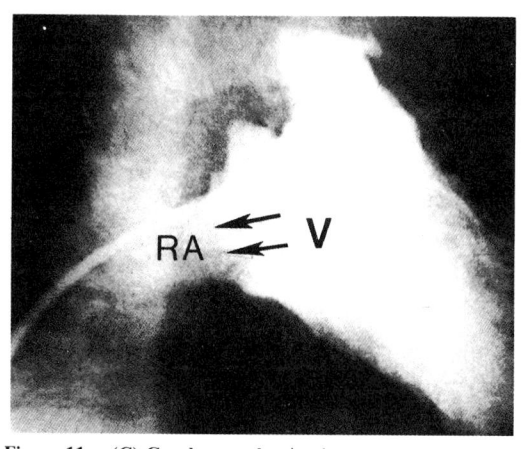

Figure 11. (C) Good example: Angiogram.

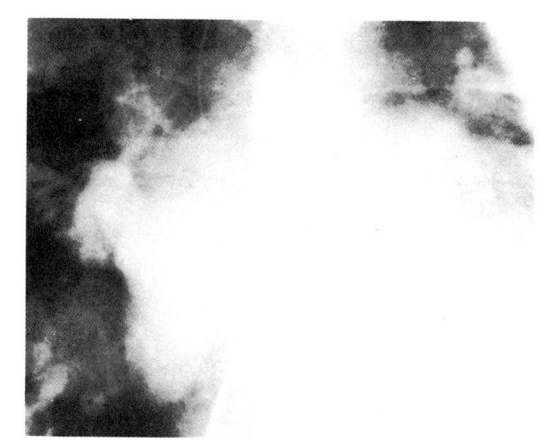

Figure 11. (D) Poor example: Angiogram.

STS Audiovisual Brochure © The Society of Thoracic Surgeons, reprinted by permission.

7

Writing for Publication

N.J.B. Wiggin, J.C. Bailar III, C.B. Mueller, W.O. Spitzer, and B. McPeek

Introduction

The final part of research is the publication of results, and good research deserves good writing. Methods, results, conclusions, ideas, and thoughts must be published if they are to last; unless they are put into the literature they can be committed only to a small circle of colleagues or students and will lie beyond recall once verbal communciation ceases. The great body of recorded surgical knowledge is in the permanent collection of books and journals prepared by individuals so that others may read, reread, contemplate, refute, or accept them. Writing and publishing is more than an obligation of every sophisticated scholar or clinician; it is an essential part of any definition of a productive investigation.

It is helpful to discuss scientific writing in terms of *substance, content,* and *form.* All three are critical to communication, and hence to good writing. By substance we mean the subject matter of the writing, considered at several different levels: the subject of a book, a paper, a paragraph, a sentence or phrase. By content we mean what is said about that subject: that the author had discovered a cure for hypochondria; that Figure 1 presents thus-and-so; that two patients were lost to follow-up. Accuracy and precision are critical aspects of content. By form we mean how the content is presented: organization, clarity, economy of language, adherence to the rules of good grammar, and style.

Effective written communication requires one more thing: concern for and empathy with the reader. Too many writers believe that it is enough to send a message, but the message must also be received and properly understood. Busy readers tend to be overwhelmed with material they find on their desks; they are not likely to work very hard at understanding a poorly written offering, whatever its relevance and importance. Some potential readers will also be lazy, or tired, or distracted by other matters, and some—perhaps a majority—will not be experts in the subject matter of the writing. None, clearly, will know as much about the material they are reading as the author. If we have one point to add to the burden already borne by those who seek to write well, it is this: Pay constant attention that your message be correctly received at the other end of the communication link; the words you write have no other purpose. This puts great stress on such matters as clarity and brevity. When an interested and qualified reader misunderstands or does not attend to some point of a paper, it is the author who has failed.

The works of great and near-great clinicians nearly always meet high standards in each aspect of writing. There is of course a reason; we believe that many other clinicians may be just as great in most ways, but they have not learned to write as well. In short, good writing helps the world to recognize good work more than good work elicits good writing. Careful attention to substance, content, and form—down to the last nuances of style—will not in itself be sufficient, but it can be an invaluable professional asset. Not incidentally, it is also an asset to readers and to the discipline as a whole; that may be one reason why good writing is rewarded so well.

We note that good technical writing is not an

accident nor is ability in such writing a gift bestowed on a fortunate few. Thoughtful, conscientous, constant attention to what is—and what is not—put on paper can help much. So can courses in writing given by qualified instructors. So can careful attention to the writing successes of others. So, we dare to hope, can reading a book or chapter on the subject—but only if the new knowledge is put to use. There is no substitute for practice, objective self-criticism, and as many rounds of revision as needed to do this job well.

Scientific writing must be lucid and carry a message that leaves the reader in no doubt about the concept or idea being stated. It requires a writing style much different than that used by great writers to stimulate image formation in the minds of their readers. Style is as important in scientific work as it is in literture, but the style is diferent. The scientist should generally try to write so that the style is unobtrusive; even transparent. We read with distress of some who think that a proper "scientific" style requires pursive voice, complex sentences, words of Latin origin, and the third person. Would you rather read, "Specimens were individually developed by exposure to the atmosphere at ambient temperatures", or, "I dried each sample in room air." And which, do you think is most likely to be found in a research report? Hemingway, in "Snows of Kilmanjaro" or "The Old Man and the Sea", deliberately sought to evoke many images that would be unique to the individual reader. The intent of scientific writing is the direct antithesis, i.e., to transmit a message with such clarity that all readers will receive the same information and arrive at the same conclusion. It demands that the writer be so precise that no one will be confused and no reader will be permitted the privilege of developing his own concept about what the writer wished to say.

Many books are available to instruct the novice or the expert author in "how to write"; a few are listed in the bibliography (1–10). Some deal with organization and logic; some cover style and the use of biologic words and abbreviations; some tell you how to use words and phrases to clarify, amplify, and communicate a clear message, and to bring power to your writing. For thirty years, the ultimate reference work has been Strunk and White (8). Every author who writes in English should obtain a copy of this little book and read it carefully—many times.

It is always advisable to develop the overall scope of your message by thinking in terms of paragraphs of 5–20 sentences, with each paragraph containing a coherent concept that is developed sequentially. Some writers paste their paragraphs on the wall as they write. They can thus see the whole as they put technical procedures, data, ideas, or results into the appropriate paragraphs, and they can easily re-arrange the paragraphs in a sequence that allows the reader's thoughts to flow from research question, to study design, to data, to analysis, to conclusions.

Good scientific writing requires that your words say exactly what you mean and that you construct sentences that are direct and pungent. The subject of every sentence must be easily identified and the verb readily visible. Each sentence must have a noun or pronoun as its subject, and each transitive verb must have a clearly stated object. Sentences often are most powerful when they begin with nouns accompanied by few adjectives and have action verbs with few qualifiers. Avoid the passive voice. Sentences that begin with clauses or dangling phrases referring to elements within the sentence are confusing and generally fail to convey a clear message. Eschew verbosity. Keep sentences short; half a dozen typewritten lines is usually too long. Write in good English, rather than jargon, and your ideas will stand out clearly. Multiple drafts before submission are always more rewarding than multiple drafts after a rejection.

Each communication must convey a significant message, such as a report of an original research study, a critical analysis and review of the work of others, or a brief appraisal of something that has been observed or written. The content and format of a written article depend on your purpose in writing it. Some of the common formats, arranged in an order that is didactically useful rather than a reflection of their relative importance, are:

Monographs
Research Papers
Review Articles
Editorials
Letters-to-the-Editor

Monographs

Senior clinicians in various academic posts often serve as leaders or members of research groups or task forces formed to study scientific problems of particular concern to some institution or to the public. The terms of reference of such research assignments, whether they are supported by a conventional research grant or undertaken in response to government or agency contract requests, often require that a lengthy monogaph be written. The final product may comprise several hundred pages of double-spaced typewritten material, with numerous tables, figures, conclusions, recommendations, and references. One can easily see why the commissioning agency may require such a document. It constitutes not only an archival record of the deliberative process, research methods, results, and conclusions, but also a basis for policy-making.

Unfortunately, much valuable research or scholarly work is lost to the scientific community because it is buried in monographs that are replicated in very limited numbers and not subsequently published in peer-reviewed, indexed journals. Readers will find it difficult, or even impossible, to discover the existence of publications with such limited circulation. The net result, too often, is the creation of an obstruction to the normal widespread diffusion of good research. If you have a choice between writing a monograph or writing a series of research papers for publication in journals, choose the latter. An indexed journal is cited in the national and international biomedical indexing systems available in most academic libraries. The cross referencing of key words and key ideas in such research resources make it relatively easy for your colleagues and other investigators throughout the world to discover your work.

Sometimes you may find that the potential value of a monograph for you, or for the sponsoring agency, or for the public is great enough to justify a substantial investment of your time and effort. If you have accepted a contractural or professional obligation to write a monograph, you can still take advantage of having a principal volume of reports that can be referred to by your research team as they prepare other articles for publication in journals. If you must write monographs, write only those that will be published in archival sysems that provide ready access to them.

Scientists sometimes fear that the stringently limited space available for many journal articles will prevent adequate reporting of a large data set or the extensive deliberations of an expert task force. Yet monographs, journal articles, and book chapters are not mutually exclusive; monographs can be created, if necessary, as supplements to brief and focused shorter articles. The shorter articles in journals can reveal the source of supplementary data banks in footnotes and references. The availability of the longer documents can be enhanced by using microfiche and commercial microfilm firms to duplicate the information for those who need it at nominal cost.

The traditional sequence, which you may alter if there is some reason to do so, is to discuss your research findings with your peers; prepare a draft of your paper; revise your draft to take account of the constructive criticisms you have received; submit your paper for publication in a peer-reviwed journal; follow up with book chapters when your findings have been validated and accepted; and make reference to the foregoing in any monographs or journal articles you write on the same subject. A major research project or expert inquiry can easily generate several original, related, yet distinctive publications. As a final world on monographs, avoid contracts and grants that emphasize a requirement for a confidential report that will be given only limited circulation. If you are an autonomous academic or professional investigator, it is wise to refuse an assignment if there is no guarantee that your finished work will be released for open publication within a period of 6 months at most.

Research Papers

The most valuable advice anyone can give you as a prospective author of a research paper is to devote adequate time, thought, and expert collaboration to the refinement of your research question, the design of your study (including appropriate outcome measures), its careful performance, and the correct analysis and interpretaton of the data. If you have fulfilled these requirements, you can easily get help in writing your paper, if you need it. If your study was poorly conceived and executed, no one can help you. No amount of analytical or writing skill can convert poor data into a good paper.

Getting started is a major hurdle for most of us. Although your paper will eventually end up in the standard format of introduction, methods, results, discussion, and abstract, you are not required to write it in that sequence. Start with whatever you find it easiest to write about, e.g., your methods or results. Another approach is to write and rewrite the first sentence, then the first two, and finally the first three sentences however many times it takes to get them into a form that you feel is exactly right. You may then discover, to your surprise and delight, that you can draft the rest of the paper without difficulty. As you write, your effort will often gather a momentum of its own that will carry you through the parts you considered most intimidating at the outset.

Remember that your intended reader is not only intelligent but also hard-pressed for reading time. You need state something only once, as clearly and directly as possible. Circling around what you want to say or saying it two or three times is more likely to drive your reader away than to drive your point home. Don't coin new words or define new meanings until you have assured yourself that the word and meaning you want do not exist already. A dictionary, Fowler's "Modern English Usage" (11), and a thesaurus are useful aids. Be careful not to employ elegant variation where it might confuse your reader.

The *Introduction* should be a straightforward account of why you embarked on your study, what you hoped to learn or achieve by doing it, and what others who have studied the same or a closely related problem have reported. Your review of other research reports need not be as exhaustive as it would be for a review article. A few significant and directly relevant articles may be enough. Review articles are often cited in Introductions, and should be cited more often, because they can facilitate writing, reduce length, and still give interested readers a guided entry to the relevant literature.

When you are giving your reasons for carrying out the study, it is important to confine yourself to the questions or the hypothesis you had in mind when you started. Additional questions prompted by your results should be left for the discussion section of your paper.

The *Methods* portion of your paper is very important to every sophisticated reader who wishes to be satisfied about the appropriateness of what you did and the validity or reliability of the results your methods produced. An adequate and precise description of the population you studied, your approach to randomization, the experimental intervention, your choice of outcome measures, etc., will enable readers to compare your results with those obtained by other investigators. Adequate description of methods is also needed if others are to contrast or combine your results with their own to gain new insights. This matter is discussed in an earlier chapter.

If your research project has involved a clinical trial, you will need to describe eligibility criteria, admission of patients to your study before allocation, random allocation to different treatment or control groups, the mechanisms you used to generate your random assignments, patients' blindness as to which treatment they received, blindness of the person assessing the outcome as to which treatment the patient received, the methods of statistical analysis included in your design, and how you determined your sample size or the size of detectable differences (12).

All of the foregoing are discussed later in this chapter or in other chapters of this textbook. They are listed here to remind you that you will need to deal with them in your paper.

The appropriate level of detail regarding statistical matters varies from one paper to another and even within one paper. Fully detailed descriptions of statistical dsign and methods are seldom required because few readers will need them or wish to replicate your study exactly. It is usually sufficient to cite standard works on statistical design for important details and to provide technical references whenever the design is unusual or particularly complex. Your report should emphasize such features of your design as "partially balanced incomplete blocks", "treatments assigned by using a random number table, with numbers supplied in sealed opaque envelopes", or "status before and after treatment, as assessed and recorded by a person blind to the assigned treatment". You must, however, supply enough detail to allow readers to assess the most important potential sources of bias in your results. The omission of such basic information is a frequent and serious deficiency in published reports (13).

Although much technical detail should be omitted, your paper must still be self-contained with respect to general aspects of your study's design, even if you repeat information provided in earlier reports on other aspects of your investigation. If the specific details are essential and require considerable space to present them, consider reporting them once as a separate paper in a methodology journal, or make them available on request from your laboratory, hospital, or university.

A good example of how to report the statistical design of your study is:

Three hundred female patients were assigned to a control or a treatment group on the basis of the last digit of their hospital admission numbers. If the last digit was even, the patient was assigned to the control group; if odd, to the treatment group. Treatment patients were given two 250-mg. tablets every 6 hours; control patients were given two lactose tablets, identical in appearance and taste to the drug tables, q6h.

(While this description is good, the method it describes is not. Someone who knows the allocation method can know the treatment group to which a specific patient will be allocated. Whether and when a patient is admitted to the study may then be influenced by a referring physician. The result can be a biased, non-random allocation of patients among treatment groups of the study.)

Detailed statistical consideration of the data collection phase of a study, including quality control, is rarely needed in journals whose primary purpose is to report results. If your paper is accepted by and published in a respected, peer-reviewed/scientific journal, its readers should have just enough information to know that your study was competently performed, that your data are accurate to the degree of precision you have specified, and that careful independent repetition of your work would produce essentially the same data within the limits of random variation.

In the *Results* section of your paper, the appropriate level of statistical details, including means, variances or standard errors, P-values, regression coefficients, and the like, depends on the nature of your subject and the purposes of your paper. Whatever statistical measures you use, they should be clearly labeled. A mean of precisely which set of observations? A variance of what statistic? A P-value for what statistical method, testing what specific null hypothesis against what alternative(s), under what assumptions? A regression coefficient in what units of observations? An example of appropriate detail is:

Pulse rate was measured for all 36 subjects immediately before and 10 minutes after the 3-minute infusion of the drug. The mean increase was 19.6 pulses per minute, with a standard error of the mean of 4.3. Although earlier studies suggested that pulse rate does not change, we found a consistent increase, with a two-sided P-value of 0.023 on the basis of a matched-pairs t-test analysis that assumes the differences are approximately normally distributed.

Sufficient detail should be given regarding your methods of statistical analysis to enable a knowledgeable reader to reproduce your result if supplied with your raw data. This level of detail is particularly needed if your method of analysis is likely to be unfamiliar to most readers. Clinical journals will not often ask you to provide statistical computations that are familiar to most of their readers and they will rarely wish to publish computational formulas. When references are required or appropriate, standard works (e.g., 14, 15) are preferable to original sources because they are usually more readily available and easier to understand. Although it may be essential that you analyze your data in several ways, you should present only the most easily understood analysis that is technically correct. You may then state that, although other kinds of analyses were performed, the results obtained were in accord with those presented. If, however, different analyses lead to substantially different conclusions, the differences must be described and an attempt to reconcile them must be presented.

In most papers, the descriptions of statistical methods are best assigned to the appropriate parts of the Results and Discussion sections. Mosteller (16) has covered many additional aspects of reporting statistical studies, including construction of tables; presenting numeric values; overlap among text, tables, and figures; and standard statistical notation. Communication about statistical matters is often so important, and problems can be so frequent and subtle, that you should cultivate a close tie with an experienced professional statistician. A statistical review of your paper by such an individual, before you submit it, will often lead to suggestions that will improve it significantly.

Other matters must also be addressed in the results section of your paper. Demogaphic and clinical data on the patients in different treatment groups must be provided to demonstrate that they were in fact similar. You must also supply data on the complications experienced by your patients after treatment, the numbers of patients who were lost to follow-up, and the reasons why they were lost.

Carefully constructed tables offer you a way to present a large amount of data clearly and concisely. To avoid overly complex tables, divide your data into sets that convey information related to one or two specific points. Resist the temptation to present all the same data again in your written text. Once is enough!

In the *Discussion* section, you will want to discuss potential sources of error and bias in your study, the conclusions that can be validly drawn from your data, the applicability of your findings to other patient groups, and any specific directions for future research suggested by your work. Do not overdo these matters, though. Few readers will need to know everything you have learned or speculated about. Discussion sections often offer more scope for creativity than Introduction, Methods, or Results, but they should be kept short and pungent.

Now that your paper is written, writing the *Abstract* is in order, regardless of whether it will appear at the beginning or the end of your paper. You must be brief, and you must not put anything in it that is not in your paper. In as few words as possible, tell the reader what your study is about, the essential features of its design, and the main results. Short Abstracts are more likely to be read than long ones, and the Abstract for a paper should be just long enough for a reader to decide whether to go on to the full text. ("Abstracts" for publication in the proceedings of a meeting are another matter that we do not discuss in this chapter.)

Finally, go through your paper and pick out 4 to 8 *KeyWords* or phrases that will enable others who are interested in your findings to discover your paper by searching indexes to the literature using the words you have chosen.

Review Articles

Review articles are written to give perspective to previously published work. They are not original publications although they may contain new findings from old data if they are based on meta-analysis rather than the traditional approach, as described in Section III, Chapter 1. Writing a review may appear to be dull work, but if it is well done you will gain an extensive knowledge and a comprehensive view of the subject. A good review paper is usually 10–50 manuscript pages in length. The subject may vary in breadth according to the extent of current knowledge; i.e., the more voluminous the related literature, the more narrowly focused your review should be. The accompanying bibliography should be comprehensive, and sometimes exhaustive. A good review offers critical evaluation of the literature and considered conclusions about the state of affairs in a special area. It is usually expected to include comments about every item in the bibliography. Reviews generally go beyond a historical account of a field to an exposition of the current state of knowledge and understanding in the subject area. As a consequence, attention to recent literature is usually more important than retracing of historical development.

It is wise to contact the editor of the journal in which you wish to publish your review before you begin work on it. You will need to know whether the topic is suitable and acceptable, whether the proposed scope is appropriate, and whether you, the author, have the required credentials. Some journals stress bibliogaphic completeness, others stress critical evaluation; you should know exactly what is expected.

Organization of your review paper is important. Once you have assembled the bibliography, the preparation of an outline is essential. Although there is no prescribed order for traditional reviews, and the format of reviews employing meta-analysis varies, an appropriate outline is mandatory before writing starts. The outline imposes substantial structure on the intellectual content of the review, and it is not rare for the outline itself to be the main contribution to a confused and confusing field. If your outline is carefully thought out, the scope of your review will be defined, the logic of your sequence will be apparent, and the content of its sections can be easily deduced. This outline, which is so important to you as the author, is also important to the reader. It may be included as a quasi-index at the beginning of your review or be incorporated within the text as topic and sub-topic headings.

The anticipated readership of your review must be considered. Research papers are read by peers, i.e., individuals who are expert in the topic area; review papers are read by a wider readershp from various backgrounds. You will have to take special care to avoid jargon and abbreviations and to use a writing style that is expansive and clear rather than telegraphic.

A special introductory paragraph is required for each section because many review readers pick and choose rather than read the entire article. This paragraph must cater to the readers, skimmers, and skippers by providing a comprehensive statement that leads logically into the material contained in the section.

A critical review always requires conclusions while an annotated bibliography often does not. A Conclusion section is a truly comprehensive summary that is succinctly stated and obviously drawn from the material under review. An authoritative conclusion is unique to you, the author, and it may be the most rewarding part of the review process, not only because your readers and their patients gain from it but also because your obligation to write it means that you will have to develop a consummate understanding of the topic.

Editorials

An editorial is usually a signed expression of personal opinion composed either at the request of the editor or as a free-standing unsolicited set of comments. As opinion, it carries an implicit weight of authority and need not concur with the general position of the journal, the authors of papers it discusses, or any one else. It frequently accompanies or follows a paper that has already been published; if so, it must relate closely to the same subject. A few sentences of historical background can set the topic in perspective, restate the content or conclusion of the work being discussed, and lead into your own comments. In general, editorial comments should amplify, expand, or give a sense of perspective to the major topic. You should rarely or never, attack the manuscript under discussion although you may express reservations about the conclusions that can be drawn from it.

An invited editorial usually carries weight because of the established credibility of its author whose name should be well-known to the expected readership. If you are not well-known, you may establish your credibility by referring briefly to some special experience or expertise that gives you license to express your ideas with a minimum of referenced support. The supporting bibliography is always short, perhaps no more than half a dozen well chosen citations. Editorials are usually supportive, broad in scope, and designed for a readership that may not be especially expert in the topic area. If your editorial is too long or wordy, you will lose your readers. If you devote thought to your subject and express your views clearly, you can make a significant contribution to current thinking on the chosen topic.

Letters-to-the-Editor

The "letters" portion of a medical or surgical journal is usually one of its best read sections. As a result, letters have become important elements in communication. Letters must be brief and lively. They are often controversial, but never unfriendly. Occasionally, original studies appear first in the letter section. Brief case reports with a little interpretaton, comments on previously published material, or statements of opinion may appear as letters. A good letter has one major constraint—it must deal with only one topic. To write a good letter, put the topic into perspective with two or three sentences that state or refer to the issue. Then, make observations or present ideas that may be new or may rebut material previously published. Close with a clear statement of your conclusions so that the readers will know what position you have taken.

Your letter may be accepted by the editor if it is appropriate for publication and it suits the mission of the journal. If it refers to work that has been published, it is likely to be sent to the author of the original paper for his comments or rebuttal, which may be published with your letter. Be very careful to review his data and quote his observations correctly. Be prepared to have him take issue with your position—a position you are obliged to justify in a minimum of space.

References

1. CBE Style Manual Committee. CBE style manual: A guide for authors, editors and publishers in the biologic sciences, 5th Ed. Bethesda: Council of Biology Editors Inc., 1983.

   Designed by the Council of Biology Editors this book gives ideas about writing in acceptable format, tables, graphs, illustrations, abbreviations and standard terminology. It discusses editors, the review process, and copyrights and contains all the required features to make it a reference work for everyone who writes in the biological field.

2. Day RA. How to write and publish a scientific paper. Philadelphia: ISI Press, 1983.

   Easily read, homorous, well-annotated and full of helpful admonitions about the entire process of writing in the scientific world.

3. Gowers E. The complete plain words. Baltimore: Penguin Books, 1970.

   An excellent paperback guide concerned with the choice and arrangement of words to get an idea from one mind and to another, as exactly as possible.

4. Hewitt RM. The physician writer's book. Philadelphia: W.B. Saunders, 1957.

   A gentle overview on how to put thoughts and ideas into manuscripts and papers—a classic for many years.

5. Huth EJ. How to write and publish papers in the medical sciences. Philadelphia: ISI Press, 1982.

   A small paperback published by the Science Information Service that is easily readable, well annotated, cryptic and full of helpful ideas about writing and submitting papers and the review process.

6. King LS, Roland CG. Scientific writing. Chicago: Am Med Assn 1968.

   A sophisticated, small paperback that assists the expert in organization, the subtle use of words and phrases, opening sentences, and avoidance of cliches. It extends the basic English of Strunk and White into the world of science.

7. O'Connor M, Woodford FP. Writing scientific papers in English. N.Y.C.: Elsevier/Excerpta Medica, 1976.

   A small volume filled with information about writing scientific papers for authors whose first language is not English. It covers the review and editing process as well as the construction of manuscripts.

8. Strunk WM Jr., White EB. The elements of style, 3rd ed. N.Y.: MacMillan Publishing Co., 1979.

   A small paperback which has been a classic for thirty years. It gives excellent advice about how to eliminate redundant words and phrases, construct clear messages, and achieve a clear, graceful prose style.

9. Research: How to plan, speak and write about it. Hawkins Fliffor and Sogi, Mario, editors. Berlin-Heidelberg-New York-Tokyo: Springer-Verlag, 1985.

10. Graves R, Hodge A. The reader over your shoulder: a handbook for the writing of English prose. N.Y.: Random House, 1979.

11. Fowler H W. Dictionary of modern English usage. 2nd ed. N.Y.: Oxford University Press, 1965.

12. DerSimonian R, Charette, LJ, McPeek B, Mosteller F. Reporting on methods in clinical trials. New Engl J Med 1982;306:1332–1337.

13. Emerson J.D., McPeek, B, Mosteller, F. Reporting clinical trials in general surgical journals. Surgery 95: 572–579, 1984.

14. Snedecor GW, Cochran WG. Statistical methods. 7th ed. Ames, Iowa: The Iowa State College Press, 1980.

15. Colton T. Statistics in medicine. Boston: Little, Brown and Co., Inc, 1974.

16. Mosteller F. Medical uses of statistics. Bailar J, Mosteller F. Editors. Waltham, Mass. New Engl J Med, 1986.

8

What to Do When You Are Asked to Write a Chapter for a Book

B. Lewerich and D. Götze

When you receive an invitation to contribute a chapter or section of a book, allow yourself 10 minutes to feel flattered. Then, read the letter again and try to figure out exactly what the editor or senior author wants you to do. Most invitation letters are rather vague because, for understandable reasons, the inviting editor does not want to give away too much information about his project before he gains the author's agreement to participate in the effort.

Before you answer the invitation, ask yourself a few specific questions and try to answer them honestly.

Do I really have the time to take on another obligation?
Is it likely that I will be able to complete the required work by the stipulated deadline?
Do I want to write about the topic suggested, or will the editor permit me to alter the given subject in some satisfactory way?

Only if you are able to answer all the questions with "yes", should you accept the invitation.

A good friend may feel offended if you reject such a request, but your friendship will suffer much more if you have to ask for repeated extensions beyond the deadline. Be aware that experts in delaying contributions soon earn a "special" reputation among editors and publishers.

Before you agree to write a chapter for a book, make sure you ask the inviting editor the following questions, at least:

What kind of readership do you want to reach?
What is the complete outline of the book like?
(Ask for as much detailed information as is available.)
How many pages will your publisher allow for my chapter?
How many figures, and how many tables am I allowed to use?
How many references are allowed?
Do I have to prepare ready-for-print figures?
Is the use of color figures permitted?
Is there a sample chapter that would help to clarify any further questions?

Since some editors feel that their job is finished when the outline of the book has been drawn up and the authors have been invited, ask your editor for a detailed explanation of how your chapter should be structured.

The more detailed the editor's advance instructions are regarding your chapter, the less difficulty there will be in incorporating your contribution into the book and the fewer will be the revisions you will have to make. An editor is well-advised to send participating authors a sample chapter at the beginning to give them some idea of what their work should look like. It can be taken as a general rule that, the less specific and the less strict a book editor is in approaching authors, the less acceptable the book will be.

When you have received answers to all the foregoing questions, start work on the manuscript as soon as possible. Good authors have many demands on their time and energy. Do not postpone writing the article until two days after the deadline. The excuse that you can only work under pressure is a very bad one. Grapes and cheese produce excellent results when put under pressure, but brains behave differently.

There are several things you can easily do as soon as you agree to prepare a contribution:

- Develop your own manuscript outline and check it with the editor(s) to make sure you really understand your assignment.
- Start a bibliographic search and collect relevant reprints.
- Speak with other experts for fresh ideas or recent work you are not aware of.
- Look into other books on the subject to see whether a similar contribution has been published before.
- Find out what could be done better.
- At an early stage, start developing sketches of the figures you are going to use.
- If you want to use figures that have already been published, seek permission for their reproduction from the author or publisher, now.
- Obtain author's instructions for the preparation of manuscripts from the editor or publisher to avoid inconsistencies of format within the book as a whole.

Technical Considerations

- Type the text of your contribution double-spaced with broad margins on both sides to allow space for the editor's and the copy editor's corrections. The typist in the printing company will have fewer difficulties when your text is not crammed together too closely.
- If you plan to type your manuscript on a word processor, contact the publisher before you start to obtain advice on how to proceed.
- Attach figures, diagrams, and tables on separate sheets—these parts are handled separately in the production process and the will make things easy for the printer.
- Make sure that each page and each figure carry your name. It may happen that some figures will get mixed up, but yours never will be.
- See that all your figures and tables are cited in your text with numbers. The book editor may change the numbering if necessary but your material can always be identified.
- Be sure that the way you cite references complies with the instructions given by the publisher. Be even more careful about giving correct page numbers, volume numbers and publication years.
- See that all the references listed at the end of your chapter are mentioned in the text, and vice versa. Make sure that all references are complete with names of all authors, title, publication date, volume, pages. If books are quoted supply authors' names, editors' names where appropriate, book title, pages referred to, publication date, and publisher's name and location. Ask your editor or publisher which citation system you should use: e.g., Vancouver or Harvard guidelines for the preparation of manuscripts.
- No one else can verify the sources you have used as well as you can. Readers who order a reprint of a paper you have referred to will be anything but pleased when they receive a photocopy of an article on water pollution, when your article was about surgery of the pancreas.
- When you have a near-to-final draft of your manuscript, ask a friendly co-worker to read and review it critically with you. Ask the same help from a friend who works in another area.

A final important rule to be heeded when you are involved in the writing of a book is: **Do not tell the readers what you know about the matter; tell them what they should know about it.**

When you have delivered the complete manuscript to the editor or publisher, you are not quite clear of your committment, yet. Your manuscript will be checked by the editor and publisher for its content, consistency, completeness and clarity. You may get your manuscript back, marked with queries and flags. Even if you consider the queries inappropriate, try to answer them as clearly and postively as possible. If someone has misunderstood a point, do not attack the messenger; accept the opportunity to explain the point more lucidly. In most instances, this will improve the book's readability, promote readers' understanding, and smooth production. Make sure to adhere to the deadline set for the return of the revised manuscript. The manuscript that comes in last sets the pace for the whole publication.

When the final copy-edited manuscripts of all contributors are in the hands of the publisher and everything is ready for type-setting, the publisher will notify you of the appropriate date on which you can expect to receive galley and/or page proofs so that you can plan your time for proof-reading. If you will be unable to do the proof-reading at the indicated time, (you may be on holiday, at a congress, etc.) let the publisher and editor know immediately so that some alternate date can be arranged.

When you receive the proofs:

- Check them carefully for correct spelling, completeness, correct structuring (headings, sections, paragraphs), and optimal arrangement of text, figures, and tables.
- Answer *all* queries even if you think some of them require no comment.
- Do not add new material (text, figures, or tables) since this may necessitate a complete new "paste-up" of the whole book. This will not only delay the publication date but will probably cause you to be billed for the extra costs so incurred.
- Return proofs by the requested time, i.e., usually 48 hours after you received them. Publishing a book is a team effort that involves not only the author(s), editor(s) and publisher, but also the less visible and equally important typesetters, printers and binders. If anyone's work is not delivered on time, the schedule of everyone else is delayed, progress comes to a halt, publication is delayed, and costs soar, sometimes astronomically.

Summary

Do not agree to contribute to a book unless you honestly believe you will be able to complete the task by the stipulated deadline. Moreover, do not agree until you have received, from the editor, a detailed outline of the planned book as well as sufficient information about the intended readership and the type of material desired. Write exactly what you have been asked to write. Show understanding toward your readers and mercy toward your co-workers in the production of the book.

SECTION V

International Perspectives on Surgical Research

Introduction

This book was born in the course of a series of consultations about barriers to surgical research, unattained but attainable goals for investigators, and training opportunities for aspiring academic clinicians.

The informal and enlightening international pilgrimage of one of the editors, described in the introduction of this textbook, progressed to a more formal consultation in a planning conference convened at Eppan in the Italian Tyrol during the autumn of 1984. The participants were from nine countries. There was no intent or pretense that the planning process could involve an extensive representation of nationalities. However, the architecture of the book was adopted at this conference and the book has subsequently been written for the international community of established and training university surgeons and their scientific partners. Preceding sections dealt with the methodological and practical aspects of clinical research; this section is a "tour d'horizon" of real-life settings in which the principles of surgical research can be and are being translated into research accomplishment. In many ways, this is the "soul" of the book. It has also been one of the most difficult to assemble. Reports from senior academic surgeons in nine countries are presented. The status of surgical research is presented from the individual viewpoint of each author, not as a summary of all available information from each country. We did not impose a rigid format on each chapter, nor did we attempt to standardize the language. Instead, we have preserved the unique style and flavor of each contribution within the limits of translation requirements.

In Chapter 10, the editors have pooled some of the information supplied by the authors to allow more direct comparisons to be made between the postgraduate educational programs in surgery. Data on the funding of research from the (Fogarty) foundation, presented in this chapter, help establish a framework for comparison of the level of interest and accomplishment in biomedical research.

1

Surgical Research in Canada

D.S. Mulder

This chapter provides a brief overview of the development and present status of surgical research in Canada. It reflects the personal experience and observations of the author and makes no attempt to be a comprehensive discussion of the contribution of every university department in Canada.

The science of surgery has made tremendous strides in Canada since Sir William Olser stated in the late 1880's. "The physic of the men who are really surgeons, is better than the surgery of the men who are really physicians; which is the best that can be said of a very bad arrangement" (1). Since that provocative statement was made, surgery at McGill University has evolved quickly, primarily on the basis of clinical activities. The personality, wisdom and forward thinking of George Armstrong, Thomas Roddick, James Bell, and Edward Archibald, brought high clinical standards to surgery at McGill by the late 1930's.

Dr. Archibald made monumental contributions and was influential in the establishment of the American Board of Surgery in 1937. In addition to his efforts in graduate surgical education, he had a life-long interest in promoting both basic and clinical research. He lead in the investigation of gastric, biliary, and pulmonary physiology, and more importantly, inspired and encouraged several young surgeons to obtain additional training in laboratory science. He was instrumental in sending Donald R. Webster to work on gastric physiology with Boris Babkin in 1928.

The tremendous advances in surgery during World War II set the scene for rapid developments in clinical and basic laboratory surgery in Montreal. Dr. Fraser B. Gurd established the McGill residency training program and developed the Department of Experimental Surgery and the Donner Building Laboratories on campus. These were the beginnings of laboratory research in surgery at McGill University.

In Toronto, Professor Gallie was a leader in establishing a training program that placed academic surgeons in most university centers across Canada.

Wilder Penfield established the Montreal Neurological Institute on a solid base of clinical and surgical research. His basic surgical investigations led to the current surgical management of epilepsy and the training of several generations of neurosurgeons who have assumed positions of academic leadership throughout North America.

William Bigelow in Toronto, Fraser Gurd and Lloyd D. MacLean in Montreal, and Walter McKenzie in Alberta lead the development of research in university surgical departments in Canada.

Bigelow's innovations in the use of hypothermia and the development of effective cardiac pacing were landmarks in the progress of cardiovascular-thoracic surgery. The observations of Gurd and MacLean in the area of shock and low-flow states led to improved nutrition in the surgical patient and to an objective assessment of patients' immune status in many surgical illnesses.

The development of surgical science in Canada has been greatly influenced by the proximity of the United States. The opportunities afforded to Canadians to participate in the scientific forums of most major U.S. surgical societies, was invaluable in the development of surgical science in Canada. Exposure to such giants in surgery such as Blalock, Ravdin, Graham, Wagensteen, Francis Moore and Gibbon left their mark on many of the young Canadian surgeons who have become today's surgical leaders.

It is paradoxical that virtually every university department of surgery in Canada conducts significant basic and clinical research in the 1980's, and concern for the status of surgical research in Canada has reached a peak. This is reflected in three recent studies of research grants to clinical scientists. A research committee established by The Canadian Association of General Surgeons held a retreat, in 1985, to examine the problems confronting surgical research in Canada and the possible solutions. On the basis of a preliminary questionnaire sent to university departments of surgery in Canada, Dr. John Duff was able to identify requests for $2 million to support research that was not approved for funding by granting agencies and applications for a further $500,000 for projects that were approved by peer-review although funds were not available. The acute lack of research funds on both the federal and provincial level, identified at The Canadian Association of General Surgeons' research conference, was attributed to a general shortage of biomedical research funds and a particularly pronounced decline in the funds specifically allocated to surgical research (2).

Twenty-five scientists identified the following five problems facing surgical research over the next decade:

1. *Failure to recruit the most scholarly individuals into surgical programs.* "Universities are not actively encouraging the most scholarly students to consider surgical careers. Instead, application for surgical training tends to be left to the individual, and those who might accomplish the most outstanding research results do not always apply."
2. *Training programs are not designed to train the surgical scientist.* "Cooperation from universities and department heads is necessary to ensure that provision is made within surgical training programs to encourage research and to train researchers."
3. *Surgical investigators are not held in high esteem by clinical surgeons.* "Practicing clinical surgeons, in general, do not yet realize the importance of surgical investigators to the profession as a whole, or to their own day-to-day work."
4. *A critical shortage of adequate funding of research and researchers.* "If more funding is not made available for surgical researchers in Canada, not only will general surgery be deprived of the new findings it needs to meet the patients' requirements, but Canada will lose its research talent to other countries, particularly the United States."
5. *Demands of research, teaching and practice produce time constraints, that cannot always be resolved.* "In Canada, research funding does not permit the researcher to devote his full-time attention to his investigations. This places a great limitation on research productivity, and makes it more difficult to acquire the excellence that can only be developed through sustained research activity."

In 1982, Dr. Pierre Bois established a second joint Task Force of the Medical Research Council (MRC) and the Royal College of Physicians and Surgeons of Canada [(RCPS(C)] to examine the apparent continuing decline in the number of clinicians engaged in research. This followed a similar study by Dr. Robert Salter (3), in 1981, whose committee emphasized the need for clinician-scientists and noted the problems in attracting, recruiting, training and supporting them. Salter's study recommended an overall increase in funding for biomedical research and particularly for the support of M.D. scientists. It also urged the Royal College of Physicians and Surgeons of Canada to increase its emphasis on, and recognition of, the research component of specialty training.

An earlier MRC sub-committee, under the chairmanship of Dr. David Sackett (4), had drawn attention to the need to improve the clinical application of new scientific knowledge. Dr. Sackett identified the lack of human and financial resources required for epidemiological studies and clinical trials as one of the most important barriers to the application of new knowledge to clinical care. Such expertise is almost non-existent in Canadian departments of surgery.

In 1984, the joint Task Force, chaired by Dr. Henry B. Dinsdale, made several important recommendations (5). The Task Force defined the "clinician–scientist as an M.D. who is engaged, both in research and patient-care" and noted that the amount of patient-care and responsibility will vary between individuals and disciplines, and may change during any one professional career. The Task Force emphasized the importance of continuing exposure of medical students to research and suggested an evaluation of the impact of summer research traineeships on the subsequent development of M.D.'s basic researchers following graduation from medical school. Research training following the M.D. degree was also carefully assessed.

The Medical Research Council Fellowship program has been a major source of financial support for research training in Canada. Table I shows the number of M.D. and Ph.D. applicants for MRC fellowships. The low success rate of 50%, in the 1980's, is undoubtedly a factor in encouraging medical graduates to consider a direct route to full-time practice. The Task Force stressed the importance of post-M.D. fellowships for research training remaining a high priority program for the Medical Council. It also recommended that MRC consider the establishment of a program to augment research training for all M.D.'s considering careers as clinician-scientist that would include salary support for fellowship training and initial faculty appointments (5 years).

The Task Force felt that the Royal College [RCPS(C)] must assume greater responsibility for encouraging research training in all medical and surgical specialties. It recommended that the accreditation of specialty training programs be made conditional on satisfactory levels of research activity and that all disciplines be encouraged to include at least one year of research training in their specialty training requirements.

The chairmen of surgery departments have instituted a study to examine the level and funding of research activity in Canadian departments of surgery. It is estimated that the current level of surgical research in two thirds of Canada's 16 medical schools is lower than desirable.

The Medical Research Council does not have a separate surgical committee; all grant applications are submitted to standing committees for adjudication of their scientific merit. The desirability of creating a separate surgical committee to review all grants submitted by surgical scientists has been debated for a long time but the consensus, to date, is that all medical surgical scientists should compete solely on the basis of scientific merit. However, Dr. Pierre Bois, President of the Medical Research Council, has responded positively to a recommendation by the surgical chairman and has been most helpful in encouraging more surgical scientists to sit on MRC review panels. This increase in surgical representation on the various scientific committees will improve the peer-review process for surgical grants.

Another source of concern is that, while surgical research is proceeding at varying levels of effectiveness in every department in Canada, current fee schedules, particularly in Quebec, exert growing pressure on surgeons to increase clinical productivity at the expense of research and teaching. Maintaining an environment for effective surgical research is the major challenge facing any surgical department chairman.

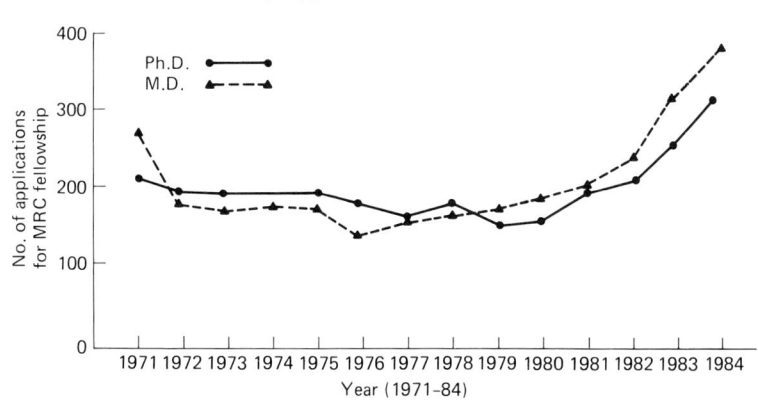

TABLE I. MRC fellowship applications.

Attitudes

Canadians have a very positive attitude toward medical research in general. Public knowledge and understanding of specific advances in surgical research are increasing rapidly, quite apart from such dramatic developments as heart and liver transplantations. The public interest in biomedical research is convincingly demonstrated by its voluntary contribution of $50 million to biomedical research in Canadian faculties of medicine in 1984 (Table II). Well-organized lay groups not only participate in fund-raising and volunteer care of patients, but also donate their expertise in management, budget control, computer science, etc. This type of support is invaluable, particularly when governmental health-care funding is constantly being reduced.

Surgeons' attitude towards surgical research has changed dramatically over the past 10–15 years; surgical research is non significantly more important in the eyes of most practicing surgeons and trainees in surgery. The development of outstanding role models in every university department of surgery has been a highly significant factor in bringing about this change of attitude. To be such role models, surgical scientists have to maintain a high level of excellence in the clinical arena, provide research leadership, and be productive surgical investigators.

Funding of Surgical Research

Biomedical research expenditure in Canadian medical faculties during each of the 5 years between 1979 and 1984 have been documented in a study by Ryten (7). Table II is a summary of the essential data, which confirm that the financial support of biomedical research comes mainly from federal or provincial governmental agencies. The Medical Research Council of Canada is the major funding agency at the federal level; the F.R.S.Q. (Fonds de la recherche en sante du Quebec) functions at the provincial level in Quebec.

Overall, Canada spends approximately 0.11% of its gross domestic product on biomedical research and development.

It is virtually impossible to identify funds that are dedicated specifically to surgical research. A detailed, department by department study of surgical research budgets was done some years ago by Dr. Robert McBeth, but a new survey is required to obtain data for a valid comparison.

MRC provides personnel support for research training through its fellowship program and for new and established investigators through its scholarship program (Table III). The F.R.S.Q. provides similar support Quebec. Operating grants, awarded by the MRC on the basis of annual competitions, usually provide for a 3-year period of support during which annual progress reports are required. The low success rate of applications for operating grants (25%) often discourages young surgical investigators, and leads to interuptions in valuable research programs or a return to full-time clinical surgery.

Monies voluntary donated by the public are channelled through such organizations as the Canadian Cancer Society and the Canadian Cardiovascular Society or their provincial counterparts. In addition to supporting basic and applied research on a competitive peer-reviewed

TABLE II. Expenditures for bio-medical research by Canadian faculties of medicine (1980–84) (thousands of Canadian dollars).

Source	1983–84	1982–83	1981–82	1980–81	1979–80
Federal Gov't.	118,000	105,000	94,000	77,000	68,000
Provincial Gov'ts.	63,000	52,000	43,000	21,000	15,500
Charitable Agencies:					
National	46,500	44,000	38,000	34,000	29,000
Provincial	6,000	6,000	6,000	12,500	7,000
Private Industry	8,000	4,600	4,700	4,500	2,500
University Sources	15,800	10,000	10,700	4,000	3,000
Foreign Sources	9,700	9,500	10,750	10,980	8,200
Miscellaneous	12,000	11,500	5,600	10,500	8,400
	279,000	242,600	212,750	174,480	141,600

Modified from Eva Ryten.

basis, these organizations actively educate the public about the importance and results of biomedical research.

The relatively meagre funding of biomedical research by private industry in Canada comes primarily from the pharmaceutical sector. Much of this support takes the form of "contract research" for specific clinical studies on the efficacy of particular drugs or antibiotics organized by university departments of medicine or surgery.

Virtually every department of surgery is provided with space and other indirect financial support for research activity that is channelled through hospitals and universities. These sources have grown in importance, particularly in the province of Quebec. Such support is frequently administered through the establishment of a research institute closely associated with a university teaching hospital. University salaries are an important but shrinking means of support for full-time clinician scientists in every department of surgery in Canada. Identicification of the precise level of support for research is often difficult because clinical activities, teaching and research are so often blended in the daily lives of clinical scientists.

The MRC is the principal source of funding for research training for surgical residents and its program is directed individuals who wish to pursue 2 or 3 years of research training culminating in a Ph.D. So far, provincial ministries of health have not provided funding for shorter periods of research training during surgical residency.

A significant level of financial support for surgical research is generated by virtually every surgical department through the "excess earnings" of its full-time university staff, or donations made by individual academic surgeons. These funds are important to the chairman because they provide "seed money" for launching research projects and travel expenses for surgical residents and surgical scientists who present papers at scientific meetings. The current low fee schedules in Quebec have considerably reduced this form of financial support for surgical scholarship.

The Royal College of Physicians and Surgeons of Canada provides limited funds for research training in the form of scholarships, travel grants, and research awards. The Canadian Association of General Surgeons has established a scholarship program for surgical research and intends to generate fund to support surgical research in Canada, but the level of support currently available is small.

The Education of the Academic Surgeon

Most doctors who intend to be surgical residents now proceed through a straight internship following graduation from medical school at about age 25. The straight internship combined with a variety of surgical rotations in the second year, constitutes a 2-year core training period that is designed to include exposure to the basic principles and techniques common to all surgical disciplines. On successful completion of this 2-year period, the candidate is eligible to write

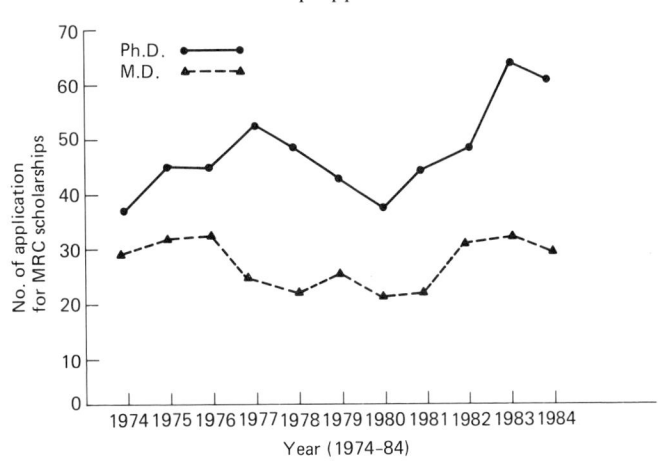

TABLE III. MRC scholarship applications.

the examination in basic science in surgery set by the Royal College of Physicians and Surgeons of Canada. This training meets the requirements for virtually every surgical discipline.

The McGill training program in general surgery is 5 years in length. The weekly schedule of the clinical surgical service is outlined in Table IV. A sabbatical-type year of surgical scholarship is encouraged following the 2-year core training. This year may be spent in the basic surgical laboratory, in a basic science department on the university campus, or in another hospital department such as the Department of Pathology. It allows the surgical resident time, not only to read and reflect, but also to acquire some of the methodological skills common to all research, such as statistical analysis and experimental design. Some surgical residents are extremely productive during this year, but the basic purpose is to ensure their active involvement in laboratory research and to give the program director an opportunity to select potential candidates for more intensive research training or Ph.D.'s in basic science disciplines.

Two further years of senior surgical responsibility are required to become eligible to try the written and oral examinations in general surgery of the Royal College. Successful candidates are allowed to become consultants in general surgery in community-based or university centers. University-based surgeons tend to acquire further skills in more specialized areas of surgery or additional research training in areas of particular personal interest. The certificates of special competence in vascular or thoracic surgery, recently approved, usually require 1 or 2 additional years of specialty training. Specialization in cardiovascular thoracic surgery requires a minimum of 2 additional years of training beyond completion of the requirements in general surgery.

Every surgical trainee is required to participate in historical or prospective controlled clinical research studies under the supervision of a staff surgeon. Virtually every university department of surgery in Canada is well supported in terms of library facilities, computerized literature searches, and audio visual aids.

TABLE IV. Weekly schedule general surgical resident (Montreal General Hospital).

	Monday	Tuesday	Wednesday	Thursday	Friday	Saturday	Sunday
06:00 07:00		Ward Rounds Structural Literature Review					
07:00 08:00	Ward Rounds		Ward Rounds	Ward Rounds	Ward Rounds		
08:00	Out Patient Clinic	Operating Room	Operating Room	Operating Room	Operating Room	Ward Rounds	Ward Rounds
11:00 12:00	Endoscopy		Oncology Rounds		Oncology Rounds		
14:00 15:00	G.I. Rounds Service Chief Rounds Ward work			Teaching Afternoon a. formal Ward Rounds & all staff b. informal case presentations c. Combined pathology, radiology, Rounds		On call for all Emergencies every third night and every third weekend	
16:00 17:00		Attending Staff Rounds	Mortality & Morbidity Rounds		Attending Staff Rounds		
17:00 18:00	Surgical Research Seminar						
18:00 19:00			Basic Science Seminar Monthly Practice Oral Examinations				

Ample opportunities to present the results of studies are provided at surgical meetings throughout North America. Canadian surgical residents can present their research findings at the annual meeting of the Royal College or at any of its sub-specialty meetings. The most prestigious achievement for a surgical resident is to have a paper accepted for presentation at the American College of Surgeons' forum on fundamental surgical research. Most surgical training programs sponsor an end-of-the-year surgical residents' day, to give recognition to both the clinical and basic research performed by residents during the preceding academic year. The considerable variation in the quantity and quality of research usually reflects the attitudes of the faculty in the various surgical discipline.

Few privileges and responsibilities can be greater than being the research advisor of a budding surgical scientist. A close one-to-one relationship develops during the period of at least one year when the research advisor is not only a role model but also the principal source of guidance in the formulation of a problem and how to undertake its rigorous investigation. Advisors must create an environment that is conducive to research by providing adequate laboratory facilities, effective personnel support, and advise on how to obtain operating funds and choose suitable didactic courses to supplement the research activities. It is imperative that, in the process of giving such support and guidance, the research advisor still allows the candidate sufficient flexibility to branch off into his or her own independent research.

Legal and Cultural Considerations

Although an opposition movement against animal experimentation is growing in Canada, as it is elsewhere, public education has been effective in convincing most citizens the value of basic surgical research and the direct contribution made to it by animal experimentation. Emphasis has been placed on the humane care and attention given to every animal used in a hospital laboratory. The rigid standards enforced by hospital research institutes and by Medical Research Council accreditation visits have done much to improve the standards of animal care throughout Canadian laboratories. The care of animals of virtually every university department of surgery is supervised by a veterinarian.

Interest in clinical trials in surgery is increasing in Canada and the urgent need for improvement in the quality of such studies is evident. Sackett has drawn attention to the deficiency of basic epidemiological and statistical techniques in most Canadian clinical trials (4). Canadian surgeons are awakening to the need to acquire such skills to enhance their success rate in competing for MRC grants. Most university hospitals now have well established clinical trials committees that carefully examine the ethics of any human study. The value of clinical trials carried out in intensive care units, wards, surgical operating rooms may be one of the greatest oversight of academic surgeons in Canada. The unique opportunities these areas present for studying cost-effectiveness in the delivery of surgical care, have received minimal attention in Canada.

Conclusion

Surgical scholarship has made great progress in Canada since Osler's assessment in 1880. Basic surgical research has blossomed in many university centers since World War II, but disparities in the quality and quantity or surgical research in Canada's 16 medical schools is still cause for concern. As many as two-thirds of the university departments of surgery fail to meet the level of research activity required for accreditation by the Royal College of Physicians and Surgeons of Canada. Studies carried out by the Canadian Association of General Surgeons and the chairman of surgical departments have identified a serious inadequacy in the funding for training in surgical research and the insecurity of personnel support for young surgical scientists (7). Implementation of the recommendations of the MRC/RCPS Task Force (1984) (5,8) would go a long way towards guaranteeing the continued growth and development of surgical research and would allow the production of the individuals needed to fill the depleted ranks of surgical scientists (9).

References

1. Cushing H. In: The life of Sir William Osler. Gryphon, editor. Birmingham, The Classics of Medicine Library, 1982.

2. Cohen M. Chairman of Canadian Association of General Surgeons Research Committee—personal communication.
3. Salter RB. Report of the M.R.C. Committee on clinician scientists in Canada. M.R.C., June 1981.
4. Sackett D. The application of biomedical research to health care. M.R.C., December 1980.
5. Dinsdale H. Medical Research Council Royal Joint Task Force on clinician scientists. M.R.C., 1984.
6. Frederickson DS. Biomedical research in the 1980's. N Engl J Med 304:509–517, 1981.
7. Ryten E. The funding of research activities of canadian faculties of medicine (1983–84). A.C.M.C. Forum December 1985;18:9–14.
8. Roncari DAK, Salter RB, Till JE, Loey FH. Is the clinician scientist really vanishing? encouraging results from a Canadian Institute of Medical Science. C.M.A.J. 1984;130:977–979.
9. Mulder DS. "Entre Amis". Presidential address, 45th Annual Meeting of the Association for the Surgery of Trauma, Boston, Mass: Published in the Journal of Trauma, March 1986.

2

Contributions from France

J-H. Alexandre

Introduction

Surgical research in France is carried out principally at the largest university affiliated hospitals. Most of the major French surgical departments have active research programs. The results of research activities in the surgical specialties are the mainstay of national meetings and international conferences conducted in France under the sponsorship of European surgical associations, such as the French Surgical Association, the Plastic Surgery Society, the National Vascular Surgery College, the Bone Surgery Study Group, the Hand Study Group, the International Organization for Statistical Studies of Esophageal disease, and the research group on Abdominal Wall Studies. Each surgical department organizes at least one convocation annually for the presentation of the results of innovations and surgical accomplishments of the service.

Since 1960, experimental surgery chairs associated with anatomy and physiology departments have been created as an adjunct to surgical services at the teaching hospitals. Most hospital-based surgeons complete a rotation in the department of anatomy during internship, comprised of lectures to medical students, cadaver dissections, and fundamental research in surgical anatomy. I followed this path in my training, and eventually became professor of anatomy as well as professor of surgery.

In addition to collaborative research with anatomists and other basic scientists, surgical research projects are carried out in our community in conjunction with biostatisticians, radiologists, ultrasonographers, and other clinical scientists.

Surgical research provided the basis for Lortat-Jacob's successful completion of the first right hepatic lobectomy, Dubost's replacement of aortic aneurysm by prosthesis, and Henry's successful completion of a cardiac transplantation in a recipient still alive now 20 years following surgery. The development of Carpentier's cardiac value bioprostheses, the transplantation of the kidney by Degaudart d'Allines, Dubost, and Kuss, and the development of hip prosthesis by Juede and Merle D'Aubigne are among France's contributions to surgery which developed from research programs.

The Surgeon's Curriculum, and the Role of Research

Internship in France has a somewhat different meaning from its traditional understanding in many Western countries. The internship or "internat" lasts four years somewhat like a general surgical residency program in North America. A typical week for a French surgical resident is outlined in Table I. It is followed by two to six years as an assistant to the chief of the surgical department, as occurs in the German, English, Swedish, and Japanese systems, among others. This latter category may soon be replaced by the designation as "practicien internat" a more permanent position achieved after six years of internship and successful completion of examinations subject to the approval of the chief of service.

Candidates for surgical training are selected for the residency on the basis of their standings

TABLE I. Weekly schedule.

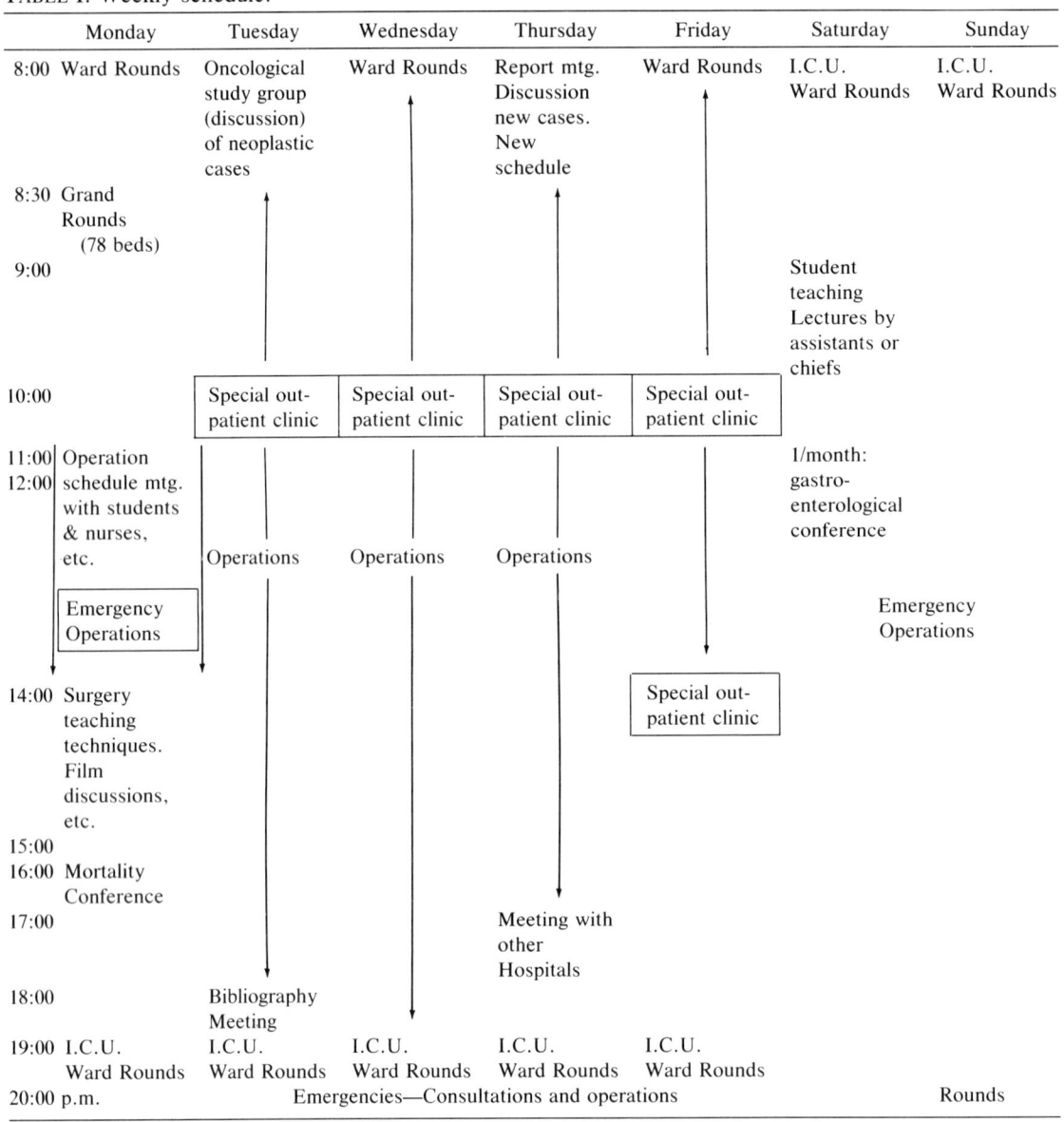

	Monday	Tuesday	Wednesday	Thursday	Friday	Saturday	Sunday
8:00	Ward Rounds	Oncological study group (discussion) of neoplastic cases	Ward Rounds	Report mtg. Discussion new cases. New schedule	Ward Rounds	I.C.U. Ward Rounds	I.C.U. Ward Rounds
8:30	Grand Rounds (78 beds)						
9:00						Student teaching Lectures by assistants or chiefs	
10:00		Special out-patient clinic	Special out-patient clinic	Special out-patient clinic	Special out-patient clinic		
11:00 12:00	Operation schedule mtg. with students & nurses, etc.	Operations	Operations	Operations		1/month: gastro-enterological conference	
	Emergency Operations						Emergency Operations
14:00	Surgery teaching techniques. Film discussions, etc.				Special out-patient clinic		
15:00 16:00	Mortality Conference						
17:00				Meeting with other Hospitals			
18:00		Bibliography Meeting					
19:00	I.C.U. Ward Rounds	I.C.U. Ward Rounds	I.C.U. Ward Rounds	I.C.U. Ward Rounds	I.C.U. Ward Rounds		
20:00 p.m.		Emergencies—Consultations and operations					Rounds

in highly competitive examinations taken by candidates between the ages of 22 and 27 years, and after four or five years of medical school. From the beginning of the residency, the surgeon in training finds a place on a research team on a voluntary basis and commits one or two afternoons a week to attending a laboratory in experimental surgery, or less frequently in anatomy, immunology, or physiology.

Approximately one of four residents seek further, more concentrated training in surgical research. The future cardiac, hepatic, or transplantation surgeon has a higher probability of linking his training directly to research. Because of the unresolved technical and biological problems in this fields, there seems to be immediate tangible benefit for the candidate's future practice and career to achieve proficiency in research.

Residents who do not pursue training in surgical research may choose programs leading to a university certificate of proficiency in statistics, anatomy, or legal or occupational medicine. For those who pursue a career in research, original experimental or basic scientific publications definitely promote the advancement of their academic careers. The quality of the work, the number of publications, and the reputation of the journal where the publication appears are important considerations in advancement.

The amount of time spent on research during surgical training has been variable in the past. As of 1985, a general decision has been reached that each surgeon who seeks to be a hospital physician will dedicate one full year of his residency to surgical research. Those who envision a university career may spend a longer period leading to a specialized diploma. A resident must necessarily spend at least one year of his surgical training in research in order to learn how to set up a project, including formulation of the original idea, obtaining financial support, assembling a research team, learning to work as a team member and to work competitively in the field. Statistics and other related skills should be developed during this period which should be between the third and fourth year of the residency. It seems desirable that the researcher be exempted from clinical work for this period. When integrated into a clinical unit the surgeon who has received adequate training in surgical research can devise other projects, and will be sufficiently competent in the research process to direct a team or supervise it personally one or two afternoons a week.

In my opinion, a steady commitment to research should be maintained throughout the university surgeon's academic career, i.e., during residency, assistantship and later as head of a surgical department. This commitment need not be as binding for those destined for community hospitals or private practice.

There were approximately 6,000 surgeons in France in 1985, among 130,000 physicians in a total population of 55 million. Fifty percent of surgeons work in the private sector, 25% work part time in hospitals, and 25% are full time hospital surgeons. The majority of full time hospital surgeons are university surgeons who are committed to a career that includes surgical research, teaching, and patient care.

Although surgical research is theoretically possible in a large number of hospital centers in France, it is really the prerogative of university centers. These centers have the staff and equipment to facilitate the conduct of surgical research, such as laboratory facilities, support personnel, and computerized access to literature searches for the accumulation of a bibliography of French and foreign articles.

The surgeon in training in surgical research has the opportunity to present his work at the French Surgical Association's Annual Research Forum. There are a variety of other annual meetings in France and Europe where research data can be presented after appropriate committee review. Nearly all of these meetings use the English language as the common language. Accordingly, a foreign exchange program appears highly desirable for the surgeon in training for a university career. We consider it mandatory that a French researcher spend at least six months in a country where he will be able to perfect his mastery of the English language.

Animal experimentation is conducted in French laboratories under ethical surveillance. The public is sensitive to animal suffering, but for the most part accepts the need for experiments on animals. The advantage of using animals for development of proficiency in surgical procedures is well illustrated by the Amphitheatre des Hopitaux Fer a Moulin directed by Professor Cabral in Lyon. This special institute for teaching surgery and anatomy provides the setting for learning advanced techniques in surgery from films, demonstrations, and direct personal experience in performing new surgical procedures in experimental animals. Through this mechanism new advanced techniques of surgery can be made available to the population at a high level of efficiency through effective use of the surgical research laboratory. For example, the techniques of replacement of the ascending thoracic aorta with coronary reimplantation, and the regimen of immunosuppression currently used throughout the world for cardiac transplantation were developed in the experimental surgical laboratory in France by Cabral and his colleagues.

Research institutes offer the only full time research opportunities for surgeons. Nearly all surgical researchers are paid by hospitals or universities as full time university hospital employees to fulfill the threefold objective stated in the Debre Law of 1960: caring for patients, teaching, and conducting research. Research objectives and finding are determined by the national granting agencies such as The National Scientific Institute for Medical Studies and Research (INSERM) which provides some limited funding for surgical studies; and the National Centre for Scientific Research (CNRS) which is more oriented toward basic science.

Funds are also awarded from the 24 universities in France, and from the municipalities through Public Assistance. For example, some of the support for surgical research at my hospital comes from the Public Assistance of Paris, a large organization employing over 70,000 people, which supervises the management and funding of 22 hospitals in Paris.

Detailed research proposals are submitted to these bodies for support of research through an established research institute such as the Gustave Roussy in Paris-Ville, the Curie Institute in Paris, the Rene Huguenin Cancer Center in Saint-Cloud or the International Center for the Fight Against Cancer in Lyon or Montpellier. The choice of a research subject for the young surgical researcher is somewhat dependent on the availability of funding from the research institutes, and on the chief of service, who serves in a supervisory role, assisting and establishing research goals, obtaining research grants, work space, manpower and help in the analysis of data and presentation of results. The chief of service can oversee a number of researchers involved in several projects and is responsible for the quality and quantity of the work performed. The government has recently proposed a more complex integrated structure to combine autonomous surgical units under large surgical departments, whose chief and department council will determine policy and report to the university dean to assure that the goals of teaching and research activity are attained.

Funding for Surgical Research

Overall, France spends approximately 0.18% of its gross domestic product on biomedical research and development. Government funding is responsible for the bulk of research in France but the allocation for surgery remains a very small fraction of the research budget. In addition to the CNRS, INSERM, the Ministry of Welfare, and the Ministry of Education and Municipal Governments also allocate money for research. It is of great interest to note that 20% of the research budget allocated by the City of Paris is set aside for surgical research projects. This is a unique resource.

Certain university departments or hospitals receive private, anonymous donations for research, but the funds from these sources are relatively limited compared to their counterparts in the United States, for example. Some pharmaceutical companies participate in research projects involving their products, such as anticoagulants, antibiotics, or analgesics when the substance under evaluation will become the object of upcoming marketing campaigns. Most funding from pharmaceutical companies goes to their own research departments or to the departments of internal medicine because surgeons use only a few highly specialized drugs.

Because of recent reductions in funding of surgical research from CRNS, INTERM, and the Ministry of Education some surgical research units have been disbanded. Others have been forced to develop private sources of funding to support scientific projects and travel to scientific meetings.

In some hospital centers, academic surgeons or professors are asked for personal donations to create bursaries to support research. Curiously, tax credits are not allowed for such gifts. Funds or facilities for foreign surgical researchers to visit French laboratories are minimal. The Ministry of Research plans to establish a system of bursaries for exchange programs.

French surgical research, though embattled for priority and funding has a proud record of accomplishment and a prospect of continued contribution to the advancement of surgical science.

3

Traditions and Transitions in Germany

H. Troidl and N. Boenninghoff

Introduction

This description of surgical research in the Federal Republic of Germany, is the expression of a personal view, rather than a survey of all institutions. It is based on the senior author's experience during several years of training at three different university surgical departments—Munich, Marburg, and Kiel and as the incumbent of the second chair of surgery at the University of Cologne.

Brendel (1) describes three levels of surgical research:

1. **Basic research** that attempts to gain basic knowledge without regard to its applicability for man;
2. **Applied research** that explores possible new treatments using all the available methods of research;
3. **Clinical research,** whose goal is to extend our knowledge of disease and to test new methods of diagnosis and treatment.

Surgical research is conducted at all three levels only in university departments of surgery, but not always in each of them. In West Germany, including West Berlin, university departments retain the old, traditional structure, with one responsible chairman heading the entire department. These university departments provide surgical care for patients and engage in teaching and research. The chairmen of such departments have a remarkable and enduring responsibility, since they may hold their positions for as long as twenty-five years. The chairman or "Ordinarius", is expected to operate almost every day and to have a very broad practical knowledge of surgery. To be selected for a chair, he has to be broadly trained in all aspects of operative surgery and be respected for both his surgical skills and his scientific activities. In the final selection process, a candidate must prove his practical abilities by performing surgery in front of a commission. Consequently, a narrow focus in clinical surgery is not desirable for academic surgeons-in-training. The chairman is also expected to have the administration skills required to run a large department, even though his previous experience generally provides little preparation for such broad teaching, research and administrative responsibilities of the Chair of Surgery.

Because the traditional chairs have such extensive responsibilities for administration, health care, and teaching, some have established more or less independant, theoretical or experimental units to assist in the better fulfillment of the traditional research responsibilities. Well known examples of these exist at the Universities of Munich, Cologne, Heidelberg and Marburg. These units pioneered the development of this approach to surgical research in Germany. The physician who is head of the theoretical or experimental division has usually had special training in a biomedical science, such as biochemistry or physiology. These relatively independant divisions of experimental surgery need the capacity to address broad issues of surgical research. Occasionally, however, their small size and relative independence of their directors make it difficult for clinical surgeons to pursue their own research ideas. As a result, some surgical chairmen are establishing their own experimental groups in addition to the existing surgical research divisions. One solution to this dilemma is the so-called "Marburg Experiment" which is explained in Section 3, Chapter 1. It is a highly interactive program of collaboration that links each academic surgeon to a specific preclinical scientist in a continuing "partnership". At quite a few universities, surgical research is carried out without a structured research department, by surgeons with different levels of training—sometimes without any help, sometimes in cooperation with scientists from such fields as anatomy, pathology, chemistry, biochemistry, etc.

The attitude of the German population toward surgical research, is somewhat indifferent or skeptical. Much of the public has no idea that surgical research exists, except when a sensational surgical event, such as the implantation of an artificial heart, gets media coverage. There are virtually no spontaneous or organized financial donations for surgical research. The outstanding exception is the "Deutsche Krebshilfe", a public initiative founded to raise money for cancer research, treatment, and rehabilitation.

Information on surgical research in the media is rather scant and naive, with a few exceptions like the one mentioned earlier. In this atmosphere, clinical trials must be carried out very carefully, if at all. We must deal with the suspicion that we are "experimenting on the patient" by devising ways to inform patients about planned treatment or research without increasing their anxiety. There is a tension between patients' desire to be fully informed and their not wanting to be frightened by undesired detail.

Some surgeons are suspicious of clinical trials, and mock them because of the requirement that there be an explicit expression of doubt concerning the best choice of medical treatment. The admission by a surgeon of any element of doubt in his decision making is unfavorably regarded. "A surgeon should always know everything!" is the traditional expectation of the general public. But, only God is omniscient!

Even in universities, surgical research is not as highly valued as surgical practice. Scientists in other disciplines take a critical view of surgeons as researchers. The chance of a habilitation thesis about purely clinical issues in everyday surgery being accepted is severly limited or non-existent! For a thesis, the young surgeon must spend a lot of time in a theoretical institute, if sometimes only to add a "scientific veneer" to the thesis project.

Even in university surgery departments, the attitude towards surgical research may not always be enthusiastic. Many professors of surgery think of surgical research as a major part of their responsibility, have done serious work, and are keenly interested. Advancement depends more on numbers of papers and presentations than on original ideas and their careful analysis and validation. Sometimes, interest in research ceases with the acquisition of the title of professor. In spite of their administrative burdens, masses of students, and persistent struggles with the administration, these chairmen remain enthusiastic about new ideas and aware of the worldwide influence Germany continues to exert in such areas as gastric surgery, orthopedics, vascular surgery, and endoscopy.

Surgical research certainly does not rank first in the minds of practicing surgeons. "Practical experience" and "excellent technique" are at the top. As a result, German technical standards are very high in any comparison among countries. This applies to the smaller hospitals, the universities, and the larger community hospitals.

Outside the university departments, the academically oriented surgeon is regarded with some suspicion and frequently encounters the view that if he is scholarly, he may be able to analyze and discuss surgical problems, but be unable to operate! Stelzner summarized this attitude as: "The nightingale doesn't win a prize at the poultry competition". It is important to recognize that there can be excesses in either direction, including the possibility that some practical surgeons may employ the best techniques but perform the wrong operations.

The attitude of German surgical residents towards surgical research is not different from those in other western countries. Few enter a university surgical department to carry out research exclusively. Most of them choose a department based on its ability to teach them good surgical practice. If, along the way, they are given an opportunity to take part in a research program, they gladly embrace it because research productivity leads to an academic title, and the possibility of a better position later on.

Research Funding

Overall, the Federal Republic of Germany spends approximately 0.28% of its gross domestic product on biomedical research and development. After the prosperous 1960's, financial support for research began to diminish slowly in Germany. The resources that are generally available, are examplified by what happens in our department at Cologne.

The university provides each surgical chairman with an annual budget derived from a grant from the provincial (Bundesland) government to carry out teaching and research. The amount of such budgets varies considerably between different provincial governments and universities. At Kiel, the annual amount was D.M. 30,000, at Cologne, the amount for our experimental unit is D.M. 60,000 per year. This annual amount is independently managed by the chairmen to support research and teaching activities. The experimental unit of the second chair for surgery in Cologne is comprised of nineteen persons, employed on a full-time basis for research; four are academic professional colleagues. This means that only D.M. 2,200 ($1,000.00 U.S.) per assistant per year is covered by current, university provided funding. This example shows how small the basic budget for surgical research is and how important it is to raise additional money from federal and private sources.

Except for university grants, and some industry and private money, funds are awarded on the basis of competitive research grant applications for the support of specific research projects. Most are reviewed by a commission that requires progress reports at defined intervals during the grant period and for competitive renewal. From 1975 through 1985, the German Research Foundation (Deutsche Forschungs Gemeinschaft or DFG) received from 38 to 51 grant applications from surgical departments; approximately 50% of the requested sums were approved and funded (Table I).

Local conferences and workshops are financed either by the surgical societies, (e.g., Lower Rhein-Westphalian Surgical Society) by their membership dues with additional support from industry, or exclusively by industry. Private donations are a rare source of research support.

Local community budgets for hospitals do not provide money for research at all, but cover only patient care. Travelling expenses to conferences, both inside and outside of Germany, must be financed out of one's own pocket or by seeking sponsors from industry. As an investigation of a provincial ministry found out, there has been remarkable variance in the allocation of university-distributed federal research money to different colleagues at the seven universities of North Rhein Westfalia ranging from DM. 27,000 to DM. 6,000! It might be interesting to correlate these allocations with a citation or productivity index. The same analysis could make interesting international comparisons, e.g., funds per researcher per entry in the Citation Index, number of doctoral theses, number of supervised Ph.D.'s, or number of publications in respected journals.

Training

The educational programs for a clinical surgeon and a surgeon with scientific ambitions, are outlined in Table I (Section V, Chapter 10). In West

TABLE I. DFG grant history of general surgical departments.

Year	Grant applications submitted n (DM)	Grant applications approved n	Grant applications withdrawn n (DM)	Percentage of requested sums approved
1983	36 (5,593,100)	26	1 (115,496)	50.7
1984	46 (5,160,355)	32	3 (49,225)	51.4
1985*	28 (4,754,137)	22	3 (12,758)	52.7

*January 1, 1985–August 31, 1985.

Germany, there is no uniform concept for the training of an academic surgeon. The ideas vary from university to university, within a single university at any time, and from time to time. There is no universal agreement about when surgeons should obtain research training, and whether they should do only experimental research, only clinical research or a combination of both. We prefer that a young colleague should spend 1 to 2 years in a basic scientific discipline before becoming a resident at a surgical university department. It is certainly advantageous for the assistant to be able to communicate in an additional language such as English or French.

Young residents in a university department often join an on-going research project, devote a limited amount of time during the week's routine to it, and gradually progress to their own projects that may eventually lead to habilitation.

Time Management

Adequate time is an essential precondition for research. The schedule in our department is fairly typical for Germany (Table II). The need for efficiency in patient care leaves little time for research. In fact, our calculations indicate that we need two more assistants to staff our clinical program without including time for research! After a 6-hour operating day and taking care of a ward, a surgeon has difficulty in changing his focus of concentration from a bleeding gastric ulcer or a difficult anastomosis to the planning of an experiment or discussing

TABLE II. Weekly schedule.

Time	Monday	Tuesday	Wednesday	Thursday	Friday	Sat/Sun
A.M.						
7:00	Ward Rounds	Ward Rounds	Ward Rounds	Ward Rounds	Ward Rounds	
7:30	Report/Meeting	Report/Meeting	Report/Meeting	Report/Meeting	Report/Meeting	
8:00	I.C.U. Ward Rounds	I.C.U. Ward Rounds	General Surgery Research Meeting	I.C.U.	I.C.U. Ward Rounds	Ward Rounds
8:30	Operations	Operations	Operations	Operations	Operations	Report/I.C.U.—Ward Rounds (9:15)
P.M.	Special Out-Patient Clinics	Special Out-Patient Clinics	Special Out-Patient Clinics	Special Out-Patient Clinics	Special Out-Patient Clinics	
2:00		Chief's Ward Rounds				Non-elective Operations
2:30	Operation—schedule mtg.		Operation—schedule mtg.	Operation schedule mtg.	Operation schedule mtg.	
4:30	X-Ray mtg.		Lectures and Grand Rounds	X-Ray mtg.	X-Ray mtg.	
5:00	Report of Op/Gen. mtg.			Report of Op/Gen. mtg.	Report of Op/Gen. mtg.	
5:30	Interdisc. Angiology Conf.			Journal Club & Case-F Conf.		
6:00	I.C.U. Ward Rounds	I.C.U. Ward Rounds	I.C.U. Ward Rounds	I.C.U. Ward Rounds	I.C.U. Ward Rounds	I.C.U. Ward Rounds
6:30	Interdisc. Gastroenterology Conference					

scientific problems with freshness and enthusiasm. The toll of night duty, usually twice per week, is another problem that a surgical resident has to cope with. In addition, there is the German compulsion to master surgery from head to toe. Possible solutions to these problems include: (1) arranging days without an elective operating list,(2) providing a larger number of residents, (3) granting some residents a complete exemption from clinical obligations for some period of months, and, (4) a combination of these with the establishment of an experimental unit adapted to the local situation. Setting aside an additional day without operations will require a reduction in the bed occupancy, which, in our country, would bring a reduction in budget and in surgical personnel. On the other side, an increased number of residents reduces the ratio of cases per surgeon and prolongs the length of residency training because a resident needs a defined number of operations to take the examination for certification as a surgeon.

Debate continues in Germany about the ideal way to combine research and surgical training. Some believe that surgeons should be out of daily clinical practice for a year or two to carry out their research projects. Others argue that surgeons, and especially junior surgeons, need constant surgical practice to develop and maintain their skills. This need is comparable to the situation of a serious athlete, who must workout continuously to "stay in shape." A novel approach to this dilemma is offered by the Marburg experiment that allows the clinical surgeon to combine his skills with those of a theoretical surgeon in a continuing scientific collaboration. Other models exist in Munich, Berlin and Cologne, especially in Cologne-Merheim where Professor Heberer has established a somewhat similar organization. What is specific about the "Marburg Experiment" is the integration of clinical surgery with experimental surgery. *Integration* is the key word for without it, a gap generally develops between clinical surgery and research. The legitimate independence of the theoretical or basic scientist does not always lead to greater efficiency in surgical research. Professor Heberer commented on this in 1974, as follows, "The contact of the researchers with the clinic can be loosened by institutionalization. As a result, special fields can become the primary foci to the extent that creative impulses arising from clinical practice are not accepted anymore." The Marburg experiment requires the basic scientists to accept responsibility for participation in medical decision-making, even for individual patients. The theoretical surgeon must help to answer such questions as, "How important is a gastrin assay for the patient in this bed?" Recent advances in experimental methodology are brought into the department by the theoretical surgeon, such as the planning of controlled clinical trials, and the use of new ways to quantify outcomes like "reduction in pain". The theoretical surgeon in the Marburg arrangement also assumes a major responsibility and administration of both clinical and experimental research, although conducting research remains primary role.

The "small research group" is an essential feature of the Marburg experiment. We demand the fullest exchange of ideas and integration of clinical and basic research, not only until surgeons achieve a habilitation degree, but for life. The "small research group" is characterized by the following:

Purpose Integration of clinical and theoretical research on the basis of long-term, personal and practical cooperation.
Composition One theoretical surgeon, one or two clinical surgeons, one technical assistant, one or two students.
Assignments A weekly meeting.
Planning and discussing experiments.
Systematic follow-up.
Special clinical examinations.
Conduct of experiments.
Special services for the department.

The discussion and exchange of information gleaned from the literature is part of the planning and discussion of experiments. The "small research group" jointly examines patients included in clinical trials for a systematic follow-up. The rapid exchange of ideas that develops between the clinicians and the theoretical researchers makes it possible to carry out effective basic and clinical research, in our opinion. The relative smallness of each group does limit its capacity to cover all aspects of research work. The theoretical partner, for example, cannot always provide effective help to an enthusiastic surgeon who wishes to explore his own ideas if they involve areas of scientific knowledge that lie outside the theoretical scientist's field of expertise. Other questions that arise are:

Is it feasible to apply The Marburg approach in a large department?
How does it cater to a large variety of research projects?
Can research on both clinical and experimental surgery be carried out at one place without difficulty?

In closing, we feel that the role of the academic surgeon who is an active, effective clinical surgeon and a researcher is a challenging but achievable one. The first and most important qualification is that genuine concern and compassion for patients.

The second is practical, technical ability to perform operative surgery well. The academic surgeon should not be perceived as a biochemist or statistician with surgical training, but as a surgeon.

Third, but essential to the successful performance of surgical research is a fascination with ideas and the ability to develop, analyze and validate them. To fulfill this role the surgical researcher must be physically strong, energetic and psychologically resilient.

References

1. Brendel W. Medizinische Forschung an Mensch und Tier. Gesundheitsforum S.Z. 1985;154:8.

4

Japan's Integration of Eastern Values and Modern Science

T. Aoki, K. Hioki, and T. Muto

Introduction

Japan is a small nation comprised of many islands and populated by 120 million people. There are nearly 150 physicians per 100,000 population, and the number of physicians continues to rise. They are concentrated in the larger, populous cities. The remote mountainous regions, and outlying islands still have few doctors. The country has well developed science and biomedical research programs. It is now generally accepted in Japan that research is absolutely necessary for the advance of medicine and surgery. Japanese surgeons recognize that both clinical practice and surgical research are equally important, like the wheels of a car.

Research projects are formulated in each surgical department, and sometimes by a cooperative team formed with the other clinical and academic departments in the university. In most universities, there are several research groups in a surgical department, and each surgeon generally belongs to one of the research groups.

Despite heavy clinical commitments, many full-time surgeons are able to find time for surgical research, because they belong to a group of two or three surgeons who share the responsibilities for treating their common patients. Some senior residents can spend a period doing full-time research. This generally occurs in the third year of surgical training, when the resident is 26 to 32 years old.

History of Surgical Research in Japan

From the seventh century, medicine in Japan had been based on Chinese Medicine. In the mid-nineteenth century, Western medicine was introduced. The government invited scholars from Germany to establish the national medical colleges and dispatched young doctors to Germany to study medicine. As a result of this policy, Japanese medicine became completely German, from the academic system and facilities, to the methods of diagnosis and treatment. This continued even after Japanese physicians assumed the leading professorships. The Japan Surgical Society was founded in 1897 and German surgery completely predominated until 1945. Just after the end of the World War II, American surgery, together with American culture, became the prevailing influence, replacing the German approach to Medicine, with its emphasis on theory. The American approach, emphasized empiricism and innovations in practice. A change was observed in surgical research, from the European style predominated by that of Germany to a mixed style including American methods, with particularly obvious progress seen after 1950. Advances in anesthesia, including excellent equipment imported from the U.S.A., England and Germany facilitated the gradual spread of general endotracheal anesthesia. Drastic improvements were made in operating room equipment, instruments, and the equipment and techniques for pre- and post-operative management. Further invasive surgery became possible for malignant tumors. The survival rate in operations for cancer of the esophagus, stomach, rectum, lung, pancreas and liver improved. Dramatic advances occured in the specialized fields of thoracic surgery, especially in open-heart surgery, in microsurgical techniques of neurosurgery, and in pediatric surgery.

Advances in both clinical and laboratory research were achieved through cooperative efforts among scholars in all areas of medicine, including pathology, physiology and biochemistry.

Although Professor Ohsawa had reported successful resection of carcinoma of the esophagus in 1933, following the work of Torek and Kirschner, Nakayama established the effectiveness of resection of carcinoma of the thoracic esophagus through his performance of over 2,000 operations between 1964 and 1970. Through their surgical research, Nakayama and his students lowered the mortality while enhancing the resectability and the survival rate. To attain this goal, they studied pathological physiology and nutritional management. They emphasized the importance of staged operations and examined the significance of preoperative irradiation. Nakayama was famous for his rigorous instruction in clinical research. Most of the present Japanese leaders in this field, were his students.

Professor Honjo, formerly of Kyoto University, now Chairman of the Board of Directors of Kansai Medical University, successfully performed a total excision of the pancreas in a case of pancreatic cancer for the first time in Japan in 1949. In the same year he performed a right hepatic lobectomy for metastatic liver cancer following an operation for rectal cancer, the first successful case of its kind in the world. Research by Honjo and his students elucidated the pathophysiology and treatment of diabetes following pancreatic resection. They carried out experimental and clinical research on hepatoenterostomy in cases of inoperable cholangioma and interruption of the hepatic artery and branches of the portal vein in inoperable liver cancer. They carefully conducted animal experiments to resolve questions arising from their clinical research. Their specialized knowledge of pathology, physiology and biochemistry was indispensable.

The present distinguished chief of The Cancer Institute Hospital in Tokyo, Dr. Kajitani, established systematic lymphadenectomy for gastric cancer through investigations in the pathology laboratory and the operating rooms. He conducted this research over a period spanning 47 years while he was on the Surgical Staff of a hospital affiliated with the Cancer Institute, a private foundation for cancer research. Many foreign surgeons visit his hospital to observe surgical procedures and many university surgeons in Japan have been his students.

Japanese surgical research developed endoscopic diagnosis and treatment of diseases of the airway and digestive tract. This has revolutionized surgical treatment throughout the world.

Current surgical research in Japan is focussed primarily on:

1. Elucidating **general problems** such as wound healing. Examples include studies of the mirocirculation, fibrin glue and the chemistry of fibronectin.

   Nutrition, include home hyperalimentation, infusions of branched chain amino acids or eicosopentanoic acid, and new methods for nutritional assessment.

   Shock: The pathophysiology and treatment of endotoxin shock, surgical infection and disseminated intravascular coagulation are among the major research projects.

2. Research aimed at elevating the level of success in **cancer treatment** or eradication;

   Hepatectomy for liver cancer, a major problem in Japan, requires development of improved surgical techniques, for intraoperative diagnostic evaluation, and postoperative care.

   Composite resections and **reconstruction** problems in advanced cancers of the airway, lung, esophagus including extensive lymphadenectomy.

   Techniques for early detection and treatment of lung, esophageal, gastric and hepatic cancer.

   Adjuvant therapy such as chemotherapy hyperthermia or immunotherapy.

3. Research in the field of **organ transplantation.**

   Kidney transplantation in Japan is established to a comparable degree as that in other advanced countries, however, **heart** transplantation and **liver** transplantation are markedly delayed. Due to strong religious feelings, public debate continues on the determination of death, and there is not yet a consensus. Liver transplantation candidates are currently sent overseas for treatment. In 1968, Professor Wada performed a human heart-transplant operation. Strong public feelings about the definition of brain death were aroused, and strict criteria have only recently been developed by a commission of the Ministry of Health and Welfare. We can expect that major organ transplantation will rapidly develop in

Japan. Scholars are vigorously performing basic and animal research.

Research During Residency Training

The residency system is adopted in only a few medical institutions in Japan. Graduates from medical school obtain a medical license for the first time when they have passed the national examination, but they can practice only after a training period of 2 years. Only medical institutions authorized by the government may provide this training. Most candidates for surgical training, after passing the national examination enter the hospital associated with the university from which they graduated. In some cases they must pass an additional entrance examination. These young surgeons in training may enter research after 2 years of basic surgical training. Research may lead to the title, Doctor of Medicine, a special academic title, held by fewer than 30% of medical graduates in Japan. During the pursuit of the M.D., the candidate serves as an unpaid assistant at the university, and indeed, pays tuition for the "post graduate course in surgery". To provide for living expenses, most young surgeons work part-time in private hospitals assisting in the operating room.

There are two possible tracks to become an "M.D." in a surgical field:

1. Following completion of 2 years clinical training, the candidate attends a post graduate course, after passing the school entrance examination, and starts surgical research. It takes 4–5 years for a candidate to publish a research thesis to obtain the "M.D.". In this track, the fresh M.D., then receives clinical surgical training.
2. After 4–5 years clinical training, the candidate enters surgical research under the instruction of the chief professor, and publishes an M.D. thesis 8 to 10 years after graduation. Young surgeons are motivated to carry out research, in part, to obtain the title "M.D.", which is required or advantageous for gaining a teaching staff position in a medical school, or a position as chief in another medical institution, or even for the purpose of operating a private clinic.

Since surgical research is carried out to resolve questions facing daily clinical situations we think it best that the research training be started only after at least two or more years of surgical training. Young surgeons who embark on research at this time are motivated by a desire to solve clinical problems, to advance their surgical careers, or to advance a career in clinical surgery. We estimate that over 75% of young surgeons enter surgical research for at least a period. However, it may be disadvantageous for them if the period of research training is too long or if the training lacks opportunities for clinical surgical experience. Ideally, young surgeons should choose their own research problems. However, when an institution cannot fully provide the required staff or facilities for a particular project, residents are sometimes exchanged with another institution, otherwise they must limit the scope of their research to what that their own institution can accommodate. In Japan, generally the chief professor selects research topics for residents. In most institutions, young surgeons chosen to enter research continue for at least 2 years free of clinical responsibility during the day, but sharing night duty with the other residents. During research training, young surgeons do not always stay in one department, but may move to another department or even to another institution if necessary.

Although it is disadvantageous for young surgeons to be isolated from clinical surgery training for two or more consecutive years, this is considered an inevitable consequence in Japan. During clinical training, it is difficult to find time for research. In our institution only young surgeons involved in research with the aim of acquiring the "M.D." are relieved of clinical responsibility. No exemption is made for other surgeons in research, in order to maintain the cooperative arrangement of cross-coverage among the staff. The typical week for a Japanese resident is outlined in Table I.

General Comments About Research

In the private medical school in Osaka Prefecture, each department maintains its own research unit. Also there is a larger, general research facility furnished with equipment and technicians available to every scholar. It is possible to collaborate with other clinical or basic

TABLE I. Weekly schedule.

	Monday	Tuesday	Wednesday	Thursday	Friday	Saturday/Sunday
07:30	Residents' Ward Rounds	Residents' Ward Rounds	Residents' Ward Rounds	Residents' Ward Rounds	Residents' Ward Rounds	Residents' Ward Rounds
08:00	Preoperative Patient Conference			Preoperative Patient Conference		
09:00	Elective Surgery	Grand Rounds Walking Rounds with Professor of Surgery	Care of Ward Patients	Elective Surgery	Grand Rounds Walking Rounds with Professor of Surgery	Care of Ward Patients
10:00	Care of Ward Patients		Endoscopy Radiology	Care of Ward Patients		
	Out-Patient Clinic	Out-Patient Clinic	Out-Patient Clinic	Out-Patient Clinic	Out-Patient Clinic	Out-Patient Clinic
11:00		Chest Conference	Hepato Biliary Conference		G.I. Conference	
12:00		Case Study Conference			Care of Ward Patients	Departmental Staff Meeting
13:00		Out-Patient Clinic				
14:00	Special Out-Patient Clinic for Follow-Up Studies	Death Conference	Special Out-Patient Clinic	Special Out-Patient Clinic	Special Endoscopy Radiology	
15:00					Special Out-Patient Clinic	
16:00						
17:00						
18:00	G.I. Conference					
19:00			Research Work/Emergency Operations			

science departments if more specialized knowledge or techniques are necessary.

Most university surgeons participate in research. Their clinical work and teaching responsibilities force them to allocate time for research in the early morning or at night. Research training vary widely in Japan. Community hospitals generally provide only clinical training. Young surgeons who seek academic careers generally return to the university to do research after completing a few years of clinical training in community hospitals.

In Japan, literature searches are computerized by an on-line information system available in the library of each university. Each library stocks not only journals in Japanese but also foreign journals, most of which are published in English. Accordingly, it is an indispensable qualification for physicians to be able to read papers written in English. Most journals published in Japan are written in Japanese. Among them, The Journal of the Japan Surgical Society enjoys the largest circulation.

In the past, medical education was conducted through the use of German textbooks, and patients' medical histories were generally recorded in both Japanese and German, in mixed style. Recently, this custom has changed and most young doctors use English. Since the textbooks for clinical training and the references needed for research are written in English, skill in this language is important.

The time has come to introduce new and different ideas and methods in every field in Japan, Fellowships for residents from other countries to study in Japan are an important means for promoting this exchange. A few institutions, including ours, have already put this into practice. We firmly believe that the exchange through personnel will be beneficial to all countries involved. We all must support this important development in surgical education.

The Research Advisor

Many of the hospitals attached to research institutes are university affiliated and have a large number of research fellows. Since the acquisition of an M.D. or a Ph.D. degree is a basic requirement for obtaining a position or advancing academically, Japanese academic surgeons must have their own research programs and also serve as research advisors to their assistants.

One research advisor may be responsible for varying numbers of research fellows depending on the university, hospital or department. The number may differ among individual advisors within the same department. On average, 4 or 5 fellows are attached to one advisor, but that number ranges from 0 to 10. Research advisors usually provide guidance to their fellows throughout their careers. Advisors help assistants find sources of research funding, and part time jobs for living expenses. The overall group research program frequently proceeds with the advisor's work as its core and each assistant undertakes projects related with the advisor's theme. The ability to look to the needs of others is a desirable characteristic for the ideal advisor in Japan. Research fellows prefer to be affiliated with the research group of an advisor possessing such qualities.

Funding

Government funds administered by the Ministry of Education are the main source of support of scientific research, including biomedical research. The national universities and research institutes depend exclusively on this source. Grants for research are awarded on the basis of peer review, and are equally available to all public and private universities or institutes. Prefectural, municipal and private universities may receive additional support for research from university or hospital funds and from the pharmaceutical companies. Funds are also available from the Ministry of Health and Welfare for Health Services Research. Awards for Surgical Research funded from the National Government are reviewed by **surgeons** chosen to serve for two years as referees. A typical research budget for our surgical departments is presented in Table II.

The allotment of the grants for scientific research by the Ministry of Education is announced annually in the "List of Research Subjects Adopted for Grants for Scientific Research by the Ministry of Education" by the Society for the Study of Scientific Research Funds. The "Japanese Scientific Monthly," published by the Japan Society for the Promotion of Science, carries a survey of organizations supporting re-

TABLE II. Budget for surgical research for a typical Japanese department of surgery.

University funds	Y 3,000,000	$U.S. 15,000
Ministry of Education	3,000,000	15,000
Ministry of Health	3,000,000	15,000
Pharmaceutical Industry	5,000,000	25,000
Municipal Government	2,000,000	10,000
Prefectural Government	2,000,000	10,000
Private foundations	2,000,000	10,000
Total	20,000,000	100,000

search, listing various fundations providing grants for participants in international conferences, and for scholarships. Surgeons have not participated extensively in these grants and scholarships, which are intended to cover a wide range of scientific domains.

The Surgical Societies do not provide financial support for research or travel to scientific meetings. Surgical researchers usually carry out clinical work and serve on the teaching staff concurrently; there is no institution at which a specialized scholars can receive a salary only for research work.

In surgical research, granting agencies rarely attempt to influence research activities themselves; however, grants obtained for specific research can not be spent for any other project, and spending of equipment funds for travel expenses or salary is not permitted.

Legal and Cultural Considerations

The Japanese public attitude toward animal experimentation is rather positive, though consideration must be given to the improvement of cages for laboratory animals and the assignment of a specialized veterinarian to breed and care for the animals, in response to appeals of certain societies for the prevention of cruelty to animals. Researchers, as well as the general public, think that developmental work through animal experimentation is an indispensable step before controlled study in healthy human volunteers. At the same time, the public attitude toward clinical trials is extremely negative in that patients will not permit themselves to be used as "material" for clinical experiments. The reason for this attitude is a basic public consensus that a certain treatment should be applied to specific patients only after its efficacy has been fully confirmed through animal experimentation, and after the physician is fully convinced that it is the *only* and *best* treatment available. The percent that *giving to the patient what the physician believes best is the basis of the physician–patient relationship* is widely accepted in medical education. Therefore, physicians who acknowledge that they are incapable of judging what is the best for their patients may lose the confidence of both patients and peers.

As a natural consequence of the belief that humans should not be used for experimentation, it is very difficult to obtain consent from a patient for participation in a clinical trial using the accepted North American and Western European method. Our medical legislation does, however, grant a patient the right to have sufficient explanation about the treatment to be given, and requires informed consent before any sugical operation. In Japan, eligible patients are generally admitted to a clinical trial, allocated to a treatment and, then, consent for treatment is sought without reference to the method of allocation.

At present, the number of medical malpractice suits is rapidly increasing in Japan. In 1985 a "Declaration of Patient Rights" was announced by a group of volunteers including lawyers. The physician–patient relationship is losing its traditional basis and a new basis, requiring more direct communication of detailed medical information is developing. Yet, patients have tradionally been protected from the diagnosis of cancer. Under such circumstances, clinical trials in surgical research require thorough legal and cultural consideration by research advisors. Because the direct method of obtaining "informed consent," as it is done in U.S. is still not generally accepted and might incur trouble in Japan, careful consideration is especially necessary.

In Japan, there are no organizations or courses of instruction in surgical research save for these developed in each individual surgical department or in cooperation with other academic departments of a university. A formal program of instruction for surgical research would be very useful. Perhaps it might be provided on an international or national basis. A book on a academic management for surgeons would be very useful. Most of the chairmen of surgical departments are concerned about the future financial support.

Nevertheless, the future of surgical research is brightened by the many young surgeons who have committed themselves to academic training. We anticipate that Japanese surgery will contribute innovative research solutions and future leaders to the international community of surgical scholars.

Acknowledgement

The authors wish to thank Professor Masakatsa Yamamoto, Director of the Department of Surgery at Kansai Medical University in Osaka, and Professor Fusahiro Nagao, Director of the Department of Surgery at Jikei University School of Medicine in Tokyo for advice and support during the preparation of this chapter.

5

New Initiatives and Ideas in Spain

P.A. Sánchez

Spanish medicine has shared in the changes that have characterized developments in Western medical communities since the 1930's—the introduction of a great deal of advanced technology; increasing and irreversible collectivization of health care services; deeper appreciation and extension of the concept of individuality within the framework of scientific pathology; and prevention of disease and promotion of health (1). As a result of marked social disparities, progress has not been uniform, and major differences in health care delivery have co-existed in different regions and according to social class until recently.

At the end of the civil war (1936–39), the devastation of many areas and a very poor supporting economy made the rebuilding of medical facilities both costly and slow. Attention had to be directed toward the most urgent needs, such as coping with epidemics and alimentary problems. The personal efforts of doctors contributed greatly to the improvement of community health in the face of precarious conditions and a considerable degree of sanitary disorganization. Shortly thereafter, in 1944, the National Health Act established the underlying principles of the Social Security System, changed the organization of medical care delivery, and strongly influenced the subsequent development of medicine. Historical and political circumstances conditioned the birth and growth of the system, and some of the errors and pitfalls introduced in the initial phases are still with us.

Traditional public and private beneficence has slowly disappeared and been replaced by the social security services. These have grown enormously and have generated a giant bureaucratic machine whose budget approximates that of the country. At present, the social security medical care program covers virtually all the 38-million inhabitants of Spain.

Primary care was incorrectly organized at the outset and the consequences are still evident—overloaded outpatient clinics, poor medical care and maldistribution of resources. Nevertheless, a good network of public hospitals has been built and, although its geographical disposition is not completely adequate, it has brought evident benefits to the population and contributed to the modernization of medical practice. Although *teaching* and *research* were not considered among the primary goals of the system, residency programs have been progressively incorporated in hospitals since the middle 1960's with great success. Research, however, has remained the "poor sister" of the system and only a few centers have limited facilities and extremely poor financial support.

The Social Security Health Service permeates the whole entire system and influences not only medical care but everything related to it by virtue of the economic resources it commands—even a high percentage of the beds in private hospitals and other institutions is under its control as the result of certain financial arrangements. This brief outline of the weaknesses and successes of the health care system is a prerequisite to understanding the practice of medicine in Spain and the modest role played by research.

An acute problem that has a great impact on the present situation is the existence of over *20,000 unemployed,* or under-employed, medical graduates. The number of medical doctors in 1984 was 106,537—297% more than in 1965. The resulting density of one doctor per 350 inhabitants is one of highest in Europe, being exceeded only in Italy and the German Democratic Republic. The ratio will be even higher within the next 6–8 years.

In addition, political concessions allowed new medical schools to open during the 1960's and 1970's without any serious planning study, and in spite of a lack of necessary financial supper for some of the existing schools, (with the exception of the University-Clinical of Navarra, all medical schools belong to the State Administration). Budgets have been maintained at a very low level, much below the requirements of modern medical schools. As an example, only 630 US dollars per student were spent in 1982 in contrast to 4,500 in the United Kingdom and 2,500 in France.

The problem, however, is not only economic but also organizational. Medical curricula remain anchored in the past; subjects like bioengineering, preventive and social medicine, electronics, epidemiology, and research methodology are not taught during the 6 years of medical school. Spanish universities have not kept pace with the deep changes within society. Locked up inside themselves, the universities have maintained rigid personalistic structures and have lost, with few exceptions, the beat of time. New surgical areas, like cardiac or neurosurgery, have developed almost completely outside the university environment. Security of privileges, a closed atmosphere, and strong archaic corporatism have caused them to turn their backs to reality in many instances. The result is a dangerous disconnection from society.

Only a few of the medical graduates of the recent years have had access residency programs. Official public posts as general practitioners are also scarce. The immediate future for thousands of young doctors is, therefore, rather dismal. *Numerus clausus* has been introduced in medical schools recently, but it was not drastic enough. Some 3,000 new medical students continue to be admitted each year and the effects of this administrative decision will not alleviate the situation appreciably until another decade has passed.

Political attention has been focused on solving these urgent and sometimes dramatic problems, but research remains in a deferred position. The enormous rise in health care costs combined, in many instances, with inadequate management of the public sector has led to real financial difficulties which, in turn, have had an obvious repercussion on the funding of research. At present, the number of investigators is proportionately one tenth that in other countries in Western Europe. *"Brain drain"* mainly to the USA, has been a constant fact of Spanish scientific life during the past 30–40 years.

Research has generally and traditionally been confined to isolated groups with little or no government help. Personal efforts have occasionally produced some continuity and such splendid results as those achieved in histology and neurology by Ramon y Cajal's school. This, however, has not been the general rule and scientific research has had little influence in or on Spanish society.

The general population has been indifferent to research, including surgical research and is unaware of its importance to the real progress and development of the country; only in a very few exceptional circumstances has a plea been made for greater support. Things have changed slightly in the last 8–10 years due, not to a change in the general attitude, but to occasional collaboration by the mass media to emphasize the need for research. Through the media, the man on the street is beginning to be aware of the chronic absence of a coherent policy toward research. Some professionals and scientists (Ortega y Gasset and Marañón in the past; Ochoa, Grisolía, Mayor Zaragoza, Sols, Rof Carballo, and others, now) are trying to influence public opinion through the media but their efforts appear to have evoked little or no response from the general population.

To reduce the country's great dependency on foreign technology (almost 80% of medical equipment and supplies are imported), the State Administration has announced some national programs mainly in the field of services. They appear to be directed more at covering some of the big deficiencies rather than to stimulating the creative capacity of young scientists—traditionally, more attention has been paid to the humanities than to the sciences. The entry of Spain into the European Economic Community opens new channels of international cooperation, specially in the field of high technology, and will produce obvious benefits in the immediate future.

There are no facilities for research by *community surgeons*. Their daily efforts are devoted exclusively to clinical activities and most of them have had no training in surgical research.

The small amount of surgical research that is performed is carried out only in University or large hospitals to which patients are sent for special diagnosis and treatment. There are few facilities and it is always difficult to find the adequate funds. With few exceptions, research is not an obligatory part of departmental commitments although it is partly necessary for a university career. Attitudes vary greatly from one department to another, and it is very difficult to make any generalizations.

In contrast to this negative panorama of research, the quality of health has risen spectacularly during this century; the mean life expectancy was 73.4 years, in 1980, compared with only 34.76 years, in 1900. Spain currently has the lowest overall mortality of the European Common Market countries and 11.3% of the population are over 65 years of age. Cardiocirculatory disease (45%), tumors (20%) and respiratory disease (8%) are the main causes of mortality. However, the mortality from intestinal infection, which is 3 times higher than in other Common Market countries, reveals big deficiencies in the organization of the health system and poor public education regarding sanitation and hygiene (2).

Funding of Surgical Research

Spain's position as last among European countries in terms of research funding, only 0.4–0.5% of the gross national product goes to research and development, contrasts sharply with its level of industrialization. Contributions to research by the private sector is also very low—only 20% compared to 55% in other industrialized countries. The technological import/export ratio is 10:1. Mean expenses per investigator/year are around $76,000 (USA)—sensibly less than in other European countries.

Surgical research units are supported by the budgets of their own hospitals as far as staff and facilities are concerned, but grants to finance programs and fellowships are also available. The main sources of such funds are the CAIC y T (Advisory Committee on Scientific and Technical Research) which is closely connected to the Ministry of Education and Science, and the FIS (Health Research Fund) which is an organ of the Ministry of Health. Both organizations support research programs, including fellowships within and outside Spain, after presentation of successful project proposals.

The FIS (until recently the Social Security Research Fund—FISS) is a government funding program that receives considerable support from the pharmaceutical industry. Its resources come mainly from the *complimentary discount* granted by the industrial companies when they sell their products to the Social Security Services. In addition, it receives a specified amount from the budget of the National Health Institute as well as private and institutional contributions. At present, the funds are assigned directly in the national general budget, but in fact the pharmacological industry supports this interesting fund indirectly, even though it is administered by the government.

The main areas financed by the FIS are summarized in Table I. The total budget in 1984 was 1,000 million pesetas and it is expected that, after approval of the new Health Act, this amount will rise to 10,000 million per year. Almost 43% was spent on research grants in 1984, 25% on personnel training and 2% on administration of the budget. Each area has a Technical and Scientific Advisory Committee, composed of experts in the field. They review the projects, but

TABLE I. Main areas supported by the Health Research Fund (FIS).

1. Research
    Biomedical
    Preventive and community medicine, sanitation planning, medical computers, public health, epidemiology, and prospective studies.
    Pharmaceutical
    Sanitary systems, economy and health, sanitary management
2. Training and education (fellowships)
    Initiation into research
    Studies in foreign countries
    Traveling fellowships
    Foreign medical graduates
3. Scientific meetings
4. Publications
5. Scientific equipment and supplies

final approval is in the hands of the Administrative Committee.

The major grants to research in the past have gone to the following hospitals: Clinica Puerta de Hierro, Centro Ramón y Cajal, Fundación Jiménez Díaz, Universidad Autónoma Hospital La Paz in Madrid; Hospital Clínico y Hospital Santa Cruz y San Pablo in Barcelona; and Hospital La Fe in Valencia. About 10–15% of the projects supported by these grants deal with surgical research.

The main surgical research laboratories in Spain are those of Clinica Puerta de Hierro, Centro Ramón y Cajal and Hospital La Paz in Madrid. In these centers, there are full time research staffs. The Hospital Provincial in Madrid also has a new surgical research unit (Jose Baros). Surgical units in university hospitals and in other Social Security hospitals in different cities usually have part-time research workers, especially in microsurgery.

Very few private foundations specifically support surgical research—the main ones with funds for biomedical research are listed in Table II. The National Council for Scientific Research does not have a section dedicated specifically to surgical research. Industrial companies seldom make grants for biomedical research and pharmaceutical firms are mainly interested in trials of new drugs.

Surgical associations do not have enough funds to support research projects, although in recent years some of them have offered certain grants to cover travel expenses to present papers at scientific meetings. This particular activity has also been supported by the pharmaceutical and biomedical companies.

Surgeons in Spanish-speaking countries in Central and South America can apply for financial support through the *Institute of Iberoamerican Cooperation,* an agency associated with the Ministry of Foreign Affairs. In fact, several hundred Iberoamerican students and graduates receive financial assistance every year through the different grants offered by this Institute. Its funds are distributed among many different areas, of which medicine is one of the most demanding and most favored. As well, 5% of the positions offered in residency programs each year are reserved for Iberoamerican medical graduates.

TABLE II. Main private foundations with funds for medical research

1. FUNDACION RAMON ARECES
   Avda. del Generalísimo, 25 - planta 5°
   Edificio Cadagua
   28046 MADRID
2. FUNDACION BALEAR
   UNIPSA
   c/ Pedro Muñoz Seca, 2
   28001 MADRID
3. FUNDACION PEDRO BARRIE DE LA MAZA
   (Conde de Fenosa)
   Cantón Pequeño, 1
   15003 LA CORUÑA
4. FUNDACION CIENTIFICA DE LA ASOCIACION ESPAÑOLA CONTA EL CANCER
   Amador de los Ríos, 5
   28010 MADRID
5. FUNDACION GENERAL MEDITERRANEA
   Velázquez, 12
   28001 MADRID
6. FUNDACION JIMENEZ DIAZ
   Avda. de los Reyes Católicos, 2
   28040 MADRID
7. FUNDACION MAPFRE
   Carretera de Majadahona a Pozuelo, Km. 3,500
   MAJADAHONA.- (Madrid)
8. FUNDACION JUAN MARCH
   Castelló, 77
   28006 MADRID
9. FUNDACION PUBLICA DE SERVICIOS HOSPITALARIOS Y ASISTENCIALES "MARQUES DE VALDECILLA"
   Avda. de Valdecilla s/n
   39006 SANTANDER
10. FUNDACION PUIGVERT
    Cartagena, 340-350
    Apartado 24.005
    08025 BARCELONA
11. FUNDACION CONCHITA RABAGO DE JIMENEZ DIAZ
    Avda. de los Reyes Católicos, 2
    28040 MADRID
12. FUNDACION EUGENIO RODRIGUEZ PASCUAL
    Espalter, 6 - 8°
    28014 MADRID
13. FUNDACION UNIVERSITARIA AGUSTIN PEDRO Y PONS
    Facultad de Medicina
    Casanova, 143
    08036 BARCELONA
14. FUNDACION FERRER INVESTIGACION
    Gran Vía Carlos III, 94-98 ento.
    08028 BARCELONA
15. FUNDACION HISPANA DE CARDIOLOGIA
    Murcia, 11 entlo.
    28045 MADRID

A considerable number of students (mainly undergraduates) from Arab countries are also favored by special grants offered by the government. In regard to surgeons from other countries, conditions differ greatly according to existing bilateral cultural and exchange programs. The National Health Institute and the Department of Cultural Relationships, a section of the Ministry of Foreign Affairs, are the agencies providing most of the funds.

Achievements in Surgical Research

In spite of the inadequacy of financial support and of a true research atmosphere, the personal efforts of some surgeons have made possible the development of original contributions through the years. It is a fact of history that it was the work of some surgeons that was decisive in introducing European medical ideas and advances as well as experimental research into Spain in the last third of 19th century. The institution founded by the surgeon, F. Rubio (1827–1902) provided a model that was widely imitated thereafter. The work of J. Cardenal, J. Ribera and A. San Martin reached international recognition in the following generation (3).

The worldwide recognition of the significance of Cajal's investigations in the early years of this century was an incentive to many institutions to integrate research into their curricula. The powerful influence of the Institución Libre de Enseñanza (Free Teaching Institution) on several generations of investigators, including a number of renowned surgeons, is particularly noteworthy. The tremendous trauma of the civil war interrupted the advance of research in a number of different schools since many investigators disappeared or went into exile leaving a large void behind them. During the reconstruction of the country, there were other more urgent medical needs and research was again dependent on the determination of a few. Since then, a constant flow of young investigators to industrial areas (England, Germany and mainly the USA) has taken place.

During the late 1950's and early 1960's, new surgical specialties needed the support of research for their clinical work. Interesting laboratories were rudimentary in structure and equipment; neurosurgery expanded thanks to the pioneering works of men like Ley, Tolosa, Barcia Goyanes and Obrador. Pallencephalography was one of the original diagnostic techniques described in those years (4), as summarized by Obrador (5), founder of the Institute of Neurological Science were a considerable amount of the experimental surgery was carried out. In recent years, Rodríguez Delgado has continued the experimental studies in neurophysiology that he started while at Yale University; his collaboration in the field of functional neurosurgery has been significant.

In the early years of experimental cardiovascular surgery in Spain, surgeons had to improvise experimental laboratories in order to evaluate new techniques of extracorporeal circulation and, in some units, residents rotated through them as part of their training. Important and original contributions were made by C. Gómez-Durán (homologous and heterologous cardiac valves) (6,7) and F. Alvarez Díaz (first low profile valvular prosthesis) (8). The tricuspid annuloplasty described by N.G. de Vega (9) had universal acceptance. Cardiovascular surgery has maintained a number of ongoing research programs and some of the best known results are flexible valvular rings (10,11), the use of heterologous pericardium (12), and some innovations in prostheses (13,14). The main interest in now focused on surgery for arrhythmias (15), heart transplantation and the development of new techniques for dealing with congenital heart problems (16–19).

Clinical research has generated important advances in most surgical specialties. For example, Spanish contributions in ophthalmology (Barraquer, Arruga, Carreras, Murube, etc.) and in urology have achieved international recognition. In urology, the following are of considerable interest: S. Gil Vernet's investigation on the structure and morphogenesis of prostatic carcinoma (20); A. Puigvert's demonstration of non-obstructive calyx dilation, (now known as megacaliosis or Puigvert's disease (21); and L. Cifuentes' demonstration of vaginal epithelium in the trigonum vesicae that undergoes the same changes as the vaginal epithelium during the menstrual cycle (22). More recent contributions include those of Ruano-Gil (23) in embryology and of Páramo (24) and Vela Navarrete (25) on polycystic disease and the technique of constant pressure flow pyelography (26). The outstanding studies on lithogenesis by L. Cifuentes (27), the important innovations introduced by J.M. Gil Vernet in surgery of renal calculi and renal transplantations (28,29) transverse ureterorenoscopy (30) and the transection of spermatic vessels in carcinoma of the prostate (31) have also received general acceptance.

In traumatology and orthopedics, interesting clinical investigations have been carried out mainly in the areas of prostheses and transplants, arthroscopic surgery, electric stimulation in consolidation and pseudoarthrosis, and immunological studies (32).

The foregoing examples demonstrate our organizational existing and potential capacity to open new paths if the chronic organizational problems afflicting Spanish medicine are solved. A detailed description of all the achievements in surgical research in the different specialties is beyond the scope of this summary. A multidisciplinary approach has been noticed in recent years, and the first results of collaboration with basic sciences investigators are beginning to be seen in different fields. One example is the current increase in interest in organ transplantation research that has developed in centers with well-equipped experimental laboratories (33–37).

Legal and Cultural Considerations

In general, animal experimentation presents no problem from a legal point of view. The public's attitude is not negative as long as the proper set-up is provided. So far, the *antivivisection movement* is feeble and has almost no influence on public opinion. The present legal void in this specific area is partly covered by the recommendations of the International Council on Animal Experimentation, as stated by the Spanish Society on Animal Experimentation.

Different laws regulate human clinical trials. Until recently, it was not difficult to carry out such trials and few legal controls were applied. Now, a committee in each hospital has to approve any clinical trial and the local or regional health authorities have to know about it. This is the theory, but in practice, there is a certain degree of general permissiveness.

Consent is now required for any clinical trial as well as for the special explorations, surgery, etc. The new Health Act stipulates patients rights, including the right to be properly informed about diagnostic and therapeutic procedures. In general, patients' and families' attitudes toward the professional behavior of hospital doctors are good, but an increasing resistance to the system itself can be noticed. Criticism of the functioning of the Social Security system is a daily feature in the press and it has had the effect of turning public opinion against doctors too. The out-patient clinics, in particular, are a source of constant conflict; their huge size and primitive diagnostic and treatment methods require major transformations. Although there is increasing dissatisfaction with public medicine, recent polls have revealed a growing appreciation of doctors' work, especially where hospitals are involved. Although almost the total population (98%) is covered by public medicine (social security), many social sectors still prefer private consultants or use the services of private insurance companies.

Although changes are now occurring very rapidly, not all are in line with real progress and better quality. The long-standing disorganization within the complex health care system certainly requires improved management, but the State Administration—a giant bureaucratic machine, reinforced under the current socialist government seems to be obsessed with exercising its control at all levels, including such obviously independent areas as research. Politicians' distrust of the medical profession has grown to a dangerous point. Physicians are dissatisfied with their daily work and the way they have to perform it, and fear the possibility of being turned into regular civil servants. Professional, economic and social incentives are disappearing rapidly and a great confusion about the immediate future has replaced the enthusiasm of past decades.

The process of socialization in medicine is irreversible, but no sincere attempts have been made to find constructive solutions to the big problems posed by the transformation of the health care system. Medical associations' points of view are not taken into consideration and an image of the physician as a nostalgic defender of outdated privileges is often offered to the public. In this "ceremony of confusion" embroidered with dangerous demagogic statements, a general *politicization* of medicine, even in daily practice, has taken place in recent years. The temptation to complete the nationalization of health care with a consequent loss of freedom and independence hovers over the whole medical profession in paradoxical contrast to the undoubted rise of freedom in public life. Physicians working for the public health care system are bound to fixed salaries and regulated working hours, regardless of the quality of their work; professional activities are restricted or forbidden outside working hours; patients' choice of physician is strongly limited to geographical areas and certain health centers; the prescription of drugs is limited; political influence has a growing impact on the appointment of individuals to such responsible posts, as hospital directors, membership in research granting committees, etc. The necessary deep medical reforms are now arriving after much delay, but they include the incorporation of some of the big mistakes made a long time ago in other Western countries (38). Progressive "proletarianization" of the medical profession is going to affect the development of medicine negatively from the doctor–patient relationship to the highest levels of research. The tendency to equalize, no matter what the commitment may be, has started to operate and its first consequences are already being felt: routine mediocrity is, in many instances, evaluated as being at the same level and in the same category as a creative effort to bring about improvement.

Some of these problems do not belong exclusively to Spanish society, but an outline of them is essential to a better understanding of the poor position in which medical research is situated. In spite of all the inconveniences and difficulties, investigation has grown in recent years (50% more projects in the period 1978–82 than in 1973–77) and some areas, like biochemistry, have reached a level of achievement that is high above the mean for the country. The Spanish investigator is suffering from a lack of organized support, that results in an unfortunate lack of continuity in his endeavors.

Few hospitals have surgical investigators on their staff. When they are, they are usually part of the Department of Surgery, Physiology or Basic Sciences. If the Research Department is independent, conflicts occasionally arise because they surgical projects are not always of interest to the persons in charge.

Existing administrative regulations oblige hospitals to have a Research Committee. Most projects have to be submitted for its approval, but there is a certain flexibility outside pure experimental work.

The preferences of granting agencies exert considerable influence on general research activities and the main lines of investigation (epidemiology, at present, for State Administration grants, hypertension in the case of certain drug companies, etc.). Most surgical research depends on government grants.

The meetings of surgical societies are the usual places to present research data and results. Each society holds at least one meeting a year. The Spanish Society for Surgical Research, founded a few years ago, has recently agreed to a joint annual meeting with the Spanish Surgeon's Society.

Languages skills are considered a prerequisite for surgical research. More attention is now paid to their development at all educational levels, and the younger generations are better equipped in this area. As in many other countries, English dominates, particularly in the scientific literature, while French and German have dropped markedly in comparison with their use in the first half of this century. Research results are usually published in Spanish surgical journals, but authors try to get their best work published in prestigious international periodicals to achieve recognition and reach larger scientific communities.

Surgical Training and Research

Surgical training and training in other medical areas were not well organized until recently. Certain hospitals maintained high standards in their residency programs with requirements in time and quality similar to other Western countries, but this was not the general rule. In addition to the big disparity among the different programs and the lack of control over them, the official title of specialist could be obtained in a shorter time, regardless of the training followed. In certain cases, a certificate from the head of a department or service was enough to allow a candidate to obtain the official title without any strict verification of the appropriate training by the administrative health authorities. Medical associations opposed this practice and repeatedly recommended procedures that would end not only the confusion but also the frequent injustices it gives rise to when candidates were appointed staff positions.

In the meantime, certain centers made considerable efforts to improve their residency programs, but the negative consequences of the inadequate quality control and planning were soon felt. In some hospitals, residents were needed to handle the daily work-load, but they were also considered a "cheap labor force"; their training was faulty in many areas and the experience they received fell far short of the desired objective. Some medical and surgical specialties became oversaturated after a few years, and many specialists could not find a job in their field at the end of their residency training. This bitter situation has obviously generated a great deal of frustration among young doctors, particularly in those who followed long serious programs.

This situation has been greatly alleviated by the Medical Specialties Act (1978), that codified the previously dispersed requirements and regulated access to, and the content and requirements of postgraduate training. Forty-three different medical and surgical specialties requiring basic hospital training were officially recognized in addition to another 6 that did not require hospital practice*. Twelve of the specialties are surgical (see Table III).

Each medical specialty has a National committee, composed of certified specialists who represent the Health Ministry, Education Ministry, Medical Association and Specialty Societies. Each National Committee sets the requirements for its specific area (theoretical and practical programs), selects and controls the teaching units, regulates the number of residents to be admitted each year, judges the final examination, etc. The title or certificate of the specialty is given by the Ministry of Education and Science. This certificate is required to take

TABLE III. Surgical specialties with training programs and official certificates (1985)

Angiology and Vascular Surgery
Cardiovascular Surgery
Ear, Nose and Throat Surgery
General Surgery
Maxillary and Facial Surgery
Ophthalmology
Pediatric Surgery
Plastic and Reparative Surgery
Neurosurgery
Thoracic Surgery
Traumatology and Orthopedic Surgery
Urology

up any hospital position but not for strictly private practice.

Under the Medical Specialties Act, all surgical residency programs must provide a 5-year period of training, of which 1 or 2 years are devoted to a general surgery program and the remainder to a specific area. Some specialties (cardiovascular, plastic) considered this 5-year program insufficient and demanded a longer period of training. A new Act (1985) has allowed them to present new plans and, starting in 1986, some programs will probably have longer durations depending on the content of the specialties. Some are even considering the possibility of requiring complete training in general surgery before entering the specific area. A re-evaluation of some branches of surgery is currently taking place so that the certificate can be unified (for instance, thoracic, cardiac and vascular surgery, with an additional period of training to get specific qualification in one of the areas). A general consensus has been reached to adapt the different programs to those of the Western European countries although the latter are far from being uniform. Accordingly, the present can be regarded as a transitional period leading to more serious and exacting training and the desirable possibility of a common European certificate.

The Medical Specialties Act of 1985 introduced some positive innovations: flexible programs; higher standards for obtaining teaching credit; a tendency to unify programs and provide opportunities for broader training in basic medicine or surgery; and residents' representatives in the National Committees, etc. it perpetuates, however, some general failures, particularly in quality control, and eliminated the final oblig-

---

*Hydrotherapy, space medicine, physical education and sports medicine, legal and forensic medicine, work or occupational medicine, and stomatology. Until 1985, dentists had to graduate in Medicine and Surgery before entering the Stomatology School for 2 years. Under present regulations, dentists will require a 5-year period of training in special schools and will not need to graduate from a medical school. Twelve of the specialties are surgical (see Table III).

atory examination to obtain a specialty certificate—a situation that all the National Committees or Boards have systematically opposed (it was really a populist administrative concession to the residents' associations's increased unrest). Annual evaluations are supposedly done by the local teaching committees; in practice, this is equivalent to the automatic awarding of the specialist certificate at the end of the residency period, regardless of the quality of the training received.

Candidates for the residency programs are selected through a highly competitive national examination (over 22,000 candidates in 1985 for only 1,300 resident posts throughout the country). Those who obtain the highest scores have a choice of specialty and center; opportunities diminishing according to rank order. The number of places has been progressively reduced in recent years due partly to the oversaturation in certain specialties and partly to a decrease in the funds provided by the National Institute of Health for those that are possible, but some major shortcomings are generally recognized—mainly those derived from the impossibility for many to select their desired specialty. Teaching and training capacity is obviously underused and is only partly taken up by foreign doctors. Studies of alternatives methods of training are in progress, mainly in such specialties as radiology, rheumatology, and anesthesiology where high demand is expected within the next decade.

Research is not an obligatory part of surgical training except in a very few institutions. In these, residents usually spend part of their third or fourth year in the research laboratory. During this time, they maintain contact with the clinical section by taking calls, attending medical–surgical meetings, etc. Although it is difficult to estimate how many receive such training due to the big differences among institutions, the percentage of surgical residents obtaining some training in surgical research is not over 5%.

Big hospitals usually have some research programs, particularly in certain surgical specialties. In general, surgical residents are more attracted by the practical aspects of the training program; those who wish to dedicate themselves to research careers are the exceptions. Although reluctant to spend any time in the research laboratory, many feel pleased that they did it. Most of them state that the experience they acquired will be of great benefit to them in their future careers as clinical surgeons. During the period of research, the resident is paid the salary previously established for his training, which is the same throughout the whole country without regard to the institution.

It is very seldom that a resident can choose his own research problem. Usually he is engaged in the project that is currently in progress. In some rare instances, he is permitted to choose a subject within a general area followed by the Department. When the research project is part of the requirements for a doctorate or Ph.D. degree, he is freer to choose a particular problem, but he must always be under the supervision of a tutor. To obtain the degree of doctor of medicine, a written thesis is mandatory but it does not always have to deal with an original research project—it can be dedicated to the review of a particular problem. For many physicians, this is the only time in their career that they are in contact with research.

In spite of the tremendous lack of facilities, most surgical national committees recommend the inclusion of some sort of training in surgical research in their programs. A suggestion has been made that some qualified residents should rotate through the centers that have research laboratories, but this is very difficult to accomplish in practice.

The surgical residency program is fully oriented toward clinical practice. The obligatory inclusion of experimental surgical research in a residency program is not possible, at present, since many of the centers with approved training programs do not offer research opportunities. The availability of only a few research fellowships that are usually poorly funded hinders the dedication of some time to research at the end of the residency program.

The main motivation for a resident to obtain training in research is usually to advance a surgical career within the academic community. Unfortunately, much of the work done in the laboratory, even at University level, is aimed at reproducing, in animals, surgical techniques (or variations) that are used in humans. For some reason, this is considered a way of getting experience and developing skill with a particular technique. Lack of proper basic science support precludes engagement in big research projects in many instances.

It is mandatory to accomplish some sort of research if an academic career within a university is planned. Sad to say, much of it is only performed to fulfill certain curriculum vitae requirements. Due to strongly rooted University corporatism, it is almost impossible to get a high teaching position as a professor by working outside the university hospitals. For this reason, selection does not always take place among the most experienced or best prepared surgeons and many excellent surgical specialists have no chance of reaching professorial rank even if they are engaged in teaching programs at postgraduate level.

Surgical residents participate more often in clinical research. There are more in this area and many residents appear as co-workers in papers published by a department. Such collaboration is an asset when they apply for a hospital position.

Possible Solutions

The same general considerations apply to surgical investigation as to research in general. First of all, it is necessary to put aside Utopian plans. With her present feeble economy, Spain cannot approach, in short term, the expansion in research and development of the Western industrial countries. It is mandatory, however, to consider scientific research as a national priority under present circumstances. "Since society and politicians do not realize that industrial development, quality of life, and professional standards depend directly on the national scientific capacity, it will be very difficult to get the means and stimulation that Spanish science requires"(39).

Most Spanish scientists are agreed that one of the worst impediments to research is bureaucratic stagnation. A good basic structure is essential for future development and the lack of a coherent organization is felt at all levels. This has to be put in the hands of persons with acceptable track records in research and with the capacity to find solutions without having to depend on obscure bureaucratic decisions. Obviously, responsibility in the administration of public funds should be a strict requirement.

Better coordination of public and private financial agencies is also necessary. Free enterprise should not be regarded with suspicion by the State Administration. More financial support is desperately needed but the State General Budget has assigned 20% less to health care in 1986 than in 1984. Finding appropriate incentives to promote the expansion of research activity in the private sector, which at the moment is really minimal, is urgent. The recent Science Act is too ambiguous in this respect although it envisages greater administrative flexibility.

Along with such important organizational changes, biomedical research needs to make better use of the available resources, both human and material. Priorities should be fixed without stifling the enthusiasm and independence needed by the investigator to maintain his ability to perform valuable scientific work. Clinical research also needs better control and coordination which at the first level, can be done by the hospital or center itself. Quality and productivity requirements have to be exacting, so that the number of non-productive persons can be reduced. The present high costs of research require that the opportunities to pursue research careers be reserved for those who are really motivated and demonstrate a dedication to continuity in their work. The limited resources available for research must not be wasted when the results are really disappointing. In addition to reinforcing the existing centers, careful planning is required to ensure that anomalies and external pressures do not interfere with investigators' freedom and spontaneity (39). Part of the budget should be dedicated to the maintenance of the infrastructure (40), which is so often neglected in the Spanish system.

Access to medical schools has to be reserved for those who are really capable, rather then on the basis of the disastrous political populistic concessions of the past. Somehow, in spite of the current time limitations, contact and dialogue between professor and student must be re-established. Otherwise, the medical school can turn into an officially designated office for the conferring of titles and certificates. The system for selecting faculty members is also in need of a real overhaul. A post should not be tenable for life if the quality of the work performed over a period of years is not at a high level.

Only a small amount of surgical research is currently performed in the universities. To recover its true path and rhythm, and maintain its connection with the society it serves, scientific research must be one of the primary aims of each university. The abandonment of the ivory tower mentality is one of the first actions to be taken if a true transformation is desired.

Medical students should be taught the *methods* of surgical research. During their training period, residents must have contact with experimental surgery, must be seriously involved in clinical investigation, and must not be regarded or treated only as simple data collectors. The possibility for clinical surgical staff to dedicate some portion of their careers to research should also be contemplated (40), even though the present rigid administrative schemes are a serious obstacle.

With few exceptions, the libraries of medical schools and hospitals are not good enough. Modern systems of information retrieval are urgently needed to give trainees easy access to the international medical literature.

Adequate salaries are unknown in public medicine today. An experienced surgeon working for the Social Security System earns less than a specialized worker. As a result, many physicians hold a second post or have to dedicate extra hours to find a supplementary income. Mental and emotional dedication to scientific research is not possible if a decent living is not guaranteed.

Physicians were not accorded any active role in the organization of the health care system and were hardly consulted about it. Distrust and a certain resentment against them have continued through the years as reforms were introduced. Physicians are not good at organizing for the defense of their profession; trade unions and other organizations are filling the gaps even if they only represent a minority of the medical community. An improvement in financial support and working conditions affecting surgical research will definitely not occur without constant pressure on the health administrative authorities and an effort to ensure that the public is properly informed.

This outline is not intended as a catalogue of complaints, but the complexity of the present health care organization gives rise to enormous problems for scientific research in Spain that are different than those in many Western countries. They can only be solved by escaping from demagogic deceits. Little surgical research is done, at present, and the structural organization does not permit rapid changes. A solid supportive research atmosphere has to be created within the spanish society so that the absence of *intellectual daring* (41) disappears. Critical thinking, a sound methodological approach to research, and motivation for scientific endeavor will then be accorded appropriate recognition and many of our investigators will not have to abandon research or leave the country.

References

1. Laín Entralgo P. Historia Universal de la Medicina. Barcelona: Medicina Actual, Introduccion: 1964;VII:XVII.
2. Diez Dominguez P: España, una salud europea. El Pais Futuro, Dec, 12, 1985.
3. López Piñero JM, García Ballester L, Faus Sevilla P. Medicina y sociedad en la España del siglo XIX. Madrid: Soc. de Estudios y Publicaciones, 1964:105.
4. Barcia Goyanes JJ, Calvo W, Barcia Salorio JL. Un nuevo método de exploración del encéfalo: la palencefalografía. Rev Esp Oto-Neuro Oftalm, 1956:83–84.
5. Obrado Alcalde S: Evolución de la neurocirugía española en los últimos treinta años. Neurocirugía Luso-Esp. 1977;17:75.
6. A method for placing a total homologous aortic value in the subcoronary position. Lancet 1962;2:488–489.
7. Binet JP, Durán CMG, Carpentier A, Langlois J. Heterologous aortic valve transplantation. Lancet 1965;1275.
8. Alvarez F, Rábago G, Urguía M, Castillón L. Eccentric mitral valve prosthesis with a rigid hinge. Experimental observation. J Cardiovasc Surg 1966;7:226–231.
9. de Vega NG. La anuloplastía selectiva, regulable y permanente. Una técnica original para el tratamiento de la insuficiencia tricúspide. Rev Esp Cardiol 1972;25:555–556.
10. Gomez Duran C. Clinical and hemodynamic performance of a totally flexible prosthetic ring for atrioventricular reconstruction. Ann Thorac Surg 1976;22:458–463.
11. Puig Massana M. Conservative surgery of the mitral valve. Annuloplasty on a new adjustable ring. In: Cardiovascular Surgery 1980, edited by Bircks W, Ostermeyer J and Schultes HD. New York: Springer Verlag, 1981:30.
12. Gallo JI, Pomar JL, Artiñao E, Durán CMG. Heterologous pericardium for the closure of pericardial defects. Ann Thoracic Surg 1978;26:149–154.
13. Castillo-Olivares JL, Goiti JJ, O'Connor F, Nojek C, Téllez G, Figuera D. Válvulva supra-anular de

bajo perfil para reemplazamiento mitral. Rev Esp Cardiol 1977;30:23–26.
14. Montero C, Castillo-Olivares JL, Cienfuegos JA, Figuera D. Xenogenic cervical duramater; a new anisotropic tissue for heart-valve prosthesis. Life Support Syst. 1985;3:233–246.
15. Cabo C, Gonzálex MA, Linacero G, et al. Acquisition, processing and stimulation system in cardiac arrhythmias surgery.
16. Alvarez Díaz F, Hurtado del Hoyo E, de León JP, et al. Técnica de correción anatómica de la transposición completa de grandes vasos. Comunicación preliminar. Rev Esp Cardiol 1975;28:255.
17. Alvarez Díaz F, Cabo J, Alvarez A. Neuva técnica cerrada de ampliación del tracto de saléda del ventrículo derecho. Rev Esp Cardiol 1981;34:293.
18. Alvarez Díaz F, Cabo Salvador J, Cordovilla Zurdo G. Partial reconstruction of right ventricular outflow track without cardiopulmonary bypass. J Thorac Cardiovasc Surg (letter) 1982;83:149.
19. Arcas R, Herreros J, Llorens R. Neueva técnica quirúrgica experimental para la transposición de grandes arterias. XV Congreso Nacional de la Sociedad Española de Cardiología, Santander (Abstract Book). 1977:61.
20. Gil Vernet S. Enfermedades de la Próstata. Madrid: Ed Pas Montalvo: 1955.
21. Puigvert A. La Megacaliosis (Disembrioplasia de las pirámides de Malpighio). Rev Clin Esp 1963;91:69.
22. Cifuentes L: Cistitis y cistopatías. Madrid: Ed Paz Montalvo; 1947.
23. Ruano-Gil D, Coca Payeras A, Tejedo Mateu A. Obstruction and normal recanalization of the ureter in the human embryo. Eur Urol 1975;1:287.
24. Páramo P, Segura A: Hilioquistosis renal. Rev Clin Esp 1972;126:387.
25. Vela Navarrete R, Robledo A. Polycystic disease of the renal sinus. J Urol 1983;129:700.
26. Vela Navarrete R. Constant pressure flow controlled antegrade pyelography. Eur Urol 1982;8:265.
27. Cifuentes L. Composición y estructura de los cálculos renales. Barcelona: Ed Salvat, 1984.
28. Gil Vernet JM, Caralps A. Human renal homotransplantation: new surgical technique. Urol Int 1968;23:201.
29. Gil Vernet J. New surgical concepts in removing renal calculi. Urol Int 1965;20:255.
30. Pérez Castro E, Martínez Piñeiro JA. La ureterorrenoscopia transuretral. Arch Esp Urol 1980;33:3.
31. Romero Maroto J, Nistal M, González Gancedo P, Bellas C, Aranas A. Transection of spermatic vessels (Bevan's technique): experimental study. J Urol 1983;130:1232.
32. Jiménez Cisneros A: personal communication, 1985.
33. Cuervas-Mons V, Maganto P, Cienfuegos JA, et al. Ectopic liver using dispersed liver cells as a support measure in acute fulminant hepatic failure. Hepatology 1982;2:183.
34. Eroles G, Maganto P, Pinedo I, et al. Development of an experimental model of cirrhosis and its treatment by syngeneic hepatocyte transplantation into the rat spleen. Eur Surg Res 1983;15:26-27.
35. Abascal J. Aislamiento, perservación e isotransplante de islotes de Langerhans. Doctoral Thesis. Madrid: Universidad Atuónoma, 1981.
36. Casanova A. Estudio del autotransplante del tejido insular pancreático sin aislamiento específico en el sistema portal extraportal en perros totalmente pancreatizados. Doctoral Thesis. Santander: Universidad de Santander, 1982.
37. Golitsin A, Pinedo I, Cienfuegos JA, Chamorro JL, Ortiz Berrocal J, Castillo-Olivares JL. Study of the early rejection of the heterotopic transplanted heart by using 201-Thallium. Experimental study. Eur Surg Res 1983;5:41.
38. Biörck G. How to be a clinician in a socialist country. Ann Intern Med 1977;86:813–817.
39. Toledo González J. Investigación contra burocracia. Interview with S. Ochoa, F. Mayor Zaragoza, A. García Bellido, E. Vinuela and D. Vázquez, El Pais Futuro, October 16, 1985.
40. Mariño C. Interview with F.J. Rubio, El Médico, November, 1985.
41. Laín Entralgo P. La ausencia de osadía de la inteligencia, El País, July 16, 1985.

6

Orderly Evolution to a Better Future in Sweden

S. Fasth and L. Hultén

Introduction

Surgical research in Sweden has a long tradition of excellence which has been enhanced by the positive attitude of governmental authorities towards medical and surgical research during the last 40 years. Significant investments made during the 1950's created a solid foundation for the rapid and extensive expansion in research that took place during the 1960's, in parallel with industrial and economical development in Sweden. External contacts, particularly with Western Europe and the United States, flourished during the 1960's as part of the growth in the international exchange of research information. The resulting increase in awareness of international research activity had a significant impact on internal standards for research quality and validity.

In the early 1970's a temporary slow-down was evident. Limitations on state funding of research were introduced, and it was generally understood that society's interest in research had abated and been replaced by suspicion in some quarters. This trend has now reversed completely and research is generally accorded a positive and important role in the development of Swedish society. In 1980 Sweden spent approximately 0.26% of its gross domestic product on biomedical research and development.

Surgical Research Training

It is widely acknowledged that advanced surgical research must be based on an extensive and effective training program. A comprehensive analysis of research training made by governmental authorities during the 1950's and 1960's, concluded that too little organized instruction and supervision in combination with excessive clinical work demands resulted in a lack of effectiveness. The lack of collaborators and the isolation of research fellows in surgery was particularly noted. The commission recommended that surgical research training programs should be more structured, should be of four years duration, and should give research trainees the opportunity to produce four or five original papers with their supervisors or other collaborators. The papers should be published in international scientific periodicals of high standards and brought together and discussed in a thesis, for subsequent defense at a public dissertation. The choice of scientific subject should be open and the topic of the dissertation need not be surgically or clinically oriented. It could encompass basic research in physiology or biochemistry or other related scientific disciplines. When the thesis is approved, the degree of "doctor of medicine in surgery" is conferred on the researcher. The degree is analogous to the Ph.D., and makes the graduate eligible to apply for an appointment as a "docent" in surgery. The applicant is evaluated by a special board which reviews clinical independence and competence, scientific ability, general character and qualifications for such an academic position. An approved dissertation, including four or five original papers, is not considered sufficient qualification in itself. Other scientific publications must establish the candidates breadth of knowledge and independence. Evidence demonstrating ability to teach, and to supervise research trainees are also required.

A shorter training program, for example, two years, is still discussed because the present system only gives a small proportion of the total number of surgeons an opportunity to do research. Arguments against shortening the training period include the inherent dangers of lowering the quality and revising the general aims of the research training. The current aims of surgical research training are:

1. to inculcate an in-depth knowledge of surgery, foster a systematic approach to working, and develop a capacity to think critically and creatively that will characterize the graduate as an individual capable of performing independent scientific work;
2. to encourage research that will contribute to the overall development of science;
3. to reinforce the establishment of international contacts between research scientists; and
4. to meet society's need for highly qualified surgeons in key positions of surgical leadership.

Training in research can be initiated at three stages in a surgical career.

1. *During medical school.* Medical students who intend to become surgeons sometimes undertake research training in a biomedical science such as physiology. Alternatively, a "docentur" in physiology can, after a few years of surgical residency and surgical research be converted into a "docentur" in surgery. Those who follow this route usually embark on it between the ages of 20–24 years as the result of deciding to pursue an academic career in surgery in a university department.
2. *Immediately following graduation from medical school.* Embarking on research training at this stage has become uncommon because it puts the research fellow in the position of having neither clinical experience nor scientific education.
3. *After three to five years of surgical residency in a county hospital.* Those who choose this path start their research training at age 32–34 years. With recommendations from a chief surgeon at a county hospital, the young surgeon will be employed as a resident in a surgical department of a university hospital. Table I outlines the weekly schedule for a university hospital resident in Sweden. This is the most common choice, and probably the most appropriate, because the young surgeon will have the opportunity to assess the sur-

TABLE I. Weekly working scheme for a resident in research training in a Swedish surgical university department.

	Monday	Tuesday	Wednesday	Thursday	Friday	Saturday	Sunday
07:45–08:30			Staff Meeting, X-Ray Demonstrations				
08:30–10:00	Ward Rounds with the Consultants		Ward Rounds with the Consultants	Ward Rounds	Ward Rounds with the Consultants		
10:00–11:00							
11:00–12:00	Ward Work	Operations	Ward Work	Operations	Outpatient Clinical Ward Work		
12:00–13:00						Literature studies, preparing of manuscripts, etc.	
13:00–14:00	Research				Meeting with the Research Advisers	On duty at the hospital every 5th Saturday or Sunday.	
14:00–15:00	Work		Out-Patient Clinic		Research Work		
15:00–16:00	Ward Rounds	Ward Rounds					
16:00–17:00	Research Education Course	Scheduled Student Teaching	Staff Meeting	Research Work			

gical techniques and management procedures that he has been taught. A county hospital residency is considered an extremely important part of the fundamental training of a Swedish surgeon. The surgery performed in most university hospitals in Sweden is so highly specialized that common operations, such as hernia repairs and cholecystectomies are usually excluded.

The Research Advisor

It is a part of the duty of all members of the surgical staff of a university hospital to teach medical students and supervise research trainees. The number of trainees supervised varies, but is generally limited to protect the quality of supervision. The importance of supervising research trainees in surgical subspecialities has gained increasing recognition in recent years, particularly in the selection of candidates for positions such as assistant professor or professor. The supervision of research trainees carries considerable responsibility since it is the adviser's duty to discuss possible research topics, participate in designing an individual plan of research training, and contribute to the development of a research protocol. The adviser is supposed to maintain continuous contact with the research trainee in order to discuss the work in progress and offer constructive criticism while taking care to encourage the trainees independence and creativity. The advisor is responsible for ensuring the availability of adequate resources for the research trainee from the host institution and accepts ultimate responsibility for the design of the thesis, the quality of the dissertation, and the nomination of an appropriate opponent for the public dissertation.

Funding of Surgical Research

The Medical Research Council of Sweden usually provides support for the employment of research nurses or laboratory assistants in surgical research. Such funds are applied for by surgeons-in-chief who are scientifically and administratively responsible for their expenditure.

Funding can be obtained from *pharmaceutical companies* for projects of particular interest to them. Such funds can be used for staff employment during a specified period, but cannot normally be used to pay the salary of the surgeon. Other industries make limited contributions and insurance companies support research projects on traffic and occupational accidents.

Private foundations give significant support to surgical research by providing funds for the purchase of laboratory animals and supplies and the compensation of human subjects. The awarding of such funds is usually administrated by medical societies.

Hospital and University Funds: Hospitals support clinical research but basic research is regarded as the responsibility of the universities; medical schools supply funds to research trainees for laboratory animals and materials and for the compensation of human subjects. The universities also arrange and finance research training courses. Significant *national funding* is given directly to hospitals to reimburse them for the research and teaching performed by surgeons. The distribution of the surgeons time between research, student teaching and clinical work is not clearly defined, but research probably accounts for 10–15 % of the total. As a result, the research trainee can usually perform part of his research in parallel with his clinical duties while receiving financial support from national funds.

The financial resources available to the individual researcher are satisfactory. There is freedom of choice among many possible projects and no interference or control is normally exercised provided agreed scientific and financial reporting schedules are respected. *Surgical societies* in Sweden provide some financial support for research projects and for participation in national and international conferences. They do not contribute to any research fellowship.

The medical research council of Sweden provides scholarships and stipends for the support of foreign researchers and their families to come to work in Sweden. The researcher can use whatever resources and funds can be spared from this basic support for the project in question. The medical research council publishes announcements of available awards and eligibility requirements, regularly, and distributes them to all registered research trainees. Similar announcements are made by the medical schools and medical and surgical societies. Funding available from the pharmaceutical industry is advertised in national scientific periodicals. With the exception of the pharmaceutical industry, which expect a direct or indirect economic return from a research project, no topic preferences or biases are expressed by granting agencies.

The Effect of Research Training on the Surgeon

The overall objective of research training for the surgeon is to instill an extensive knowledge of surgery, develop a methodical approach to work and encourage critical thinking. Enhancement of personal creativity is normally noticeable after one or two years of concentrated scientific studies. Most individuals who undergo such research training will continue in some sort of clinical research after they have left the university hospital. A surgeon who has completed research training and achieved an appointment as "docent" has a high social status.

Research training, an approved dissertation, and a position as a "docent" are now prerequisites for a consultant position in surgery, e.g., a chief surgeon at a county hospital or any academic position at a university hospital. The paucity of private surgical units in Sweden makes the number of surgical appointments smaller than in many other countries and increases the competitive pressure on candidates for them.

There are few disadvantages in combining research training with fulltime surgical work in Sweden. Although students get an insight into scientific methodology during their basic medical studies, the high demands placed on scientific competence by surgical research make such introductory courses inadequate. No form of undergraduate scientific training could produce the level of scientific sophistication required for surgical research. A surgical resident in a county hospital who develops an interest in a particular surgical topic can apply to any university or to any group of researchers with the same interest for research training. In this sense, the resident's choice of topic for research is completely free. A resident who has no specific topic of research in mind but who wishes to undertake research training, is given an overview of the different projects in progress at the institution in question to enable him to make a choice. Although the usual duration of formal research training is four years, it may vary according to the nature of the project and the difficulties arising during execution of the research. Projects involving animal experiments can sometimes be completed in a shorter period than clinical projects involving patient follow-up.

The research trainee is usually employed as a registrar or junior staff member and can use part of each day or part of each week for research activities. Because time spent "on call" is compensated by a corresponding amount of time off, the research trainee can take every fifth or sixth week off and devote part or all of it to research. Although the research trainee can also be relieved of clinical practice duties during limited periods of time he normally dedicates a significant portion of his nights and week-ends to research work that does not have to be performed in hospital, e.g., literature reviews and the working up of results. University hospital surgeons have a duty not only to provide clinical service but also to teach medical students, conduct research, and supervise research. University regulations require that 30 % of the total working hours be devoted to research supervision.

Organization of Library Service

All county hospitals and university hospitals have well equipped medical libraries that provide for literature reviews and immediate access to most national and international medical periodicals. Swedish and Scandinavian surgical societies meet several times a year for the presentation of the results of surgical research. Swedish surgeons also participate frequently in international surgical conferences.

Since Sweden is a small country, the research trainee will be completely dependent on the international literature, which is predominantly in English, French or German. To fulfill the requirement to publish his work in highly reputable international periodicals, the research trainee must have a good command of English and, to some extent, of German and French. Because English tends to dominate most international conferences and the research trainee often has to present his results orally, he must be able not only to make such oral presentations but also be able to conduct the subsequent discussion in English.

Permission to perform animal experiments has been restricted in Sweden during recent years as it has in many other countries. Acute (nonsurvival) experiments and some chronic animal experiments can still be performed provided the protocol has been approved by the local ethics committee which includes lay people. The regulations covering human experiments are also clearly defined and the public attitude towards such experiments is mainly positive. Informed consent is mandatory. The written information provided to individuals prior to obtaining consent must be approved by the local ethics committee.

Since the socialized health care system in Sweden relieves the patient of any medical or surgical fees, it is comparatively easy to perform clinical research. A high level of continuity with regular and frequent follow-up visits makes it possible to carry out reliable studies with a low percentage of drop-outs. A great number of randomized clinical investigations of the comparative merits of different surgical procedures for peptic ulcer, for the treatment of cancer of the colon and rectum, and for the treatment of inflammatory bowel disease, have been performed in Swedish hospitals in recent years.

Attitudes Toward Surgical Research

Although the public's attitude toward surgical research is generally positive, criticism has been directed at animal experiments for either surgical or medical research. Patients who are asked to participate in research projects, however, generally display a positive attitude and it is usually not difficult to obtain informed consent for clinical trials or to find "healthy control subjects" for research studies.

Most universities and scientific societies regard surgical research in the same light as research in physiology biochemistry, and collaboration is common between surgical and basic science departments in Sweden. Surgical staffs in university clinics generally view research favorably because it is considered as important a prerequisite for appointment to university clinical positions as teaching and clinical work.

Chief surgeons in county hospitals are, with very few exceptions, "docents", which automatically signifies that they have had extensive research training and have produced a successful dissertation. The same is often true of their surgical colleagues in consultant positions because they too regard research training as a prerequisite for appointment to their positions. As a consequence, residents in such county hospitals are encouraged to perform clinical research such as follow-up studies for the assessment of surgical results. The attitude among residents toward continuing their research training at a university hospital to the "doctor of medicine" level is generally positive, but changes in the social and economic structure during recent decades tends to interfere with this ambition. For example, the resident's spouse often has a full time job, and moving from a county to a university hospital may entail significant or even insurmountable personal or financial problems.

Achievements and Prospects for Surgical Research

Pioneering contributions to vascular surgery were made early in the 20th century by Professor Einar Kay at the Karolinska Hospital. Dr. Clarence Crafoord won an international reputation in cardiac surgery by developing a method for surgical treatment of coarctation of the aorta, and introducing the use of heparin prophylaxis against postoperative thromboembolism. Professor Herbert Olivercrona made significant contributions to the diagnosis and surgical treatment of brain tumors. Lund's test, developed in 1952, is now used all over the world to assess the exocrine function of the pancreas; it is an excellent example of how collaboration between clinical chemistry and surgery can contribute to the development of diagnostic tests of wide clinical importance beyond the bounds of surgery.

Professor N.G. Kock gained international renown when he presented a method for the construction of a continent ileostomy in 1969. This advance could not have been made without the extensive experimental studies in animals that he initiated and performed in the department of physiology.

Investigation is now well established in all surgical subspecialities in Sweden and generally meets high international standards. It encompasses both basic and clinical studies carried out in collaboration with other clinical specialties and academic institutions. The very positive attitude toward surgical research expressed by governmental authorities during the 1980's indicates that it will probably retain its good health and high status for some time.

7

The Confluence of Private and Public Resources in Switzerland

F. Largiadèr

Introduction

Switzerland is a small country; 6.2 million inhabitants live in an area of 40 000 km (2) that is partially covered by high mountains. Medical care is of very high quality and is organized according to liberal principles. The current ratio of medical doctors to inhabitants is high at 1:500 and, if the present trend continues, it will be 1:300 in a few years.

The general attitude of the population towards surgical research is friendly, but not engaged. At the university level, research is considered a natural part of surgery, but the average standard is not very high. Research is often equated with publishing, in which quality and originality are by no means stressed by the whole surgical community.

Practicing surgeons take a rather reserved stance towards research in a country with a conservative attitude and a tendency to adhere to traditional values. A humanitarian attitude, strength of character, and surgical craftsmanship are still considered the most important characteristics for a surgeon. Clinicians in practice have a tendency to see surgical research as an activity that contradicts these values as if it were not possible to unite both in one person!

An emphasis on practical medical work is expected by the majority of medical students, whereas interest in research is rather limited.

This by and large friendly, but by no means enthusiastic, support for surgical research has been subjected to several negative influences during recent years. The baby boom before 1965 has induced a rapid expansion in the universities and a general concern in the population about a possible over-abundance of graduates. This concern has been transferred to research, in general. There has been an enormous rise in health care costs and many politicians are tempted to reduce these costs by reducing research funding. General financial restrictions in the public sector have led to a significant decline in government funding of research. The "antivivisection movement" is also getting more and more attention and animal experimentation is meeting with increasing resistance.

Achievements of Surgical Research

There is no exclusively Swiss development in medical or surgical research. Research has always been dependent on single individuals and as a result, has lacked continuity and has developed differently from one university to another. Surgical research, especially experimental surgical research, has only been supported systematically since 1950. Lenggenhager and Maurice Mueller in Bern, Allgoewer in Basel, and Senning in Zuerich established surgical research programs in Switzerland.

Purely Swiss contributions to surgical research are difficult to enumerate, because of the close ties between our surgical researchers and those in neighboring countries. The work of Cesar Roux in Lausanne and Theodor Kocher in Bern, in the early days of surgical research, have to be mentioned. Theodor Bilroth and Ferdinand Sauerbruch, who were professors of surgery in Zuerich, made important contributions to surgical research before coming to

Switzerland and after leaving Zuerich for Austria and Germany. The "Arbeitsgemienschaft fuer Osteosynthese" has gained, and currently enjoys, an international reputation for its research in bone-fracture healing (1). Another example of a new development is pancreatic transplantation, in which Zuerich was one of the first centers of clinical and experimental investigation in the world (2).

Institutions for surgical research are now associated with universities, with only a few exceptions, such as the laboratory for surgical research in Davos and an institution in Bern, both of which are privately funded.

Clinical research in university departments, such as controlled randomized studies, is not separated, administratively, from clinical routine and is not performed by special personnel. There are no positions devoted permanently and exclusively to clinical surgical studies in any university.

Experimental surgical research is an independent division in only one university, Lausanne. In the other four—Basel, Bern, Geneva, and Zuerich—experimental surgical research is part of the surgery department. The head of surgical research is not a faculty member and has the position of a "Leitender Arzt" in Zuerich and Basel and of "Oberarzt" in Bern. He is in charge of 1 or 2 residents and technical personnel comprising 2 to 4 laboratory technicians and 2 to 6 nurses. In Bern, the group is completed by a veterinarian; in other places, a veterinarian is in charge of the animal facilities. Most of the research in the laboratories is performed by surgeons who occupy the positions of clinical residents or receive salaries from research foundations.

Funding of Surgical Research

Various amounts of government funding are available for experimental research. In Basel, government funding covers only a small part of costs; in Bern, it makes up half of the budget; and in Zuerich, it is the principal source in the amount of $SFr 200 000 per year. Overall, approximately 0.46% of the gross domestic product of Switzerland is devoted to biomedical research. Practically no money is available for surgical research from pharmaceutical firms and industries. These sponsors concentrate mainly on trials of new drugs. Surgical fees do not form an important part of research funding. Surgical associations do not have the means to finance fellowships or travel to scientific meetings. Research performed by the "Arbeitsgemeinschaft fuer Osteosynthese" is outside the universities and belongs in a special category since it is funded by profits from the sale of materials for osteosynthesis.

There are many private foundations that support medical and, to some extent, surgical research. These foundations are administrated by universities, industries or private boards, but the grants received from them are rather small $ SFr 5000–20,000 per project. There is no comprehensive register of these foundations, but incomplete lists are available from the administration departments of the universities and from the "Schweizerischer Wissenschaftsrat, Wildhainweg 20, 3000 Bern".

The most important federal institution for support of research is the Swiss National Foundation (Schweizerischer Nationalfonds zur Foederung der Wissenschaftlichen Forschung, Bern). This institution has a government budget and supports research projects according to internationally accepted standards.

Research During Residency Training

Acceptance criteria for residency training in surgery have been set by the Swiss Medical Federation (FMH) and accepted by the government. Approved residency programs require a curriculum of 6 years, spent partially in large and partially in small surgical units. Most surgeons voluntarily prolong the residency period to 8–9 years. There is a precise catalogue of required clinical and operative activities in which research, and especially experimental research, are not included. A typical work day for a Swiss resident is outlined in Table I. Board certification in surgery is possible after residency programs outside the university hospitals.

The inclusion of experimental surgical research in such a residency program is impossible, because even large institutions with no connections to universities do not offer research opportunities. Research training for residents is

TABLE I. A normal clinical day for a Swiss resident.

07:30	Morning conference
07:50	Rounds on emergency patients
08:15	
	Operations
14:00	
15:00	Daily conference of the sections
15:30	Departmental conference: Review operations of the day, programs for the following day
16:10	
16:15	Rounds and ward work, followed by:
	Monday: Scientific conference
	Tuesday: Student teaching
	Wednesday: Mortality conference
	Thursday: Postgraduate teaching conference
18:30	Friday: Grand Rounds

offered in all university hospitals, but the number of positions and the facilities available for research are limited. Research fellowships are tenable during the residency program (for instance, in Bern) or at the end of the residency program as the start to an academic career (for instance, in Basel).

Research During Residency Program

Surgical research is an indispensable part of surgery at the academic level, because it teaches the surgeon how to think scientifically and enhances the surgeon's ability to develop new concepts and techniques. Only selected individuals identified as future academic surgeons at the universities, should embark on surgical research, and the limited resource available for research should be reserved for them. Including research in the program of every resident has been tried, but the results were disappointing and bore no adequate relation to the effort and money invested. It was hardly ever possible to motivate a surgeon to do research unless he had previously expressed the wish to do this type of work. To obtain the degree of Doctor of Medicine in Switzerland, it is necessary to write a thesis. Thus every candidate has to write one publication that is scientific in style, although not necessarily in content. This is sufficient for most physicians.

Scientific work in the form of surgical research should be reserved for an elite. Motivation for scientific work is an important criterion for the selection of candidates. Scientific interest and the will to solve problems usually coincide with ambition and the concept of using scientific work as a means of improving career development. These two motivations are almost inseparable and no effort should be made to separate them.

About 35% of our residency positions are filled by young physicians who have been selected according to principles just described, and we expect them to become scientifically oriented surgeons with high technical skill. Continuing selection is necessary, and inept candidates are eliminated during the course of their residency program. We project that 20% of our residents will complete their training, as planned.

During the curriculum laid out for these specially selected surgeons, they will spend six months to a year in research. During the day, they will not be involved in clinical routine, but they have to fulfill regular night and week-end duties. Since six months or a year is not enough to complete scientific work of some value, these surgeons will do research in addition to their regular clinical routines during the rest of their residency periods, during off-hours if necessary. The privilege of being selected for a career in academic surgery is considered to be worth such an extraordinary effort in Switzerland.

References

1. Mueller ME, Allgoewer M, Willeneger H. Manual der Osteosynthese. Berlin/Heidelberg/New York; Springer, 1969.
2. Largiader F, Baumgaertner D, Kolb E, Uhlschmid G. Technique and results of combined pancreatic and renal allotransplantation in man. In: Segmental pancreatic transplantation. Stuttgart/New York; Thieme, 1983.

8

Historical and Organizational Influences Upon Surgical Research in the United Kingdom

R. Shields

Surgical research in the United Kingdom presents an interesting paradox in the 1980's. On the one hand, there is hardly a surgical trainee who is not engaged in some form of clinical investigation, and it would be a rare occasion for a trainee devoid of research experience to be promoted to the senior ranks of the profession. Many surgical specialties have founded their own research societies, and the Surgical Research Society receives three to four times more abstracts than it can present at its twice yearly meetings. Yet in the last decade, the resources to support surgical research have been greatly reduced. In 1981, the University Grants Committee, which portions government funds for higher education to the individual universities, cut the financial support of the universities by 15% and for the first time, instructed the universities that medical schools should not be protected from the reductions. The budgets of the government funded research councils, such as the Medical Research Council, were considerably reduced, and many projects considered to be of high scientific merit could not be funded. Overall, the United Kingdom spends approximately 0.16% of its gross domestic product on biomedical research and development.

Increased productivity in the face of reduced resources may superficially suggest a high degree of efficiency but conceals a disturbing state of affairs. Several elements of the situation may be unique to the United Kingdom. For example, a relatively poor economic performance and a government committed to reducing public expenditure. Nevertheless, there are underlying problems shared with many western countries such as manpower problems, over production of doctors and especially surgeons, greater allocation of resources to community medicine for the aged and mentally ill or handicapped. The annual budget for heatlh care requires an annual increase of about 2–5% in western countries merely to cope with an aging population and to keep up with advances in ordinary medical care.

History of Surgical Research in the United Kingdom

The names of Hunter and Lister stand out of the earlier pages of medical history as surgeons whose research contributions have saved the lives of countless patients, but in their time, surgical advances generally sprang from careful clinical observations and deductions. It had not been appreciated, except by a few, that advances could originate from controlled observations or modifications in physiological and pathological processes in man or in animals. Surgical research, as we would recognize it today, began in the United Kingdom about fifty years ago. In 1933, the Royal College of Surgeons of England established the Buxton Brown Farm for experimental research, indicating clearly their perception that surgical progress was dependent on research, not least upon experiments in animals. At that time, two surgical department chairmen, Wilke in Edinburg and Illingworth in Glasgow, created in their surgical departments, an environment conducive to the rapid development of surgical research. They encouraged attitudes of scientific discipline in the laboratory and at the bedside, encouraging their trainees to question current surgical views.

The scene was set for a rapid burgeoning of surgical research which took place in the immediate postwar years.

At the end of World War II, many highly experienced young surgeons returned from the armed services wishing to participate in the rapid advances of surgical care which they saw during the war. The establishment of the National Health Service in 1948 initiated a massive growth in hospital services, especially teaching hospitals, and a great increase in the number of full-time specialists within the hospital service. Academic clinicians staffed the university departments and provided clinical service to the National Health Service patients. They were not involved in private practice and therefore, could devote their energies to teaching and research. The influence of the United States during this phase of development of British surgical research cannot be exaggerated. The close links forged during the second World War and easier travel thereafter allowed many British department heads and young academic surgeons to visit and to study in surgical departments in the United States. The research of Blalock, Wagensteen, Moore, Dunphy, Code and others created a ferment among British surgeons who returned with the determination that British surgery would share in the rapid growth of research.

During the 1960's, medical schools shared in an unparalleled expansion which universities enjoyed following the publication, and governmental acceptance of the Robbins Report, which advocated that university education should be provided for all of those able to satisfy the suitable entrance requirements and who wished to be admitted. New buildings were constructed, existing departments were expanded. Increased staffing in departments of surgery allowed greater concentration on surgical research.

However, in the last decade, partly because of economic stagnation, and more so, because of the Government's avowed policy to reduce public expenditure and curtail higher education and research, financial resources, directly and indirectly derived from the State, have been greatly reduced. As a result, in the period 1973–80, Britain's world share of publications in biomedical sciences fell by 11%, and its citation share by 27%. The relatively generous funding of universities has been abandoned. However, after three to four years of equal misery across the board, the University Grants Committee is introducing *selective* funding for research, so that those institutions and departments which are active in research will receive additional income, above a basic income for teaching. Superficially such an arrangement seems attractive, but there is a fear that a central organization will not be able to pick its way through the complexities of funding of research, with the result that only established and powerful research groups will be funded and that perhaps exciting and important new initiatives may go unrecognized. There is good evidence that neither the University Grants Committee nor the Medical Research Council understand the complexities of the funding of medical schools nor the difficulties of clinical research. The bulk of Research Council funding is directed to the big battalions of the basic sciences especially the glamour of molecular biology. It is left to the charitable agencies, such as the Wellcome Foundation, to provide the more imaginative initiatives in clinical research.

If surgical research is defined as research which is undertaken by surgeons and directed toward improvement in surgical care, some hint of the make-up of surgical research was given in the paper by Chetty and Forest (1981). They examined the contributions, over a five year period, to the major surgical research societies in the United Kingdom and Europe. At the Surgical Research Society, which is the main generalist society for the presentation of surgical research in the United Kingdom, 97% of the papers were presented by university departments of surgery, with gastroenterology predominating. Almost two thirds of the papers were orientated towards clinical practice and one third were rated as "surgical" (Table I). At its sister society in continental Europe—the European Society for Surgical Research—85% of the papers came from departments of surgery, with cardiac surgical topics being the more numerous. While fewer papers were dedicated to clinical research than with the Surgical Research Society, more papers were devoted to surgical topics.

The Surgical Research Society tends to concentrate on gastroenterology and vascular surgery because, for historical reasons, these have been the major interests of senior staff in uni-

TABLE I. Research classified as "surgical research".

Preoperative:	indications for surgery. preoperative monitoring and preparation.
Operative:	technique, suture material: prostheses; instruments: results of surgery.
Postoperative:	
Care	haemodynamic and respiratory monitoring metabolism, fluid and electrolyte balance, parenteral nutrition.
Complications	
Immediate	thrombosis and embolism; wound infection and dehiscence; cardiopulmonary and renal failure; intestinal dysfunction.
Long-term	malabsorption; metabolic problems: mortality.

From Chetty and Forrest, 1981.

versity departments. However, because many younger surgeons have received basic training in molecular biology, immunology etc., one can identify within the contributions to the society, a swing away from surgical physiology to molecular biology. Moreover, other surgical disciplines, e.g., urology, orthopedic surgery, otorhinolaryngology, neurosurgery, have all established their own research societies. Certain multidisciplinary societies, e.g., the British Transplant Society and the British Society of gastroenterology, constitute the main national forum for surgeons undertaking research in these particular fields.

Attitudes and Opportunities in Surgical Research

The Surgical Resident

Although the primary aims of the surgical trainee are to develop clinical acumen and to acquire operative experience, many wish to have experience in surgical research. There is an obvious desire to participate in surgical advances and to improve the standard of surgical care of their patients. There are many who are excited by the investigations and enjoy the pleasure and enhance prestige of the delivery and publication, of a well-prepared paper. However, the fierce competition, which now faces surgical trainees in the United Kingdom, has been the main stimulus to surgical research and many, if not all, trainees take up a full-time post in research during their surgical training. These posts are sought partly while the trainee marks time awaiting promotion to more senior posts, and also partly to improve career prospects in a very competitive field.

The United Kingdom doctor qualifies at an earlier age than in several other countries, especially the United States (Table I in Chapter 10).

The majority of those aspiring to a surgical career take the first step on the promotional ladder immediately after internship. The young trainee quite properly wishes to acquire critical experience in the wards and operating theatre and therefore it is unusual for a trainee to take time off for surgical research before the age of thirty, by which time he has passed the examination for the diploma of Fellowship of a Royal College. The Fellowship (e.g., F.R.C.S.), an early milestone along the surgical road, indicates a certain standard of knowledge and training of surgery in general. It is an entry qualification to the more intensive higher surgical training, which is taken at the senior registrar/lecturer level. Surgical research is usually undertaken by a trainee after the Fellowship, in a registrar post, at the age of 30–33.

Less commonly, the trainee becomes involved in surgical research at an earlier stage in his career. Some, indeed, may have been introduced to research during their student days, when they have intercalated a year of study to obtain a science degree. Others may, during the early years of their surgical training, take 1–3 years off to obtain experience in a basic science subject, often reading to a Ph.D. These are usually young surgeons who are research-oriented and academically inclined who have, been attracted to research, at an early stage by working in an academic surgical. It can be a difficult decision to embark on research at such an early stage in their career, because of the understandable desire to pass the difficult examinations of the Royal College and, to become directly involved in clinical and operative work. There is therefore a conflict in career aims. Without doubt, this is an ideal time to enter surgical research, because the young surgeon is usually bright, curious and inquisitive, with a mind unfilled by surgical dogmatism. At this stage, the surgical trainee must receive considerable support from his seniors to allay fears that his surgical promotion may be delayed. Such reassurance, however, is readily given, because these people are usually of the highest calibre.

More usually, entry into surgical research is delayed until the trainee obtains his fellowship at about the age of thirty. At this time, the trainee comes up against a severe narrowing in the path toward higher surgical training. There is an inordinate delay at this stage. The trainee does not obtain much further experience or responsibility until appointment to a senior registrar or lecturer post. Generally these posts cannot be applied for with any chance of success until ten years after qualification and at least five years after obtaining the Fellowship. It is not unusual for there to be 60–70 applicants, of which only 5–8 will be short-listed for interview. A review of the successful applicant for these posts (Taylor and Clyne, 1985) shows that nearly all have had 1–2 years in surgical research, published, on average, 6 papers and made ten presentations at research meetings. Almost all of these trainees possess a higher university degree, such as a doctorate of medicine (the basic British qualification is Batchelor of Medicine), Master of Surgery (Ch.M. or M.S.), or a Ph.D. At one time these were qualifications which would ensure entry to a consultant post in a prestigious teaching hospital; now they have become common currency for appointment to a senior registrar post. Surgical research obviously benefits from these circumstances, but it is perhaps the only good by-product of a wasteful and increasingly unacceptable system.

A recent survey (Dehn, Blacklay and Taylor, 1985) of registrars undertaking surgical research in the United Kingdom, brought up some surprising information. In more than a quarter of the cases, the salaries of these registrars were met by the National Health Service, twice as many as the research councils, indicating perhaps the relatively low level of funding of clinical research by the Medical Research Council. The individual's enjoyment and success of the research was related to the quality of supervision. Over half the respondents to the questionnaire spoke highly of the direction of the research. Only half of those undertaking the research had any previous experience, or indeed an interest, in the subject of the research, indicating that the choice of topic was dictated largely by the departmental interest and facilities, rather than the individual concerned. The importance of good supervision cannot be over-emphasized and recently the British Science and Engineering Research Council issued valuable guidelines for research supervision which have been taken up by most research-oriented departments (Christopherson, Boyd, Fleming et al, 1983). Most of those questioned considered that the experience had been worthwhile, with a positive gain in logical and critical thought and increased awareness of scientific methods. Not surprisingly, many expressed the view that they had learned how *not* to do research. The conclusion of the survey was that the majority of trainees enjoyed their time in research, had been adequately supervised, and would probably continue to undertake some form of research throughout their career. Few however, wished to continue in academic work, suggesting that the research had been used mainly for career advancement.

Programmes of higher surgical training—for senior registrars and lecturers—extend over 4 years, but experience in surgical research in an approved centre at home or abroad, of up to one year, will be recognized toward accreditation. Training programmes are, by their nature, restrictive, but they do not materially affect surgical research greatly, because at present they extend largely over the 32–36 year period. Most trainees have already participated in research by this age. However, the rigidity of the training programmes makes it difficult for these lecturers, who underpin the research activity of most departments, to move freely from one centre to another, especially to take a year off clinical service for more basic laboratory work.

Lecturer and Senior Lecturer

The holders of these full-time university posts have honorary contractual duties within the National Health Service. Equivalent in status to senior registrar and consultant respectively, they fill key positions in the university departments and represent the main source of research activity. In addition to heavy teaching commitments, they have to contribute a considerable amount of service work to the hospitals to which they are attached. This is usually represented as six service sessions, approximately six half days, out of the conventional eleven sessions per week. Most university clinicians devote more than their contractual sessions to clinical care, often because of the demand upon the particular expertise which they may possess, and because of the heavy clinical load which is a common feature of British hospitals. Such an arrangement affords a stimulating and satisfying professional life, but inevitably, the time that the university clinician devotes to research becomes increasingly eroded. A typical timetable of two of the lecturers in my own department, each working in different hospitals, is attached in Table II. In general, in what seems to be a seventy hour week, eight hours are spent in administration (for university and health ser-

TABLE II. Weekly schedule.

	Monday	Tuesday	Wednesday	Thursday	Friday	Saturday	Sunday
08:00		Clinical Rounds with		Clinical Rounds with			
08:15		Junior NHS Staff	Clinical Rounds with	Junior NHS Staff			
08:30	Clinical Rounds with	Operating Theatre	Consultants	Operating Theatre	Dept. Business		
09:00	Junior NHS Staff				mtg. Hospital Grant Rounds	48-hour Emergency Intake Every Fourth Weekend.	
10:00	Bedside Teaching		Department Surgical			Morning Clinical Round Alternate Weekends.	
10:30	of undergrads Med. Students		Rounds		Endoscopy Clinic		
11:00	Administration discharge		Department Research				
11:30	letters arrange		Meeting				
12:00	admissions select patients for student seminar		Department X-Ray Meeting				
12:15	Grand Round						
12:30							
13:00				Research			
13:30	Clinical Rounds with Consultant	Services/ Research Sessions in	Outpatient Clinic		Outpatient Clinic		
14:00	Outpatient Clinic	Gastroent. unit, incl. Endoscopy,					
15:00		Oesophageal Manometry, etc.					
16:00		Clinical Rounds with			Ward Rounds		
16:30		Consultants					
17:00		Pathology Meeting					
17:30	Postgraduate Surgical						
18:00	Meeting Organized by University						
19:00	Departments						

vice), four hours in teaching, thirty hours in research (mainly in the evenings and at weekends) and twenty eight hours in clinical service. A lecturer performs personally about thirty operations each month, the magnitude of the operation depending on his clinical experience.

The university surgeon can often find himself in a professional dilemma. He must engage effectively and fruitfully in research and failure to do so can lead to a reduction in resources and failure to advance his career. Yet his professional surgical colleagues will not hold in high regard a university surgeon whose clinical practice is meager and narrowly restricted and whose research is divorced completely from surgical practice. The pressures on the university surgeons are undoubtedly heavy.

Professors and Chairmen

Clinical professors are for the most part full-time employees of the university medical school, but also have an honorary clinical contract with the National Health Service. Like a senior lecturer, they spend more than half their working week as hospital consultants involved with patient-care and other NHS service commitments. In teaching hospitals, surgical staff are usually grouped into service units or "firms". The university staff usually form one service firm, consisting of junior NHS staff (e.g., registrars), lecturer, senior lecturer (or reader) and professor. The university unit may be one of 3–5 firms in the hospital, providing an equal share of clinical service. The administrative task of directing the hospital firm, as well as the academic department, takes up a good deal of the professor's time, over and above his clinical service and therefore tends to encroach upon research. In general, clinical professors spend little time at the bench in the laboratory and tend to direct their own research teams, for whom they have to obtain resources from the grant-awarding agencies and foundations.

The university department is expected to spearhead clinical research. Surgical trainees in the Health Service look to the university department for formal training in research. While there is no shortage of recruits, the chairmen and other directors of research who are accountable to grant-awarding agencies, must ensure that the research is well done and therefore have to distinguish between those aspirants who are competent, curious, with drive and initiative, from those whose only interest in research may be to advance their career prospects.

In medical schools, there may be a variety of other surgical departments apart from general surgery, e.g., urology, orthopaedic surgery, neurosurgery, cardiothoracic surgery. In smaller medical schools there may not be separate departments for these disciplines, but within the main department there is a senior lecturer/reader devoted to the specialty. The main departments of surgery, for historical reasons, tend to have their research and clinical interests mainly in the fields of gastroenterology, vascular surgery, oncology, transplantation and endocrine surgery. It is not usual for a professor, or other senior member of the university clinical staff, to devote his clinical practice and research to quite a narrow specialty within these broad disciplines, e.g., colorectal surgery, diseases of the breast, etc. This contributes to the development of focussed clinical research.

Among departments, two clear patterns of research activity can be identified. An entire department may be devoted to a single clinical and research topic. For example, all members of the staff may be directed to research within the single theme of transplantation. Alternatively, senior members of a university department may have quite separate clinical and research interests and form their own research teams. In this way, the departmental interests can extend over a wide range of surgery. One member of the department may be interested in colorectal surgery, a second in vascular surgery, a third in transplantation. Each system seems to have its advantages and disadvantages. An entire department devoting all its resources of men and material to one major theme can, with good leadership, be highly effective, participating in major advances and attracting funds from the major grant-awarding authorities. On the other hand, it can be difficult for the non-professional members of the department clearly to demonstrate their own particular contributions to the work of the department. Appointments, or search committees may have difficulty in deciding if a senior lecturer of the department would be able to direct major research teams on his own.

National Health Service Surgeons

The majority of surgeons are employed by the State and receive a salary as either a full-time or part-time consultant. The NHS surgeon can play a greater or lesser part in surgical research, depending upon individual opportunities and preferences. Although there are considerable opportunities for clinical research, the National Health Service does not allocate laboratory space for research and therefore accommodation usually has to be found within the university department or other such space that the researcher may find. The NHS staff, however, have an access equal to university surgeons to the major grant-awarding authorities, such as the Medical Research Council, and may have been renowned for the considerable valuable contributions which they have made to surgical care. These consultants usually have a considerable clinical service load. To devote time to effective research with a busy NHS practice and a private practice can present considerable difficulties.

There are many surgeons, especially in district general hospitals, who have neither the time nor facilities for prosecuting clinical or experimental research. However, among them, there is a general awareness that improvement in patient care will only be achieved by investigative work and most are only too willing to join in multi-centre trials, or to refer patients with problems to university units for further investigation. Although private practice has increased in the United Kingdom, the bulk of the clinical work is carried out in the National Health Service. Since there is no direct payment from patients, and staff are salaried, there is no restriction to referral of patients to centres and individuals for further investigations. There is usually a close relationship between university employed clinical and NHS staffs. Both work closely together in the same hospital and each has responsibilities for teaching. In general, there has grown up a considerable respect between university and NHS staff for one another's abilities and dedication.

Attitude of the Public

As a result of the media, especially television and the popular press, there is a very active interest in medical matters among the public, but the public is more fascinated by glamorous and exciting surgical research, e.g., heart surgery and transplantation. Both the television and the press have shown considerable responsibility in their presentation of research topics, so that the public possesses a remarkably broad knowledge of significant advances in surgery. Members of the public are obviously not entirely clear who carries out the research and how it may be funded, but they expect that surgical research will be carried out in major teaching hospitals and have an admiration and respect for those making major contributions.

For the most part, the medical profession in the U.K. enjoys the respect of the public and is rated highly for its integrity and dedication. This respect shows itself in an easy cooperation and collaboration by the public in research. Patients understand that research and teaching is carried out in major hospitals and very readily give informed consent for participation in trials of treatment and clinical investigation in which they themselves may not be an immediate or direct beneficiary. This cooperation is sustained by the establishment in each hospital of ethical committees in which lay members of the public are involved.

Major legislation is underway in the United Kingdom concerning the use *of animals in experimental work*. Hitherto animals could not be used for research unless the investigation received a certificate from the Home Office, the responsible Government agency. A laboratory can, at any time, be visited by Home Office inspectors who have right of access. All animals can be inspected and current work reviewed. Any breaches of the regulations can lead to withdrawal of a license and occasionally prosecution. As far as surgical research is concerned, the current arrangements are, on the whole, satisfactory. Animals receive good care and investigators have demonstrated responsibility. However, criticisms of the use of animals for testing of cosmetics, and protests amongst the self-styled animal liberators, has led to legislation now being presented before Parliament to tighten up the regulations.

Financing of Surgical Research

In the United Kingdom, surgical research is mainly financed from Governmental sources, directly or indirectly. A smaller, but important, contribution also comes from grant-awarding foundations and only a small proportion comes from legacies, donations and private practice.

Within British universities, research has been funded through the dual support system. One arm of the system is the provision, by the universities of buildings, major apparatus and senior staff. The other limb is the provision of some capital and recurrent funding for specific research projects by the Medical Research Council. The Medical Research Council does not wish to provide universities with the salaries of senior staff or the erection of major institutes or buildings within medical schools. The Council expects to find, in those areas which it will support, well-equipped laboratories and highly trained staff. Although the system of dual support is under considerable stress and strain with recent Governmental cuts, the principle has been most effective.

For its buildings and staff, a university medical school is largely funded by Government, through the agency of the University Grants Committee, whose members are senior university people, selected for their expertise and knowledge. The Committee decides on the allocation of these funds to individual universities, each of whom assigns a proportion of its resources to its constituent Faculties for equipment, staffing and recurrent costs. In this way, a faculty of medicine will be provided with buildings, laboratories, academic, technical and secretarial staff. There will also be modest grant for running costs and for the purchase of equipment. The allocation contains very little to support research directly.

The main Government support of medical research is the Medical Research Council. This organization has two major institutions of its own, one for basic science and the other for clinical research, but in neither is surgical research represented. The Medical Research Council supports institutes and units in universities throughout the United Kingdom, but none is devoted to surgical research.

A surgical research worker can, however, hope to obtain financial support by a successful application to the Medical Research Council for a project grant, which lasts for three years, or a programme grant, which lasts up to five years. The latter are more substantial grants, but are given to only a relatively few workers. Over the last decade, only a few have been awarded for surgical research. In recent years, clinical research workers, have criticized the Medical Research Council for what they see as a bias towards the basic sciences, e.g., molecular biology, genetics, and immunology.

Fortunately there are several other bodies in the United Kingdom, mainly charitable foundations, which not only provide considerable funding of clinical research, but seem to be more sensitive to the problems which face clinical research workers. Chief amongst these is the Wellcome Foundation, which has responded to diminishing governmental support for research by increasing considerably its own allocation. It has identified the particular problems of surgical research with great foresight. For example, a young surgeon in training who has shown aptitude for research may not wish to commit himself too early to an academic career and may be reluctant to apply for a post such as a lecturer, indeed he may have neither the basic qualifications or record of publications to enable him to do so. Wellcome Surgical Fellowships allow a young surgeon, at the level of a third or fourth year resident, to spend one or two years in obtaining a training and experience in surgical research. These awards are among the most prestigious that a young surgeon can receive and are an important first step on the academic ladder. There are other charitable foundations, especially in the field of cancer, e.g., Imperial Cancer Research Fund, Cancer Research Campaign, etc., which support research in departments of surgery but the scope of their support is limited by their terms of reference.

There are two other small sources of indirect Government funding which deserve mention. The Department of Health and Social Security assigns to each NHS Region funding to support medical research. These grants are usually meant to fund research which would not normally receive support from the Medical Research Council teaching hospitals and university departments receive a substantial proportion of their expertise and research orientation. This system of funding is sensitive to local initiatives and serves very usefully as pump-priming for pilot research projects.

Another source of funding is endowment, or trust funds, derived from monies and other donations which had been bequeathed or donated, mainly to large teaching hospitals before the establishment of the National Health Service. These sums have not been absorbed by Government agencies nor can they be used for financing the Health Service, and provide the teaching hospitals with considerable flexibility in supporting various initiatives, including research.

Most departments of surgery obtain funds to support research from legacies, gifts, etc. In addition, some support can also be obtained from drug companies, but such support is usually related to the drug in which the company has a specific interest. Some departments of surgery also depend for research funds on an income from the treatment of private patients. Many patients, both in the United Kingdom and from abroad, seek medical care as private patients from university staff, because of their national or international reputation. There are usually two restrictions on such private practice by university staff; first that it is carried out within NHS hospitals rather than private hospitals, and that the income earned is not for the personal remuneration of the member of staff, but is added to the income of the department, to be used largely for research purposes.

Conclusion

The opportunities to undertake surgical research in the United Kingdom remain good. It is doubtful how long the present situation will last, because of the reduction in the funding of the universities and the National Health Service. There does seem to be still sufficient sources of finance for good projects. Among surgical trainees, there is a greater realization that experience in research will be most helpful to their career advancement. There is generally among surgical trainees and consultants, an appreciation that advancement in patient-care will depend largely on clinically based investigations.

The opportunities to present surgical research are ample. The main platform for the presentation of research papers of the established investigator and the surgical trainee is the Surgical Research Society. This Society, which meets twice a year, has a membership open to anyone, surgeon or otherwise, actually engaged in surgical research. Many associated surgical disciplines have now established their own research society, many of whose meetings are arranged to coincide with meetings of the main Surgical Research Society.

The main organ of publication of surgical research in the United Kingdom is the British Journal of Surgery. For several decades, this journal confined its publications to retrospective reviews and reports of interesting cases, but vigorous editorship, combined with strict peer-review, has undoubtedly lifted this journal into the ranks of the major journals of surgery in the world. The journal is the official organ of the Surgical Research Society and twice a year, papers which have been read at the Society are published in the journal.

The British National Health Service, whatever its short-comings (and many of these are shared by many health-care systems), offers considerable opportunity for clinical research. Easy referral of patients with specific problems to surgeons with a particular interest and high expertise, and the absence of pecuniary interest and financial competition, facilitates the referral of patients and involvement in multi-centre trials. Despite the considerable clinical load of individual surgeons, the general atmosphere, especially in teaching hospitals, is conducive to research. Indeed it is often surprising how much support there is for research from the hard-pressed NHS health authorities.

Nevertheless, considerable dismay is felt among clinical researchers. In the past, planning had largely been based on an expectation of economic growth. However, economic stagnation in the 1980's coupled with Governmental emphasis on the cutting of public expenditure, has thrown both the universities and the Health Service into a frenzy of activity, based on a drive for increased efficiency. The current aim is to treat, teach, and research at the same level of activity as heretofore with very much reduced resources.

9

Research Challenges and Solutions in the United States

M.F. McKneally

Introduction

In the United States, surgical research is learned and conducted almost exclusively in university programs. While many of the 311 surgical training programs encourage residents to pursue a period of research, only a small minority of programs require research, and even fewer have well-developed curricula that provide reliable training in scientific methodology, organization of research projects, funding, analysis of data, and publication.

Surgical research training is largely tutorial, centered around individual surgeons who are proficient at research and who gravitate toward surgical departments with a strong emphasis on research. Such mentors are also sought by smaller departments to impart academic luster to otherwise largely clinical programs.

Surgical research was initiated in a small number of institutions under the strong influence of Alfred Blalock at The Johns Hopkins University, Evarts Graham at the University of Washington at St. Louis, Isidore Roudin at the University of Pennsylvania, and Owen Wangensteen at the University of Minnesota. These surgeons and their students recognized and emphasized the importance of research to the expansion of surgical knowledge and to the development of technical solutions to unresolved surgical problems. There was a significant increase in surgical research during World War II, especially on blood substitutes, wound care in general, and heart wounds in particular. This latter experience led to the development of heart surgery as a major American surgical research theme and contribution to surgical progress.

Following the launch of the Soviet space satellite "Sputnik" in 1957, a broad commitment of Federal funds to the support of scientific research lead to an expansion of surgical research in many institutions. Both the public and the government recognized the need to support scientific activity to keep American science abreast of scientific advances in other countries. During the past decade, funding for scientific research, including surgical research, diminished.

There has been a study section for surgical research within the National Institutes of Health, the principal U.S. agency for research support, since its formation in 1947. This surgical study section provides separate peer review for grant applications in fields related to surgery. There are now two such study sections: the "Surgery, Anesthesiology and Trauma" Section and the "Surgery and Bioengineering" Section; together they review 400 to 500 grant applications per year and fund approximately 25%.

The American public's attitude toward surgical research has generally been positive. The success of surgical research in the development of techniques for cardiopulmonary bypass, cardiac valve replacement, coronary artery surgery, support or substitution for the failing heart, and major organ transplantation has fascinated most people. Surgical research enjoys less esteem within the university community, partly as the result of deficiencies in the scientific training of surgical researchers during the period of most rapid expansion. Preclinical scientists have been critical of the level of scientific rigor of much surgical research, particularly studies conducted in human subjects where a multiplicity of uncontrolled patient variables may confound scientific analysis.

The attitude of surgeons, themselves, ranges from the denigrating view held by some community surgeons that surgical researchers are "mouse doctors," to the high level of respect accorded to the best surgical investigators within the university surgical community. Surgical residents usually reflect the attitudes of their mentors. The majority of residency candidates regard training in surgical research as a delay in their progress toward clinical practice, but this is becoming more readily accepted as the number of attractive post residency positions for surgeons diminishes. The interest of a small minority in the scientific analysis of surgical problems prompts them to seek highly academic residency programs offering a substantial period of training in the research laboratory such as developed by Sabiston and Moore. The introduction of mandatory surgical research rotations into predominently clinical institutions is frequently associated with friction and discontent.

Achievements of Surgical Research

Surgical research in the United States began with empirical attempts to improve the care of surgical patients. American surgeons eagerly pursued the application of the various techniques of inducing anesthesia to ease or eliminate the pain of surgical operations. This period of activity was characterized by active surgical scholarship that emphasized the acquisition of knowledge by direct experience, spirited discussion, and observation of the techniques of other surgeons. The French surgeon Alexis Carrel (1873–1944) emigrated to the United States to perform experimental surgery at the Rockefeller Institute in New York City early in the twentieth century. Carrel imparted a major impetus to the application of the scientific method to the solution of surgical problems. His animal experimentation on wound healing, vascular anastomoses, and transplantation provided a dazzling illustration of the contributions scientific surgeons could make, but it took almost a century for a full appreciation of Carrel's work to penetrate and be applied by the surgical community (1).

Alfred Blalock at The Johns Hopkins University followed the tradition of John Hunter in attempting to devise surgical solutions to naturally occurring problems by taking advantage of anomalies and variants seen in nature, e.g., the creation of a patient ductus arteriosus to increase pulmonary blood flow in patients with pulmonic stenosis and tetralogy of Fallot (2). The clinical application of Blalock's experimental work caused a revolution in the care of patients with congenital heart disease, and accelerated the development of laboratories in which large animal experiments could be conducted to familiarize surgeons with the techniques of cardiac and vascular surgery.

Wangensteen and his students at the University of Minnesota studied obstruction and decompression of the gastrointestinal tract (3), and applied gastric physiology in partnership with the Physiology Department under the direction of Maurice Visscher. Visscher and Wangensteen devised a training program that included a year of pure surgical research in the laboratory and a year of more abstract preclinical research in the Physiology Department. The surgeons brought a refreshing vigor, a tendency to rise early, and enthusiasm for the expeditious completion of experiments to the environment of the physiologists. Conversely, the intellectual rigor of the physiologists had a positive impact on the scientific thinking of the surgeons. Wangensteen's mandatory laboratory rotations provided the setting for very active participation by young residents in experimental surgery on the heart during the 1950's. The development of the heart-lung machine by Dewall and Lillehei at Minnesota and by Gibbon at Jefferson Medical College represents one of the highest accomplishments of surgeons working in the laboratory and emphasizes the uniqueness of surgical research. Surgeons who attempted to suture the beating heart were uniquely aware of the necessity of stopping the heart to allow repair of complex defects. As a result, they worked tirelessly to develop a means of perfusing the body with oxygenated blood during periods of induced cardiac arrest.

Funding for Surgical Research

The Federal government, through the National Institutes of Health provides a total of over $3.6 billion per year for the support of original programs of biomedical research, awarded on a highly competitive, peer reviewed basis (4). Approximately 0.25% of the gross domestic product in the United States is devoted to biomedical research. It is estimated that 5% is devoted to surgical research although the overlap with other areas, such as cancer and immunology makes this estimate uncertain (5). National foundations such as The American Cancer Society and The American Heart Association, supported by public solicitations, provide another major source of funding.

Drug companies and the biomedical technology industries contribute funds to research laboratories for the testing of new applications of patented pharmaceuticals or devices. Private foundations have recently made increasing amounts available for scientific research. The U.S. tax laws are designed to encourage industry and private individuals to contribute to biomedical research.

Surgeons themselves have directly supported surgical research by paying for laboratory personnel, animals, and equipment from their own surgical practice incomes. The creation of the Orthopedic Research and Education Foundation (6), supported by direct contributions from practicing orthopedic surgeons, is a highly significant development. This foundation awarded over one million dollars to residents and young academic orthopedic surgeons in 1985 to undertake research on problems targeted by surgeons as being appropriate areas for research activity. Such initiatives protect the young surgical investigator from the discouraging experience of competing unsuccessfully with full-time laboratory scientists.

Some surgical departments make direct appeals for funds to support their research by mailings to post-surgical patients or by presentations to industry. This approach has the advantage of immediacy and gives the donors a keen sense of direct participation in the surgical research project. In some centers, faculty surgeons contribute a fixed percentage of their private practice income to an educational or research fund for residents. Such funds provide important support for initiating research projects but are insufficient to run a surgical laboratory. However, they provide tangible evidence of senior surgeons' commitment to research and their concern for their juniors' careers.

Surgical societies provide research fellowships for advanced residents or surgeons immediately out of residency training to spend time in laboratories where there is an emphasis on research. The American College of Surgeons provides two such awards and administers another award supported by a drug company. The American Association for Thoracic Surgery and the American Surgical Association have recently initiated two similar awards for American applicants. Surgical societies generally do not support travel to scientific meetings; this is regarded as the financial responsibility of training programs.

Fogarty Fellowships, available through the National Institutes of Health and the Graham Traveling Fellowships of the American Association for Thoracic Surgery, sponsor surgical research by foreign visitors in the United States.

Career investigator salary awards are available in the United States for research in such specifically designated areas as cardiology, cancer, etc. Although they are not generically designated for surgeons, surgeons do apply. These awards substantially supplement the salaries of young investigators and require that they be relieved of clinical responsibilities while pursuing career development through research and educational projects. The National Institutes of Health also provide opportunities for surgeons to work as salaried members of the surgery branch of the Institute for a period of several years or as career investigators in the Institute.

The granting agencies emphasize particular areas in their selection of research programs for support, but use the peer-review system for awarding grants and do not interfere significantly with the conduct of the research. Drug companies and companies manufacturing medical devices tend to be far more proprietary in their interaction with surgical researchers evaluating their products.

Surgeons in the United States under the auspices of the American College of Surgeons and the leadership of Dr. William P. Longmire have formed the Conjoint Council on Surgical Research to document the level and quality of surgical research in North America. The Conjoint Council developed because of the concern about the diminishing success of surgeons competing with Ph.D. scientists for research funds at the National Institue of Health level. This group has defined surgical research as "research done by surgeons, but also research related to surgical diseases and perhaps specifically, that form of research which benefits from a surgeon's recognition of a relevant clinical problem and the transition of knwoledge into its solution". Surgeons in Canada will work with the Conjoint Council in data collection and in developing methods of improving the level of surgical scholarship.

The Conjoint Council has established committees of special interest in the areas of gastroenterology, trauma, burns, transplantation, cardiovascular disease, metabolism and nutrition and cancer. The Council is presently working on data collection as a first step in its long-range aims to increase the quality and quantity of surgical research.

Research During Residency Training

A surgical resident who spends a period in surgical research develops a more comprehensive knowledge of a specific area of surgical science, learn to appreciate the limits and pitfalls of data collection and analysis, masters the rudiments of manuscript preparation, adds surgical publications to his resume, and enhances the likelihood of his obtaining a desirable clinical or academic position on completion of training.

During the 1960's graduates of research-oriented surgical training programs in the United States could readily find clinical and academic opportunities in other parts of the country. During the subsequent two decades, the demand for surgeons with research training has decreased, except in rapidly developing fields such as liver or heart-lung transplantation. Surgical residents trained in the theoretical and practical aspects of these techniques are highly desirable exports of the surgical programs where they were learned. These and similar exceptions aside, most surgical training programs cannot afford to have more residents than are justified by the post-residency clinical opportunities. Consequently, inclusion of a research rotation in the surgical training program becomes a special consideration requiring careful integration of the needs of the resident, the surgical community, and society at large.

The salaries of residents during periods of surgical research were once funded fairly generously by the National Institutes of Health through training fellowships and research grants. Cutbacks in these programs have put severe constraints on this source of support. Special fellowships, such as the National Institutes of Health Fellowship Program in Academic Surgery, need to be restored to allow surgical departments to provide salary support for a resident who is not contributing to the generation of income for the department. Hospitals that depend on income from insurance payors or the Federal government are feeling increasing pressure from these sources to eliminate the allocation of any of the health care dollar for the training of residents, even when they are performing exclusively clinical work. As a result, the hospital as a source of funding for the surgical trainee during his research period is disappearing. In general, residents do not receive any special financial incentive to dedicate part of their training period to surgical research; the principal incentive is career advancement through exposure at local or national scientific meetings where the results of the resident's research project are presented or when they are published. Exposure to national meetings and scientific presentations at an early level in residency increases awareness and interest in an academic career.

Residents generally enter into a period of research after the two year core curriculum of surgical training, if research is to be an integral part of their training program. This seems to be an excellent time for participation in surgical research, although it does interfere with orderly progress toward proficiency in clinical surgery if the research is conducted in total isolation from the clinic. The ideal arrangement for the academic surgeon may be a program of research that is integrated into the schedule of each week. Complete isolation of the resident from clinical pressure for prolonged periods of research allows consecutive thinking and full concentration, but tends to create the mistaken impression that research is incompatible with the daily life of a practicing surgeon. At some institutions, the resident is advised to go to the laboratory to pursue a research topic after residency training is completed. This seems particularly unwise because it disables the resident as a clinician and forces him or her to re-enter practice at an advanced level with inadequate immediate preparation.

Residents are motivated to pursue research careers when they perceive a positive effect of the knowledge and skills acquired in the laboratory on the performance and personal satisfaction of their clinical role models. Surgical researchers who are fumbling, incompetent, or impractical clinicians have a negative impact on the resident. Skillful surgeons who have a keen sense of the value of scientific research impart a powerful stimulus to residents to pursue research as a developmental step in their surgical careers. A positive experience in research training alters the practice of surgeons inasmuch as it makes them more cautious about accepting folkloric remedies and authoritarian prescriptions of treatment, and kindles an enthusiasm for increasing knowledge in their chosen field of surgery.

Young surgeons who have learned the scientific approach to surgery through research and who have published scientific articles are much more likely to secure attractive clinical and academic positions. This latter benefit is probably the most significant motivating factor in convincing residents to include a period of surgical research in their training. At our institution, residents who undertake training in surgical research are carefully selected on the basis of their promise, aptitude, and enthusiasm in relation to research support for the surgical resident during his research training is provided from clinical funds derived from patient care, and through a National Institute of Health (NIH) training grant specifically targeted at teaching surgeons basic scientific research skills in the physiology department.

The training required to make a surgical resident into a scientific surgeon is similar to what is needed to develop other research scientists. The usual undergraduate curriculum of premedical students rarely includes exposure to the thinking process of the research scientist, reducing unsolved scientific problem to answerable questions. This qualitative difference is even more striking in medical school and residency where the accumulation of factual knowledge and its clinical correlations are emphasized. Acquisition of the scientific expertise needed for the effective execution of research requires active participation in research; it cannot be obtained by reading about the accomplishments of others or by replicating their experiments.

Part of the motivation to pursue research arises from the satisfaction derived from solving a personally formulated question based on ones own observations and mental processing of existing knowledge, a rare privilege enjoyed by only a small minority of scientists. Fewer than 1% of scientists in industry are allowed to formulate their own research projects. Even medical research conducted in the more open milieu of the university generally follows broad outlines laid down by a seasoned investigator with proven competence to direct the expenditure of society's investment in obtaining answers to the questions he or she has formulated. It is generally unrealistic and possibly frightening to surgical residents to allow or force them to create their own research programs before they enter a research setting. Like all junior members of the scientific community, they tend to gravitate toward laboratories that are active in research areas of interest to them, and their training is enhanced if they are allowed to choose a component of the program that is most intriguing to them. When they have learned the methodology of science in such a setting, they often go on to develop and test hypotheses that are variants of, or logical sequels to, the studies they participated in initially. The ability to choose one's own research problem and to defend the scientific approach adopted for its solution is generally the result of, rather than a prerequisite for, research training.

The research component of most training programs in surgery is generally a block period of one year; some academic programs allocate two or more years to research. The concept of devoting a part of each day or each week to research is foreign to North American surgical training programs. Because the call of a patient in distress is an irresistible summons away from the research laboratory or scholarly pursuits, isolation of the surgical trainee from clinical work has been a standard method of making time available for surgical scholarship. Nevertheless, the development of a program incorporating research into the clinical work week would teach residents how to integrate research activities into their subsequent careers as practicing scientific surgeons. Within the clinical context, the protection afforded to residents when they are assigned to the operating room for long surgical procedures is a good model. It is well established in the minds of colleagues, nurses, and patients that surgeons and residents must be cross-covered and protected to allow concentrated attention and consecutive thinking as well as sterility in the operating room during such periods. Application of the same principle in resolving the problem of how to perform research in a clinical setting seems highly desirable. Resolution of the conflict between the service needs of the surgical program for house staff and the temporal requirements for training in surgical research, will depend on the active participation of residents.

Teaching and Presenting Research

A faculty of surgeons, all equally engaged in scientific research, is often presented as an ideal, but is unusual in practice. There are real advantages in diversity. The clinical surgeon in an academic department is often a valuable partner in the support of research and a role model for the residents interested primarily in clinical surgery. It seems reasonable to expect that only a minority of residents will follow the example of the minority of their mentors who are active participants in research. At our institution, a small private medical college affiliated with a private and county hospital and a Veteran's hospital, surgical research is performed by 4 of 10 general surgeons, 3 of 7 cardio-thoracic surgeons, 2 of 3 neurosurgeons, 1 of 3 orthopaedic surgeons, 1 of 3 urologists, and 1 of 3 ear, nose, and throat surgeons. Many of our physiologists in a well-funded, research-oriented physiology department are active in collaborative and independent research projects related to surgery.

In the United States, literature searches are readily conducted through computerized programs available at university libraries and by subscription to information retrieval services. Although such searches provide immediate access to much of the information in the literature, they deprive the researcher of the experience of serendipitously finding related material during the course of a personal library search. They give the resident a false sense of having thoroughly covered a subject because the review technology employed connotes an ability to encompass all available data on the subject.

The results of surgical research by young investigators are presented at the Surgical Forum of the American College of Surgeons, an annual research meeting regarded as the first choice among venues for the presentation of residents' work. The Forum attracts a fairly large international attendance and is accessible to residents and faculty members who submit their abstracts on a competitive basis. As many as 250 are accepted for presentation each year.

Other opportunities for the presentation of surgical research projects are offered by such societies as The Society of University Surgeons, The American Association for Academic Surgery, The American Surgical Association. Regional and speciality organizations provide another category of local or specialized forums at which research-oriented papers are generally welcomed.

In training programs which lead to a Ph.D. in surgery or basic science, an acceptable level of knowledge of two foreign languages is required in addition to successful completion of a thesis and course work in surgery and a basic science. Statistics is occasionally allowed as an alternative to a second foreign language. American surgical researchers often have difficulty in evaluating the accomplishments of those who publish their work in other languages. International exchange of research data and personnel would be greatly facilitated by an increase in the foreign language proficiency of American surgical scholars. Foreign scholars studying in the United States are at a great disadvantage in securing positions and communicating with surgeons in the United States if they are not proficient in English.

The Immigration Service of the Federal Government generally requires visiting researchers to return to their country of origin after a defined period of research in the United States. The likelihood of a foreign visitor securing a position to carry out research in the United States is usually enhanced if the applicant has an academic position to return to following the visit to the United States; this is a specific requirement of eligibility for the Graham Travelling Fellowship of the American Association for Thoracic Surgery.

The Research Advisor

The surgical research advisor is responsible for providing perspective and insight in the selection of residents for research training. Some residents are best suited for a period of surgical scholarship that does not involve extensive experience at the laboratory bench. Research advisors feel privileged to participate in the scientific work of the residents who come under their tutelage and benefit from the residents' industry and intellectual energy in extending the advisor's own research, and in seeking answers to other scientific questions of mutual interest.

The number of fellows a single mentor can effectively advise depends on the time constraints imposed on the mentor. An active clinical surgeon with an active research program can rarely handle more than one or two advisees. Research fellow can reasonably expect that their advisor will offer guidance and counselling during the period of research and in the months immediately preceding it. The research fellow is generally given an opportunity to participate in ongoing, productive research programs that involve exposure to the process of conducting research in a setting where many of the start-up problems have been solved. In addition to allowing the research fellow to step onto a "moving train" that is making progress toward a defined research goal, the advisor challenges the fellow to learn the basic process of developing new solutions to scientific problems. With rare exceptions, research advisors maintain a keen interest in the subsequent careers of their advisees and facilitate their access to subsequent academic opportunities.

Legal and Cultural Considerations

The public attitude toward animal experimentation in the United States has become progressively more negative in recent years. Legislation, lobbyists, and very active protest groups limit the conduct of acute experiments in domestic animals. Well-defined guidelines for the care of experimental animals are rigidly enforced by research institutions; compliance with these rules is an absolute requirement for funding by most granting agencies.

In contrast, open discussion of the potential benefits of participation in human clinical trials and wide publicity in the lay press about the knowledge gained through such trials have produced widespread and increasing acceptance of the controlled clinical trial. The trials of coronary surgery (7) and segmental mastectomy (8) were particularly important in this regard. Informed individual consent is a strict requirment for clinical research. Extensive documentation of the background for the clinical trial is generally incorporated in the informed consent document; a careful personal explanation of the purpose, risks, and gains of participation is mandatory and is generally regarded as the responsibility of the researcher. In practice, the required information and explanations are often given to the patient and family with the active participation of a research nurse or research fellow. This experience benefits the residents as well as the patients.

Most human clinical trials are conducted as two-armed comparisons between the best available treatment and a new treatment for which the reasonable scientific argument can be made that it may offer some improvement over standard therapy. Review boards composed of physicians, preclinical scientists, and such laymen as clergymen and lawyers review proposed trials in human subjects at most institutions throughout the United States. It is the responsibility of these institutionally-appointed review boards to protect both the participants and the institution from ill-conceived or unethical research.

Problems and Opportunities for Surgical Research Directors

Only a few organizations have courses devoted to instructing surgeons in the management of research programs. Such courses as are offered for the training of academic personnel in the management aspects of chairing an academic department generally emphasize contemporary management techniques. A unique program, specifically for the training of academic chairmen, is offered by Harvard University. A formal program of instruction in surgical research training would be extremely valuable for advisors and possibly for research fellows. The curriculum of such a program should include instruction in scientific methodology, statistical training, and a well developed section on grants and publications. This book represents a step toward the development of such a program.

The achievements of surgical research in the United States are the result of diverse, energetic, and devoted scholarly efforts at many levels in many centers. Despite the problems presented, we can celebrate the improvements in surgical care derived from the experimental laboratory and from controlled clinical trials in surgery. They warrant a firm commitment from our citizens to support and extend this productive enterprise (9).

References

1. Carrel A. Results of the transplantation of blood vessels, organs and limbs. JAMA 1908;51(20):1622–1667
2. Blalock A, Taussia HB. The surgical treatment of malformations of the heart in which there is pulmonary stenosis or pulmonary artesia. JAMA 1945;128:189-
3. Wangensteen OH, Wangensteen SD. The rise of surgery: from empiric craft to scientific discipline. Chapter 6, Intestinal obstructions. Minneapolis: University of Minnesota Press, 1987:106–141.
4. NIH Data Book, NIH Publication NO. 85-1261, June 1985.
5. Rikkers LF, Bland KI, Kinder BK, et al. Funding of surgical research: the roles of government and industry. J Surg Res 1985;39:209–215.
6. Orthopaedic Research and Education Foundation, 444 North Michigan Avenue, Suite 1550, Chicago, IL 60611.
7. CASS Principal Investigators. Myocardial infarction and mortality in the coronary artery surgery study (CASS) randomized trial. N Engl J Med 1984;310:750–758.
8. Fisher B, Bauer M, Margolese R, et al. Five-year results of a randomized clinical trial comparing total mastectomy and segmental mastectomy with or without radiation in the treatment of breast cancer. N Engl J Med 1985;312:665–681.
9. Thompson JC. The role of research in the surgery of tomorrow. Am J Surg 1984;147:2–8.

10
Common Characteristics and Distinctive Diversity in Surgical Research: An International Analysis

M.F. McKneally, H. Troidl, D.S. Mulder, W.O. Spitzer, and B. McPeek

Introduction

While there is general agreement that surgical research can make a substantial contribution to the education of surgeons, the care of patients and the advancement of knowledge, there is considerable diversity in the approaches used to teach, conduct and fund research in different countries throughout the world.

Time Management

Surgeons confront unique logistical problems when they are learning research methods and when they are attempting to practice research. Since excellence in surgery requires good performance *both* in clinical judgment *and* technique, the problem of integrating scholarly activities and clinical practice is usually more difficult for the surgeon than for academic physicians in other disciplines (see Section I, Chapter 3). Clinical investigators in medical subspecialties may spend 70% of their time in the laboratory, and two or three half-days per week in the ward or the outpatient clinic. There may be one or two months of "rounding" in a university hospital. Such a distribution of activities enables reasonably credible performance of academic internists and other physicians both as clinicians and scientists. A surgeon cannot retain clinical credibility without operating and caring for patients for an appreciably larger number of working hours every week, yet a surgeon cannot succeed as an investigator without a substantial investment of time and intellectual energy in "hands on" research, especially during the first several years. The increasing complexity of hypotheses and methodology demands several years of non-clinical postgraduate education in basic sciences, statistics or clinical epidemiology, and even social sciences. A common denominator in many of the chapters of this section is the acute dilemma of the chairman, the investigator and the trainee: how to reconcile the irreconcilable. For the established academic, the only solutions advanced by implication in most countries is Osler's formula: "Work . . . hard work . . . and more work" (see Section I, Chapter 4). Generally, excellence seems to be reserved to those willing to do two full careers in one lifetime. For the trainee, the solutions involve not only the same magnitude of work, but greater risks in career choices, financial loss due to lengthening of the training period and the need to master two or more disciplines in order to achieve personal academic goals as bridge scientists.

Some of the patterns which have evolved in the countries surveyed may lead us to a better resolution. The early identification with a research team described in France, Canada, Germany and Japan suggests that the awakening of awareness of the scientific method can begin early in clinical training. The weekly research rounds for all surgeons held at McGill provide a continuing stimulus for the clinical residents. Protected time in the laboratory during the clinical rotations appears to approach the ideal, but may require a larger number of residents to meet service needs. The manpower needed to staff research programs without interrupting the residents' ongoing clinical responsibility seems to be available in England and Sweden. The remarkable excess of doctors in Spain has not lead to a glut of research manpower, but research program development and funding could not absorb more personnel there at this time. The increasing number of physicians and surgeons being educated throughout the world may lead to a queue of able candidates waiting for research posts in the future. At the present time, except for brief six-month or twelve-month electives in research, trainees must also fit their investigation into a busy service and didactic learning schedule. The examples of trainee's daily schedules show this clearly. Generally, research work is of subordinate priority in the eye of the residents' chiefs and that of service oriented hospitals and health agencies.

Financial realities do not explain the whole problem, but in all the countries contributing to this overview, resources are very important determinants of outcome in the clinical investigator's unending war, waged simultaneously against insufficient time, against the consequences of trying to serve both the patient and science, and against the disadvantage of competing for research funds with Ph.D.'s who have more extensive scientific preparation and who are unencumbered by heavy clinical commitments. Interesting solutions to the time-management problem of accomplishing surgical research in the schedules of the busy academic clinician include the relatively independent experimental surgical departments in Munich and Cologne, and the more integrated "small research group" of the Marburg experiment. A narrowing of the spectrum of clinical responsibility to more easily coincide with the research thrust of the investigator has been favorably reported from England, Sweden and the United States, but is apparently incompatible with German tradition at this time. The dilemma of restricted university funds to support research personnel is well presented in the German experience, and echoed by most other authors.

We now examine some of the economic determinants of biomedical research and the known implications for clinical investigation.

Investment in Research

Everyone recognizes that knowledge knows no frontier and that the leading journals have articles reporting the results of reseach from most of the countries on the globe. As we think of our own fields, we can recall important work from colleagues around the world. While there are always problems generalizing results found in one institution to the patients in another, we are as interested in research results from Budapest as we are in those from Edinburgh; techniques developed in Winnipeg are as valuable as those from Miami. Despite the universality of research and our desire to reap its benefits, there are marked differences between countries in the opportunities available for surgical research.

Recognizing that countries differ markedly in the resources they allocate to research, we attempted to make international comparisons of funds for research in surgery. We must report that we were unable to locate comparable data across countries that would permit us to do this, for in no country were we able to find reliable data on surgical research alone. At least some financial data are available for almost all countries, but it is aggregated in such a way that it is impossible to tease out research related to surgery. Definitional artifacts also produce difficulty in comparing data from one country to the next. The best that we have been able to do is to locate information concerning overall biomedical research expenditures. Obviously, surgical research will consume varying amounts of the total biomedical research budget in various countries but we have no data suggesting how this varies or by how much.

For many countries of the world, there is scant information about the extent of research expenditures, perhaps due to peculiarities in reporting. For example, the U.S.S.R. and the Democratic Republic of Germany (D.D.R., East Germany) have extensive research and development investment but publish very little data as to the extent or intensity of research efforts. So-called third world nations perform little research, and rely on the more developed nations to pioneer science and technology. Some countries, like China, do perform research but centralized information does not appear to be collected and maintained about the extent of the effort. Available data is, therefore, largely confined to the industrialized western European countries, Canada, the United States, Australia, New Zealand and Japan. These countries are member states of the Organization for Economic

Cooperation and Development (O.E.C.D.). Yugoslavia participates in the O.E.C.D. to a limited extent. Even within the O.E.C.D. data there are problems sorting out medical research. For example, in Germany and Switzerland research budgets of pharmaceutical and chemical firms are pooled in a single category because the large firms in both of these countries produce industrial chemicals as well as pharmaceuticals. For them, such an aggregation makes sense, but it complicates comparisons of support for biomedical research between countries. Among international organizations, only the O.E.C.D. seems to gather data across its member countries systematically. Despite some problems of definition these results appear to be the best available (1).

The O.E.C.D. encompasses three defined areas of research and development; basic research, applied research and experimental development. **Basic research** is experimental work undertaken primarily to acquire knowledge without any particular application or use in view. **Applied research** is also original investigation undertaken to acquire new knowledge. It is, however, directed primarily toward a specific practical aim or objective. **Experimental development** is systematic work drawing on existing knowledge that is directed towards producing new materials, products or devices or to improving those already in use. The O.E.C.D. defines *biomedical research* as the study of specific diseases and conditions including detection, cause, prophylaxis, treatment and rehabilitation. They also include the design of methods, drugs and devices used for diagnosis or treatment, and broad areas of scientific research undertaken to obtain a basic understanding of the life processes that affect disease and human well-being. The definition also includes clinical trials and epidemiologic studies, but not research in fields like health education.

In the data reported, the effects of inflation and differing national currency exchange rates are controlled by converting all prices to 1975 prices and all funds to U.S. dollars using the 1975 exchange rates. Since exchange rates are based on supply and demand for internationally traded goods, one might expect the purchasing power of a constant U.S. dollar to be similar in terms of equipment. Salaries of research workers present a problem. The purchasing power is likely to be greater in countries with a lower per capita domestic product.

Data for the United States and for Switzerland were available for every year from 1970 through 1980. For other countries, data were available only for varying subsets of those years. For this reason, the reported data converted to 1975 U.S. dollars was fit to an ordinary least squares curve and some of the values reported for 1975 and 1980 represent such smoothed data projections.

Table I shows the domestic biomedical research and development funds per capita in 1975 and 1980 for each of the nine countries discussed in this section of the book. The United States of America has the largest absolute funding for biomedical research and development. In 1975 this amounted to $3,874,800,000 yet the United States is only fourth highest in spending per capita. Switzerland, the highest per capita contributor to biomedical research and development, spent a total of $250,900,000,000. in 1975. The Spanish, who spent less than the others per capita, still had a total biomedical research expenditure of $42,800,000. Overall public funds account for roughly half of the total. But for some individual countries the private sector contributes the larger share. The most striking case is Switzerland which has by far the highest private funding per capita due in great measure to the presence of major pharmaceutical firms in a relatively small country. Switzerland's public funding level is only a little above the mean for the nine countries and below that of Sweden, United States, and Germany. Sweden with a public biomedical and research development funding of $20.10 per capita leads the public sector funding.

Figure 1 shows public domestic biomedical

TABLE I. Domestic BMRD funds per capita (1975 U.S. dollars).

	1975	1980
Switzerland	39.17	38.99
Sweden	22.43	29.12
Germany	19.08	21.81
United States	17.94	19.95
France	11.49	13.37
Japan	10.42	13.35
Canada	8.13	9.25
United Kingdom	6.77	8.06
Spain	1.21	1.36

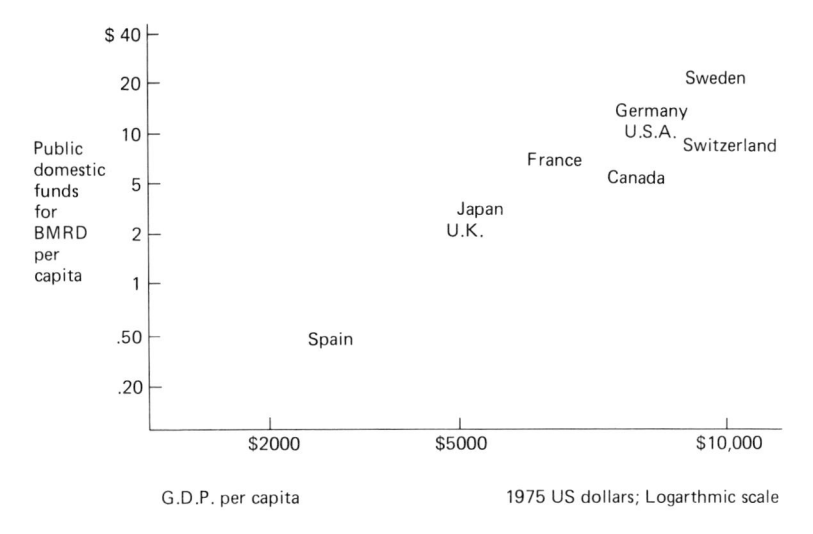

10. Common Characteristics and Distinctive Diversity in Surgical Research

FIGURE 1. Public domestic funds for BMRD per capita and GDP per capita.

research and development funds per capita compared with gross domestic product per capita. The gross domestic product per capita is a standard indicator of national economic activity. The strong, positive correlation we see demonstrates that in general biomedical research and development is funded at a higher rate in higher income countries.

Public domestic biomedical research and development as a percent of gross domestic product also correlates strongly with gross domestic product per capita. Not only do the richer countries have more money to spend on biomedical research, they tend to spend relatively more of what they have.

These data can also be used to suggest how much biomedical research, a country "ought" to fund. National income measured in gross domestic product per capita is an important predictor of biomedical research funding. Of course, this relationship provides no normative basis for determining how much biomedical research should be funded by any individual country. One can measure the level of actual funding in relation to what the gross domestic product would predict based on the pattern for all countries. Public domestic biomedical research and development funding, actual and expected are used to calculate a relative effort as shown in Table II. Notice that the relative effort ranges from almost 1.5 for Sweden down to almost 0.5 for Spain. The United Kingdom spends close to what one might expect based on the overall pattern for all countries.

Because of the difficulty of obtaining absolutely comparable data across countries due to the definitional problems discussed earlier, we recognize the true values of these numbers may vary somewhat from those given. At the same time, they do provide an interesting view of how the various countries we discuss compare with each other in terms of their biomedical research funding. It would be even more interesting if we were able to extract the data for surgery alone.

The analysis of research activities should, of course, be carried further. We have discussed

TABLE II. Relative effort in public domestic funding on BMRD: 1980.

Country	Relative effort*	Public domestic BMRD funds per capita (1975 US dlrs)	
		Actual (Smoothed)	Expected
Sweden	1.44	20.10	13.99
United States	1.31	13.36	10.17
Germany	1.15	11.92	10.40
Japan	1.14	5.27	4.62
United Kingdom	1.03	3.12	3.01
France	.93	8.15	8.74
Switzerland	.72	10.05	13.95
Canada	.66	6.71	10.22
Spain	.52	.72	1.38

*Smoothed Actual/Expected.

the financial resources used in biomedical research. It would be interesting to be able to consider the products of research. Numbers of publications, publications in particularly prestigious journals, or citation indexes are sometimes used to measure the immediate products of research. At the same time, the real product of the system ought to be improvement in health, perhaps life expectancy or some measure of reduction of morbidity. The editors fear that valid links between research investment and health outcomes will only be possible some years in the future.

A Comparison of Research Training for Surgeons

The general education of students who eventually enter a surgical career varies in the intensity of preparation for university studies. American and Canadian graduates of secondary schools generally enter the university for a four year pre-medical training program at age 18. At that point, they are approximately 18-24 months behind their European counterparts in terms of general and scientific education. Medical school begins earlier for European students and extends for a longer period of time. Table III, prepared from the descriptions of the education of an academic surgeon in each country, provides a comparative outline of the training programs. Research may be commenced in medical school and is required in some countries for an academic medical degree, but is not required for the practice of medicine. For example, in Germany, Japan and England, a doctorate in medicine is a special degree which requires a thesis based on research performed by the medical student. Residency in surgery begins as early as age 24 in England and as late as age 27 in Sweden, where a compulsory period of practice in the health service adds two years to the surgeons overall training period. A six month rotation in general surgery is included during this period of service.

In Germany, Switzerland and Sweden, there is a clearly defined pathway for the academic surgeon which includes a requirement for extensive participation in clinical and experimental research, stringent criteria to qualify for examination by the faculty and a clear designation as a "docent" who has demonstrated his broad knowledge of surgery. The most rigorous requirements appear to be those in the German system which demands about 25 publications, 15 oral presentations, and a clinical and experimental thesis defended in an oral examination. Only a small fraction of surgical residents pursue the lengthy pathway leading to full qualification for the academic life at approximately the age of 40 in all three countries. This course brings the candidate to a point which is approximately analogous to a publication and productivity record which would qualify an academic surgeon for promotion to the rank of associate professor in many North American universities. The "habilitation" or thesis project in the German system may be started within the six years of general surgery training. It usually prolongs this period because it reduces the opportunity for the candidate to accumulate the list of surgical cases required to qualify for completion of the residency program. In German university hospitals, the assistants who are chosen to become an "oberarzt" after 6 years or more of training usually have completed the "habilitation" process and bear a responsibility for the day-to-day administrative management of the operating room and surgical floors considerably in excess of the administrative responsibilities of senior North American surgical residents. Four years following approval of the thesis and certification as a "docent", surgeons are eligible to be promoted to the rank of professor. They may then proceed up the academic ladder at the university hospital, or take a position as chief of surgery at a major community hospital.

Swedish residents may complete clinical training in county hospitals where they have extensive exposure to the common problems of general surgery. Those interested in an academic career then return to a university hospital for advanced training in complex areas of surgery such as transplantation. During this interval they prepare their dissertations, conduct research, and establish the publication record required to qualify for examination. The French system offers a shorter period of 5 years of residency training without a chief residency at the end. Research is carried out intermittently during the course of the residency programme; a recent modification of the French residency in surgery has been the addition of a dedicated year of surgical research at some institutions.

In the United States and Canada, medical students graduate and qualify for entry into surgical training at approximately the same age as their European counterparts. During surgical residency, some may spend one year in research as part of their general education in surgery. Residents who show a particular aptitude for an academic career select programs which offer one or more years of additional research to develop a solid foundation in clinical and basic science, including a knowledge of research design, statistics and familiarity with the methods of securing extramural funding for research. Research in North America is generally concentrated in a period of study isolated from the pressures of clinical surgery in order to allow the resident to concentrate on scientific development. This period of research is often placed after a two-year core curriculum of surgery. Following the research rotation the resident returns to the heavy clinical responsibilities of senior residency, but may attempt to keep the research project going through a team of collaborators developed during the laboratory years. This period introduces the tension between research and clinical care that dominates the lives of most academic surgeons. Residents who are entering surgical sub-specialties leave the general surgery program after the core-curriculum to specialize for 3 to 4 years in otolaryngology, urology, neurosurgery or orthopedic surgery. Specialists in plastic surgery, cardiovascular and thoracic surgery, or vascular surgery first complete the minimum of five clinical years of general surgery training before seeking further sub-specialty training. Academic graduates of the North American programs generally finish their formal residency training at 32 to 35 years of age depending on the amount of subspecialty training they pursue. At that time, they may be selected to join the faculty of a medical school and to serve on the surgical staff of a university hospital where they usually begin their climb up the academic ladder as an instructor. In this role, they are analogous in many ways to the university "oberarzt" but they do not stay in the hospital at night to take calls as they did during their residency. Academic rank, requirements for promotion and the ages at which they are attained vary from university to university. The ages cited in Table III are approximate for the minimum at each rank.

In England, medical school graduates enter surgical training at a younger age than their counterparts in many other countries. Trainees are fully qualified for the Fellowship of the Royal College of Surgeons and for surgical practice by the age of 29. They may well have participated in research during residency training, however because of a lack of opportunities to enter the practice of surgery, there is a large number of registrars who continue in a resident-like role in the National Health Service. While they contribute to patient care and research in the academic setting at this level, registrars may wait 10–20 years before the next advance of their academic careers.

Japanese academic surgeons enter the university for pre-clinical medical science at approximately the same age as their counterparts in Europe. After two years of basic science and four years of clinical science, they are eligible for certification as a physician at the age of 24. They may then enter surgical residency in a community hospital, where there is no opportunity to perform research or for academic promotion. Those who are interested in the academic track affiliate with a university hospital in the role of an unpaid assistant or may enroll as a postgraduate student of surgery, paying tuition to the university clinic in order to participate in the lectures and conferences of the university surgical service. Assistants support themselves by working part-time in the operating room at private hospitals for one half day per week. This period of activity as a doctor-in-training or a "university clinic student" may last for four years or more. If an opening becomes available and these assistants have performed well they may qualify for a position as "assistant doctor" in the university hospital. Some applicants for the position spend 1–2 years in fundamental research in the laboratory in order to qualify academically for this position. At the age of thirty one, after a considerable period in the role of student, and two years in the role of laboratory researcher, the candidate enters a program analogous to a European or North American university hospital senior residency or

TABLE III. Comparative outline of training programs.

Age	Germany	Switzerland	Sweden	France
4	Kindergarten	Kindergarten		
5				Ecole maternale
6	Elementary school	Primary school		
7				Primary school
8			Comprehensive school	
9				
10	Gymnasium			
11				
12				Secondary school
13		Gymnasium		
14				
15				
16			Gymnasium	"Lycee"
17				
18				
19	Basic medical science (2 Yrs)	Basic medical science (2 Yrs)	Medical school	Faculty of Science (1 Yr)
20				Faculty of Medicine (4 Yrs)
21	Clinical science (4 Yrs)	Clinical science (4 Yrs)		
22				
23				
24				
25	"Physician in training" (2 Yrs)			
26		"Licensed physician" General surgery training (6–8 Yrs prolonged by intercurrent military service)	Compulsory health service (2 Yrs, including 6 mths in general medicine)	"Certification" Internship/General Medicine (2 Yrs)
27	General surgery training (6 Yrs)		General surgery training County Hospital (4½ Yrs)	Residency in surgery (5 Yrs) (+1 yr research for university career)
28	University or Community Hospital (research)			
29		University or Community (research) Hospital		
30				
31				
32	Oberarzt Oberarzt		Oberarzt	
33			Research training (5 Yrs) Leading to Doctorate in Surgery	
34		Oberarzt		
35				"Professeur d'Universite"
36				
37				
38	Habilitation			
39			Docent in Surgery	
40	"Private Dozent"	Dozent		
41	Chefarzt			
42				
43				
44				
45	Professor			Chief of Surgery
46	Ordinarius			
47	**Where there is a range in age those given are generally minimums.			
48				
49				
50				

10. Common Characteristics and Distinctive Diversity in Surgical Research

Age	United States	Canada	England	Japan	Spain
4	Kindergarten	Kindergarten		Kindergarten	
5			Elementary school		
6	Elementary school	Elementary school		Elementary school	Elementary education
7					
8					
9					
10					Secondary school
11	Junior high school	Junior high school			
12			Secondary school	Junior high school	
13					
14	High school	High school			
15				Senior high school	
16					
17					University medical school (5 Yrs) Unlimited enrollment, high attrition
18	Premedical college	Premedical college	Medical school	Medical school Premedical Course (2 Yrs)	
19					
20				Basic science (2 Yrs)	
21	Medical school Basic science 2 Yrs	Preclinical science (2 Yrs)			
22				Clinical science (2 Yrs)	
23	Clinical science 2 Yrs	Clinical science (2 Yrs)	Internship		Internship (License to practice)
24			General surgical training (Includes 6–12 mths Basic Science	Medical Doctor, Basic Surgical Training (2 Yrs)	University or Community Hospital Clinical Assistant
25	Doctor of Medicine (M.D.)	Doctor of Medicine (M.D.)			Clinical Apprenticeship (2 Yrs) Assistant with course work
26	Surgical Residency (2 Yrs) Core Curriculum	Rotating Internship		Postgraduate ←or→ Surgical Course (4 Yrs) Training (6 Yrs) (2–3 Yrs research (Senior 1 Yr clinical Course) training) (may include surgical research 2–3 Yrs)	
27	University Hospital Research (1 Yr)	Community Hospital Surgical Sub-Specialty (3 Yrs)	Core training—surgery (2 Yrs)		
28			Registrar		
29		Surgical scholarship (1 Yr)			Research (2–4 Yrs) Thesis leading to Phd in Basic Science	General Surgery (5 Yrs) Self arranged
30	Senior Surgical Residency (2 Yrs)	Surgical Residency Senior clinical years (2 Yrs)	FRCS Diploma "Post FRCS" University and NHS Medical School	Doctor of Medicine	Assistant Doctor
31	Chief Resident	Chief Resident			Doctor of Medicine	Surgical Assistant
32		Cardiothoracic, Plastic Residency			
33			Lecturer Senior Registrar	Instructor	
34	Assistant Professor	Assistant Professor	Senior Lecturer		
35					
36			Reader Consultant		
37					
38					
39			Professor		
40				Assistant Professor	
41	Associate Professor	Associate Professor			
42					
43					
44	Professor of Surgery	Professor of Surgery		Associate Professor	Chief of Surgery
45					
46					
47					
48					
49					
50				Professor of Surgery	

assistantship. During this period the academic surgeon performs in a role similar to the role of senior registrar in England, or instructor in North America. He may stay in this role until he is in his fifties, although successful candidates move up the academic ladder to the rank of assistant and associate professor and, perhaps eventually, to chairmanship. Assistant doctors and academic surgeons in general are not well paid and are expected to work one day per week in private hospitals in order to supplement their income. They may go into practice in the community if their prospects for advancement do not appear to be promising.

We asked our contributors to diagram a representative day in the life of a young academic surgeon. The time commitments for operating, out-patient care, ward rounds, research, and teaching are illustrated in the particular chapters. There was a striking difference in the availability of time for research among the countries reporting. Because of the availability of funding for research, the large number of academic assistants, and the time schedule of the National Health Service in Sweden, a substantial amount of time is dedicated to research within the working day. In most of the other reporting countries, the dilemma of the academic surgeon is always the same, finding enough time to perform research.

Attitudes Toward Surgical Research

The attitude of the public toward surgical research seems to parallel the attitude of community-based and university surgeons, and is reflected by the legislative bodies and the public's giving in their level of funding for research in general and surgical research in particular. In general, the public's understanding about the benefits of medical research has improved in the past two decades. Information regarding surgical research has often emphasized spectacular high technology procedures such as implantation of the mechanical heart or liver transplantation. There is a need for further public education in the area of applied clinical research and health services cost-effectiveness.

A survey from nine countries presented in this book reveals a wide spectrum of attitudes by the public and of surgeons toward research. In Spain there is little surgical research outside of technical exercises to develop the proficiency of clinical surgical teams in new surgical techniques such as organ transplantation. Formal scientific studies to analyze surgical problems are unusual at the clinical or laboratory level. This low level of activity in surgical research is not related to the number of physicians who are available to perform it since Spain has a striking excess of physicians and surgeons, many of whom are forced to seek employment outside of the medical community to survive. The intensity and organization of surgical research in Spain seems to reflect the attitude of the populace, which the authors characterize as indifferent. Only 0.04% of the gross national product of Spain is devoted to biomedical research and so the atmosphere, support personnel and organized programs of investigation have not been developed to allow easy access of surgeons to training in research. A fascinating funding mechanism for research exists in Spain where a surcharge is added to each prescription drug and set aside for a medical research fund managed through the social security system.

The public's attitude toward research in Germany and France seems to be "positive but skeptical". That is, effective research programs which result in notable clinical success (for example, cardiac transplantation) are beginning to reduce public skepticism about the application of the scientific method to the solution of clinical problems. Nevertheless, there is a strong residual feeling that the doctor, particularly the surgeon, should be an authority on his subject who is able to prescribe and carry out appropriate treatment without any element of doubt. The success of the European Organization for Research and Treatment of Cancer (EORTC) in promoting randomized trials of cancer chemotherapy throughout Europe has been a positive influence in spreading the understanding of the application of the scientific method as opposed to authoritarian prescription for the resolution of clinical problems. A unique funding mechanism described by our French and Japanese colleagues is a specific allocation in the budget of some municipalities for the support of surgical research.

In the United States, Canada, Switzerland, and Sweden the application of the scientific method to the resolution of surgical problems is fairly well accepted within the general population and is regarded as appropriate by many physicians and surgeons. In these countries, as elsewhere, the position of surgical research within the scientific community is not as advanced as it might be. The precise level of funding for surgical research is difficult to isolate due to anatomic, or disease-oriented panels which award and record funds dispersed in most governmental agencies. There is a general feeling that surgical research, as illustrated by injury research, receives a low level of funding related to its importance as a health problem (2). We need more accurate data on the funding of surgical research, a goal currently pursued by the Canadian Association of General Surgeons and by the Conjoint Council on Surgical Research in the United States.

In Japan, scientific research is supported at an increasing level each year in the national budget. The solution of clinical problems by analysis of outcomes in groups of patients who are randomly assigned to a variety of treatments is still perceived as a culturally-shocking Western approach to patient care. Experimental trials of new treatments are generally characterized by low accrual when randomization is a requirement for patient entry. The attitude of clinicians towards surgical research, however, is positive.

The close relationship between levels of funding and public attitude demands that surgeons become involved in education of the public, governments at all levels, and granting agencies. Surgical leaders armed with data must develop a more effective interface with government and industry in order to assume an influential role in determining priorities for the delivery of clinical care as well as excellent execution of basic and applied research.

Lessons Learned, Problems Identified and Goals

Review of the reports from the nine nations reveals the need for increased *support* among citizens of most countries for biomedical research, particularly investigation involving intact human beings. The crucial role research plays in improving the length and the quality of patient's lives not sufficiently understood. Everyone involved in clinical research, from world reknowned scholars to first year registrars must be involved in the process of public education to encourage better participation in research and more financial support through governmental agencies, private foundations, and individual gifts.

Funding for surgical research must be won in a increasingly competitive market. The issues of whether separate funds should be set aside by granting agencies for surgical research is unresolved. Improved instruments for quantifying the input and output of surgical research are required. It would be helpful in analyzing and justifying funding for research projects in surgery if the expenditure for surgical research per capita, or as a function of gross domestic product could be related to outcome measures, for example, in terms of production of research papers in prestigious journals, citation indices and, finally, on health care outcomes.

Academic surgical leaders must include among their responsibilities public education and dynamic personal interaction with the political process to protect their patient constituency, and to secure adequate funding for research education and for the scientific analysis of the consequences of health policy changes. We recognize a special need for surgical leadership in health services research on problems of manpower, specialization, and health care organization.

The society that demands improvements in medical care, not just sympathy for the sick, must get behind the effort in a tangible way. There is no more tangible support for research to be given than willingness to be a participant in a clinical trial. Surgeons, more than most clinicians, are keenly aware of the imperfections of their knowledge because the outcomes of their interventions are frequently manifest in the short term. Surgeons closely monitor their outcomes in morbidity and mortality conferences and tissue committees. Instinctively, surgeons wish to submit competing treatments in their armamentarium to rigorous scientific scrutiny. They are encumbered in their intent by the instincts of their patients who want to consider their surgeon infallible and incapable of doubt. Such tensions are not easy to resolve in any society. They are especially troublesome in countries where the projected certainty of the doctor is considered to be an intrinsic part of the therapeutic manoeuvre. This task of public education by clinicians is facilitated by responsible journalism which reinforces the benefits of patient participation in the development of improved treatments. Surgeons with access to political leaders and opinion-shapers must exercise their responsibility to inform and judiciously persuade whenever possible.

Our sample of opinions from academic surgeons in nine countries identifies *time management* as a major problem in the training of surgical scientists, in the maintenance of operative skills to keep them competitive. Some of the solutions include:

1. The development of a *team* with sufficient clinical manpower to allow the surgical scientists to return to the laboratory and complete scientific task unencumbered by clinical responsibility during defined periods of time.
2. The *integration* of scientific collaborators into the surgical program, as in the Marburg Experiment, so that a surgeon's viewpoint is brought to bear on research problem throughout even thought the surgeon may not necessarily participate in "hands-on" laboratory execution of the research.
3. Narrowing each surgeon's field of specialization sufficiently to allow intensification of scientific study of the field is an additional, useful mechanism for protecting surgeons from the overwhelming demands of a broad spectrum of responsibility. For example, concentration on pancreatic transplantation can facilitate the development of a focussed clinical and laboratory research program that is highly interactive, and intensive, yet the scholar is protected from the demand of covering the full breadth of general surgery. The development of focussed programs of clinical and experimental resarch of this nature requires the collaboration of clinical colleagues and the support of the surgical chiefs.

Rigidity in the educational framework of training programs militates against an exchange of teachers and students among countries. We support attempts of academic and political leaders to correct such artificial barriers to progress. North Americans and others should emulate countries in the European Economic Community who have started taking tangible steps to facilitate educational and research exchanges.

We encourage program directors and chairmen to arrange adequate training in research for talented residents and registrars. At the same time we recognize the importance of maintaining the credibility of surgeons as superb clinicians. We welcome and encourage the increasing trend of surgical scholars involvement in methodological trainings for laboratory, clinical and epidemiologic research. From such a process will emerge future leaders, the independent bridge scientists, sophisticated collaborators in large trials, productive partners in laboratory inquiry, and knowledgeable contributors to health services research.

The development of increasing methodological skills among surgeons conducting research on surgical problems is illustrated by the well designed and executed randomized trials of surgical versus medical treatment in coronary artery disease conducted in Europe (3) and North America (4). Similarly, the definition of the role of limited resection in the surgical treatment of breast cancer illustrate a happy combination of careful scientific methodology and disciplined surgical practice (5). A surgeon who presents reliable data in precise and technically sophisticated statistical terms is a powerful new voice in surgery. The future surgical scholars must develop skills in writing and public speaking. Those who aspire to leadership in the academic world must work hard to communicate with scholars in other countries. Americans, especially, must study to overcome their lack of language skills, a major impediment to true international exchange. Surgical chairmen must remember that a surgeon with one or two years of experience in a sister discipline is only able to facilitate collaborative research rather than practice that other discipline independently. A half-trained statistician may be almost as lethal as a half-trained surgeon.

The universal desire of each of our patients is to get the best possible care. We can achieve the best standards if the leadership in academic surgery engages in research and focuses on problems that arise in patient care. If widespread involvement of academic surgeons in research is thwarted by review mechanisms that fail to give proper weight to the relevance of research questions put forward by clinicians, then the review system requires revision to promote cinically-related research. The success of the surgical study sections in the United States provide convincing support for this strategy. If funding mechanisms or local customs in any country fail to foster relevant research about problems that matter to surgeons and their patients, educational steps should be taken to correct the problem. For example, Japanese academic surgeons might insist that the medical curriculum include a strong orientation to scientific methods that have direct relevance to the choice of treatment for patients. Modern students must learn that decisions should be based on evidence and not on opinion, no matter how eminent the source. Students everywhere should learn how to weigh evidence from various types of design and should know enough about statistics to be informed consumers of quantitative information, and judicious teachers of the public.

We have identified a small number of prominent issues that need to be addressed. Resource allocation for research must increase. Citizens must join with clinicians in taking responsibility to advance the knowledge that ultimately benefits each individual member of society. Clinicians and the public alike must learn how to deal with uncertainty and work to improve treatments, not pretend we know more than we do. In the short run it means application of the highest order of clinical judgement and technical skill. In the longer run it requires imagination, diligence, and excellence in the pursuit of new knowledge.

We can celebrate the fact that in spite of ostensibly insurmountable obstacles the science of surgery advances and patients everywhere benefit from the achievements of those who will not be discouraged or defeated.

Each country can point to important contributions in recent years. Open heart surgery, pioneered in the United States, inaugurated a new era of effective intervention for a large number of disorders hitherto irreversible and often terminal. Investigators in France advanced the surgical treatment of the aorta. In the United Kingdom, controlled trials were first applied in surgery by Goligher; total hip replacements were introduced and rigorously evaluated and changed the lives of advanced arthritis victims. Spain has contributed technical advances in open heart surgery, while Canadians contributed innovations in pediatric surgery, and developed hypothermia and cardiac pacemakers. Research in Switzerland enabled osteosynthetic surgery. The Swedes combined outstanding clinical investigation with rigorous population science to advance an understanding of the natural history of low back pain and to discriminate effective from worthless interventions in all stages of that disorder. Endoscopy was made possible in its present sophisticated modalities by Japanese research. In Germany, a combination of judicious program development and health services research established the world's exemplary prehospital trauma services for entire regions of that country.

We look forward to exciting new contributions in the closing decades of this century. We must study our problems together and work out joint solutions across interdisciplinary and international boundaries. The editors and authors of this text have had a stimulating and encouraging experience exchanging ideas about the solution to research problems. We look forward with enthusiasm to continued and increasing international cooperation and progress in this adventure.

The first step on the long road is *excellence in methods*. We have attempted to make it easier to take the first step for those committed to these goals wherever they live and work.

References

1. Our data on research funding are adopted from: Shepard DS, Durch JS. International comparison of research allocation in health sciences: an analysis of expenditures on biomedical research in 19 industrialized countries. Boston, Mass.: Harvard School of Public Health Institutes for Health Research, 1984.
2. Foege WH. Committee on trauma research. Commission on life sciences national research council and the institute of medicine. Washington, D.C.: National Academy Press, 1985.
3. European Coronary Surgery Study Group. Long-term results of prospective randomized study of coronary artery bypass surgery in stable anging pectoris. Lancet (8309) 1982;2:1173–1180.
4. Kaiser GC, Davis KB, Fisher LD, et al. Survival following coronary artery bypass grafting in patients with severe angina pectoris (CASS). J Thor Cardiovasc Surg 89;1985:513–524.
5. Fisher B, Baur M, Wickerham DL, et al. Relation of number of positive axillary nodes to the prognosis of patients with primary breast cancer. An N.S.A.B.P. Update. Cancer 1983;52(2):51–57.

SECTION VI

Opportunities in Surgical Research

1
Future Horizons in Surgical Research

F.D. Moore

". . . and a horizon is nothing save the limit of our sight"

Rossiter Worthington Raymond,
A Commendatory Prayer

To estimate what lies beyond your horizon, it is wise to examine the terrain from whence you came. Over the past four decades, since World War II, surgical research has functioned in four modes.

1. *New Procedures.* New surgical procedures have been developed where there was none before. Examples include open heart operations using a pump oxygenator, organ transplantation, microsurgery of the brain and middle ear, laser surgery of the detached retina, repair or replacement of aortic aneurysm, and prosthetic replacement of major joints.
2. *A Bridge to the Basic Sciences.* Providing a bridge of research brings basic science directly to the bedside of the surgical patient. Examples include advances in understanding surgical metabolism, intravenous feeding, the biology of convalescence, metabolic care in surgery, new use of anticoagulants and antibiotics, and the beginnings of immunology in surgery.
3. *Collaboration with Clinical Colleagues.* The surgeon now joins with other clinical colleagues to make surgical care more effective and sophisticated. Examples include the blossoming of cancer surgery into multi-modality collaborative treatment involving several other disciplines, the improved orthopedic management of rheumatoid arthritis, the use of pacemakers, the use of ultrasound and computed axial tomography.
4. *Improving the Old by Surgical Engineering.* The self-improvement of surgery is often triggered by holding up the mirror of self-examination and criticism. This is the ancient means by which surgery has improved; now hastened by incisive research. The evolution of surgery in the care of cancer of the breast, liver resection, prostatectomy, pituitary neoplasms (combined with irradiation), fracture stabilization, are examples of how surgery has improved itself through repeated performance and by a clearer understanding of its own shortcomings. Advances in the evaluation of new procedures, or "technology assessment", belong in this category.

The use of these four modalities in surgical research has required *two basic inputs*.

1. *People, institutions.* The recruitment and academic support of young people interested in surgical research require the establishment of surgical laboratories and their expansion and integration. This mandates the building of collaborative bridges with basic science departments and the support of surgical research by Boards of Trustees and hospital Directors, university Deans, and science colleagues. It requires an understanding that surgical research has a significant mission, and that its accomplishments are some of the most remarkable biomedical advances of this century.
2. *Financial support.* This includes personal and family financial support for the young investigator, "seed money" for young people and their ideas. As they get started, they do not yet have the bibliography or background to command outside support. Later they must

have full backing in seeking funds from the large donors, foundations, and institutions. The backing of the home university and its non-surgical faculty is often the most important, and in some areas, the most difficult to obtain.

With these *four operational modes,* and their *two basic inputs,* there remain *two questions* to be answered about special aspects of surgical research, by each surgical department head.

1. *What is the role of modern basic quantitative biology* in surgical research? Very few surgeons are basic biologists. But this limitation is not confined to surgery. It is true also of medicine, pediatrics, psychiatry, and radiology. As the methods of modern science have become progressively more challenging, fewer expert clinicians have mastered those skills.
2. *Where does health policy fit in surgical research?* Health policy research includes the role of surgical care in social rehabilitation, cost-benefit analysis, surgical manpower, law and ethics, the organization of surgical departments, establishment of new practice patterns, the burden of malpractice litigation, and the application of highly technical methods to life support in critical illness. All of these enter into the practice of surgery. They cannot be neglected by research even though they have not in the past been considered important aspects of classical surgical investigation. If surgical research neglects them, critical decisions about surgery are made by ill-informed sociologists and legislators.

Finally, in all aspects of surgical research we have an *underlying basic mandate:*

To have an ideal impact on the care of the sick, surgical research must be done by surgeons or under their guidance. The surgical investigator may play the key role or a more modest one. The surgical presence, its inspiration, and the driving force of its scientific and clinical insight is essential for the success of surgical research.

Now, returning to the four modes by which surgical research operates, we might take a quick glance—not quite in focus—at that future horizon that is the limit of our sight.

New Procedures

In 1935, very few people would have predicted perfection of the pump oxygenator to support surgery on the open heart; in 1952, it was termed impossible. As recently as 1953, it was stated that the transplantation of organs between unrelated individuals would be impossible. Both these negative predictions were made by experts in their fields. Surgical upbringing from the turn of the century onward had always taught that large foreign bodies in the wound were a sure recipe for disaster, let alone artificial heart valves or large plastic prostheses to make a new hip joint; success is now the rule.

These examples demonstrate how false negative predictions can be in the field of new surgical procedures. One must be quite presumptuous in 1986 to imagine what might be on the surgeon's operating list in the year 2000—and that's only 14 years away.

It would be my guess that further perfection of transplantation and extension to other organs and tissues will occur. These will hardly be called "new" operations, although many (pancreas, small bowel) still pose unsolved problems.

Head injury remains the commonest cause of death from trauma, whether automobile, home, child abuse, or military. Microvascular operations for various types of intracranial bleeding or infarction in head injury might become a reality. The sorting of head injuries to discern which ones might be salvageable by early direct treatment of the brain and its vasculature remains an important future horizon. New imaging modalities, such as nuclear magnetic resonance and positron emmission tomography may be crucial.

The development of artificial organs is in a vigorous phase at the time of this writing, and will surely continue for many decades. In general, these fall into two categories.

First are those artificial organs that are physiologically outside the body and perform some function for the body, albeit implanted under the skin in some cases. This includes the extracorporeal pump oxygenator (the first effective artificial organ ever developed), the artificial kidney, the artificial pancreas, and the pacemaker. The pump oxygenator and the pacemaker are now so widely used that we scarcely think of them as artificial organs.

The second group are those artificial organs truly *in situ*. The artificial heart is an example and at present it is suffering from a surpassing difficulty. In animal models, the tendency to cerebral microembolism may have been masked by the lack of behavioral knowledge of the animal itself (speech, affect), or by actual differences in coaguiability of the blood. In any event, microembolism, usually to the brain but possibly also to other organs, has been a major complication in most of the patients in whom artificial hearts have been implanted. This unfortunate complication has deprived this expensive, bulky, and awkward form of life support from providing a life of acceptable quality for such patients.

In this regard, the recent developments of an endothelium- stimulating substance (angiogenin) holds great promise. It seems reasonable to expect that implantable hearts and other left ventricular assist devices may have endothelial linings grown within them that make them essentially physiologic as regards coagulation induction. Were this to be possible, the use of artificial hearts would be limited only by the awkwardness of the extracorporeal power source. The work of several investigators in attempting to develop an implantable power source, whether electrical, magnetic, or nuclear, remains an important aspect of research that should occupy the time and attention of several capable collaborative groups encompassing energy conversion, engineering, medicine, and surgery.

The heart transplant requires poisonous immunosuppressive drugs; the artificial heart requires capricious anticoagulants. The trade-off has not been as simple as it appeared.

Will there be some new form of operation that might at one stroke be applicable to many forms of cancer? It might involve an organ implant, such as lymph nodes or spleen containing "educated" lymphocytes that would assault the tumor, or a micro filter implant containing gene-implanted microorganisms that synthesize diffusible substances such as interleukin II or anti-angiogenin. Though these might be new operations, they would basically be the product of bringing new immunologic science to surgical care.

A remarkable loss of surgical "turf" has occurred in the past decades. When mastoidectomy yielded to antibiotics and polio reconstruction disappeared with the vaccine, no surgeon and no patient objected! All were elated. But there are other losses of territory—the ultrasound-guided deep needle biopsy, angiographic embolization in hemorrhage, percutaneous angioplasty, colonoscopic polyp removal. Many such developments need a steady surgical hand and the longstanding "field familiarity" of surgeons with the problem. Surgery (chirurgie) is "doing with the hands" which others can learn. In some cases the surgeon should insist on participation. More turf will be lost over the horizon; in some cases the surgeon must "keep a hand in" and master new techniques from other fields. At the same time, the surgeon will take over the territory of others as he has, for example, in deafness and coronary disease—and here, in return, he must learn new concepts to bolster and validate his techniques.

A Bridge to the Basic Sciences

It is in this area—the bridge to basic science—that immunology looms so large. The birth of molecular immunology should surely be applicable to cancer, to transplantation, and to surgical infection. Most immunologists who worked through the difficult decades of the '40s, '50s, and '60s, readily acknowledge their indebtedness to surgery. The growth of tissue transplantation, the description of the HLA groups, a better understanding of the events of tissue rejection, were all a central part of the rebirth of immunology. They helped move it from a field of pragmatic clinical testing to basic molecular biology. Several Nobel laureates (Burnet, Medawar, Benacerraf) have worked in these areas of tissue types, immune competence, histocompatibility, and antigen genetics.

At present time, many young surgeons are entering immunology just as in the past they may have selected physiology, metabolism, neurology, microbiology, or biomaterials, as basic science fields. And yet, viewed in the harsh light of 1986, the message of molecular immunology has not yet revolutionized anything in surgery. Looking to the future of immunologic applications in surgery, there is a sensation of unfounded hopefulness and of plotting strategies as yet unrealized. My own scientific faith affirms the tremendous surgical potential of molecular immunology.

In the field of cancer, the reality of immune surveillance seems to be borne out by the occurrence of Kaposi's sarcoma, and other mesenchymal tumors in patients suffering from acquired immune deficiency syndrome. There is an increased incidence of these viral-induced tumors in patients on immunosuppressive drugs, though the incidence varies according to the drug and certain other demographic or genetic factors of the patient. Despite this suggestive information, the immunologic treatment of cancer remains in its infancy. The hope that some sort of nonspecific immune stimulus, such as BCG or C-parvum, would assist in clinical cancer care has not been borne out. Interferon has not proven effective in more than a handful of instances. Considering the possibility that induction of lymphocytes to specific immune capabilities has been established in several *in vitro* and animal systems, cancer treatment possibilities remain inviting. The exposure of a sibling donor to a purified specific cancer cell surface antigen might make it possible to transplant that subject's spleen or lymph nodes into the cancer patient later with possibly beneficial results.

As applied to surgical sepsis, increasing immunologic knowledge seems to be providing the basis for specific therapy, much as it did in the early days of the application of metabolic knowledge to surgery. But clinical case-management has not yet altered much. It now seems clear that certain types of surgical trauma inhibit the production of immunoreactive globulins and may have adverse effects (possibly through an overload mechanism) on the activity of specific lymphocyte subpopulations. All clinicians are familiar with the phenomenon of death from sepsis after trauma or surgery, with multiple treatment modalities, successively changed antibiotics, and finally the failure of several organs in sequence. This sequence suggests that repair of the patient's immune system, were it possible, might be life-saving. The terminal events suggest widespread immune deficiency.

The syndrome of "multiple organ failure" (like the syndrome of "adult respiratory distress syndrome") is merely putting words that sound specific on a wide variety of clinical phenomena that often have little relationship to each other. The recent era may well go down in history as one in which the mishandling of antibiotics was a prime characteristic. Adverse effects include overdose of antibiotics that are in themselves immunosuppressive and the acquisition of antibiotic resistance by successive strains of organisms. The patient is converted into a bacteriologicaly sterile but immunologicaly suppressed setting for overgrowth of ordinary commensals, such as the fungi and cytomegalic virus infections. This is suggestive not only of the misuse of antibiotics, but of a sequence that is the joint product of initial severe injury, infection, and a very adverse immune deficiency. A better knowledge of the immune sequences in such complex cases may permit the surgeon to employ new agents at his disposal, more intelligently.

As regards transplantation immunology, the induction of specific immunologic tolerance for antigens from one organ-source without global immunosuppression, remains elusive. The replacement of azothiaprine by cyclosporin has appeared significant for many transplanted organs, particularly the liver. But more careful analysis may reveal that surgical sophistication itself has been responsible for much of the improvement. In any event, cyclosporin is another immunosuppressive agent of global activity, nonspecific, and with neoplastic byproducts.

Bringing basic science to the rescue of the surgical patient in the area of physiologic support systems has several inviting possibilities. The newer knowledge of hormone mediators holds much promise. These translate the message of peripheral injury into central organ damage, nitrogen loss, energy source conversion to lipid oxidation, and activation of the basis stress response. The possibility that severe injury may have treatment modalities in the endocrine area is thus brighter than ever. If after severe injury some of this catabolic activity could be modified, and at the same time the necessary substrates could be released from within the body or provided externally, a more serene clinical course might be anticipated.

Were such methods of stress modulation to become available, one could feel almost certain, pessimistically, that they will be misused and overused. It has been observed since the beginning of surgical metabolic research that healthy young males who show a very "vigorous/brisk" response in the endocrine and catabolic areas, do very well clinically. The plentiful release of endogenous substrates for fibroplasia, leukocyte activity, and immune globulin production (from within the organism) appear to be an obvious though unproven teleologic explanation. When some hormone becomes available to mollify or abate this response, the appearances of the vigorous young male with his "brisk and florid" endocrine response will rapidly be "mollified" to resemble that of a poor and weakened old patient having his fifth operation, totally devoid of physiologic response. As with the proper use of antibiotics, the development of new hormones in this field will require a great deal of sophistication. The antibiotic record, in my opinion, is so dismal, that it provides little assurance that a large group of practitioners will be able to use such potent and dangerous new hormone preparations intelligently.

Collaboration with Clinical Colleagues

As mentioned in the introduction, one of the most spectacular examples of collaboration has been the evolution of cancer treatment in the last decade. Formerly limited to a surgical operation that was essentially "do or die", the effectiveness of which was based largely on early diagnosis, other modalities have become available and often with very good results. Their net effect has often been overrated by the public media because of enthusiasm about their very existence. This applies particularly to chemotherapy in solid tumors, and radiotheraphy with supervoltage equipment.

Despite the disappointments and the many failures, the fact is that cancer patients at the present time have a better prospect of prolonged disease-free survival with a good quality of life, than ever before. This is not due to any single "breakthrough", but rather to non-competitive collaboration in comprehensive cancer centers, where the welfare of the patient is considered more important than the specialty ambitions of any one therapist. In visiting such units, it is possible within a few hours to discern whether the various modalities, potentially competing (sometimes at such narrow quarters as different configurations of the same drug), and often involving much larger domains of sovereignty, such as surgery, radiotherapy, and chemotherapy, are truthfully collaborating for the welfare of the patient. Or are they seeking the enrollment of patients in their own "protocols" in order to get more money, more publicity, more patients, or a higher group income?

A professional is defined as a person practicing in an ambience that places the welfare of the patient or client above the social, scientific, personal, or financial advancement of the practitioner. The availability of multiple cancer therapies and therapists has truly placed the professionalism of all physicians on the line. In most instances, multiple-modality cancer treatment centers demonstrate a high order of professionalism; only in a few is it evident that research protocol-enrollment rather than the welfare of the patient, govern the outcome.

Multimodality collaborative work involving surgeons with many other disciplines will surely become a much more frequent type of surgical research, rather than less so. The surgeon at the turn of the century was often the solo actor in concert treatment, often the only person in the whole therapeutic panoply that had anything specific to offer the patient. Now, in many fields, the collaborative phenomenon prevails and the psychology of professional interaction becomes an important component as yet unanalyzed.

In addition to cancer treatment, this type of clincial collaboration promises many future rewards for the surgical patient via surgical research. The development of ultrasound and of computed axial tomography have both provided tremendous advances in surgical care. To appreciate these advances one needs only to reflect on the painful and uncertain procedures of encephalography and ventriculography to diagnose hemorrhage in the skull or disorders along the spinal column, and contrast them with the specificity and anatomic precision of tomographic scanning.

At present, nuclear magnetic resonance (NMR) and positron emission tomography (PET) hold great promise. The former seems almost devoid of adverse effect. Current apparatus does not lend itself to the scanning of extremely ill patients; the apparatus is expensive, and while not biologically dangerous, is cumbersome and awkward, and does not lend itself to any sort of emergency procedure.

PET scanning has the unique feature of demonstrating areas of functional activity within the brain. Its application to neurosurgery, to focal and stereotactic surgery for epilepsy and the development of this type of combined engineering approach to various mental, behavioral, and psychiatric problems, holds an entirely new horizon and renewed promise for neurosurgery.

The hope remains that these techniques will provide a way of salvaging at least a small fraction of formerly fatal head injuries. Very prompt attention, immediate and focal diagnosis, microsurgery or CNS excision, may save a few patients from that large group who at present are responsible for most of the mortality in civilian and military casualties.

Improving the Old by Surgical Engineering

One of the most fascinating aspects of modern surgery has been its innate capacity for self-improvement. While the majority of quantum advances in surgery in the last century have come from university centers, the gradual improvement and perfection of surgical procedures as they are routinized and made widely available, has often come from the practitioner, from clinical practicing groups, and community hospitals. Surgery is a form of applied biological science, of human engineering. It improves with practice. There are many spectacular examples of this. As one of hundreds of examples, the improvement in results of kidney transplantation between 1965 and 1978, when there was no qualitative improvement in immunosuppression, but a marked reduction in patient mortality and a tremendous increase in the fractional survival of transplanted organs, demonstrated the perfection of the technique.

The same thing has been true of open heart surgery, particularly coronary bypass operations, wherein the mortality over large areas of the United States is around 1%. This formerly imposing and immensely complex technical variety of open heart surgery and microvascular repair has become much safer, rather than more hazardous, with widespread performance.

Very few people in the clinical or scientific establishment outside of surgery understand this remarkable aspect of surgery. Many adverse views of surgical operations are based on early results before this bioengineering learning curve becomes manifest. Again, amongst the frontier group of procedures, the improvement in morbidity, mortality, and surgical perfection of liver transplantation is spectacular. This is one of the most difficult and complex operations carried out in surgery. It should only be undertaken by a master surgeon with self-confidence and specific training in this field. And yet within those limitations, its repeated performance has resulted in an improvement in results gratifying beyond expectation. These results are highly challenging to the neophyte individual or hospital starting at the low end of the learning curve.

It is important for every hospital to hold the mirror up to itself. Any hospital, clinical unit, group practice, or academic department that is carrying out surgical operations in any quantity should periodically review its results both in terms of immediate mortality and morbidity, and late survivorship and rehabilitation. While modern computer techniques render this very simple, it must be an established program adequately supported at the outset and periodically evaluated. It is of pressing importance at the horizon of surgical research.

Hospitals that cling to old operations, such as radical mastectomy in breast cancer or subtotal gastrectomy for duodenal ulcer, should have the research fortitude, often called "discipline" or "guts", to examine their own results in the light of recent advances. If indeed they can document a superior result with the time-honored procedures, they should be privileged to do so and stand up in the court of professional opinion to defend their view. The same thing applies to frequently performed standard operations such as prostatectomy, colectomy for cancer, operations on the heart valves, laminectomy for disc removal and arterial replacement of the lower limb or aorta. In all these standard areas, it should be an obligation of every surgical unit, wherever it is in the world, to know their own results, compare them with published peer groups, and set their house to rights if their results are inadequate. The support of research to do this should come from the institution itself.

The Two Basic Inputs: People and Support

Turning now to the "two basic inputs" mentioned at the start, little space need be wasted in speculation about what is over the horizon. We can say with perfect confidence that young people in surgery who are devoted to a life in science, will be as rare in the future as they have been in the past. The coercion of all young interns and residents to laboratory "projects" is positively unrewarding; it merely crowds the literature with trash. But, every young surgeon should have the door open so that if his talents call him to the laboratory, he may give them fair trial. The analogy with playing a musical instrument is too close to withhold: there is no point in forcing every young person to practice three hours a day. Only a large crashing of noise results. But there should be the instrument—a laboratory—available, and a teacher—the Professor—so that each resident in an academic unit can develop his talent, if it exists.

The backwardness of institutions in providing space for surgical research remains depressing. Surgical research is not demanding of space, although in the past animal facilities have sometimes been difficult to establish and maintain; antivivisection pressures in surgical research have been a complication for almost a century. It is an obligation of the professor of surgery to convince the Dean and the hospital Director of the necessary components of surgical research. He should be ready to call to their attention that only where research thrives and an inquiring mind is given scope, will the quality of clinical surgery be maintained at its optimal level and the hospital attract patients and residents.

Financial support for career development in surgery must increasingly come from practice income. There is an ethical aspect here that requires examination. If a practicing group—let us assume for a moment a private group clinic of the United States model (Mayo, Lahey, Crile)—sets aside professional fee income for research, one is always aware that there is here the problem of fee-splitting. The patient, or the patient's insurance company, is being charged for an activity of which they were totally unaware and unprepared to underwrite: research.

If such fee diversion becomes extensive, it is clearly unethical. This also applies to the taxation by the Dean or the University of practice income from academic clinicians. This is in essence a tax on the patient's pocketbook or the patient's insurance company, for the conduct of a medical school, an activity that the patient does not feel is intrinsic to the treatment of her breast cancer.

Counterbalancing such pressing ethical concerns is the fact that all enterprises in a free society require diversion of some income to research and development. Even the most conservative patient would assent to the diversion of some of his or her fee to improvement of surgical practice, if it were properly explained to them.

There seems to be a "reasonable" level of this sort of fee diversion, and there should be some sort of notification, in hospital publications or provided to the patient at admission, to make it clear that some of the professional costs for the patient's care are those of helping young people in education and research. Definition of a "reasonable" fraction must depend upon the scene and circumstances, but somewhere in the region of 10–15% would seem normative.

With that limitation, it is clear that surgical group practices of the academic type can provide broad support for young people to start research careers. This type of support can be used for fellowships and a few basic laboratory components for the beginner. They can never supply the sort of broadly financed support that is required for modern quantitative biology. Collaboration may help to provide some of that support, but it is only with that seed money, sometimes from practice income, that the young surgeon can possibly compete on the national scene for grant funds. And when he does go to the central source of supply for continuing grants (in the United States this is the NIH), a strong surgical voice must be there to back him up.

Where Does Basic Science Collaboration Fit in This Picture?

The future horizons of surgery will involve a more self-conscious appraisal of the role of basic science in surgical research than has been called for in the past. At the outset, the young surgeon starting in research should have a year or two to acquire the vocabulary, skills, and conceptualization of some area of basic biology, molecular immunology, genetics, or bioengineering. Following this phase, his work will often be in collaboration with scientists whose background is denoted by the Ph.D. degree. To enable this to happen, it is essential that surgical departments willingly incorporate Ph.D. scientists in their own departmental structures with appointments in surgery. While medicine, pediatrics, and psychiatry have willingly accepted Ph.D. scientists from outside their fields into their own appointment structure, this has not been so frequent in surgery. This must be allowed to occur, since it is this type of collaboration that will be so fruitful as we approach our next horizons.

Young people talented in the mechanical, spatial, and operative challenges of surgery, may not have the sort of mind that thinks in terms of molecular interactions. Now, as molecular biology has become so much more challenging, the same limitation is found in medicine and pediatrics where an increasing proportion of total research funding is held by Ph.D. scientists. Surgery must accept this same limitation, and the necessity for collaboration, if it is to move ahead.

Health Policy

Where does health policy research fit in this spectrum? Here is one of the most interesting aspects to be considered among future horizons of surgical research.

Surgical research passes through three phases: discovery, development, and delivery. The *discovery* component concerns the initial bioscience revelation of some finding of importance in surgical care; the *development* aspect is that period of surgical bioengineering improvement already alluded to. On the *delivery* side, we are concerned with new modes of surgical care delivery, the manpower, economics, and regulatory constraints within which surgery operates in every nation.

There is not space here to detail the many "delivery" components of surgical research. Quality assessment, pre-payment, collaborative delivery enterprises involving industry, quality assurance, manpower limitations, are all important.

The manpower limitation in surgery is rarely understood by other persons and in several instances in the last 25 years has been misunderstood by large national surgical organizations both in the U.S.A. and Europe. Surgeons operate upon specific disease entities; the requirement for surgeons is therefore limited by the epidemiology, the prevalence, of those diseases. The fact that this has largely escaped notice may lead to the training of an embarrassing and crippling excess of surgeons by postgraduate service programs in the United States.

While the public "appetite" for general medicine or family practitioners, has seemed insatiable, it is clear that in surgery the appetite is strictly satiable. In many fields of surgery, the predominant volume of operations (often 75% or more of total operations performed) are devoted to only a handful of specific disease entities. The requirement for such practitioners is clearly related to the epidemiology of such diseases.

The maintenance of highest quality in training and the most rigorous demands on young surgeons for quality as well as surgical talent, is an obvious corollary of this population ratio. There is no use expanding surgical training programs or recruiting additional people into surgery when the populational requirement is already met and fixed. Many young people wish to enter surgery. An absolutely strict and in many senses "brutal" mandate to weed out the incompetent, is therefore essential. If persons appear for examination before a Board of Surgical Examiners or a College of Surgeons, and cannot meet the highest standard, they should be rejected with no regrets. Because it is uneconomic and inhumane to cut people off at this late stage of their training, it is essential for in-house examinations and training entry examinations to weed out potential incompetents as early as possible. The needs for surgical manpower research in the coming decades are pressing, and unique to each country.

This book deals with international aspects of surgical research. Malpractice litigation has become a major disincentive to surgical work in the United States, and an expense for our population that approaches 3% of the total financial support for medical and surgical care. The difficulties arise from the lack of a statute of limitations in the care of children, the lack of a limitation on judgments, and the lack of a limitation on legal fees. Lawyers' concern for the welfare of the "victims" of incompetent physicians is rarely counterbalanced by the knowledge that these same victims receive only a tiny fraction of the settlements made. The need for high standards of quality assessment and constant surveillance of physicians for lifestyle disorders that may be damaging (senility, drugs, alcohol) persists. The fact remains, however, that many malpractice suits of a crippling nature are levelled against individuals who are delivering medical care of the highest quality. It is widely accepted in the press that all malpractice judgments favoring the plaintiff reveal an incompetent practitioner. This assumption has no basis in fact.

National surgical organizations in the United States have been impotent in dealing with this problem, largely because of lack of sound social research on the problem in collaboration with lawyers and judges. Other nations face, or will soon be faced with, this problem. The clear breath of fresh air leading to relief of this suffocating problem will only come from public policy based on sound social research done by surgeons.

L'envoi

This chapter has been one of peering or peeping over the horizon. We see many things promised, many challenges posed. Basing our view on the past record, we can see that many problems will be solved, but many challenges will linger on. The failures wiil be those of blindness to the power of surgical research. That blindness will be replaced by vision if the entire surgical profession in each nation supports its own native establishment in surgical research, so that surgeons may participate in every aspect of this huge and promising task.

APPENDIX A

The Declaration of Helsinki

The Declaration of Helsinki (1964), revised in Tokyo in 1975, stated the following:

Basic Principles

1. Biomedical research involving human subjects must conform to generally accepted scientific principles and should be based on adequately performed laboratory and animal experimentation and on a thorough knowledge of the scientific literature.
2. The design and performance of each experimental procedure involving human subjects should be clearly formulated in an experimental protocol which should be transmitted to a specially appointed independent committee for consideration, comment and guidance.
3. Biomedical research involving human subjects should be conducted only by scientifically qualified persons and under the supervision of a clinically competent medical person. The responsibility for the human subject must always rest with a medically qualified person and never rest on the subject of the research, even though the subject has given his or her consent.
4. Biomedical research involving human subjects cannot legitimately be carried out unless the importance of the objective is in proportion to the inherent risk to the subject.
5. Every biomedical research project involving human subjects should be preceded by careful assessment of predictable risks in comparison with foreseeable benefits to the subject or to others. Concern for the interests of the subject must always prevail over the interests of science and society.
6. The right of the research subject to safeguard his or her integrity must always be respected. Every precaution should be taken to respect the privacy of the subject to minimize the impact of the study on the subject's physical and mental integrity and on the personality of the subject.
7. Doctors should abstain from engaging in research projects involving human subjects unless they are satisfied that the hazards involved are believed to be predictable. Doctors should cease any investigation if the hazards are found to outweigh the potential benefits.
8. In publication of the results of his or her research, the doctor is obliged to preserve the accuracy of the results. Reports of experimentation not in accordance with the principles laid down in this declaration should not be accepted for publication.
9. In any research on human beings, each potential subject must be adequately informed of the aims, methods, anticipated benefits, and potential hazards of the study and the discomfort it may entail. He or she should be informed that he or she is at liberty to abstain from participation in the study and that he or she is free to withdraw his or her consent to participation at any time. The doctor should then obtain the subject's freely given informed consent, preferably in writing.
10. When obtaining informed consent for the research project the doctor should be particularly cautious if the subject is in a dependent relationship to him or her or may consent under duress. In that case the informed consent should be obtained by a doctor who is not engaged in the investi-

gation and who is completely independent of this official relationship.

11. In cases of legal incompetence, informed consent should be obtained from the legal guardian in accordance with national legislation. Where physical or mental incapacity makes it impossible to obtain informed consent, or when the subject is a minor, permission from the responsible relative replaces that of the subject in accordance with national legislation.

12. The research protocol should always contain a statement of the ethical considerations involved and should indicate that the principles enunciated in the present declaration are complied with.

Medical Research Combined with Professional Care (Clinical Research)

1. In the treatment of the sick person, the doctor must be free to use a new diagnostic and therapeutic measure if in his or her judgment it offers hope of saving life, reestablishing health, or alleviating suffering.

2. The potential benefits, hazards and discomfort of a new method should be weighed against the advantages of the best current diagnostic and therapeutic methods.

3. In any medical study, every patient including those of a control group, if any, should be assured of the best proven diagnostic and therapeutic method.

4. The refusal of the patient to participate in a study must never interfere with the doctor–patient relationship.

5. If the doctor considers it essential not to obtain informed consent, the specific reasons for this proposal should be stated in the experimental protocol for transmission to the independent committee (Section I, paragraph 2).

6. The doctor can combine medical research with professional care, the objective being the acquisition of new medical knowledge, only to the extent that medical research is justified by its potential diagnostic or therapeutic value for the patient.

APPENDIX B

Books on the Handling and Care of Animals

Title	Source
Various Species:	
Small Animal Surgery	Wingfeld WE, Rawlings CA, Philadelphia, London, Toronto, Saunders Co. 1979
Current Techniques in Small Animal Surgery	Bojrab MJ, editor. Philadelphia: Lea & Febiger, 1975
Animal Physiologic Surgery	Lang CM. New York-Heidelberg-Berlin: Springer Verlag, 1976
Experimental Surgery	Markowitz J, Archibald J, Downic HG. Baltimore: Williams & Wilkins, 1964
Schmerzausschaltung in der experimentellen Chirurgie bei Hund, Katze, Schwein, Schaf	Kupper W. In: Markenschlager M, Gartner K, editors. Schriftenreihe Versuchstierkunde, Berlin, Hamburg: Verlag P. Parey, 1984:11
Grundlagen fur Zucht und Haltung der wichtigsten Versuchstiere	Jung S, Fischer G. Stuttgart: Verlag, 1962
Biology Data Book	Altman PL, Dittmer DS. Federation of the American Society for Experimental Biology. Washington D.C.: 1964
Rodents:	
Thymusaplastische Maus (nu/nu)	Fortmeyer HP. In: Markenschlager M, Gartner K. Schriftereihe Versuchstierkunde, editors. Verlag P. Parey-Berlin-Hamburg Vol. 8, 1981
Thymusaplastische Ratte (rnu/rnu)	
The Laboratory Rat	Baker HJ, Lindberg JR, Weisbroth SH, editors. New York: Academic Press, 1980
Sheep and Pig:	
The Sheep as an Experimental Animal	Hecker JF. New York: Academic Press, 1983
Das Goettinger Miniaturschwein	Gladek P, Oldigs B. In: Markenschlager M, Gartner K: Schriftenreihe Versuchstierkunde Pare-Berlin-Hamburg: Verlag P. Vol. 7, 1981
Cat and Dog:	
An Atlas of Surgical Approaches to the Bones of the Dog and Cat	Piermattei DL, Greeleg RG, Philadelphia: Saunders Co., 1979
Anatomy of the Dog	Evens HE, Christensen GL, Philadelphia: Saunders Co., 1978

Index

A

Abstracts, writing of, 233–235, 236
Academic surgeons, 33–34, 138–139
   in Canada, 285–287
   in the United Kingdom, 330–332
   in the United States, 341–342
ADL scales, 62–63
Administrators, 22
Adverse reactions
   to anesthetics (Marburg experiment), 141–142
   to plasma substitutes (Marburg experiment), 144–145
α level, 74, 115
Analogies (in non-experimental methods), 226
Analysis of covariance, 81
Analysis of variance, 80
Analytic inference, 71
Anesthesiologists, 37
Anesthetics, adverse reactions to (Marburg experiment), 141–142
Animal experimentation, 9, 26, 142–145, 149, 291, 304, 311, 322, 333, 342
   alternative to 151–152
   benefits and necessity of, 149–150, 151
   ethics of, 124–125
   and experimental design, 155–156, 159
   guidelines for, 152
   and innovative surgery, 149–150
   and randomization, 155
   and surgical training, 150
Animal models, 152–155, 164
   criteria for, 153
   genetics of, 153–154
   and toxicity, 153
Animals
   care of, 155–158, 159–160
   diseased, 158
   killing of, 157
   optimal use of, 155
   producers of, 158–159
   quality of, 158–159
   surgery on, 156–157
Appearance, personal, at presentations, 237
Applicability (of measuring instruments), 60
Archibald, Edward, 281
Artificial organs, 360–361
Association (in non-experimental methods), 225–227
Attitude, in presentations, 237–239
Audio-visual aids, 254–267
Audio-visual presentations, 257–258
Average effect, and literature reviews, 47, 49

B

Banting, Frederick G., 30
Baseline comparability, 114
Baseline investigations, 171
Basic sciences and scientists, 19, 40–42, 137–140, 361–363, 365–366
Bayes' Theorem, 202
Before-and-after studies, 113, 227
Bernard principle, 123
Bernoulli, Jacob, 9
Bias, 14, 91, 115, 172, 181, 182, 227
   volunteer, 113–114
Bigelow, William, 281
Billroth, Theodor, 27
Binomial distribution, 83
Biological plausibility (in non-experimental methods) 226
Biomechanically activated cardiac assist device project (case study) 162–165
Biostatisticians, 176
Blalock, Alfred, 28–29
Blindness (in research studies), 113, 125, 173, 205
Brevity
   in data collection, 90
   in research proposals, 109
"Bridge tender" investigators, 21, 137

Index

Budgets, 94–95, 110, 179
  and multi-centre trials, 189–190
Buxton Brown Farm, 327

C

Canterbury v. Spence, 13
Cardiac assist devices project (case study), 162–165
Case referent studies, 225
Case series, 113
Case studies, 134
Causality (in non-experimental methods), 225–227
Cell frequency (four-fold table), 81–82, 83
Central Limit Theorem, 77, 79
Central tendency, 72
Chalmers, Thomas C, 126–127
χ^2 test, 82–83
Clarity
  and data collection, 90
  in research proposals, 109
Clerical support, 41
Clinical
  characteristics, 53–54
  significance, 75, 116
  studies, scope of, 88–89
Coding (data), 94
Coefficient of variation, 72
Coherence of evidence (in non-experimental methods), 226
Cohort analytic studies, 224
Cohorts, 134, 223–224
Co-intervention (in research studies), 114
Coisogenic strains (animal strains), 154
Collaboration, and surgical research, 162–165, 363–364
Color, in audio-visual presentation, 257–258
Combined significance tests, 50–51
Compatibility, 102, 104
Compliance, and research studies, 114–115
Computer networks, 103, 105
Computer searches, 48
Computer-to-computer exchange, 103
Computers, 96–105
  and audio-visual aids, 256
  mainframe, 101–102, 104
  minicomputers, 102, 104
  personal, 102–104
  and photography, 101
  and research, 96–97
  types of, 101–103
Conceptual definition, 89
Confidence intervals, 70
Confidentiality (of data), 95
Confounding factors, 167, 172, 227–228
  control for, 80–81, 83–84
Congenic strain (animal strains), 154
Conscience, professional, 124

Consensus conference, 253
Consistency (in non-experimental methods) 225–226
Constructs, 59
Consultants, 108
Contamination (in research studies), 93, 114
Content, in audio-visual presentations, 225
Continuity correction, 82
Control, in research studies, 49–167
Controlled clinical trials, 113, 119
  reasons for failures of, 141
Correlation, linear, 84–86
Cost analyses, 215–216
Creativity, 23
Criticism, 7–9, 112–117
Cross-over trial, 78, 114–115, 173–174, 177
Cross-sectional designs, 224–225

D

Data
  confidentiality of, 95
  data, "hard". 55–56
  data preparation of, for presentation, 236
  data security of, 95
  data "soft", 55–56
Data analysis, 46, 175–176
Data collection, 89–92
Data collectors, 94–95
Data-gathering instruments, 90–92
Data management, 191–192
Data managers, 37–38, 92, 192
Database programs, 97–98, 104
Databases, 104
Davy, Humphry, 29
Death (as outcome variable), 54
Decision-making, 144–146
Degrees of freedom, 72, 78, 82
Departmental chairmen, 38–40, 293–294, 332
Descriptive studies, 228
Diagnosis, 203
Diagnostic tests
  assessment of, 202–206
  assessment methodology, 204–205
  evaluation of, 195–206
  practicality, 198–202
  validity of, 195–198
Disability (as outcome variable), 55
Discomfort (as outcome variable), 54–55
Discriminant function analysis, 84
Discussion-periods, 246, 248–250, 252
Disease (as outcome variable), 54
Dissatisfaction (as outcome variables), 55
Documentation (of research proposals), 110
Dose-response curve (in non-experimental methods) 226
Double coding, 94

Drop-outs (research studies), 114–115
Duodenal ulcer pathogenesis (Marburg experiment), 142–143

E

Editing
  data, 93–94
  word-processing, 98–99
Editorials, 274
Effect size, 50
Effectiveness, 122–133, 213
Efficacy, 112–113, 213
Electronic mail, 103
Emergency services, 218–219
Epidemiology, 134, 207, 228, 287
Error, 8, 166–167
Ethics, 95, 108–109, 118–129
  conditional, 119–120
  in Japan, 304
Euthanasia (animals), 157
Exclusion criteria, 114–115, 170, 182
Experiment, definition of, 222
Experimental design, 23, 39, 73, 108, 112, 167, 169–177, 190
  and animal experimentation 155–159
  and ethics, 125–126
Explained variance, 85
Explanatory trials, 168, 173
Explicatory trials, 124

F

F_1 hybrids (animal strains), 154
False negative rate, 197
False negatives error, 196, 205–206
False positive rate, 197
False positives error, 196, 205–206
Fatality rates, 217
Feinstein, A., 123–124
Fincke, Martin, 15
Fisher exact probability test, 83
Fisher, Ronald Aylmer, 11
Format in audio-visual aids, 255
Formatting (word processing), 99
Forssmann, Werner, 30–31
Free paper sessions, 246
Free Standing Ambulatory Surgery Centers, 216–217
Frequency distribution, 71
Fried, Charles, 121–122
Funding, non-research, 108

G

Gastrointestinal tract haemorrhage (Marburg experiment), 145–146

Generalizability (of research studies), 116, 134
Genetics of animal models, 153–154
Gold standard, 195–196, 204–205
Gossett, William S., 77
Grammar checking programs, 100
Graphics programs, 100–101
  resolution, 105
Groups (in research studies), 70, 74–75
  and literature reviews, 47, 49

H

Health maintenance organizations, 217
Health policy research, 366–367
Health services research
  definition of, 207–208
  in Canada, 208
  and epidemiology, 207
  in the United Kingdom, 208
  in the United States, 208
Haemaccel-35 (Marburg experiment), 144–145
Haemorrhage, gastrointestinal tract (Marburg experiment, 144–146
Halsted, William Stewart, 27–28, 182–183
Hardware, 105
Harm-benefit ratio, 123, 128
Helsinki Declaration, 13, 120, 369–370
Hill, Sir Austin Bradford, 12, 225–227
Histamine (Marburg experiment), 141–145
Histograms, 71, 73
  in audio-visual aids, 256, 265
Historical controls, 10, 181–182, 228
Holmes, Oliver Wendell, 226
Human resources, in surgical research, 364–365
Hunter, John, 18, 26–27
Hypothesis, 7, 24, 43, 46–47, 73, 75, 89, 112, 162–163
  in abstracts, 234
  alternative, 76
  directional, 75
  multiple, 74–75
  non-directional, 75
  in research papers, 271
Hypothesis generation, 222, 228

I

Illogical values, 94
In vitro studies, 151–152, 159
In vivo studies, 151–152, 159
Inbred strains (animal models), 153
Inclusion criteria, 114–115, 169–170, 182
Inferential statistics
  of means, 77–81
  of Rates and Proportion, 81–84
Information needs of surgical research, 218

Informed consent, 12–14, 122–123
  in Germany, 294
  in Japan, 304
  and randomization, 127–128
  in Spain, 311
  in Sweden, 322
  as two-way transaction, 122
  in the United Kingdom, 333
  in the United States, 342
Innovative treatments, 119, 126–127
Interactions, and literature reviews, 47, 49
Interim analysis, 14–15, 176, 178
Internal consistency (in measuring instruments), 57–58
International meetings, 238, 246–248, 250
Interventional trials, 124
Investment in research, 345–348

J
Jenner, Edward, 26, 152

K
Karnofsky Performance Status, 63–64
Katz Index of ADL, 62, 64
Keypunching, 94
Key terms, 89
Keywords, 273
Knee scale, 62–64
Koch, Robert, 153
Kocher, Theodor, 27
Kuhn, Thomas, 7, 8

L
Langenbeck, Bernhard von, 26–27
Langerhans, Paul, 30
Languages and language barriers, 246–248, 291, 296, 303, 312, 321–322, 341
Language interface, 87–98, 105
Lead-time bias, 181
Length bias, 181
Lettering in audio-visual aids, 255, 262–263
Letters-to-the-Editor, 274–275
Libraries, 48, 286, 303
Line graphs, in audio-visual aids, 256, 265
List processing programs, 100
Lister, Joseph, 26–27
Literature
  reviews, 43–51, 107–108, 163–164
  searches, 48
Litigation, 366
Living matter, differentiation of, 150–151
Local area networks, 103–105
Louis, Pierre-Charles-Alexander, 10

M
McGill Pain Questionnaire, 59, 61–62
McGill University, 281, 286
McGill University project on cardiac arrest devices (case study), 162–165
MacLean, Jay, 30
McNemar test, 84
Magnitudes, 80
Malpractice, 366
Management trials, 168–173
Mann–Whitney U Test, 80, 83
Mantel–Haenszel χ^2 test, 84
Manuscripts, 23, 237, 243
  preparation of, 277
Marburg experiment, 40, 137–146, 162, 297–298
Mathematical modelling, 229
mean, 70, 72–73, 77
Means, difference in, 78–79
Measuring instruments, 57–64
Median, 72
Medical records, 91
Medical Research Council of Canada, 282–284, 287
Medical Research Council of Sweden, 320
Medical students, 29–31, 34
Medicine and the sciences, 29, 33
Melzack, R., 61–62
Meta-analysis, 46–47, 49, 51
Methodology, 113, 120–121
Milan Group (multi-center trial), 186, 188
Mode, 72
Models, in audio-visual presentations, 259
Modem, 103
Moderators, 249–253
Monitoring, 203
Monographs, 270
  preparing manuscripts for, 276–278
Morton, William T.G., 30
Muench, Hugo, 49
Multi-centre trials, 92, 180–193
  and ethics, 120, 193
Multiple comparisons problem, 115
Multiple linear regression, 86
Multiple logistic regression, 84
Myocardial assist devices project (case study) 162–165

N
National Health Services (UK), 328, 333
National Institutes of Health (US), 336–339
Nausea, measuring instruments for, 62
Nausea Questionnaire, 62, 64
National Surgical Adjuvant Breast Project, 183–189, 213–214
Negative findings, 109, 115
Negative predictive value, 198–199, 201–202

Non-experimental methods, 222–229
Non-parametric testing, 79–80
Non-random control trials, 11
Normal distribution, 72, 77–78
Nuclear magnetic resonance, 363–364
Null hypothesis, 73–77, 80–82
Nuremberg Code, 120

O

Observation, 7, 10, 29, 91–92, 223
   and error, 115, 166–167

P

Pain, measuring instruments for, 61–62
Paired t-test, 164, 177
Panel discussion, 251–252
PAP test, diagnostic evaluation of, 197–202
Paradigms, 7, 8
Parameters, 70
Parametric estimation, 70
Parametric testing, 80
Pare, Ambroise, 26–27
Pathological specimens, in audio-visual presentations, 256–257, 264
Patient compliance (and measuring instruments), 60–61
Patient variables, 53–54
Pearson correlation coefficient, 84–86
Peer review, 22–23
Penfield, Wilder, 281
Percentile ranges, 72
Perfusionists, 37
Pharmaceutical companies, 285, 321, 325
Photography and computers, 101
Physical function, measuring instruments for, 62–63
Physiologic characteristics, 55
Placebo effect, 166–167
   and ethics, 125–126
Plasma substitutes, adverse reactions to (Marburg experiment), 144–145
"Play-the-winner" randomization, 15
Plotters, 100–101, 105
Poisson, Simon-Denis, 10
Popper, Karl, 7–9
Positive predictive value, 198–199, 201–202
Positron emission tomography, 363–364
Post-test probability
   of a negative result, 199, 201–202
   of a positive result, 198–199, 201–202
Poster sessions, 260
Practicality (of measuring instruments), 60–61, 90
Pre-analysis (of data), 94
Precision (of measuring instruments), 59, 60, 177
Pre-coding (in data collection), 90

Presentation,
   at international meetings, 246–248
   techniques of, 237
Presentations
   longer, 240–245
   shorter, 236–239
Pre-tests, 93, 178
Prevalence, 198
Printers, 99–100, 105
Printing (word processing), 99–100
Prognostic stratification, 113–114, 172, 185
Programs, 96, 101
Proof-reading, 278
Proportion of variance, 85, 86
Proportional spacing, 105
Proportionality ethics, 123
Proportions, 81
Protocols, 39, 168–171, 173, 177–178, 190
Public opinion and surgical research, 352–353
   in Canada, 284
   in Germany, 294
   in Japan, 304
   in Sweden, 322
   in the United Kingdom, 333
   in the United States, 336–337
Publication, 22–23, 74, 76, 178, 193, 326
   writing for, 268–275, 276–278
Publication bias, 49
p value, 50, 74–77, 80

Q

Quality control, 191
   in multi-center trials, 185
Quality of life measuring instruments for, 63–64
Quality of Life Index, 63, 64
Quasi-random allocation, 113
Questionnaires, 91

R

Random control clinical trials, 12–16, 134, 180–181, 213–214
Random sampling, 70
Randomization, 113, 126–127, 171–173, 222–223
   and animal experimentation, 155
   central, 12
   and ethics, 119, 121, 123–124, 126
   and informed consent, 14, 127–128
   and therapeutic relationships, 123–124
   timing of, 173
Randomly-mating populations (animal models), 153
Range, 72
Rate, 70, 73
   in cohort studies, 223–224
Reference management programs, 101

Reference centers, 41
Regression, linear, 85, 86
Regression coefficient, 85–86
Regression of variables, 85
Regression toward the mean, and clinical practice, 167
Reibl versus Hughes, 122
Relational database systems, 97
Relationships
  dependent (between variables), 84–85
  non-dependent (between variables), 84–85
Relative odds, 227
Relative risk, 227
Reliability (of measuring instruments), 56–58, 90–92
Repeated measures (data collection), 92
Repetitive sampling, 77
Research, philosophy of, 7–9, 118
Research advisors, 303, 320, 341–342
Research funding, 20–23, 106, 108, 345–348, 353
  applications, 23, 41, 43, 106–111
  in Canada, 284–285
  in France, 292
  in Germany, 295
  in Japan, 303–304
  in Spain, 308–310
  in Sweden, 320–321
  in Switzerland, 325
  in the United Kingdom, 333–335
  in the United States, 337–339
Research laboratories, 38
Research proposals, 106–111
  criteria for success of, 109
Research questions, 89, 106–107
Research staff
  evaluation of, 93
  training of, 93
Research teams, 92
Resources (outlined in research proposals), 110
Response rate (questionnaires), 91
Response time, 101, 102, 105
Reversible association (in non-experimental methods), 226
Review articles
  and literature reviews, 273–274
  and readers, 274
  and research papers, 271
Review committees, 23
  for abstracts, 234
"Revolutions" in science, 8
Risk ratio, 227
Rutstein, David R., 121

S
Salary supplements (for technicians assisting in research), 38
Sample mean, 77

Sample size, 50, 70, 76–86, 115, 164, 185
  calculation of, 79, 83, 176–177
Sample variation, 47
Samples, selection of, 169–171
Sampling, 10
  convenience, 70
  distribution, 77
  systematic, 70
  variation, 70
Sandstrom, Ivar, 30
Scientific method, 7
  and practice of surgery, 36
Scientific statement, definition of, 7
Scientific writing, 268–275
  and abstracts, 233–235, 273
  and monographs, 270
  and reader, 268
  and research papers, 270–273
  and review articles, 273–274
  style in, 269
Scoring, 89
Screening, 199, 201–204
Second opinions, and surgical services, 216
Security
  and computers, 103
  and data, 95
Seminars, 252
Sensitivity, 195, 196–198
Sensitivity
  and construct validity, 59
  and precision, distinction between, 60
Sequential measurements (in non-experimental methods), 227
Sickness Impact Profile, 63–64
Side effects, 114
Significance testing, 70, 78, 79
Simultaneous translation, 248, 250
Skeletal muscles, synchronously stimulated, for myocardial assist device (case study), 162–165
Slides, 254–258, 262–267
  preparation of, 237, 238
Sociodemographic characteristics, 53–54
Sociopersonal characteristics, 53–54
Software, 105
Speakers, at panel discussions, etc. 250, 251
Spearman rank correlation coefficient, 86
Specialization, 19, 138, 354
  in Canada, 283, 286
  in France, 290
  in Spain, 313–314
Specificity, 195, 197–198
Specificity of association (in non-experimental methods), 226
Spelling-checking programs, 100
Spread, 72
Stage fright, 244

Staging, 181–182, 203
Standard deviation, 72
Standard error of the mean, 72–73
Standards, and surgical research, 125
Statistical analysis programs, 98, 105
Statistical, power, 50, 76–77, 79, 115
Statistical significance, 74–76, 86, 115–116
   and clinical importance, 75
   and meta-analysis, 47, 50, 51
Statistics
   descriptive, 70–73
   development of, 9–10
   inferential, 70–71
   in research papers, 272
   and the surgical investigator, 69, 86–87
Stipends, 31
Strength of association (in non-experimental methods), 225
Student's *t*-test, 78, 79
Study base (non-experimental method), 227
Study manuals, 178
Study objectives, 106–107, 112, 167–169
Study on Surgical Services for the United States, 207, 209
Style, in oral presentations, 237–239
Surgeons
   and confirmation of diagnoses, 36
   and the sciences, 19, 29, 33
   as surgical investigators, justification for, 167
   and surgical research, 284, 337
   theoretical, 139–141
Surgical assistants, and surgical research, 37–38
Surgical care
   and ethics, 119
   levels of, 216–217
   quality of, 55
Surgical departments, 24, 29
Surgical education, 19, 23, 24, 138, 140, 348–352
   and animal experimentation, 150
   in Canada, 285–287
   in Germany, 295–296
   history of, 26–34
   in Japan, 301–302
   in Spain, 312–315
   in Sweden, 318–321
   in Switzerland, 325–326
   in the United Kingdom, 329–330
   in the United States, 339–341
Surgical investigation, definition of, 21
Surgical investigators
   and basic science and scientists, 19, 22, 38, 137–148
   and biostatisticians, 39
   ideals of, 24
   and integrity, 24–25
   and peers, 22–23
   problems of, 19–21
   and research funding, 20–23
   and surgery departments, 24, 29
   and surgical education, 23
   types of, 21–22
Surgical problems, 1–2
Surgical research 28–29, 137–145
   attitudes toward, 352–353
   and basic science, 361–363, 365–366
   in Canada, American influences on 281–282
      attitudes toward, 284
      funding for, 284–285
      problems of 282–283
   case study of, 162–165
   and collaboration, 36, 39–40, 42, 363–364
   in France, 289–292
      achievements of, 289
   in Germany, 137–148, 293–298
      attitudes towards, 294
   history of, 9–10, 26–32
   human relationship aspect of, 121–122
   and individual scholar, 34, 36, 39–40, 42
   in Japan, 299–305
      attitude towards, 304
      history of, 299–300
   justification for, 18–19, 120, 166
   levels of, 293
   new procedures in, 360
   and patient care, 37
   and practice of surgery, 31–33
   in Spain, 306–316
      achievements of, 310–311
      funding for, 308–310
      history of, 306–308
   and standards, 125
   and surgical education, 23–24, 40–41, 348–352
   in Sweden, 318–323
      achievements of, 322–323
      attitudes toward, 322
      funding for, 320–321
   in Switzerland, 324–326
      achievements of, 324–325
   and team work, 37
   therapeutic relationship aspect of, 13, 123–124
   in the United Kingdom, 327–335
      American influences on, 328
      attitudes toward, 333
      funding for, 333–335
      history of, 327–329
   in the United States, 336–343
      achievements of, 337
      attitudes toward, 336–337
      funding for, 337–339
Surgical residents, 329–330, 339–341
   in France, 289–290
   in Germany, 294
   in Switzerland, 326
   in Canada, 281–287

Surgical services
  accessibility of, 209–210
  availability of, 209
  in Canada, 209, 211–212
  costs of, 216–217
  effects of, 212–214
  fatality rates of, 217
  information needs of, 218
  monitoring of, 217
  quality control, 217–218
  patient satisfaction and, 210
  utilization of, 210–212
Surgical students, and international meetings, 41, 287
Surgical techniques
  and animal experimentation, 149–150
  and multi-centre trials, 189
Swammerdam, Jan, 29
Symptoms, measuring instruments for, 61–62

T

Target disease, 195, 204–205
Target populations, 70, 77, 114
Team leaders, 22, 165, 190–191
Terminals, 105
Theoretical surgeons, 138–139
Time management, 344–345
Toulmin, Stephen, 119
Toxicity, and animal models, 153
Transformations (on statistical analysis programs), 98
Transparencies, 258
Transplantation, 360–361
Trauma services, 218–219
Treatment impact (in studies), 50
Triage, 203
Trials, aborting of, 176, 192
True negatives, 196
True positives, 196
2 x 2 tables, 81–82
Type I error, 74–76, 79, 176–177
Type II error, 76–77, 79, 115, 176–177

V

Validity
  in measuring instruments, 58–59, 90–91
  of research studies, 112–115
Variability of data, 76
Variables, 53, 69–73
  categorical, 69, 73
  continuous, 69, 71–73, 76, 84–85
  dependent, 84–85
  dichotomous, 69
  independent, 54, 84–85
  nominal, 69
  ordinal, 69, 86
  outcome, 54–57, 60
  polychotomous, 69
  treatment, 53–54
Variance, 72, 80, 85
Vesalius, Andreas, 29–30
Video display units, 100–101, 105
Videodiscs, 259
Video-tape and film, 258–259
Visick scale, 62, 64

W

Wangensteen, Owen H., 28
Wilcoxon Signed Rank Test, 80
Wellcome Foundation, 328, 334
Withdrawals (and research studies), 114–115, 174–175
Word processing programs, 98–100

X

X-ray films (in audio-visual presentations) 256, 267

Z

Z-scores, 50–51
Zelen, M. 14

Invitation to Critique

The editors and authors hope that revisions of this book will be justified by the interest it stimulates and its usefulness to colleagues. Further editions will be enriched beyond what our efforts alone could accomplish with critique from the readers. Accordingly, we ask that you write to us with constructive feedback under any or all of the following headings or questions:

Does the plan of the book incorporate most issues in research of importance to surgeons?

Strong chapters

Chapters that could benefit with change (specifics are important)

New chapter titles suggested

Errors of fact, interpretation, spelling, or style

Existing sections, chapters, or passages which are particularly well done and deserving expansion or emulation in other parts of the book

Other topics

All suggestions will be carefully considered by the editors. Please mail them to:

>Dr. David S. Mulder
>Professor of Surgery
>McGill University
>Montreal General Hospital
>1650 Cedar Avenue
>Montreal, Canada H3G 1A4

LESLEY COLLEGE
RD29 .P75 1986

Principles and practice of res

0 1139 0064292 8

Principles and practice of research

DATE DUE

LESLEY COLLEGE LIBRARY
30 MELLEN STREET
CAMBRIDGE, MA 02138-2790

WITHDRAWN

FEB 5 '88